T0179963

Bugs
as
Drugs

Bugs
as
Drugs

**THERAPEUTIC MICROBES
FOR THE PREVENTION AND
TREATMENT OF DISEASE**

EDITED BY
Robert A. Britton
Baylor College of Medicine, Molecular Virology and Microbiology,
Houston, Texas

Patrice D. Cani
Université catholique de Louvain, Louvain Drug Research Institute,
WELBIO–Walloon Excellence in Life Sciences, Brussels, Belgium

ASM
PRESS

Washington, DC

Library of Congress Cataloging-in-Publication Data

Names: Britton, Robert A. (Robert Allen), editor. | Cani, Patrice D., editor.
Title: Bugs as drugs : therapeutic microbes for the prevention and treatment
   of disease / edited by Robert A. Britton, Baylor College of Medicine,
   Molecular Virology and Microbiology, Houston, Texas; Patrice D. Cani,
   Universit?e Catholique de Louvain, Louvain Drug Research Institute,
   WELBIO, Walloon Excellence in Life Sciences, Brussels, Belgium.
Description: Washington, DC : ASM Press, [2018] | Includes index.
Identifiers: LCCN 2017045971 (print) | LCCN 2017046421 (ebook) |
   ISBN 9781555819705 (ebook) | ISBN 9781555819699 (print)
Subjects: LCSH: Microorganisms--Therapeutic use. | Bacteria--Therapeutic use.
   | Medical microbiology. | Probiotics.
Classification: LCC QR46 (ebook) | LCC QR46 .B775 2018 (print) |
   DDC 572/.472--dc23
LC record available at https://lccn.loc.gov/2017045971

doi:10.1128/9781555819705

Printed in Canada

10 9 8 7 6 5 4 3 2 1

Address editorial correspondence to:
ASM Press, 1752 N St., NW, Washington, DC 20036-2904, USA.
Send orders to: ASM Press, P.O. Box 605, Herndon, VA 20172, USA.
Phone: 800-546-2416; 703-661-1593. Fax: 703-661-1501.
E-mail: books@asmusa.org
Online: http://www.asmscience.org

Contents

Contributors

Stephen T. Abedon
Department of Microbiology, The Ohio State University, Mansfield, Ohio

Emma Allen-Vercoe
Molecular and Cellular Biology, University of Guelph, 50 Stone Road East,
Guelph, Ontario, Canada

Anissa M. Armet
Department of Agricultural, Nutritional and Food Science, University
of Alberta, Edmonton, Alberta, Canada

Jennifer M. Auchtung
Alkek Center for Metagenomics and Microbiome Research and Department
of Molecular Virology and Microbiology, Baylor College of Medicine,
Houston, Texas

Guido J. Bakker
Department of Internal and Vascular Medicine, Academic Medical Center,
Amsterdam, The Netherlands

Rodolphe Barrangou
Department of Food, Bioprocessing and Nutrition Sciences, North Carolina
State University, Raleigh, North Carolina

Luis G. Bermúdez-Humarán
Micalis Institute, INRA, AgroParisTech, Université Paris-Saclay,
Jouy-en-Josas, France

Robert A. Britton
Baylor College of Medicine, Molecular Virology and Microbiology,
Houston, Texas

Patrice D. Cani
Université catholique de Louvain, Louvain Drug Research Institute,
WELBIO – Walloon Excellence in Life Sciences, Brussels, Belgium

Paul E. Carlson, Jr.
Division of Bacterial, Parasitic, and Allergenic Products, Office of Vaccines
Research and Review, Center for Biologics Evaluations and Research,
Food and Drug Administration, Silver Spring, Maryland

Anne-Marie Cassard
INSERM U996 Inflammation, Chemokines and Immunopathology,
DHU Hepatinov, Univ Paris-Sud, Université Paris-Saclay,
Clamart, France

Fraser L. Collins
Department of Physiology, Michigan State University, East Lansing, Michigan

James Collins
Alkek Center for Metagenomics and Microbiome Research and Department
of Molecular Virology and Microbiology, Baylor College of Medicine,
Houston, Texas

Edward C. Deehan
Department of Agricultural, Nutritional and Food Science, University of
Alberta, Edmonton, Alberta, Canada

Susana Delgado
Department of Microbiology and Biochemistry of Dairy Products,
Dairy Research Institute of Asturias, Spanish National Research
Council (IPLA-CSIC), Villaviciosa, Asturias, Spain

Patricia I. Diaz
Division of Periodontology, Department of Oral Health and Diagnostic Sciences,
University of Connecticut Health, Farmington, Connecticut

Sheila M. Dreher-Resnick
Division of Bacterial, Parasitic, and Allergenic Products, Office of Vaccines
Research and Review, Center for Biologics Evaluations and Research,
Food and Drug Administration, Silver Spring, Maryland

Rebbeca M. Duar
Department of Agricultural, Nutritional and Food Science,
University of Alberta, Edmonton, Alberta, Canada

Krista Dubin
Immunology Program and Infectious Disease Service, Memorial
Sloan-Kettering Cancer Center, and Immunology and Microbial
Pathogenesis Program, Weill Cornell Graduate School of Medical
Sciences, New York, New York

Melinda A. Engevik
Department of Pathology and Immunology, Baylor College of Medicine, and
Department of Pathology, Texas Children's Hospital, Houston, Texas

Philippe Gérard
Micalis Institute, INRA, AgroParisTech, Université Paris-Saclay,
Jouy-en-Josas, France

Claudio Hidalgo-Cantabrana
Department of Microbiology and Biochemistry of Dairy Products,
Dairy Research Institute of Asturias, Spanish National Research
Council (IPLA-CSIC), Villaviciosa, Asturias, Spain

Anilei Hoare
Division of Periodontology, Department of Oral Health and Diagnostic Sciences, University of Connecticut Health, Farmington, Connecticut

Mingliang Jin
Department of Microbiology and Immunology, Northwestern Polytechnical University, Xi'an, Shaanxi, China

Brian P. Landry
Department of Bioengineering, Rice University, Houston, Texas

Philippe Langella
Micalis Institute, INRA, AgroParisTech, Université Paris-Saclay, 78350 Jouy-en-Josas, France

Abelardo Margolles
Department of Microbiology and Biochemistry of Dairy Products, Dairy Research Institute of Asturias, Spanish National Research Council (IPLA-CSIC), Villaviciosa, Asturias, Spain

Philip D. Marsh
Division of Oral Biology, School of Dentistry, University of Leeds, Leeds, United Kingdom

Laura R. McCabe
Department of Physiology, Department of Radiology, and Biomedical Imaging Research Center, Michigan State University, East Lansing, Michigan

Max Nieuwdorp
Dept. of Internal & Vascular Medicine, Academic Medical Center, and Dept. of Internal Medicine, VU Univ. Medical Center, Amsterdam, The Netherlands; Wallenberg Laboratory, Dept. of Molecular and Clinical Medicine, Univ. of Gothenburg, Gothenburg, Sweden

Laura Ortiz-Velez
Baylor College of Medicine, Molecular Virology and Microbiology, Houston, Texas

Paul W. O'Toole
School of Microbiology and APC Microbiome Institute, University College Cork, Ireland

Eric G. Pamer
Memorial Sloan-Kettering Cancer Center and Weill Cornell Graduate School of Medical Sciences, New York, New York

Narayanan Parameswaran
Department of Physiology, Michigan State University, East Lansing, Michigan

Maria Elisa Perez-Muñoz
Department of Agricultural, Nutritional and Food Science, University of Alberta, Edmonton, Alberta, Canada

Gabriel Perlemuter
INSERM U996 Inflammation, Chemokines and Immunopathology,
DHU Hepatinov, Univ Paris-Sud, Université Paris-Saclay, and AP-HP,
Hepatogastroenterology and Nutrition, Hôpital Antoine-Béclère,
Clamart, France

Hubert Plovier
WELBIO-Walloon Excellence in Life Sciences and Biotechnology, and
Metabolism and Nutrition Research Group, Louvain Drug Research Institute,
Université Catholique de Louvain, Brussels, Belgium

Gregor Reid
Lawson Health Research Institute, Human Microbiome and Probiotics,
F3-106, 268 Grosvenor Street, London, Ontario, Canada

Naiomy D. Rios-Arce
Department of Physiology, Michigan State University, East Lansing, Michigan

Patricia Ruas-Madiedo
Department of Microbiology and Biochemistry of Dairy Products,
Dairy Research Institute of Asturias, Spanish National Research
Council (IPLA-CSIC), Villaviciosa, Asturias, Spain

Lorena Ruiz
Department of Microbiology and Biochemistry of Dairy Products,
Dairy Research Institute of Asturias, Spanish National Research
Council (IPLA-CSIC), Villaviciosa, Asturias, Spain

Elisa Salvetti
School of Microbiology and APC Microbiome Institute, University College
Cork, Ireland

Borja Sánchez
Department of Microbiology and Biochemistry of Dairy Products,
Dairy Research Institute of Asturias, Spanish National Research
Council (IPLA-CSIC), Villaviciosa, Asturias, Spain

Jonathan D. Schepper
Department of Physiology, Michigan State University, East Lansing, Michigan

Leopoldo N. Segal
Department of Medicine, NYU Division of Pulmonary, Critical Care,
& Sleep Medicine, New York, New York

Scott Stibitz
Division of Bacterial, Parasitic, and Allergenic Products, Office of Vaccines
Research and Review, Center for Biologics Evaluations and Research,
Food and Drug Administration, Silver Spring, Maryland

Jeffrey J. Tabor
Department of Bioengineering and Department of Biosciences, Rice University,
Houston, Texas

Jan-Peter van Pijkeren
Department of Food Science, University of Wisconsin-Madison, Madison, Wisconsin

Terence Van Raay
Molecular and Cellular Biology, University of Guelph, 50 Stone Road East, Guelph, Ontario, Canada

James Versalovic
Department of Pathology and Immunology, Baylor College of Medicine, and Department of Pathology, Texas Children's Hospital, Houston, Texas

Jens Walter
Department of Agricultural, Nutritional and Food Science and Department of Biological Sciences, University of Alberta, Edmonton, Alberta, Canada

Benjamin G. Wu
Department of Medicine, NYU Division of Pulmonary, Critical Care, & Sleep Medicine, New York, New York

About the Editors

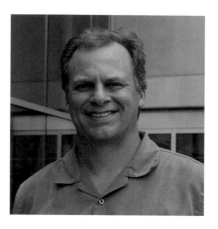

Dr. Robert Britton is a Professor in the Department of Molecular Virology and Microbiology and is a Member of the Alkek Center for Metagenomics and Microbiome Research at Baylor College of Medicine. He presently directs a Therapeutic Microbiology laboratory that is focused on the use of microbes to prevent and treat human disease. Currently funded research projects in the laboratory range from the study of how traditional probiotic strains can ameliorate osteoporosis to how intestinal microbial communities resist invasion by the diarrheal pathogen *Clostridium difficile*. His laboratory has made several advances in the development of genetic and microbial growth platforms to aid in the understanding of how microbes promote health and disease. These include the development of precision genome engineering technologies for lactic acid bacteria and the development of human fecal minibioreactor arrays to study the function of microbial communities in a high-throughput manner.

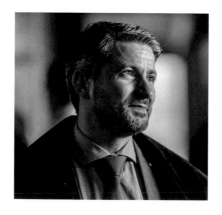

Dr. Patrice D. Cani is a Professor at the Université catholique de Louvain (UCL) and investigator for WELBIO (Walloon Excellence in Lifesciences Biotechnology) and the Fund for Scientific Research (FRS-FNRS). He is a member of the Royal Academy of Medicine of Belgium and the recipient of prestigious grants and prizes. He has published more than 200 papers, reviews, and chapter books in the field of gut microbiota, prebiotics/probiotics, and metabolism. In the early 2000s, he started to investigate the interactions between gut microbes and complex biological systems (endocannabinoids, immunity) by using prebiotics. In 2007, he discovered the concept of metabolic endotoxemia and more recently the role of specific bacteria (e.g., *Akkermansia*). Twitter: @MicrObesity.

Preface

The reinvigoration of research into the human microbiome—the collection of microbes that reside within and on our body—has resulted in novel insights into the role of these microorganisms in health and disease. Associations between the composition of the intestinal microbiome and many human diseases, including inflammatory bowel disease, cardiovascular disease, metabolic disorders, and cancer, have been elegantly described in the past decade. Because of these seminal discoveries and the increased public interest in the use of probiotics and prebiotics to impact health, many researchers and entrepreneurs are working toward translating the human microbiome into novel diagnostics and therapeutics. Thus, one of the main objectives of this volume is to provide insights into how one may capitalize on the enormous amount of knowledge being generated in microbe-human interactions for the translation into products that will benefit humankind.

We note that microbiome research, and the use of microbes as therapeutics, is not of recent origin. Elie Metchnikoff posited over 100 years ago that lactic acid bacteria found in fermented milk were beneficial to health and prevented intestinal "putrefaction." Ben Eiseman and colleagues began using fecal enema as an adjunct therapy in the treatment of pseudomembranous enterocolitis in 1958, a full 20 years prior to *Clostridium difficile* being identified as one of the main causative agents of this disease. Indeed, fecal transplantation for the treatment of disease dates back centuries to the 4th century, when Ge Hong, a well-known traditional Chinese medicine doctor, described the use of human fecal material by mouth to treat his patients with severe diarrhea.

Why, then, the increase in developing novel therapeutics and diagnostics using microbes now? Significant improvements in genetic engineering of non-model organisms, next-generation sequencing technology, and metabolic profiling have certainly stimulated much confidence in being able to harness microbes to improve health. In addition, systems biology approaches and synthetic engineering of microbes are now high-throughput and cost-effective enough to explore a much wider range of therapeutic possibilities to be vetted.

Finally, we note there is much hype and enthusiasm over the use of microbes—not only classical probiotics but also future next-generation beneficial microbes and engineered bacteria—to make significant impacts on many human diseases and to restore healthy microbial communities. However, our understanding of how microbial communities function to influence health is still quite shallow, and translation to therapeutics will require patience and basic research. For example, the linking of many diseases to altered microbial communities is only by association, and in many cases these correlations have only been uncovered in mouse models. We must acknowledge that despite the explosion of science in the gut microbiome in the past decade, much of the work has described associations between the microbiome and disease with few instances of causation. Until microbiome shifts that are associated with disease are shown to be truly driving disease manifestation, it will be difficult to know which diseases can be tackled via microbiome manipulation. It is important to remind the scientific community that just because one or several bacteria are increased or decreased in a specific pathological situation, this does not necessarily mean they play a role in disease. Therefore, a deeper understanding of the mechanisms and functions of microbiome-human interaction will be required to fully realize the potential of developing drugs for the treatment of acute and chronic diseases. Another objective of this book is for readers to identify key gaps that exist in their respective fields that need to be closed in order to assist in moving therapeutic microbes from the bench to the bedside.

We are indebted to the authors for their contributions to this book, which we know took a considerable amount of time to produce. We hope you find the chapters informative and useful in your endeavors.

Robert A. Britton
Patrice D. Cani

A. TRADITIONAL PROBIOTIC APPROACHES

Biochemical Features of Beneficial Microbes: Foundations for Therapeutic Microbiology

1

MELINDA A. ENGEVIK[1] and JAMES VERSALOVIC[1]

BACKGROUND

The gastrointestinal tract (GIT) is a diverse and complex ecosystem shaped by continual interactions between host cells, nutrients, and the gut microbiota. The gut microbiome is estimated to contain approximately 10^{13} bacterial cells and is dominated by the major phyla Firmicutes, Bacteriodetes, Actinobacteria, Proteobacteria, and Verrucomicrobia (1, 2). Early colonizers of the GIT include bifidobacteria from the phylum *Actinobacteria*. These commensal microbes colonize immediately after birth and are speculated to prime the GIT and influence the gut-brain axis (3–5). The infant microbiota is considered to be relatively unstable. Despite dramatic changes in the microbiome structure during early life, the gut microbiota increases in diversity and stability over the first 3 years of life (6). Following this initial establishment, the microbiomes of children are generally enriched in *Bifidobacterium* spp., *Faecalibacterium* spp., and *Lachnospiraceae* compared to adults (7–9). During adulthood, the gut microbiome is considered to be stable and is dominated by the phyla Firmicutes and Bacteriodetes. While bacterial populations vary between individuals, the fecal microbiota of adults is highly stable through time (6). This

[1]Department of Pathology & Immunology, Baylor College of Medicine, Houston, TX 77030 and Department of Pathology, Texas Children's Hospital, Houston, TX 77030

Bugs as Drugs: Therapeutic Microbes for the Prevention and Treatment of Disease
Edited by Robert A. Britton and Patrice D. Cani
© 2018 American Society for Microbiology, Washington, DC
doi:10.1128/microbiolspec.BAD-0012-2016

stability is maintained until older age (>65), when the microbiome stability and function begin to decline (10, 11).

A mutualistic relationship exists between the gut microbiota and the host. Commensal microbes metabolize indigestible food components, produce vitamins, prime the immune system, modulate the enteric nervous system and potentially the central nervous system, contribute to intestinal architecture development, protect against colonization of opportunistic pathogens, and do more for the benefit of the host (12). Conversely, the host generates a stable ecosystem for the gut microbiota, providing nutrients and ecological niches. The gut selects resident commensal microbes based on their capacity to adapt to and colonize within the host.

Select commensal bacteria are able to positively alter the gut microbiome and/or host. Many of these commensal groups harbor strains that are considered to be probiotics. Probiotics are defined as microbes which confer advantages to the host and have not been implicated in conferring human disease (World Health Organization, http://www.who.int/foodsafety/fs_management/en/probiotic_guidelines.pdf), and these well-characterized organisms are known to produce a number of beneficial products which promote host health. Certain strains of *Lactobacillus*, *Bifidobacterium*, *Escherichia coli*, *Bacillus*, and *Propionibacterium* spp. have been classically used as probiotics. The value of probiotics has been supported by multiple clinical trials, which demonstrate improvements for patients receiving probiotics in response to multiple pathologies including diarrhea, inflammatory bowel disease, allergic reactions, viral infections, cancer, and others. However, a number of commensal bacteria that are not defined as probiotics are also known to produce bioactive metabolites with health-promoting effects. These commensals include *Ruminococcus*, *Eubacterium*, *Roseburia*, *Faecalibacterium*, and *Akkermansia* spp. This review seeks to identify major pathways used by commensal bacteria to benefi-

cially modulate the host, with the caveat that the majority of studies that have identified specific mechanisms tend to focus on probiotic strains.

Commensal and beneficial microbes have been hypothesized to promote health in a variety of ways: (i) exclusion of pathogens, (ii) immunomodulation, and (iii) enhancement of the intestinal barrier (Fig. 1). Several mechanisms have been proposed to explain the beneficial effects of key commensal microbes. One mechanism of great interest is the secretion of molecules which are capable of altering both the host and the microbiome (Fig. 2). Bacterial metabolites can be generated as intermediate or end products of bacterial metabolism. Secreted products can target the microbiome by acting as signaling molecules for intraspecies/strain communication (quorum sensing), for altering the intestinal environment, and for targeting certain microbes to control microbiota composition (antimicrobials). These molecules include lactic acid, hydrogen peroxide, and bacteriocins (Fig. 2). Likewise, bacterial molecules can modify the host. Metabolites can participate in functional complementation to the host metabolic capabilities, immune regulation, and improvement of intestinal barrier function. These factors include small molecule metabolites such as histamine, vitamins, short-chain fatty acids (SCFAs), polyunsaturated fatty acids, serpins, lactocepins, and secreted proteins (Fig. 2). Of note, the metabolic potential of microbes varies greatly among species and even among strains of the same species. Several studies have found that microbe-driven protective effects depend on the strains used (13–15). These differences could be due in part to the diversity of secreted metabolites. As a result, it is important to characterize the secreted products of individual microbes to identify which strains should be used for a specific disorder. Here we describe the most prominent examples of well-characterized secreted products and their documented effects on the microbiome and/or host function.

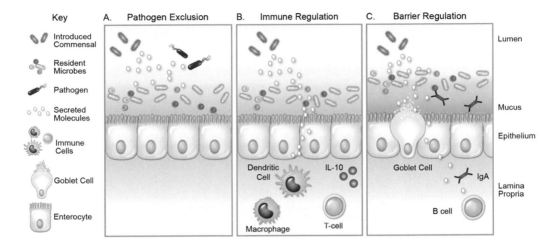

FIGURE 1 Methods utilized by commensal bacteria to beneficially modulate the intestinal environment. (A) Commensal bacteria secrete molecules which can alter the gut microbiota. By selectively inhibiting resident microbes, commensal bacteria establish an intestinal bacterial niche. Production of antimicrobial factors has also been shown to exclude pathogens. **(B)** Select commensal bacteria also secrete compounds which can modulate immune cells such as macrophages, dendritic cells, and lymphocytes such as T cells. These compounds decrease intestinal inflammation by dampening proinflammatory cytokines and promoting anti-inflammatory factors such as IL-10. **(C)** Commensal bacteria can secrete factors which modulate the functions of the epithelial barrier by enhancing the secretion of the protective mucus layer, upregulating tight junctions, and promoting secretion of molecules such as IgA.

SIGNALING COMPOUNDS

Bacteria-Host Signaling Compounds

Biogenic amine neuromodulators

Select microbes are known to produce biologically active compounds that are associated with mammalian neurotransmission and behave as neuroactive compounds. These molecules include histamine, gamma-aminobutyric acid (GABA), and tryptophan metabolites. Microbe-generated neuromodulators in the intestinal lumen likely regulate signaling within the enteric nervous system and ultimately affect the gut-brain axis. Although bacterial products such as acetate (16) and peptidoglycan (17) have been found in the central nervous system, these neuroactive compounds primarily affect the enteric part of the peripheral nervous system and are thought to act in a local manner.

Biogenic amines (BAs) are low-molecular-weight organic bases generated through decarboxylation of specific free amino acids, reductive amination of aldehydes and ketones, transamination, or hydrolytic degradation of nitrogen compounds. BAs are ubiquitously present in both pro- and eukaryotes. In bacteria, the most common mechanism of BA synthesis is the microbial decarboxylation of amino acids catalyzed by amino acid decarboxylases (18). Certain bacteria use BA production to harness the proton gradient and generate energy and/or increase the cytoplasmic pH, thereby protecting cells against acid damage (19). BAs are separated into classes based on the number of amino groups present in the structure: monoamines, diamines, and polyamines (PAs) (18). BAs are known to be key regulators of host health, particularly when acting as hormones or neurotransmitters. BAs can be classified according to their chemical structure as aliphatic (putrescine, cadaverine, spermine, spermidine), aromatic (tyramine, β-phenylethylamine), or heterocyclic (histamine, tryptamine) (20, 21). Several BAs have been associated with promoting human health.

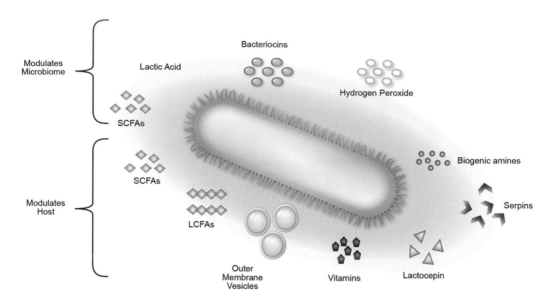

FIGURE 2 A depiction of secreted metabolites from commensal bacteria and their interactions with the microbiome or host. Lactic acid, hydrogen peroxide, short-chain fatty acids (SCFAs), and bacteriocins are all capable of serving as quorum-sensing molecules and/or directly modulating the composition of the microbiome. SCFAs, long-chain fatty acids (LCFAs), outer membrane vesicles, vitamins, lactocepins, serpins, and biogenic amines have all been demonstrated to beneficially modulate the host. Together, these bacterial products shape the intestinal environment and the host.

Histamine

Specific gut microbiota members have been reported to produce the BA histamine. Histamine is produced by decarboxylation of dietary L-histidine. Amino acid decarboxylation and BA synthesis maintain bacterial intracellular pH homeostasis (22) and can be used to generate energy using proton motive force (23). As a result, bacterial amino acid decarboxylase expression and activity are enhanced in acidic environments, leading to a locally increased pH and pH counterregulation. Bacterial amino acid decarboxylase expression is also regulated by fermentable carbohydrates, sodium chloride concentration, and oxygen saturation. Select Gram-negative and Gram-positive organisms generate histamine from histidine (24–28). The majority of histamine-producing strains belong to species of the genera *Oenococcus*, *Lactobacillus*, and *Pediococcus* (29, 30). These species harbor the gene encoding histidine decarboxylase (*hdcA*), which converts dietary histidine into hista-

mine. Histamine is known to exert proinflammatory and anti-inflammatory effects on immunoregulatory processes (Fig. 3). The type of response is dependent on the type of histamine receptor (of four known histamine receptors) that is activated. Activation of histamine receptor type 1 (H_1R) or 3 (H_3R) has been associated with proinflammatory effects; in contrast, activation of H_2R or H_4R is associated with anti-inflammatory responses.

While a number of species are capable of producing histamine, luminal histamine generated by *Lactobacillus* species has been documented to have beneficial anti-inflammatory properties. For example, several human-derived strains of *L. reuteri* contain the histidine decarboxylase gene cluster (*hdcA, hdcB, hdcP, HisS*), which is required for histamine production. *L. reuteri* ATTC PTA 6475-generated histamine suppressed the proinflammatory cytokine tumor necrosis factor (TNF) in Toll-like receptor 2 (TLR2)-activated

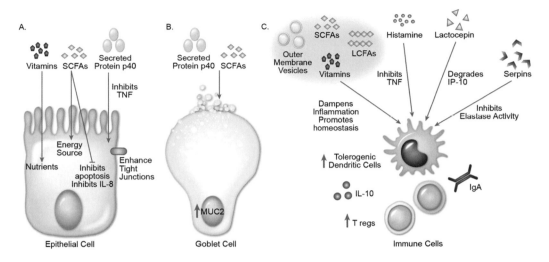

FIGURE 3 Mechanisms by which commensal secreted products beneficially modulate the host. (A) Epithelial cells. Vitamins produced by bacteria provide essential nutrients to the host. Likewise, short-chain fatty acids (SCFAs) such as butyrate are known to serve as energy sources for intestinal epithelial cells. The SCFA acetate has also been shown to inhibit IL-8 production and increase tubulin-α acetylation. Lactobacilli-produced p40 and p75 inhibit TNF-induced apoptosis and enhance tight junctions, which attenuates intestinal barrier disruption. **(B) Goblet cells.** p40 is known to transactivate the epidermal growth factor receptor, activating the downstream target Akt and stimulating Muc2 gene expression and mucin production. Acetate produced by bacteria has also been shown to increase goblet cell differentiation and expression of mucus-related genes. **(C) Immune cells.** Vitamins, outer membrane vesicles (OMVs), SCFAs, and long-chain fatty acids (LCFAs) are known to directly influence the development and function of immune cells. In general, these molecules modulate T cell and dendritic cell homeostasis and cytokine production, promoting production of anti-inflammatory IL-10 and inhibiting proinflammatory cytokines such as TNF. Biogenic amines such as histamine have also been shown to suppress proinflammatory cytokines such as TNF in immune cells, thereby ameliorating intestinal inflammation. Bacterial enzymes such as lactocepin selectively degrade lymphocyte-recruiting chemokine IP-10 and other proinflammatory chemokines such as I-TAC and eotaxin. The protease inhibitor serpin has been shown to suppress inflammatory responses by binding and inactivating neutrophil elastase. Using the highlighted mechanism, commensal bacteria produce signals that reduce intestinal inflammation and promote health.

human monocytoid cells (27). This suppression was driven by activation of the anti-inflammatory H₂R and downregulation of mitogen-activated protein kinase activation. *In vivo*, histamine-producing *L. reuteri* strains ameliorate inflammation *in vivo* in a trinitrobenzene sulfonic acid-induced mouse model of acute colitis (26, 31). Likewise, histamine from *Lactobacillus saerimneri* strain 30a (ATCC 33222) significantly lowered NF-κB activation in human monocytoid cells and suppressed interleukin 17 (IL-17) and interferon-γ secretion in wild-type mice but not in H₂R-deficient animals (32). Histamine has also

been demonstrated to alter dendritic cell (DC) responses to microbial ligands (33). Histamine was found to suppress lipopolysaccharide (LPS; TLR-4 ligand)-driven proinflammatory cytokine secretion (TNF, IL-12, CXCL10) and Pam3Cys (TLR-2 ligand)-driven TNF production. Moreover, histamine increases production of the anti-inflammatory cytokine IL-10. These responses were driven by H₂R signaling through cyclic AMP. *In vivo* addition of histamine-secreting *Lactobacillus rhamnosus* suppressed cytokine secretion (IL-2, IL-4, IL-5, IL-12, TNF-α, and granulocyte-macrophage colony-stimulating factor) secretion from

Peyer's patches in wild-type but not in H_2R-deficient mice (33).These studies indicate that bacterial histamine exerts immunoregulatory effects *in vitro* and *in vivo*.

Amino acid neurotransmitters

GABA

GABA is a four-carbon amino acid which functions as an inhibitory neurotransmitter in the mammalian nervous system and mediates diverse functions with the host. GABA can be produced by select bacterial species from the decarboxylation of glutamic acid via glutamate decarboxylase (34). GABA production is highest in microbes when the environment is acidic. Decarboxylation of glutamate consumes a proton and results in the stoichiometric release of GABA. In this manner, GABA production increases the pH of the bacteria cytosol and allows cells to resist acid stress (34). Several microbes have been demonstrated to produce GABA (35–38). Lactic acid bacteria (LAB) strains are considered to be the major group of microbes responsible for GABA production. Some examples of known GABA-producing LAB include *Lactobacillus paracasei* NFRI 7415, *Lactobacillus plantarum* C48, *L. paracasei* PF6, *Lactobacillus brevis* PM17, *Lactobacillus delbrueckii* subsp. *bulgaricus* PR1, *Lactococcus lactis* PU1, and *Bifidobacterium dentium*, to name a few (39–41). GABA is known to elicit a number of beneficial effects on the host. As an inhibitory neurotransmitter, GABA lowers the blood pressure *in vivo* in animal models and human subjects (42–44). GABA is also known to have diuretic and antidiabetic effects (45–47). In the brain, GABA enhances plasma concentration, growth hormones, and protein synthesis (48). GABA intake can regulate sensations of pain and anxiety. Mice fed *L. rhamnosus* JB-1 were shown to have region-dependent alterations in GABA receptor mRNA in the brain when compared with control-fed mice (49). *L. rhamnosus* JB-1 also reduced stress-induced corticosterone and anxiety- and depression-related behavior in treated mice (49). In human subjects, administration of a 30-day course of *Lactobacillus helveticus* and *Bifidobacterium longum* led to decreased anxiety and depression (50). Other groups have found that daily oral administration of fermented products containing microbial GABA was effective in treating the neurological disorders of sleeplessness, depression, and autonomic disorder in female subjects (51). Together, these findings indicate that gut microbes participate in the bidirectional communication of the gut-brain axis via production of neurotransmitters such as GABA. Modulation of the gut-brain axis may prove to be beneficial for stress-related disorders such as anxiety and depression.

Polyamines

PAs are small aliphatic hydrocarbon molecules with two or more amino groups (–NH2) that have a net positive charge at physiological pH (52). PAs and inorganic cations such as magnesium and calcium play an essential role in maintaining optimal conformation of negatively charged nucleic acids. Moreover, PAs are essential factors for normal cell growth, cell differentiation, and the synthesis of DNA, RNA, and proteins (53). The majority of colonic PAs are derived from commensal gut microbiota (54–56). The main PAs are spermidine, putrescine, spermine, and cadaverine. These compounds are critical for the growth and multiplication of both prokaryotic and eukaryotic cells (52, 57). In the majority of bacteria, intracellular concentrations of spermidine (1 to 3 mM) are higher than putrescine (0.1 to 0.2 mM), with the known exception of *E. coli*, which has higher putrescine (10 to 30 mM) levels (57). Cadaverine is considered to be the least prevalent bacterial PA (52, 57). In contrast, spermine is primarily produced in the presence of specific dietary sources. Consumption of pectin has been shown to increase the cecal concentrations of multiple PAs, particularly spermine (56). This effect was shown to be gut-microbe dependent because consumption of pectin- or guar-containing diets altered the concentrations and the composition of cecal PAs in conventional rats but not in germ-free rats (56). The gut residents *Bacteroides thetaiotaomicron* and *Fusobacterium varium* are major contributors of spermine and spermidine in the gnotobiotic rat cecum, suggesting that commensal bacteria can modulate PA levels (55).

Commensal bacteria can both produce and be influenced by PAs. PAs are known to possess anti-inflammatory activities, which can benefit the host. They can decrease systemic inflammation by inhibiting proinflammatory cytokine production in macrophages and intestinal epithelial cells (58, 59). Additionally, PAs function as reactive oxygen species scavengers, chemical chaperones, positive regulators of stress genes, and antimutagenic agents (60, 61). Spermine possesses anti-inflammatory activity by inhibiting NF-κB activation (62) and inflammatory cytokine synthesis (58, 63) and by selectively activating T cell protein-tyrosine phosphatase (64). In mammals, systemic PA levels decrease with age (65, 66), and decreased PAs have been associated with intestinal barrier dysfunction (67). Supplementation of middle-aged (10-month-old) mice with *Bifidobacterium animalis* subsp. *lactis* LKM512 for 6 months increased fecal spermine concentrations (67). This spermine increase correlated with increased survival, reduced skin ulcers and tumors, improved colonic barrier function, downregulation of inflammation-associated genes, and alteration of the gut microbiota composition (67). In addition, supplementation of arginine to the diets of mice and rats increased colonic concentrations of spermine and putrescine (68). A combination of both arginine and *B. animalis* subsp. *lactis* LKM512 further suppressed inflammation, improved longevity, and provided protection from age-induced memory impairment in mice (68). Several of these findings have been mirrored in patients, because addition of *B. animalis* subsp. *lactis* LKM512 increased intestinal

PAs (putrescine, spermidine, spermine, and cadaverine) (69, 70) and reduced the quantities of biomarkers of acute inflammation in hospitalized elderly patients (70).

Commensal bacteria also benefit from PA production because PAs can protect bacterial cells from reactive oxygen species (71) and mutagens (61, 72–75). PAs can also modulate gut community dynamics. Supplementation of PAs to a formula diet for neonatal BALB/c mice was found to regulate the concentrations of *Akkermansia muciniphila*, *Lactobacillus*, *Bifidobacterium*, *Bacteroides-Prevotella*, and *Clostridium* groups to levels found in the breast-fed group (76). Although PAs can be used by commensal bacteria, they can also be used by pathogens. Pathogens use PAs to promote toxin activity, bacteriocin production, biofilm formation, microbial carcinogenesis, and protection from oxidative and acid stress (77–85). While PA production and utilization are not unique to commensals, the highlighted studies provide evidence that PA synthesis by commensal bacteria may modulate the host immune response and improve patient well-being.

Tryptophan and indole

The essential amino acid L-tryptophan is used by the host to synthesize proteins and specialized molecules including the hormone and neurotransmitter serotonin (86). In addition to its use by the host, pathogens such as enteropathogenic *E. coli* and enterohemorrhagic *E. coli* can also utilize tryptophan as the sole source of carbon and nitrogen (87). As a result, conversion of tryptophan to its metabolites by commensal bacteria may effectively remove tryptophan from the amino acid pool available to pathogens. Luminal tryptophan can undergo bacterial degradation generating indole, indican, and indole acid derivatives (indolyl-3-acetic acid, indolyl-acetyl-glutamine, indolyl-propionic acid, indolyl-lactic acid, indolyl-acrylic acid, and indolyl-acryloyl-glycine). Indole is the main bacterial by-product of tryptophan. Several microbes are capable of producing indole and indole derivatives, including *Bacteroides* spp., *Bifidobacterium* spp., *Clostridium* spp., *E. coli*, *Proteus vulgaris*, *Paracolobactrum coliforme*, and *Achromobacter liquefaciens* (86, 88, 89). Bacterial tryptophanase converts tryptophan into indole, ammonia, and pyruvate. In many microbes, tryptophanase activity has been shown to be induced by tryptophan and repressible by glucose (89). Protein-rich diets have also been shown to induce bacterial tryptophanase activity (89).

Indole metabolites are noteworthy because they have been shown to provide several benefits to the host. Indole compounds secreted by commensal *E. coli* reduce attachment of pathogenic *E. coli* to epithelial cells (90). Of note, indole-3-carboxaldehyde downregulated production of pathogenic *E. coli* enterocyte effacement virulence locus and inhibited pedestal formation on mammalian cells (91). Oral administration of indole-3-carboxaldehyde was found to inhibit virulence and promote survival in a lethal mouse infection model of *Citrobacter rodentium* (91). Select indole derivatives also yielded bacteriostatic effects on Gram-negative enterobacteria, particularly pathogens such as *Salmonella* and *Shigella* (89).

In addition to the bacteriocidal effects of indole metabolites, indole itself may enhance the mucosal barrier by inducing tight junction-mediated trans-epithelial resistance and mucin production and by diminishing TNF-α-mediated activation of NF-κB (90). *In vivo*, oral administration of indole-containing capsules to germ-free mice resulted in increased quantities of tight junction- and adherens junction-associated proteins in colonic epithelial cells (92). Furthermore, germ-free mice supplemented with indole-containing capsules yielded greater resistance to dextran sodium sulfate-induced colitis (92). Indole compounds secreted by gut bacteria may be an important signal for the maintenance of intestinal epithelial homeostasis. Similar to other compounds produced by commensal microbes, indole is also utilized by several pathogens. Indole is known to regulate bio-

film formation, virulence, and production of Shiga toxins in pathogenic *E. coli* strains, as well as virulence in the rodent attaching and effacing (A/E) pathogen *C. rodentium*, and *Pseudomonas* and *Salmonella* strains (91). However, since select indole metabolites synthesized by commensals inhibit these same species, future work may focus on selecting key commensals to combat pathogens via indole metabolism.

Bacteria-Bacteria Communication

Quorum-sensing molecules

In addition to the many routes of bacterial-host communication, bacteria themselves must communicate with each other to regulate cooperative activities (93). A number of bacteria release, sense, and respond to small diffusible signal molecules, known as quorum-sensing molecules, as a method of intra- and interspecies bacterial communication. In this manner, bacteria can behave as a collective unit (94–96). Quorum sensing regulates bacterial symbiosis, formation of spore or fruiting bodies, bacteriocin production, genetic competence, programmed cell death, virulence, and biofilm formation (93, 96–99). This behavior is thought to offer significant benefits to bacteria in terms of biofilm community structure, defense against competitors, adaptation to environmental changes, and overall host colonization (93, 96, 99, 100). In general, quorum sensing relies on diffusible signaling molecules and sensors or transcriptional activators which work in concert to promote gene expression (93, 96, 99, 101, 102). Quorum sensing can be divided into three classes: (i) LuxI/LuxR-type quorum sensing in Gram-negative bacteria, (ii) oligopeptide-two-component-type quorum sensing in Gram-positive bacteria, and (iii) luxS-encoded autoinducer 2 (AI-2) quorum sensing in both Gram-negative and Gram-positive bacteria (93).

In LuxI/LuxR-type quorum sensing, acyl-homoserine lactones (AHL) act as the signaling molecules (103, 104). In this system,

AHL synthesis is dependent on a LuxI-like protein and AHLs increase in concentration in proportion to cell density. AHLs can freely diffuse across bacterial cell membranes where they are recognized and bound by the cognate LuxR-like protein, which subsequently binds specific promoter DNA elements and activates target genes. Hundreds of Gram-negative bacteria use the LuxI/LuxR-type quorum-sensing system, with each species producing a unique AHL. As a result, only similar species are able to recognize and respond to signals from their own kind (96, 99, 103, 105).

In contrast to the LuxI/LuxR system, the oligopeptide-two-component-type quorum-sensing system comprises three components: a signaling molecule and a two-component signal transduction system. The most common oligopeptide-two-component-type quorum-sensing system involves the autoinducer signaling peptide (AIP) and a corresponding two-component signal transduction system that specifically detects and responds to AIP (96, 102, 106–108). Unlike diffusible AHL signals, AIP must be transported by a dedicated oligopeptide transporter, typically an ABC transporter, to exit the cell (106–108). The AIP signal is then sensed by the two component signal transduction system, which contains a membrane-associated, histidine kinase protein and a cytoplasmic response regulator protein, which translates the signal via regulation of target gene expression (106–108). Another type of quorum sensing identified in Gram-positive streptococci is the ComRS system, which involves a small double-tryptophan signal peptide pheromone, XIP. Similar to AIP, XIP is transported inside the cell via an oligopeptide ABC transport system (Opp/Ami). Inside the cell, XIP interacts with a transcriptional regulator, ComR or ComX, thereby activating competence genes for genetic transformation (109–111). Additionally, *Streptococcus mutans* contains ComCDE and ComRS quorum-sensing systems which regulate bacteriocin production (109).

Both Gram-negative and Gram-positive bacteria can utilize the AI-2 quorum-sensing system (93, 96, 99). In contrast to the LuxI/LuxR-type and oligopeptide-two-component-type quorum-sensing systems, which provide for intraspecies signaling, AI-2 quorum sensing allows for interspecies communication. As a result, AI-2 has been termed the "universal language" (101, 102). AI-2, a furanosyl borate diester, is produced and recognized by many Gram-negative and Gram-positive bacteria (96). AI-2 synthesis depends on a luxS encoded synthase: a metabolic enzyme which converts ribosyl-homocysteine into homocysteine and 4,5-dihydroxy-2,3-pentanedione (112). AI-2 is transported inside the bacteria by the Lsr ABC-type transporter in *Enterobacteriaceae*, *Pasteurella*, *Photorhabdus*, *Haemophilus*, and *Bacillus* (113). AI-2 is then phosphorylated by LsrK and subsequently binds the transcriptional repressor protein, LsrR. Binding of phosphor-AI-2 to LsrR releases the promoter/operator region of the lsr operon, thereby promoting transcription *lsr* genes.

Since AI-2 is produced and detected by a number of diverse bacteria, it has been speculated that AI-2 facilitates interspecies communication and social interactions. This compound has been postulated to be particularly relevant in the setting of biofilms. Biofilms are considered to be structured microbial communities organized within an extracellular matrix which harness symbiotic interactions for mutual benefit of the collective (94, 95). Microbes within biofilms have diverse characteristics compared with their free-living counterparts, including enhanced resistance to antibiotics and host immune responses (93, 95, 114). Biofilms are important for both virulent pathogens and complex commensal communities within the GIT (115). For commensal microbes within the GIT, colonization of the intestinal mucus layer is a critical step in establishing ecological niches. The intestinal epithelium is covered by a continuous layer of mucus secreted by goblet cells, chiefly composed of the mucin protein MUC2 (116, 117). Mucus provides a viscoeleastic gel barrier that prevents luminal contents and microbiota from interacting directly with the epithelium and immune cells of the lamina propria. The mucin proteins are heavily O-glycosylated, and these glycans can serve as adhesion sites for commensal bacteria (118–123). Several studies have shown that intestinal communities can be visualized as biofilms of sessile microorganisms within the mucus layer (116, 124–126). High bacterial cell density within biofilms favors a mode of communication using diffusible small molecules as a mechanism for regulating biofilm formation and for social interactions (97, 127). Several studies have shown that AI-2 signaling is important for the proper development of multispecies biofilms in natural ecosystems (128–130). This signaling pathway has been particularly well documented for the oral cavity. In mixed cultures of *Actinomyces naeslundii* T14V and *Streptococcus oralis* 34, AI-2 is essential for interdigitated biofilm growth where saliva is the primary nutrient source (129). Introduction of an *S. oralis* 34 luxS mutant with *A. naeslundii* T14V diminished mutualistic growth—a defect that could be rescued with the LuxS enzyme product 4,5-dihydroxy-2,3-pentanedione. Other groups have shown luxS-dependent biofilm formation in *Streptococcus pneumoniae* (131), clinical isolates of *S. pneumoniae* D39 (132), and *L. reuteri* (133).

In the intestine, AI-2 has also been shown to play a key role in community structure and colonization. Thompson and colleagues found that AI-2 can modulate the structure of the gut microbiota by using *E. coli* to manipulate signal levels (98). In this work, AI-2 influenced bacterial behaviors to restore the balance between the major phyla of the gut microbiota, *Bacteroidetes* and *Firmicutes*, following antibiotic treatment. Although few *in vivo* studies have been conducted thus far, existing data point to the critical role of quorum sensing in the establishment of commensal communities.

METABOLITES THAT BENEFIT THE HOST

Short-Chain Fatty Acids (SCFAs)

Several bacterial species in the GIT generate SCFAs as an end product of complex carbohydrate fermentation pathways in the intestine. SCFAs are composed of one to six carbons, with the most abundant and well-characterized SCFAs being acetate, propionate, and butyrate. The composition of SCFAs in the GIT depends on microbial composition and environmental conditions, including pH, hydrogen partial pressure, and host diet (134–137). SCFAs can reach local concentrations of approximately 13 mM in the terminal ileum, 130 mM in the cecum, and 150 mM in the descending colon, making them a class of abundant colonic anions (138, 139). Most SCFAs are absorbed by the host in exchange for bicarbonate. As a result, SCFAs gradually diminish in concentrations from the proximal to the distal colon, and the luminal pH correspondingly increases from cecum to rectum (138, 140, 141). The pH reduction may alter microbial composition of the gut and prevent overgrowth by pH-sensitive pathogenic bacteria such as certain strains of *Enterobacteriaceae* and *Clostridium* (142–146). SCFAs are absorbed by intestinal enterocytes via passive diffusion or carrier-mediated transportation through SMCT1 (SLC5a8) and MCT1 (SLC16a1) transporters (147, 148). SMCT1 acts as a sodium-coupled transporter, while MCT1 is a hydrogen-coupled transporter for SCFAs and related organic acids (147–149). These transporters are found on the apical membranes of intestinal enterocytes, dendritic cells, kidney cells, and brain cells.

In addition to intestinal absorption, SCFAs can activate several G-protein-coupled cell surface receptors. SCFAs bind to G protein-coupled receptors such as GPR41, GPR43, and GPR109A, on intestinal epithelial cells and enteroendocrine cells such as colonic L cells (150–154). In addition to intestinal cells, GPR41 is also expressed in enteric neuronal cells, adipocytes, renal smooth muscle cells, and pancreatic cells (155, 156), and GPR43 is expressed by granulocytes and some myeloid cells (157–159). GPR109a is also expressed by macrophages, dendritic cells, and adipocytes. As a result of the wide distribution of receptors, SCFAs have diverse effects on the host (Fig. 3). SCFAs can regulate different aspects of host physiology, including enhanced sodium uptake and subsequent water absorption, pH regulation, chloride and mucus secretion, immune regulation, decreased bioavailability of toxic amines, and remote effects on neural activity and development (160–162).

Acetate

Acetate is the most abundant SCFA and is generated as a fermentation end product produced by enteric bacteria, as well as a product of metabolism of H_2, CO_2, or formate by acetogenic bacteria (135). *B. longum* subsp. *longum*- and *B. longum* subsp. *infantis*-secreted products suppressed epithelial cell apoptosis, ameliorated intestinal inflammation, and inhibited translocation of the *E. coli* O157:H7 Shiga toxin, thereby protecting mice against infection by enterohemorrhagic *E. coli* O157 bacteria (163). This protection correlated with fecal acetate quantities. Non-acetate-producing *Bifidobacteria* strains as well as a *B. longum* mutant with reduced acetate production were unable to mimic the protective effects of the parental strain against *E. coli* O157. Moreover, administration of acetylated starch, which increased fecal acetate, improved the survival rate. These data indicate that bacteria-produced acetate protects the host against lethal infection.

In addition to epithelial cell effects, acetate also plays an important role in immune regulation. Acetate induces T regulatory cell proliferation and accumulation (160, 164–166) and inhibits T cell histone deacetylase 6, while increasing tubulin-α acetylation (167). Ishiguro and colleagues have demonstrated that in addition to immune cells, acetate inhibits IL-8 production and increases tubulin-α acetylation within intestinal epithelial cells (167). Inoculation of germ-free

mice with the acetate producer *B. thetaiotaomicron* increased goblet cell differentiation and expression of mucus-related genes. These *in vivo* findings were confirmed *in vitro* using the mucus-producing cell line HT29-MTX, where acetate upregulated KLF4, a transcription factor involved in goblet cell differentiation (168). Mucus produced by goblet cells creates a protective barrier that prevents the epithelium and immune system from adhesion and invasion by pathogenic bacteria, microbial antigens, and other damaging agents present in the intestinal lumen (116, 127). Mucin glycans are also important sources of carbohydrate for saccharolytic bacteria, and the spatial organization and composition of mucosal communities may be influenced by variations in mucin production and glycan composition (118, 127). As a result, modulation of the mucus layer by microbial compounds such as acetate may serve to maintain a proper distance between the microbiota and host and potentially modulate the microbial community structure.

Acetate also inhibits the growth of several pathogens. Acetate alone inhibits the growth of *Pseudomonas aeruginosa* (169), while acetate in combination with propionate and butyrate inhibits the growth of pathogenic *E. coli* O157 (170), *Proteus mirabilis*, *Klebsiella pneumoniae*, and *P. aeruginosa* (169). Acetate and propionate acting via GPR43 participate in anti-inflammatory effects via the modulation of regulatory T cells (Tregs) (164, 171). *In vivo*, supplementation of acetate in germfree mice was shown to be sufficient to ameliorate the dextran sodium sulfate-driven intestinal inflammation, an effect that was not observed in Gpr43$^{-/-}$ mice (171). Interestingly, De Vuyst and Leroy demonstrated the importance of acetate as a substrate for the production of butyrate by butyrate-producing bacteria (172), implicating a crosstalk of SCFAs in microbial metabolism.

Propionate

Propionate is primarily formed via the succinate pathway by the phyla *Firmicutes* (135,

173). Propionate is principally metabolized by the liver, while acetate is metabolized by peripheral tissues. Production of acetate by the commensal *Akkermansia muciniphila* modulates mouse gene expression, particularly Fiaf, Gpr43, histone deacetylases, and peroxisome proliferator-activated receptor gamma, which are important regulators of transcription factor regulation, cell cycle control, lipolysis, and satiety (174). *In vitro* propionate inhibits several pathogens including *Salmonella enterica* serovar Typhimurium (175–178), *E. coli* O157 (170), *P. mirabilis*, *K. pneumoniae*, and *P. aeruginosa* (169). Propionate and acetate generated by microbial species stimulated the cellular function of immune cells, specifically promoting neutrophil chemotaxis (157, 171, 179, 180). In addition, propionate has been utilized for its ability to release short-term modulators of satiation and satiety, including the anorectic gut hormones peptide YY and glucagon-like peptide-1, from intestinal enteroendocrine L cells (181–185). In humans, colonic delivery of inulin-propionate esters increased plasma peptide YY and glucagon-like peptide-1 and reduced energy intake, resulting in significantly reduced weight gain, intra-abdominal adipose tissue distribution, and intrahepatocellular lipid content after 24 weeks (184). These data suggest that colonic propionate may be an important microbial metabolite in the context of host body metabolism.

Butyrate

Butyrate is generated by microbes of the phylum *Firmicutes* (including *Faecalibacterium prausnitzii*, *Roseburia* spp., *Eubacterium rectale*, *Eubacterium hallii*, and *Anaerostipes* spp.) via the butyryl-CoA:acetate CoA-transferase enzyme or phosphotransbutyrylase and butyrate kinase pathway (135, 186–188). Butyrate is primarily metabolized in the colon as an energy source utilized by intestinal epithelial cells, and this SCFA yields immunoregulatory and cancer-protective effects in the GIT. Propionate and butyrate alter immune cell function. Both propionate and butyrate inhibit stimuli-induced expression of adhesion molecules and chemokine production and suppress monocyte/macrophage and neutrophil recruitment (179). Butyrate signaling via GPR109A regulates the differentiation of regulatory Treg and IL-10-producing T cells (162) and suppresses activation of NF-κB and induction of apoptosis (189). *In vivo* production of butyrate by clostridial species induces the differentiation of Treg cells and ameliorates development of colitis (160). Apart from the major effects of butyrate on immune cell populations, this SCFA can also serve as an energy source for colonic enterocytes. Furthermore, activation of GPR43 and GPR109A by butyrate and propionate mediates cancer-protective effects associated with high fiber intake (186, 190). Butyrate also participates in antitumorigenic properties by inhibiting proliferation and selectively inducing apoptosis of colorectal cancer cells (191–194). Intracellular butyrate and propionate, but not acetate, inhibit the activity of histone deacetylases in colonocytes and immune cells. Histone deacetylase inhibition promotes the hyperacetylation of histones, effectively downregulating proinflammatory cytokines such as IL-6 and IL-12 in colonic macrophages (191, 195, 196). Together, these studies demonstrate that commensal-produced SCFAs can elicit multiple advantages for the host through the stimulation of intestinal mucus production, inhibition of inflammation, modulation of immune cell populations, and inhibition of cancer proliferation.

Long-Chain Fatty Acids (LCFAs)

While SCFAs have been thoroughly characterized with respect to intestinal biology and human health, LCFAs are gaining attention for their health-promoting activities as well (197). Similar to SCFAs, commensal bacteria are also responsible for the composition and concentration of LCFAs and subsequently contribute to LCFA-induced signaling in host cells. LCFAs are produced when dietary polyunsaturated fatty acids such as linoleic acids are converted into conjugated linoleic acids and trans-fatty acids (198–200). Germ-free mice without a gut microbiota lack detectable LCFAs (201), while inoculation of mice with the commensal *Bifidobacterium breve* in combination with a linoleic acid-supplemented diet resulted in increased conjugated linoleic acids (202). Production of conjugated linoleic acid by bacteria reduced amounts of hepatic triacylglycerols and inhibited atherosclerosis (203, 204). Although it remains unclear if LCFAs regulate host immune functions, modified polyunsaturated fatty acids are potent agonists for peroxisome proliferator-activated receptor-γ and peroxisome proliferator-activated receptor-α, which are upregulated by commensal bacteria and implicated in attenuating inflammation (197, 205–208). The role of LCFAs in intestinal homeostasis was further confirmed *in vivo* in ethanol-fed mice. Exposure of mice to alcohol resulted in an altered gut microbiota and reduced synthesis of LCFAs (209). Relative abundances of *Lactobacillus* spp., known metabolizers of saturated LCFAs, were reduced in the feces of humans with active alcohol abuse (209). The authors hypothesized that targeted approaches to restore LCFA levels might reduce ethanol-induced liver injury and restore an intact community of gut microbiota.

Vitamins

Bacteria residing in mammals are able to produce vitamins which directly benefit the host (210). Metagenomic analyses of the human microbiota from the distal colon revealed the existence of diverse clustered orthologous groups which are involved in vitamin synthesis (211). Vitamins are essential organic micronutrients which are critical for cellular function and may not be synthesized by the host. Vitamins exist as precursors of intracellular coenzymes. The majority of vitamins are produced by bacteria via the 2-methyl-D-erythritol 4-phosphate pathway. Thirteen essential vitamins for human health include the water-soluble vitamins thiamine (B_1), riboflavin (B_2), niacin (B_3), pyridoxine (B_6), pantothenic acid (B_5), biotin (B_7 or H), folate (B_{11}-B_9 or M), and cobalamin (B_{12}); vitamin C; and the fat-soluble vitamins A, D, E, and K (212). Vitamins generated by gut microbes are primarily absorbed in the colon, while dietary vitamins are absorbed mostly in the small intestine (213, 214). Data suggest that colonocytes absorb thiamine, folates, biotin, riboflavin, pantothenic acid, and menaquinones (213, 214). Vitamins provide essential nutrients to the host and directly influence the development and function of immune cells (215–218). In this manner, vitamins may promote host growth and immune homeostasis (Fig. 3).

Water-soluble vitamins

Riboflavin (vitamin B_2)
Riboflavin, or vitamin B_2, is a known component of cellular metabolism. Riboflavin is a precursor of the coenzymes flavin mononucleotide and flavin adenine dinucleotide (219). Flavin mononucleotide and flavin adenine dinucleotide are hydrogen carriers in cellular redox reactions, making B_2 critical for host metabolism. B_2 can exist in several active forms including riboflavin [7,8-dimethyl-10-(1'-D-ribityl) isoalloxazine], riboflavin-5'-phosphate (flavin mononucleotide), and riboflavin-5'-adenosyldiphosphate (flavin adenine dinucleotide). Riboflavin can be produced by both Gram-positive and Gram-negative bacteria and is well characterized in *Bacillus subtilis* and *E. coli* (220, 221). LAB strains including *L. plantarum* and *Lb. lactis* have also been identified as B_2 producers (219, 222–225). B_2 can be produced from the precursor guanosine triphosphate and D-ribulose 5-phosphate via seven enzymatic steps (220). Enhanced production of B_2 has been shown in species that are capable of simultaneously expressing four biosynthetic genes (*ribG*, *ribH*, *rib*, and *ribA*) (223, 224).

Deficiency in B_2 levels leads to ariboflavinosis, which is associated with hyperemia, edema of oral and mucous membranes, cheilosis, and glossitis (226). In rats, supplementation of a fermented milk drink containing a genetically modified B2-producing *Lb. lactis* strain was effective in reversing ariboflavinosis in a riboflavin-deficiency model (223). In humans, daily consumption of a probiotic yogurt containing *Streptococcus thermophilus*, *Lactobacillus bulgaricus*, and *Lactobacillus casei* subsp. *casei* for 2 weeks contributed to the total intake of vitamin B_2, as reflected by increased blood concentrations of plasma-free riboflavin in healthy women (227). These effects were ameliorated when subjects returned to their previous diet, implicating select supplemented probiotic bacteria in the enhanced production of vitamin B_2 (227).

Folates (B_{11}–B_9 or M)

Folates are hydrophilic anionic molecules which are produced by a number of bacteria. The generic term "folate" is typically used to include all bacterially derived folate derivatives. Folates are involved in essential cellular metabolism functions including DNA replication, DNA repair, DNA methylation, and nucleotide synthesis. Folate deficiency has been linked to a large spectrum of disorders including colorectal cancer, osteoporosis, coronary heart disease, and Alzheimer's disease, among others (228, 229). Although folate is primarily absorbed in the duodenum and jejunum, folate compounds generated by the mammalian microbiome in the colon represent a major source of host folate. Bacteria generate mono- and polyglutamylated folate, a form of folate which is easily absorbed by mammalian cells (230, 231). Multiple LAB strains such as *L. reuteri*, *Lactobacillus acidophilus*, *L. plantarum*, *L. bulgaricus*, *Lactococcus lactis*, *Bifidobacterium adolescentis*, *B. animalis*, and *B. longum* synthesize folate (228, 231–237). However, not all LAB strains are capable of generating folate. For example, *Lactobacillus gasseri*

(236), *Lactobacillus salivarius* (238), and *Lactobacillus johnsonii* (239) do not contain folate biosynthesis genes and do not produce folate. Bacterial production of folate in the presence of existing folate appears to be species dependent, with select species producing folate solely in low-folate conditions, and others continually producing folate (240). Bacteria produce folate using the precursor 6-hydroxymethyl-7,8-dihydropterin pyrophosphate and para-aminobenzoic acid (pABA, vitamin B_{10}) (25, 241).

All bacteria capable of producing folate contain the *folC* or homologous genes (231, 235). Additional genes involved in folate production include *folKE* genes, which encode 6-hydroxymethyl-dihydropterinpyrophosphokinase (*folK*), and guanosine triphosphate cyclohydrolase (*folE*) or pABA (242). Folate production relies on the combination of folate and pABA biosynthesis. Deletion of the pABA genes in *Lb. lactis* and *L. reuteri* resulted in a loss of folate production and inhibition of growth in the absence of purine nucleobases/nucleosides (242). Genetic manipulation of folate genes increased folate production in a number of species including *Lb. lactis*, *L. gasseri*, and *L. reuteri* (233, 236, 237, 242). *In vivo* addition of *Lb. lactis* overexpressing the *folC*, *folKE*, or *folC-folKE* genes improved folate status in a rat folate deficiency model (228). In *L. reuteri* ATCC PTA 6475, the gene *folC2* is required for production of 5,10-methenyltetrahydrofolic acid (5,10-CH=THF) and *folC* participates in polyglutamylation of 5,10-CH=THF. Mutations in *folC2* resulted in loss of 5,10-CH=THF and diminished the strain's ability to suppress TNF production by activated human monocytes (231). Additionally, the *L. reuteri folC2* mutant was unable to suppress inflammation to the same degree as wild-type *L. reuteri* in a trinitrobenzene sulfonic acid-induced mouse model of acute colitis (231). These studies demonstrate that select folate-producing microbes can be utilized to improve folate status and modulate the immune system in animal models.

Vitamin B_{12}

Vitamin B_{12}, also known as cobalamin, exists in its natural form as 5′-deoxyadenosylcobalamin (coenzyme B_{12}), methylcobalamin, or pseudocobalamin, and is a corrin ring or corrinoid compound. B_{12} is required for the metabolism of nucleic acids, amino acids, and fatty acids (243) and is primarily produced by anaerobic bacteria (244–246). Few bacteria are capable of producing vitamin B_{12} (247, 248). Typically, specialized bacteria found in food source animals produce vitamin B_{12}. As a result, humans must absorb the coenzyme from animal sources such as meats, fish, and eggs. However, select lactobacilli have been demonstrated to produce vitamin B_{12}. *L. reuteri* CRL1098 was found to produce a cobalamin-like compound, a form of B_{12} (249). *L. reuteri* DSM 20016 (237), JCM1112 (237), and CRL 1324 and 1327 (250) and *Lactobacillus coryniformis* (251) produced a cobalamin-type compound. These *L. reuteri* species contain an extensive cobalamin biosynthesis cluster, which is associated with the anaerobic catabolism of glycerol (or 1,2-propanediol) (252, 253). Vitamin B_{12} deficiency is associated with numerous hematopoietic, neurological, and cardiovascular pathologies. Pernicious anemia, a severe form of B_{12} deficiency, is the result of poor production of a gastric glycoprotein called intrinsic factor that facilitates the absorption of vitamin B_{12} in the small intestine (254). *In vivo* in a mouse model of vitamin B_{12}-deficient animals, supplementation of *L. reuteri* CRL 1098 reversed vitamin B_{12} deficiency (255). Gut microbes may be important in maintaining adequate body concentrations of B complex vitamins, including vitamin B_{12}.

Fat-soluble vitamins

Vitamin K

Vitamin K comprises a number of series of fat-soluble compounds which share a 2-methyl-1,4-naphthoquinone nucleus and different side chain structures at the 3-position. Vitamin K can be produced by both plants and microbes. In plants, vitamin K exists as phylloquinone (vitamin K1), which has a phytyl side chain. In contrast, bacteria generate a family of compounds known as menaquinones (vitamin K2). These compounds contain side chains based on repeating unsaturated 5-carbon (prenyl) units and are designated menaquinone-n (MK-n) according to the number (n) of prenyl units. Vitamin K is an essential cofactor in the formation of γ-carboxyglutamic acid residues in proteins which bind calcium ions. As a result, vitamin K serves a prominent role in bone formation, tissue calcification, kidney function, and blood clotting, to name a few functions (256, 257). Vitamin K deficiency has been implicated in osteoporosis-driven bone fracture and intracranial hemorrhage in newborns. The gut microbiota synthesizes large amounts of menaquinone K2, one of the forms of vitamin K (258). Quantitative measurements at different sites of the human intestine have demonstrated that most of these menaquinones are present in the distal colon (258). Specific microbes are capable of generating menaquinone K2, one of the forms of vitamin K. The genera *Lactobacillus*, *Lactococcus*, *Enterococcus*, *Leuconostoc*, and *Streptococcus* are known producers of K2 (259, 260). Other major menaquinone forms are produced by *Bacteroides* (MK-10, MK-11), *Enterobacter* (MK-8), *Veillonella* (MK-7), and *Eubacterium lentum* (MK-6). Vitamin K is predominantly absorbed in the terminal ileum of the intestine, a site where menaquinone-producing bacteria colonize as well. Collectively, the data acquired from all vitamin studies point to the selection of multivitamin-producing bacteria to compensate for common vitamin deficiencies and for promotion of gut homeostasis.

Outer Membrane Vesicles (OMVs)

Several bacteria are capable of releasing OMVs, which range in size from 20 to 300 nm in Gram-negative bacteria (261) to <20 nm in Gram-positive bacteria (262, 263).

OMV production is considered to be a common feature of Gram-negative bacteria. They are generated by membrane remodeling which occurs when the outer membrane bulges and encapsulates periplasmic components (264, 265). As a result, OMVs contain a number of soluble proteins entrapped in the OMV periplasm and multiple proteins on the external surface. Secreted OMVs can disseminate compounds to distant sites. OMVs have yielded a wide range of biological functions, from delivery of enzymes to transport of toxins, transmission of communication signals, nutrient acquisition, and induction of commensal tolerance. One beneficial role of OMVs on host homeostasis is their ability to modulate innate and adaptive immune systems (266) (Fig. 3). *Bacteroides fragilis* OMV delivery of polysaccharide capsular antigen (PSA) yielded multiple immunomodulatory effects. Monocolonization of germ-free mice with *B. fragilis* was shown to modulate CD4$^+$ T cell homeostasis and cytokine production (3). T cell modulation occurs in a PSA-dependent manner (3). OMV-delivered PSA stimulated TLR2 on Tregs and directly modulated DCs (267, 268). OMVs were internalized by DCs, and this interaction promoted tolerogenic DCs which produced IL-10 and stimulated regulatory Tregs. Furthermore, PSA production ameliorated intestinal inflammation (269), central nervous system inflammation (270, 271) and neurodegeneration (272). These studies demonstrate that OMV delivery of PSA is capable of promoting an anti-inflammatory profile which leads to tolerance and suppression of mucosal inflammation.

Serpin

Serpins are eukaryotic-type serine protease inhibitors. These molecules are synthesized by several commensal bacteria. Serpins are relatively large molecules consisting of approximately 330 to 500 amino acids (273). More than 70 serpin structures have been identified. These complex structures act as stoichiometric suicide inactivators and inhibit eukaryotic elastase-like serine proteases. Serpins are known to regulate a wide range of signaling pathways in eukaryotes. Select serpins have been shown to suppress inflammatory responses by inhibiting elastase activity (274) (Fig. 3). Several bifidobacterial species and subspecies (*B. breve*, *B. longum* subsp. *infantis*, *B. longum* subsp. *longum*, and *B. dentium*) are capable of producing serpins (275). *B. longum* NCC2705 was shown to secrete a serpin which binds and inactivates human neutrophil elastase, a product secreted by neutrophils during active inflammation (276). Moreover, bifidobacterial serpin-like proteins have been shown to reduce intestinal inflammation in a murine colitis model (277). Based on these findings, production of serpins which inhibit neutrophil elastases may be beneficial for reducing intestinal damage in the setting of overt inflammation.

Lactocepin

Lactocepins are bacterial enzymes which can degrade targeted bacteria of different genera via damage to prokaryotic cell membranes and induction of proinflammatory modulators (Fig. 3). Lactocepins can be cell wall associated or secreted, and the target specificity is strain specific (278–280). Lactocepins are mainly expressed by lactococci and lactobacilli. These enzymes are encoded by *prtP*, *prtB*, and/or *prtH*. The *prtP* genes are well documented for their caseinolytic properties. *L. paracasei* secreted *prtP*-encoded lactocepin, and this compound selectively degraded the lymphocyte-recruiting chemokine IP-10 and other proinflammatory chemokines such as I-TAC and eotaxin *in vitro* (281). Importantly, *prtP*-encoded lactocepin selectively degraded IP-10 in inflamed intestinal tissue and had no adverse effects on intestinal epithelial cell barrier function *in vivo* (281). This resulted in significantly reduced lymphocyte recruitment after intraperitoneal injection in an ileitis model. Another *Lactobacillus* strain, *L. casei*, was found to secrete lactocepin which degraded host IP-10 (282). In a murine colitis model (T cell transferred Rag2$^{-/-}$ mice), supplementation of an *L. caseiprtP*-disruption mutant resulted in more IP-10, T cell infiltration, and inflammation in cecal tissue compared to the isogenic wild-type strain. Supplementation of the probiotic VSL#3, which contains *Lactobacillus, Bifidobacterium,* and *Streptococcus*, normalized intestinal levels of IP-10 in a murine colitis model and reduced inflammation in patients with inflammatory bowel disease (282). These studies support the role of lactocepin secreted by commensal microbes as an effective treatment for chemokine-mediated diseases such as inflammatory bowel disease.

Other Secreted Proteins Known To Enhance Host Health

In addition to all the secreted products highlighted by this review, select commensal bacteria generate putative proteins which modulate the host (Fig. 3). *L. rhamnosus* GG and *L. casei* secrete two proteins designated p40 and p75 (283, 284). Lactobacilli-produced p40 and p75 were found to inhibit TNF-induced apoptosis in the intestinal epithelium. The proteins signal via the antiapoptotic Akt kinase in a phosphoinositide 3-kinase-dependent manner likely via epidermal growth factor receptor activation (283, 285). The p40 and p75 proteins also enhance tight junctions and attenuate intestinal barrier disruption via protein kinase C and extracellular signal-regulated kinase 1. Furthermore, p40 was shown to transactivate the epidermal growth factor receptor, activating the downstream target Akt and stimulating mucus Muc2 gene expression and mucin production in the human goblet cell line LS174T and wild-type mice. Intestinal mucus is a critical component of the healthy intestinal barrier, particularly in the setting of infection and inflammation (122, 286–288). Stimulation of intestinal mucus by commensal bacteria likely enhances barrier function and promotes homeostasis. Other commensal bacteria produce putative proteins with immunoregulatory

features. *F. prausnitzii* is known to produce a 15-kDa protein, termed MAM, with anti-inflammatory properties (289, 290). MAM inhibits the NF-κB pathway in intestinal epithelial cells and prevents colitis *in vivo*. Because subgroups of Crohn's disease are associated with reduced relative abundances of *F. prausnitzii*, microbial and protein (e.g., MAM) supplementation has been hypothesized to alleviate intestinal inflammation in future clinical trials. These studies highlight the need to define secreted commensal products of the mammalian microbiome.

ANTIMICROBIAL COMPOUNDS

Lactic Acid

Commensal microbes may produce organic acids such as lactic acid that may reduce local pH and suppress the growth and survival of neighboring microbes. A group of microbes known as lactic acid bacteria (LAB) produce relatively large amounts of lactic acid as a major catabolic end product of glucose fermentation. In general, LAB consist of non-spore-forming Gram-positive bacteria with a DNA base composition of less than 53 mol% G+C (291). LAB members include *Lactobacillus, Lactococcus, Leuconostoc, Enterococcus, Streptococcus, Pediococcus, Carnobacterium, Aerococcus, Oenococcus, Tetragenococcus, Vagococcus,* and *Weisella*. The generation of lactic acid results in the recycling of electron acceptors for ATP generation by bacterial species. In addition to this role in the bacteria, lactic acid production benefits the host by reducing local pH and suppressing colonization and proliferation of potential pathogens. Lactic acid is readily miscible with water due to its low hydrophobicity and low acid dissociation constant. Lactic acid is effective against Gram-negative bacteria and to a lesser extent against Gram-positive bacteria (292, 293). As a liposoluble organic acid, lactic acid in its undissociated form can penetrate the bacterial cytoplasmic membrane (294). In

Gram-negative bacteria, lactic acid transverses the outer membrane via water-filled porins and penetrates the cytoplasmic membrane. Additionally, in Gram-negative bacteria, lactic acid can act as a potent outer membrane-disintegrating agent, as evidenced by LPS release and sensitization of bacteria to detergents or lysozyme (293). Lactic acid-induced changes in cell membrane permeability can hinder substrate transport and promote further entrance of lactic acid into the cytoplasm, thereby effectively lowering the intracellular pH (293–295) (Fig. 3). Intracellular acidity can suppress NADH oxidation, altering the membrane electron transport system and transmembrane proton motive force (295). Malfunction of the electron transport system can lead to oxidative stress and generation of free radicals that damage DNA and proteins. These free radicals can then damage intracellular components as well as the extracellular membrane (296). Collectively, these mechanisms result in cell death to susceptible bacteria.

Lactic acid in sufficient quantities may inhibit the growth of a wide range of bacterial species (244, 297, 298). Addition of pure lactic acid *in vitro* has both inhibitory and biocidal effects against several pathogens, including the Gram-negative *E. coli*, *P. mirabilis*, *Salmonella enteritidis*, and *P. aeruginosa* and the Gram-positive *Staphylococcus aureus*, *Enterococcus faecalis*, *Listeria monocytogenes*, *Bacillus cereus*, and *Bacillus megaterium* and minimal fungicidal activity against the yeasts *Rhodotorula* sp., *Saccharomyces cerevisiae*, and *Candida albicans* (299). Generation of lactic acid by commensal bacteria also inhibits the growth of several pathogens including *Helicobactor pylori*, *B. subtilis*, *B. cereus*, *Staphylococcus epidermidis*, *E. coli* CB6, *Klebsiella* sp. strain CB2, *Streptococcus pyogenes*, *P. aeruginosa*, *Salmonella enterica* serovar Paratyphi, and *Salmonella enterica* serovar Typhimurium (298, 300–307). In these studies, lactic acid alters *in vivo* pH, inhibits pathogen urease activity, inhibits pathogen growth, and acts as a bactericidal agent.

Additionally L-lactic acid suppresses immune cell-mediated proinflammatory responses (308). Modulation of the immune system and alteration of local GIT pH have been speculated to selectively manipulate the gut microbiota composition (120, 121, 309), which may further promote colonization resistance and inhibition of pathogens. In addition to the antimicrobial effects of lactic acid itself, several studies have demonstrated that unidentified bacterial substances, bacteriocins, and hydrogen peroxide act in concert with lactic acid to inhibit the growth of pathogens (300, 303, 307).

Hydrogen Peroxide

Bacterially produced hydrogen peroxide (H_2O_2) is known to act synergistically with L-lactic acid (310) (Fig. 3). H_2O_2 produced by certain microbes can damage bacterial nucleic acids by creating breaks in the carbon phosphate backbone of DNA, releasing nucleotides, and preventing chromosomal replication (311, 312). Additionally, hydroxyl radicals, which can be produced from the dissociation of H_2O_2, can attack the methyl group of thymine, resulting in damaged DNA (313, 314). Anaerobic bacteria are more sensitive to H_2O_2 because they do not produce catalase, which can break down H_2O_2. In general, Gram-negative bacteria are more sensitive than Gram-positive bacteria to H_2O_2. However, select Gram-negative bacteria have developed a mechanism to deal with H_2O_2. These microbes utilize an outer LPS layer which traps active molecular oxygen (315). Lactic acid disrupts the outer membrane of Gram-negative bacteria, releasing LPS and making cells sensitive to H_2O_2 and antimicrobial agents (293). Several microbes are known to produce H_2O_2, including lactobacilli and bifidobacteria (316, 317). Many studies have demonstrated that bacterially produced H_2O_2 inhibits the growth of pathogens such as *S. aureus*, *S. enterica* serovar Typhimurium, *L. monocytogenes*, *E. faecalis*, *E. faecium*, enterotoxigenic *E. coli*,

E. coli CFT074, *Listeria ivanovii*, *S. aureus*, *Yersinia enterocolitica*, *Aeromonas hydrophila*, *Gardnerella vaginalis* DSM494, *Neisseria gonorrhoeae*, *S. mutans*, *Bacteroides forsythus*, *Capnocytophaga sputigena*, *Eikenella corrodens*, *Fusobacterium nucleatum*, *Porphyromonas gingivalis*, *Prevotella intermedia*, and *Wolinella recta* (317–328). The effect of LAB-produced H_2O_2 on pathogen inhibition was found to be significantly enhanced by lactic acid (323), supporting the role of H_2O_2 and lactic acid acting in concert to shape microbial communities. However, commensal bacteria are not the sole producers of H_2O_2. The production of H_2O_2 by the pathogen *S. pneumoniae* inhibited growth of viral *Haemophilus influenzae* and fellow bacterial pathogens *Moraxella catarrhalis*, *Neisseria meningitidis*, and *S. aureus* (329, 330). Thus, it has been speculated that pathogens use H_2O_2 production to inhibit competing organisms and secure a niche.

Bacteriocins

The production of antimicrobial compounds by bacteria provides specific microorganisms with a competitive advantage for colonization. The production of bacteriocins is a nearly universal trait, because it is projected that the majority of bacteria and archaea produce at least one bacteriocin (331–333). The ubiquity of this trait implies that bacteriocins play an important role *in vivo* as colonizing peptides, as tools for inhibiting commensal or pathogen niche occupation, or as signaling peptides (333–338). Wide variation exists in the chemical composition and mechanisms of action of different bacteriocins. Bacteriocins can be classified based on the bacteria that secrete them (Gram-negative or Gram-positive). In general, bacteriocins produced by Gram-positive bacteria have antimicrobial effects on other Gram-positive bacteria (331). Production of bacteriocins by probiotic bacteria has been speculated to promote colonization and inhibit pathogens (161, 333). In contrast, production

of bacteriocins by pathogenic bacteria has been postulated to provide a competitive edge for infection (339). Wide variation exists in the chemical composition and mechanism of action of different bacteriocins. Most bacteriocins target phosphate groups on bacterial cell membranes, deplete the transmembrane potential ($\Delta\psi$) and/or the pH gradient, and form membrane pores, resulting in membrane disruption and cellular leakage (340–342) (Fig. 4). Similar to other compounds such as H_2O_2, bacteriocins may yield synergistic effects with lactic acid and exhibit greater antibacterial activities at lower pH values. To simplify our review, we have chosen to focus primarily on bacteriocins produced by commensal bacteria, as opposed to ones produced by pathogens.

Bacteriocin diversity and classification

Gram-positive bacteriocins

Class I: the lantibiotics. Lantibiotics are small (<5 kDa) peptides characterized by the unusual amino acids lanthionine, α-methyllanthionine, dehydroalanine, and dehydrobutyrine. Within class I, molecules can be subgrouped into type A or type B according to their chemical structures and antimicrobial activities (343–345). Type A lantibiotics exhibit elongated screw-shaped peptides with a net positive charge. The shape and charge of type A molecules facilitate membrane pore formation and membrane depolarization in sensitive species. Type A molecules generally are 2 to 4 kDa in molecular weight. The best characterized of the type A lantibiotics is the *Lc. lactis*-produced nisin. Nisin inhibits the growth of a range of Gram-positive bacteria including *L. monocytogenes*, *S. aureus*, and *B. cereus* (346–349). Nisin also prevents spore germination by the pathogens *Clostridium botulinum*, *Clostridium sporogenes*, *B. cereus*, and *Bacillus anthracis* (341, 350–353). In vegetative cells, nisin binds to lipid II on targeted bacterial membranes. Nisin orients parallel to the surface of the target membrane and

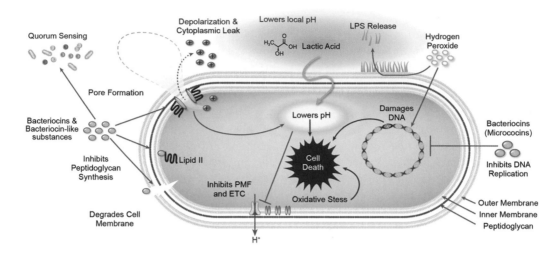

FIGURE 4 Schematic representation of the molecular mechanisms of commensal secreted products on a Gram-negative bacterium. Bacteriocins are classified based on their structure. Bacteriocins such as nisin bind to a peptidoglycan subunit transporter, thereby preventing cell wall synthesis and resulting in cell death. Furthermore, bacteriocins can initiate pore formation. Pore formation depletes the bacterial transmembrane potential (Δψ) and/or the pH gradient, resulting in membrane disruption and cellular leakage that lead to rapid cell death. Other bacteriocins insert themselves directly or degrade the target membrane, leading to depolarization and death. Bacteriocins have also been shown to serve as quorum-sensing molecules for other microbes. Lactic acid decreases local pH and suppresses the growth and survival of pathogens. Additionally, undissociated lactic acid can traverse the outer membrane via water-filled porins and penetrate the cytoplasmic membrane. This shift lowers the intracellular pH, disrupts the transmembrane proton motive force, and generates oxidative stress. Hydrogen peroxide and select bacteriocins such as microcins damage bacterial DNA and inhibit cell growth. Together, these compounds secreted by select members of the microbiota effectively target pathogens.

inserts the C terminus of the peptide into the phospholipids, thereby disrupting cell wall biosynthesis and creating a "wedge-like" pore (354). Pore formation causes a rapid non-specific amino acid and cation efflux and subsequent cell membrane rupture and cell death (355, 356). In spores, nisin also utilizes lipid II binding and pore formation in germinated spores during outgrowth, leading to membrane disruption that inhibits spore development into vegetative cells. Type A lantibiotics include lacticin (*Lc. lactis* lacticin 3147 [357], *Lc. lactis* subsp. *lactis* lacticin 481 [358]), lactocin (*L. rhamnosus* lactocin 160 [342], *Lactobacillus sake* L45 lactocin S [359]), *S. epidermidis* epidermin (360), and *Staphylococcus gallinarum* gallidermin (361).

In comparison to type A molecules, type B lantibiotics are smaller (2 to 3 kDa) globular peptides with a negative or neutral charge. Also in contrast to type A lantibiotics, type B peptides exert their antimicrobial activity via cell lysis and inhibition of essential bacterial enzymes. Type B lantibiotics increase membrane permeability and reduce ATP-dependent protein transport and ATP-dependent calcium uptake in sensitive bacterial cells, resulting in cell lysis. Cell lysis was significantly reduced when the type B lantibiotics cinnamycin and duramycin were incubated with the phospholipid phosphatidylethanolamine (362–364). The data indicate that type B lantibiotics interact with phospholipid targets. In addition to membrane effects, type B lantibiotics are also known to inhibit bacterial enzymes such as phospholipase A and peptidoglycan synthesis. Examples of type B lantibiotics include *Lactobacillus curvatus* curvacin A, *Streptomyces cinnamoneus* cinnamycin, *Streptomyces* subsp. ancovenin (365), *Streptoverticillium* R2075 duramycins B and C, and *Streptomyces griseoluteus* (R2107) duramycins B and C (366).

Class II. Class II bacteriocins are small (<10 kDa), heat stable, nonlanthionine-containing membrane-active peptides. These peptides can be further divided into subgroups based on sequence and function: a, b, c, d, and e. The subgroup class IIa comprises pediocin-like peptides containing an N-terminal consensus sequence -Tyr-Gly-Asn-Gly-Val-Xaa-Cys. Class IIa bacteriocins are produced by food-associated bacterial strains and have garnered attention due to their anti-*Listeria* activity (367, 368). Similar to class I molecules, class IIa bacteriocins kill target cells by permeabilizing the cell membrane (340, 369). Class II molecules bind to the target membrane using the cationic N-terminal beta sheet domain of the peptide, while the C-terminal regions form a hairpin-like domain which penetrates into the target cell membrane. This penetration results in leakage of cytoplasmic components through the membrane, resulting in cell death. Bacteriocins belonging to the class IIa family include *Lb. lactis* lactococcin MMFII, *Bifidobacterium bifidum* NCFB bifidocin B, *B. longum* subsp. *infantis* bifidin I, *Pediococcus acidilactici* pediocin PA-1, *Carnobacterium piscicola* carnobacteriocin B2, *Carnobacterium divergens* divercin V41, *Lactobacillus sakei* sakacin P, *L. sake* sakacin A, *Enterococcus faecium* enterocin A, *E. faecium* enterocin P, *Leuconostoc gelidum* leucocin A, *Leuconostoc mesenteroides* mesentericinY105 (280, 370–378), and *Pediococcus pentosaceus* K23-2 (379). Class IIb contains bacteriocins that require two separate peptides for activity. Similar to class IIa they act as pore-forming peptides (380). Class IIb peptides include *Lb. lactis* lactococcin G and M, *L. salivarius* UCC118 Abp118, *L. johnsonii* lactacin F, and *L. plantarum* plantaricin A, S, E, F, and JK (338, 357, 381–388). The class IIc peptides have a wide range of effects on membrane permeability and cell wall formation. One of the well-documented class IIc molecules is *E. faecalis* bacteriocin AS-48 (389). Bacteriocin AS-48 consists of five alpha helices enclosing a hydrophobic core, creating a globular structure which creates membrane pores in susceptible Gram-positive or Gram-negative bacteria. Other examples include *L. acidophilus* acidocin B, *C. piscicola* carnobacteriocin A, *C. divergens* divergicin A, and *E. faecium* enterocin P and B (390–393). Class IId bacteriocins are linear, non-pediocin-like, single-peptide bacteriocins with similar antimicrobial activity. Class IId molecules include *Lb. lactis* lactococcin A, *S. epidermidis* epidermicin NI01, and *Streptococcus cremoris* diplococcin (386, 394, 395). Class IIe bacteriocins comprise nonribosomal siderophore-type posttranslational modifications at the serine-rich carboxy-terminal region of the peptide. Class IIe molecules include *Klebsiella pneumoniae* microcin E492 (396, 397).

Class III. Class III bacteriocins comprise large-molecular-weight (>30 kDa) heat-labile proteins. This class is further divided in two subclasses: IIIa and IIIb. Subclass IIIa, also known as bacteriolysins, encompasses peptides that degrade bacterial cell membranes, resulting in cell lysis and subsequent cell death. The most well-characterized members of subclass IIIa are *Staphylococcus* spp.-produced lysostaphin. Lysostaphin is a 27-kDa peptide that cleaves cell wall cross-linking pentaglycin bridges, thereby hydrolyzing susceptible staphylococci, including the pathogen *S. aureus* (398–400). Another member of the subclass IIIa group is *E. faecium* enterolysin (401). Subclass IIIb comprises peptides which disrupt target cell membrane potential, causing ATP efflux and death. In contrast to subclass IIIa, these peptides do not cause cell lysis. Other members of class III include bacteriocins from subclass IIIb such as *L. casei* caseicin 80 and *L. helveticus* helveticin J and V-1829 (402–404).

Class IV. Class IV bacteriocins were recently described and are defined as complex bacteriocins containing lipid or carbohydrate moities. The class IV bacteriocins are cyclical due to covalent bonding of the first and last amino acids and are considered to be S-linked glycopeptides with antimicrobial activity. Examples of class IV molecules include *E. faecalis* subsp. *liquefaciens* S-48 enterocin AS-48, *E. faecalis* F4-9 enterocin F4-9, *B. subtilis* 168 sublancin (an S-linked glycopeptide), and *L. plantarum* KW30 glycocin F (GccF) (405–408). Peptides from this class exhibit a wide pH range, variable resistance to heat, and loss of antimicrobial activity when exposed to proteolytic enzymes (408–410). The cationic charges of enterocin F4-9 and glycocin F were found to be essential for interactions with charged phospholipids in target bacterial cells. These interactions did not induce cell lysis, suggesting that these bacteriocins have a bacteriostatic effect. Enterocin F4-9 yielded antimicrobial activity against *E. faecalis* and *E. coli* JM109, but not *E. faecium* and other *E. coli* members (408). In contrast, glycocin F was found to have activity against lactobacilli (410), while sublancin 168 had activity against Gram-positive bacteria, specifically *Bacillus* spp., but not *E. coli* JM101 (409). These studies indicate that class IV bacteriocins target unique epitopes.

Gram-negative bacteriocins

Microcins. Microcins are low-molecular-weight (<10 kDa) hydrophobic antimicrobial peptides synthesized on bacterial ribosomes. These molecules are primarily produced by Gram-negative *Enterobacteriaceae* (phylum *Proteobacteria*). Microcins are generally heat-, extreme pH-, and protease-tolerant (411). They exhibit a wide range of structural diversity and antimicrobial mechanisms. Microcins target other bacterial cells via pore formation, DNAse or RNAse nuclease function, inhibition of protein synthesis, or inhibition of DNA replication (412). One of the more deceptive ways microcins exert their antibacterial activity is through a "Trojan horse" strategy whereby they imitate essential nutrients (411). Microcins mimic small, high-affinity iron-chelating compounds (iron-siderophore complexes). Because iron is required for bacterial DNA synthesis, microcins resembling iron-siderophores are able to bind to outer membrane receptors on target bacteria and translocate into the periplasmic space, where they can exert their antimicrobial activity.

Despite the wide diversity, these molecules are classified in two classes depending on their molecular masses, disulfide bonds, and posttranslational modifications: class I and II. Class I microcins are plasmid-encoded and low molecular weight (<5 kDa) and are posttranslationally modified. Examples of class I microcins include *E. coli* microcin B17, C7-C51, D93, and J25. Class II microcins are larger in molecular weight (5 to 10 kDa) and produced by and active against *Enterobacteriaceae*. Class II microcins are divided into two subclasses: IIa and IIb. Class IIa microcins do not undergo posttranslational modification, while class IIb microcins exhibit posttranslational modifications in the form of a salmochelin-like siderophore motif (413). Additionally, class IIa peptides typically contain one or two disulfide bond(s). Class IIa molecules include *E. coli* microcin L, V, S, and N, all of which require three different genes to synthesize the molecule. Class IIb microcins are differentiated from class IIa by their linear structure or lack of posttranslational modifications at the C terminus (412, 414). Examples of class IIb molecules include *E. coli* Nissle 1917 microcin M, *E. coli* Nissle 1917 microcin H47, and *Klebsiella* microcin E492.

Colicins. In contrast to low-molecular-weight microcins, colicins are high-molecular-weight (25 to 80 kDa) proteins with antimicrobial activity. Colicins act by binding to outer membrane receptors, penetrating the cytoplasmic membrane, and then causing cytotoxic effects, including cytoplasmic membrane depolarization, DNase activity, RNase activity, or murein synthesis inhibition. Colicins use a two-receptor system to target cells. First, colicins bind to outer membrane receptors such as the porins OmpF, FepA, BtuB, Cir, and FhuA, which are typically used for entry of specific nutrients into the bacterial cells. Next, colicins are translocated through the outer membrane and enter the cell cytoplasm by either the Tol or Ton system, where they can exert their cytotoxic effect (415). Colicins are divided into categories based on their outer membrane translocation system (either Tol or Ton). The Ton and Tol systems are two-protein arrangements which *E. coli* uses to transfer energy from the inner membrane to the outer membrane. The systems differ in their component proteins. The Ton system consists of TonB, ExbB, and ExbD, while the Tol system consists of TolA, TolQ, and TolR. In the Ton system, ExbB and ExbD proteins make up the energy-harvesting complex, which transfers energy to the protein TonB. This arrangement causes a conformational change in TonB, which subsequently delivers energy to the outer membrane. In the Tol system, TolQ and TolR proteins compose the energy-harvesting complex, which transfers energy to TolA, resulting in a conformational change and energy to the outer membrane. The Ton system is involved in transport of compounds across the membrane, while the Tol system is involved in outer membrane maintenance. Group A colicins use the Tol protein system to traverse the outer membrane of sensitive bacteria, while group B colicins use the Ton system.

Examples of group A colicins include colicins E1 to E9 and colicins A, K, and N, and examples of group B molecules include colicins 5, 10, B, D, M, V, Ia, and Ib (412, 416). Colicins can also be classified based on their mechanism of induced cell death: (i) pore-formation colicins, (ii) nuclease-type colicins, and (iii) peptidoglycanase-type colicins. Pore-formation colicins act by creating a pore within the bacterial cytoplasmic membrane, resulting in cytoplasmic content leakage, loss of electrochemical gradients, and cell death. Examples of pore-formation colicins include colicins A, B, E1, Ia, Ib, K, and N. Nuclease-type colicins utilize DNase, 16S rRNase, and tRNase to nonspecifically digest DNA and RNA of targeted bacteria. Examples of these molecules include colicins E2 to E9. Finally, peptidoglycanase-type colicins digest peptidoglycan precursors. This digestion prevents bacteria from synthesizing peptidoglycan, a key cell wall component, and results in bacterial death (417).

Bacteriocins *in vivo*

Bacteriocin-producing strains have been shown to have an ecological advantage over nonproducing strains *in vivo*, pointing to the role of bacteriocins in niche development. For example, *E. coli* BZB1011 strains which produced colicins (A, E1, E2, E7, K, and N) were found to be persistent over time in mice compared to non-colicin-producing isogenic strains (418). Bacteriocins, particularly the lantibiotics from Gram-positive bacteria, have been shown to be effective against a number of pathogenic strains *in vivo*. The lantibiotic nisin has been shown to inhibit the pathogens *S. pneumoniae* (419), *S. aureus* (420–422), and *L. monocytogenes* in mice (123). Furthermore, lantibiotic B-Ny266 was shown to inhibit *S. aureus* (424), and planosporicin inhibited *S. pyogenes* in mice (425). The class IIa bacteriocin peptides enterocin CRL35 and divercin V41 were also shown to inhibit *L. monocytogenes* (426, 427), while bacteriocin E50-52 inhibited *Mycobacterium tuberculosis* in mice (428). Intraperitoneal injection of microcin MccJ25 reduced *Salmonella enterica* serotype Newport quantities in the spleen and liver in mice (429). As a result of these *in vivo* studies, bacteriocins have been considered for the treatment of multi-drug-resistant pathogens.

Bacteriocins as quorum-sensing molecules

For many bacteria, bacteriocin production is regulated by quorum sensing (161, 430, 431). Quorum sensing, as discussed earlier, is a cell-density-dependent regulatory system in which autoinducing signals facilitate bacterial communication. This system can sense the number of cells of the same species and synchronize the expression of key genes. Bacteriocin peptides are sensed by membrane-located histidine kinases, which transmit a signal via an intracellular response regulator, thereby activating gene transcription of the inducer bacteriocin molecule (432). The two-component signal-transduction mechanism is a key step for transcription activation and production of several bacteriocins or bacteriocin-like peptides. These include the class I lantibiotics *Lb. lactis* nisin and *B. subtilis* subtilin, as well as the class II *E. faecium* enterocin A and *L. salivarius* UCC118 Abp118 (431, 433–437). Thus, the bacteriocin peptide itself functions as a pheromone to induce its own production. When bacterial cell density is high, an autoinduction loop is activated and bacteriocins are likewise produced at high concentrations. In this manner, bacteriocins are released to target similar species only when the bacterial levels are high enough to suppress the growth of competitive strains.

Bacteriocins within biofilms are known to play important roles in bacterial competition, ecological fitness, and overall community structure (93, 438, 439). In the naturally transformable streptococci, including *S. mutans*, *Streptococcus gordonii*, *Streptococcus sanguinis*, and *Streptococcus mitis*, bacteriocin production is tightly regulated by a quorum-sensing system that also regulates genetic competence and biofilm formation (93, 438, 439). *S. mutans* has served as a well-studied example of quorum sensing and bacteriocin production. *S. mutans* uses the ComCDE quorum-sensing system to connect to bacteriocin production, stress response, genetic competence, and biofilm formation (93, 342, 438, 440–442). *S. mutans* ComC mutants do not produce the signaling molecule CSP, and these biofilms exhibit reduced biomass (93). However, supplementation of cultures with synthetic CSP restores the wild-type biofilm phenotype. *S. mutans* CSP-induced bacteriocin (CipB) can also stimulate cell lysis (443, 444). As a result, bacteriocin

production within biofilms is speculated to provide balanced competition and coexistence of multiple organisms within a microbial community (438, 439, 445).

Other Biogenic Substances

In addition to bacteriocins, select microbes are known to produce bacteriocin-like substances, which are used to describe compounds that have antimicrobial properties but are not ribosomally produced or gene-encoded precursor peptides. Examples of this class of compounds include reuterin and reutericyclin.

Reuterin

Select strains of *L. reuteri* generate reuterin (3-hydroxypropionaldehyde) during anaerobic fermentation of glycerol (446, 447). During this process glycerol is reduced to 1,3-propanediol, an event catalyzed by the coenzyme B_{12}-dependent diol dehydratase, which regenerates NAD^+ from NADH (448–450). Reuterin is water-soluble, active over a wide range of pH values, and bioactive against Gram-positive and Gram-negative bacteria, viruses, and fungi (451). The aldehyde group of reuterin is highly reactive with thiol groups and primary amines. As a result, reuterin inhibits bacterial growth by modifying protein thiol groups and inducing oxidative stress in target cells (449). Production of reuterin by *L. reuteri* was found to be enhanced by interactions with *E. coli*, indicating that cross-talk between members of the gut microbiota may regulate reuterin output (449). Reuterin has also been demonstrated to act synergistically with other bacteriocins. Nisin, lacticin 481, and enterocin AS-48 were found to enhance antimicrobial activity of reuterin against the pathogen *L. monocytogenes* (452). However, only nisin was found to increase antimicrobial activity of reuterin against *S. aureus* (452). These studies indicate that synergism between reuterin and bacteriocins is dependent on the bacteriocin and pathogen. Importantly, reuterin was found to be produced by *L. reuteri* in mono-associated germ-free mice, indicating that reuterin can be produced *in vivo* in the GIT (453).

Reutericyclin

Reutericyclin is a highly hydrophobic, negatively charged compound produced by certain *L. reuteri* strains (454, 455). Reutericyclin [(5R)-1-(2-decenoyl)-2-hydroxy-3-acetyl-5-isobutyl-Δ2-pyrroline-4-one] is an *N*-acylated tetramic acid (455), and its mode of action resembles that of weak organic acids. Reutericyclin targets the cytoplasmic membrane of sensitive bacteria by acting as a proton-ionophore. This action results in the translocation of protons across the cytoplasmic membrane and subsequent collapse of the transmembrane ΔpH (454). Reutericyclin exhibits a broad inhibitory spectrum against Gram-positive pathogens including *E. faecalis*, *Listeria innocua*, *S. aureus*, *B. subtilis*, and *B. cereus* (455). Reutericyclin has also been shown to inhibit germination of *Bacillus* spores (455). However, Gram-negative bacteria are resistant to reutericyclin due to the presence of LPS in their outer membrane. LPS is known to limit access of hydrophobic compounds, and the charged polysaccharide moieties of LPS have been proposed to bind reutericyclin, thereby rendering it inactive (454, 456).

SUMMARY AND CONCLUSIONS

This article highlighted multiple well-characterized systems that commensal bacteria use to communicate with other microbes and the mammalian host, to modify microbial communities, and to beneficially modulate the function of the mammalian host. These studies emphasize key roles of bacterial metabolites and secreted products in fine-tuning mammalian biology. Bacteria are capable of secreting multiple and chemically diverse host-modulating factors. This work has focused on commensal bacteria, but a number of these factors can also be used by pathogens. Future studies may begin to define

the secretion of products in various environments and under different conditions (i.e., inflammation, altered pH, various dietary nutrients). As we begin to understand the health-promoting compounds and metabolites generated by commensal bacteria, we will be better able to identify individual species and strains which can be tailored for specific physiological or biochemical targets of interest. The work here highlights the importance of selecting well-characterized commensal or probiotic strains with known mechanisms to address specific disease processes. The recent development of the U.S. edition of the Clinical Guide to Probiotic Products reflects the growing need for evidence-based selection of probiotics. This online database provides guidelines for probiotic products and corresponding research studies supporting the use of each specific probiotic (http://usprobioticguide.com/). These tools will likely aid clinicians in selecting disease-relevant bacterial species.

Genetic engineering of probiotic strains has also been used as a method to enhance production of molecules of interest (124). In this system bacteria could be designed to have upregulated gene synthesis or to be constitutively active. Using this model, issues of whether a given product is being secreted *in vivo* under various conditions (pH, ion composition, changing osmolarity) could be minimized. Strains have also been engineered with genes from other bacteria to create organisms capable of secreting multiple beneficial factors. Microbial engineering may lead to the production of "super" strains with the ability to release multiple factors targeted at different purposes (i.e., immunomodulation, pathogen exclusion, enhancement of the mucus barrier). Additionally, genetic engineering has been used to facilitate probiotic selection and maintenance in the host (124). This method may ensure the transient introduction of strains which are not wanted to colonize the host in the long term. Currently, social acceptance of genetically modified foods and microbes is not universal, and thus these types of modifications will likely be closely monitored in the future. An alternative approach could be to isolate and purify valuable metabolites, which themselves could also be used directly as novel therapeutics for specific disorders.

Based on studies conducted thus far, we have strong evidence to pursue the selection of probiotics and examination of specific microbial genes, proteins, and metabolites of interest. In the future we hope to use this knowledge to thoughtfully select commensal strains for a given disease treatment or prevention. Overall, these studies contribute to the rapidly expanding body of evidence demonstrating that secreted microbial metabolites can beneficially influence host physiology. In addition to probiotics, future dietary and medicinal interventions may depend on the foundations of microbial metabolite and protein discovery in the context of microbiome science.

CITATION

Engevik MA, Versalovic J. 2017. Biochemical features of beneficial microbes: foundations for therapeutic microbiology. Microbiol Spectrum 5(5):BAD-0012-2016.

REFERENCES

1. **Sender R, Fuchs S, Milo R.** 2016. Revised estimates for the number of human and bacteria cells in the body. *PLoS Biol* **14:**e1002533.

2. **Huttenhower C, et al, Human Microbiome Project Consortium.** 2012. Structure, function and diversity of the healthy human microbiome. *Nature* **486:**207–214.

3. **Mazmanian SK, Liu CH, Tzianabos AO, Kasper DL.** 2005. An immunomodulatory molecule of symbiotic bacteria directs maturation of the host immune system. *Cell* **122:**107–118.

4. **Bercik P, Park AJ, Sinclair D, Khoshdel A, Lu J, Huang X, Deng Y, Blennerhassett PA, Fahnestock M, Moine D, Berger B, Huizinga JD, Kunze W, McLean PG, Bergonzelli GE, Collins SM, Verdu EF.** 2011. The anxiolytic effect of *Bifidobacterium longum* NCC3001 involves vagal pathways for gut-brain communication. *Neurogastroenterol Motil* **23:**1132–1139.

5. **Desbonnet L, Garrett L, Clarke G, Kiely B, Cryan JF, Dinan TG.** 2010. Effects of the probiotic *Bifidobacterium infantis* in the maternal separation model of depression. *Neuroscience* **170:**1179–1188.

6. **Lozupone CA, Stombaugh JI, Gordon JI, Jansson JK, Knight R.** 2012. Diversity, stability and resilience of the human gut microbiota. *Nature* **489:**220–230.

7. **Yatsunenko T, Rey FE, Manary MJ, Trehan I, Dominguez-Bello MG, Contreras M, Magris M, Hidalgo G, Baldassano RN, Anokhin AP, Heath AC, Warner B, Reeder J, Kuczynski J, Caporaso JG, Lozupone CA, Lauber C, Clemente JC, Knights D, Knight R, Gordon JI.** 2012. Human gut microbiome viewed across age and geography. *Nature* **486:**222–227.

8. **Johnson CL, Versalovic J.** 2012. The human microbiome and its potential importance to pediatrics. *Pediatrics* **129:**950–960.

9. **Hollister EB, Riehle K, Luna RA, Weidler EM, Rubio-Gonzales M, Mistretta TA, Raza S, Doddapaneni HV, Metcalf GA, Muzny DM, Gibbs RA, Petrosino JF, Shulman RJ, Versalovic J.** 2015. Structure and function of the healthy pre-adolescent pediatric gut microbiome. *Microbiome* **3:**36.

10. **Biagi E, Candela M, Turroni S, Garagnani P, Franceschi C, Brigidi P.** 2013. Ageing and gut microbes: perspectives for health maintenance and longevity. *Pharmacol Res* **69:**11–20.

11. **Biagi E, Nylund L, Candela M, Ostan R, Bucci L, Pini E, Nikkïla J, Monti D, Satokari R, Franceschi C, Brigidi P, De Vos W.** 2010. Through ageing, and beyond: gut microbiota and inflammatory status in seniors and centenarians. *PLoS One* **5:**e10667. (Erratum, http://dx.doi.org/10.1371/annotation/df45912f-d15c-44ab-8312-e7ec0607604d.)

12. **Martín R, Miquel S, Ulmer J, Kechaou N, Langella P, Bermúdez-Humarán LG.** 2013. Role of commensal and probiotic bacteria in human health: a focus on inflammatory bowel disease. *Microb Cell Fact* **12:**71.

13. **Foligne B, Nutten S, Grangette C, Dennin V, Goudercourt D, Poiret S, Dewulf J, Brassart D, Mercenier A, Pot B.** 2007. Correlation between *in vitro* and *in vivo* immunomodulatory properties of lactic acid bacteria. *World J Gastroenterol* **13:**236–243.

14. **Marteau P, Lémann M, Seksik P, Laharie D, Colombel JF, Bouhnik Y, Cadiot G, Soulé JC, Bourreille A, Metman E, Lerebours E, Carbonnel F, Dupas JL, Veyrac M, Coffin B, Moreau J, Abitbol V, Blum-Sperisen S, Mary JY.** 2006. Ineffectiveness of *Lactobacillus johnsonii* LA1 for prophylaxis of postoperative

recurrence in Crohn's disease: a randomised, double blind, placebo controlled GETAID trial. *Gut* **55**:842–847.

15. **Maassen CB, van Holten-Neelen C, Balk F, Heijne den Bak-Glashouwer MJ, Leer RJ, Laman JD, Boersma WJ, Claassen E.** 2000. Strain-dependent induction of cytokine profiles in the gut by orally administered *Lactobacillus* strains. *Vaccine* **18**:2613–2623.

16. **Frost G, Sleeth ML, Sahuri-Arisoylu M, Lizarbe B, Cerdan S, Brody L, Anastasovska J, Ghourab S, Hankir M, Zhang S, Carling D, Swann JR, Gibson G, Viardot A, Morrison D, Louise Thomas E, Bell JD.** 2014. The short-chain fatty acid acetate reduces appetite via a central homeostatic mechanism. *Nat Commun* **5**:3611.

17. **Schrijver IA, van Meurs M, Melief MJ, Wim Ang C, Buljevac D, Ravid R, Hazenberg MP, Laman JD.** 2001. Bacterial peptidoglycan and immune reactivity in the central nervous system in multiple sclerosis. *Brain* **124**:1544–1554.

18. **Bäumlisberger M, Moellecken U, König H, Claus H.** 2015. The potential of the yeast *Debaryomyces hansenii* H525 to degrade biogenic amines in food. *Microorganisms* **3**:839–850.

19. **Pessione A, Lamberti C, Pessione E.** 2010. Proteomics as a tool for studying energy metabolism in lactic acid bacteria. *Mol Biosyst* **6**:1419–1430.

20. **Bouchereau A, Guénot P, Larher F.** 2000. Analysis of amines in plant materials. *J Chromatogr B Biomed Sci Appl* **747**:49–67.

21. **Suzzi G, Gardini F.** 2003. Biogenic amines in dry fermented sausages: a review. *Int J Food Microbiol* **88**:41–54.

22. **Tabanelli G, Torriani S, Rossi F, Rizzotti L, Gardini F.** 2012. Effect of chemico-physical parameters on the histidine decarboxylase (HdcA) enzymatic activity in *Streptococcus thermophilus* PRI60. *J Food Sci* **77**:M231–M237.

23. **Molenaar D, Bosscher JS, ten Brink B, Driessen AJ, Konings WN.** 1993. Generation of a proton motive force by histidine decarboxylation and electrogenic histidine/histamine antiport in *Lactobacillus buchneri*. *J Bacteriol* **175**:2864–2870.

24. **Rodwell AW.** 1953. The histidine decarboxylase of a species of *Lactobacillus*; apparent dispensability of pyridoxal phosphate as coenzyme. *J Gen Microbiol* **8**:233–237.

25. **Rossi F, Gardini F, Rizzotti L, La Gioia F, Tabanelli G, Torriani S.** 2011. Quantitative analysis of histidine decarboxylase gene (*hdcA*) transcription and histamine production by *Streptococcus thermophilus* PRI60 under conditions relevant to cheese making. *Appl Environ Microbiol* **77**:2817–2822.

26. **Hemarajata P, Gao C, Pflughoeft KJ, Thomas CM, Saulnier DM, Spinler JK, Versalovic J.** 2013. *Lactobacillus reuteri*-specific immunoregulatory gene rsiR modulates histamine production and immunomodulation by *Lactobacillus reuteri*. *J Bacteriol* **195**:5567–5576.

27. **Thomas CM, Hong T, van Pijkeren JP, Hemarajata P, Trinh DV, Hu W, Britton RA, Kalkum M, Versalovic J.** 2012. Histamine derived from probiotic *Lactobacillus reuteri* suppresses TNF via modulation of PKA and ERK signaling. *PLoS One* **7**:e31951.

28. **Pessione E, Mazzoli R, Giuffrida MG, Lamberti C, Garcia-Moruno E, Barello C, Conti A, Giunta C.** 2005. A proteomic approach to studying biogenic amine producing lactic acid bacteria. *Proteomics* **5**:687–698.

29. **Lucas PM, Claisse O, Lonvaud-Funel A.** 2008. High frequency of histamine-producing bacteria in the enological environment and instability of the histidine decarboxylase production phenotype. *Appl Environ Microbiol* **74**:811–817.

30. **Izquierdo Cañas PM, Gómez Alonso S, Ruiz Pérez P, Seseña Prieto S, García Romero E, Palop Herreros ML.** 2009. Biogenic amine production by *Oenococcus oeni* isolates from malolactic fermentation of Tempranillo wine. *J Food Prot* **72**:907–910.

31. **Gao C, Major A, Rendon D, Lugo M, Jackson V, Shi Z, Mori-Akiyama Y, Versalovic J.** 2015. Histamine H2 receptor-mediated suppression of intestinal inflammation by probiotic *Lactobacillus reuteri*. *MBio* **6**:e01358-15.

32. **Ferstl R, Frei R, Schiavi E, Konieczna P, Barcik W, Ziegler M, Lauener RP, Chassard C, Lacroix C, Akdis CA, O'Mahony L.** 2014. Histamine receptor 2 is a key influence in immune responses to intestinal histamine-secreting microbes. *J Allergy Clin Immunol* **134**:744–746.e3.

33. **Frei R, Ferstl R, Konieczna P, Ziegler M, Simon T, Rugeles TM, Mailand S, Watanabe T, Lauener R, Akdis CA, O'Mahony L.** 2013. Histamine receptor 2 modifies dendritic cell responses to microbial ligands. *J Allergy Clin Immunol* **132**:194–204.e12.

34. **Dhakal R, Bajpai VK, Baek KH.** 2012. Production of gaba (γ- aminobutyric acid) by microorganisms: a review. *Braz J Microbiol* **43**:1230–1241.

35. **Lu X, Chen Z, Gu Z, Han Y.** 2008. Isolation of γ-aminobutyric acid-producing bacteria and optimization of fermentative medium. *Biochem Eng J* **41**:48–52.

36. **Smith DK, Kassam T, Singh B, Elliott JF.** 1992. *Escherichia coli* has two homologous

glutamate decarboxylase genes that map to distinct loci. *J Bacteriol* **174:**5820–5826.

37. **Kono I, Himeno K.** 2000. Changes in gamma-aminobutyric acid content during beni-koji making. *Biosci Biotechnol Biochem* **64:**617–619.

38. **Barrett E, Ross RP, O'Toole PW, Fitzgerald GF, Stanton C.** 2012. γ-Aminobutyric acid production by culturable bacteria from the human intestine. *J Appl Microbiol* **113:**411–417.

39. **Komatsuzaki N, Shima J, Kawamoto S, Momose H, Kimura T.** 2005. Production of y-aminobutyric acid (GABA) by *Lactobacillus paracasei* isolated from traditional fermented foods. *Food Microbiol* **22:**497–504.

40. **Siragusa S, De Angelis M, Di Cagno R, Rizzello CG, Coda R, Gobbetti M.** 2007. Synthesis of gamma-aminobutyric acid by lactic acid bacteria isolated from a variety of Italian cheeses. *Appl Environ Microbiol* **73:**7283–7290.

41. **Pokusaeva K, Johnson C, Luk B, Uribe G7, Fu Y, Oezguen N, Matsunami RK, Lugo M, Major A, Mori-Akiyama Y, Hollister EB, Dann SM, Shi XZ, Engler DA, Savidge T, Versalovic J.** 2017. GABA-producing Bifidobacterium dentium modulates visceral sensitivity in the intestine. *Neurogastroenterol Motil.* [Epub ahead of print. http://dx.doi.org/10.1111/nmo.12904.\]

42. **Hayakawa K, Kimura M, Kasaha K, Matsumoto K, Sansawa H, Yamori Y.** 2004. Effect of a gamma-aminobutyric acid-enriched dairy product on the blood pressure of spontaneously hypertensive and normotensive Wistar-Kyoto rats. *Br J Nutr* **92:**411–417.

43. **Kimura M, Hayakawa K, Sansawa H.** 2002. Involvement of gamma-aminobutyric acid (GABA) B receptors in the hypotensive effect of systemically administered GABA in spontaneously hypertensive rats. *Jpn J Pharmacol* **89:**388–394.

44. **Izquierdo E, Marchioni E, Aoude-Werner D, Hasselmann C, Ennahar S.** 2009. Smearing of soft cheese with *Enterococcus faecium* WHE 81, a multi-bacteriocin producer, against *Listeria monocytogenes. Food Microbiol* **26:**16–20.

45. **Adeghate E, Ponery AS.** 2002. GABA in the endocrine pancreas: cellular localization and function in normal and diabetic rats. *Tissue Cell* **34:**1–6.

46. **Capitani G, De Biase D, Aurizi C, Gut H, Bossa F, Grütter MG.** 2003. Crystal structure and functional analysis of *Escherichia coli* glutamate decarboxylase. *EMBO J* **22:**4027–4037.

47. **Hagiwara H, Seki T, Ariga T.** 2004. The effect of pre-germinated brown rice intake on blood glucose and PAI-1 levels in streptozotocin-induced diabetic rats. *Biosci Biotechnol Biochem* **68:**444–447.

48. **Cho YR, Chang JY, Chang HC.** 2007. Production of gamma-aminobutyric acid (GABA) by *Lactobacillus buchneri* isolated from kimchi and its neuroprotective effect on neuronal cells. *J Microbiol Biotechnol* **17:**104–109.

49. **Bravo JA, Forsythe P, Chew MV, Escaravage E, Savignac HM, Dinan TG, Bienenstock J, Cryan JF.** 2011. Ingestion of *Lactobacillus* strain regulates emotional behavior and central GABA receptor expression in a mouse via the vagus nerve. *Proc Natl Acad Sci USA* **108:**16050–16055.

50. **Messaoudi M, Lalonde R, Violle N, Javelot H, Desor D, Nejdi A, Bisson JF, Rougeot C, Pichelin M, Cazaubiel M, Cazaubiel JM.** 2011. Assessment of psychotropic-like properties of a probiotic formulation (*Lactobacillus helveticus* R0052 and *Bifidobacterium longum* R0175) in rats and human subjects. *Br J Nutr* **105:**755–764.

51. **Okada T, Sugishita T, Murakami T, Murai H, Saikusa T, Horino T, Onoda A, Kajimoto O, Takahashi R, Takahashi T.** 2000. Effect of the defatted rice germ enriched with GABA for sleeplessness, depression, autonomic disorder by oral administration. *Nippon Shokuhin Kagaku Kogaku Kaishi* **47:**596–603.

52. **Shah P, Swiatlo E.** 2008. A multifaceted role for polyamines in bacterial pathogens. *Mol Microbiol* **68:**4–16.

53. **Pegg AE, McCann PP.** 1982. Polyamine metabolism and function. *Am J Physiol* **243:**C212–C221.

54. **Milovic V.** 2001. Polyamines in the gut lumen: bioavailability and biodistribution. *Eur J Gastroenterol Hepatol* **13:**1021–1025.

55. **Noack J, Dongowski G, Hartmann L, Blaut M.** 2000. The human gut bacteria *Bacteroides thetaiotaomicron* and *Fusobacterium varium* produce putrescine and spermidine in cecum of pectin-fed gnotobiotic rats. *J Nutr* **130:**1225–1231.

56. **Noack J, Kleessen B, Proll J, Dongowski G, Blaut M.** 1998. Dietary guar gum and pectin stimulate intestinal microbial polyamine synthesis in rats. *J Nutr* **128:**1385–1391.

57. **Cohen SS.** 1997. *A Guide to the Polyamines.* Oxford University Press, New York, NY.

58. **Zhang M, Caragine T, Wang H, Cohen PS, Botchkina G, Soda K, Bianchi M, Ulrich P, Cerami A, Sherry B, Tracey KJ.** 1997. Spermine inhibits proinflammatory cytokine synthesis in human mononuclear cells: a counterregulatory mechanism that restrains the immune response. *J Exp Med* **185:**1759–1768.

59. **Li L, Rao JN, Bass BL, Wang JY.** 2001. NF-kappaB activation and susceptibility to apoptosis after polyamine depletion in intestinal epithelial cells. *Am J Physiol Gastrointest Liver Physiol* **280:**G992–G1004.

60. **Rhee HJ, Kim EJ, Lee JK.** 2007. Physiological polyamines: simple primordial stress molecules. *J Cell Mol Med* **11:**685–703.

61. **Pillai SP, Shankel DM.** 1997. Polyamines and their potential to be antimutagens. *Mutat Res* **377:**217–224.

62. **Shah N, Thomas T, Shirahata A, Sigal LH, Thomas TJ.** 1999. Activation of nuclear factor kappaB by polyamines in breast cancer cells. *Biochemistry* **38:**14763–14774.

63. **Soda K, Kano Y, Nakamura T, Kasono K, Kawakami M, Konishi F.** 2005. Spermine, a natural polyamine, suppresses LFA-1 expression on human lymphocyte. *J Immunol* **175:**237–245.

64. **Penrose HM, Marchelletta RR, Krishnan M, McCole DF.** 2013. Spermidine stimulates T cell protein-tyrosine phosphatase-mediated protection of intestinal epithelial barrier function. *J Biol Chem* **288:**32651–32662.

65. **Das R, Kanungo MS.** 1982. Activity and modulation of ornithine decarboxylase and concentrations of polyamines in various tissues of rats as a function of age. *Exp Gerontol* **17:**95–103.

66. **Matsumoto M, Benno Y.** 2007. The relationship between microbiota and polyamine concentration in the human intestine: a pilot study. *Microbiol Immunol* **51:**25–35.

67. **Matsumoto M, Kurihara S, Kibe R, Ashida H, Benno Y.** 2011. Longevity in mice is promoted by probiotic-induced suppression of colonic senescence dependent on upregulation of gut bacterial polyamine production. *PLoS One* **6:**e23652.

68. **Kibe R, Kurihara S, Sakai Y, Suzuki H, Ooga T, Sawaki E, Muramatsu K, Nakamura A, Yamashita A, Kitada Y, Kakeyama M, Benno Y, Matsumoto M.** 2014. Upregulation of colonic luminal polyamines produced by intestinal microbiota delays senescence in mice. *Sci Rep* **4:**4548.

69. **Matsumoto M, Aranami A, Ishige A, Watanabe K, Benno Y.** 2007. LKM512 yogurt consumption improves the intestinal environment and induces the T-helper type 1 cytokine in adult patients with intractable atopic dermatitis. *Clin Exp Allergy* **37:**358–370.

70. **Matsumoto M, Ohishi H, Benno Y.** 2001. Impact of LKM512 yogurt on improvement of intestinal environment of the elderly. *FEMS Immunol Med Microbiol* **31:**181–186.

71. **Rider JE, Hacker A, Mackintosh CA, Pegg AE, Woster PM, Casero RA Jr.** 2007. Spermine and spermidine mediate protection against oxidative damage caused by hydrogen peroxide. *Amino Acids* **33:**231–240.

72. **Clarke CH, Shankel DM.** 1988. Antimutagens against spontaneous and induced reversion of a lacZ frameshift mutation in *E. coli* K-12 strain ND-160. *Mutat Res* **202:**19–23.

73. **Clarke CH, Shankel DM.** 1989. Antimutagenic specificity against spontaneous and nitrofurazone-induced mutations in *Escherichia coli* K12ND160. *Mutagenesis* **4:**31–34.

74. **Nestmann ER.** 1977. Antimutagenic effects of spermine and guanosine in continuous cultures of *Escherichia coli* mutator strain mutH. *Mol Gen Genet* **152:**109–110.

75. **Lahue RS, Au KG, Modrich P.** 1989. DNA mismatch correction in a defined system. *Science* **245:**160–164.

76. **Gómez-Gallego C, Collado MC, Pérez G, Ilo T, Jaakkola UM, Bernal MJ, Periago MJ, Frias R, Ros G, Salminen S.** 2014. Resembling breast milk: influence of polyamine-supplemented formula on neonatal BALB/cOlaHsd mouse microbiota. *Br J Nutr* **111:**1050–1058.

77. **Maurelli AT, Fernández RE, Bloch CA, Rode CK, Fasano A.** 1998. "Black holes" and bacterial pathogenicity: a large genomic deletion that enhances the virulence of *Shigella* spp. and enteroinvasive *Escherichia coli. Proc Natl Acad Sci USA* **95:**3943–3948.

78. **Goldman ME, Cregar L, Nguyen D, Simo O, O'Malley S, Humphreys T.** 2006. Cationic polyamines inhibit anthrax lethal factor protease. *BMC Pharmacol* **6:**8.

79. **Fernandez IM, Silva M, Schuch R, Walker WA, Siber AM, Maurelli AT, McCormick BA.** 2001. Cadaverine prevents the escape of *Shigella flexneri* from the phagolysosome: a connection between bacterial dissemination and neutrophil transepithelial signaling. *J Infect Dis* **184:**743–753.

80. **Torres AG, Vazquez-Juarez RC, Tutt CB, Garcia-Gallegos JG.** 2005. Pathoadaptive mutation that mediates adherence of shiga toxin-producing *Escherichia coli* O111. *Infect Immun* **73:**4766–4776.

81. **Casero RA Jr, Marton LJ.** 2007. Targeting polyamine metabolism and function in cancer and other hyperproliferative diseases. *Nat Rev Drug Discov* **6:**373–390.

82. **Gerner EW, Meyskens FL Jr.** 2004. Polyamines and cancer: old molecules, new understanding. *Nat Rev Cancer* **4:**781–792.

83. **Alam K, Arlow FL, Ma CK, Schubert TT.** 1994. Decrease in ornithine decarboxylase ac-

tivity after eradication of *Helicobacter pylori*. *Am J Gastroenterol* **89**:888–893.

84. **Patchett SE, Katelaris PH, Zhang ZW, Alstead EM, Domizio P, Farthing MJ.** 1996. Ornithine decarboxylase activity is a marker of premalignancy in longstanding *Helicobacter pylori* infection. *Gut* **39**:807–810.

85. **Fu S, Ramanujam KS, Wong A, Fantry GT, Drachenberg CB, James SP, Meltzer SJ, Wilson KT.** 1999. Increased expression and cellular localization of inducible nitric oxide synthase and cyclooxygenase 2 in *Helicobacter pylori* gastritis. *Gastroenterology* **116**:1319–1329.

86. **Keszthelyi D, Troost FJ, Masclee AA.** 2009. Understanding the role of tryptophan and serotonin metabolism in gastrointestinal function. *Neurogastroenterol Motil* **21**:1239–1249.

87. **Yanofsky C, Horn V, Gollnick P.** 1991. Physiological studies of tryptophan transport and tryptophanase operon induction in *Escherichia coli*. *J Bacteriol* **173**:6009–6017.

88. **Aragozzini F, Ferrari A, Pacini N, Gualandris R.** 1979. Indole-3-lactic acid as a tryptophan metabolite produced by *Bifidobacterium* spp. *Appl Environ Microbiol* **38**:544–546.

89. **Smith EA, Macfarlane GT.** 1997. Formation of phenolic and indolic compounds by anaerobic bacteria in the human large intestine. *Microb Ecol* **33**:180–188.

90. **Bansal T, Alaniz RC, Wood TK, Jayaraman A.** 2010. The bacterial signal indole increases epithelial-cell tight-junction resistance and attenuates indicators of inflammation. *Proc Natl Acad Sci USA* **107**:228–233.

91. **Bommarius B, Anyanful A, Izrayelit Y, Bhatt S, Cartwright E, Wang W, Swimm AI, Benian GM, Schroeder FC, Kalman D.** 2013. A family of indoles regulate virulence and Shiga toxin production in pathogenic *E. coli*. *PLoS One* **8**: e54456.

92. **Shimada Y, Kinoshita M, Harada K, Mizutani M, Masahata K, Kayama H, Takeda K.** 2013. Commensal bacteria-dependent indole production enhances epithelial barrier function in the colon. *PLoS One* **8**:e80604.

93. **Li YH, Tian X.** 2012. Quorum sensing and bacterial social interactions in biofilms. *Sensors (Basel)* **12**:2519–2538.

94. **Davey ME, O'Toole GA.** 2000. Microbial biofilms: from ecology to molecular genetics. *Microbiol Mol Biol Rev* **64**:847–867.

95. **Watnick P, Kolter R.** 2000. Biofilm, city of microbes. *J Bacteriol* **182**:2675–2679.

96. **Miller MB, Bassler BL.** 2001. Quorum sensing in bacteria. *Annu Rev Microbiol* **55**:165–199.

97. **Parsek MR, Greenberg EP.** 2005. Sociomicrobiology: the connections between quo-rum sensing and biofilms. *Trends Microbiol* **13**:27–33.

98. **Thompson JA, Oliveira RA, Xavier KB.** 2016. Chemical conversations in the gut microbiota. *Gut Microbes* **7**:163–170.

99. **Waters CM, Bassler BL.** 2005. Quorum sensing: cell-to-cell communication in bacteria. *Annu Rev Cell Dev Biol* **21**:319–346.

100. **Cvitkovitch DG, Li YH, Ellen RP.** 2003. Quorum sensing and biofilm formation in streptococcal infections. *J Clin Invest* **112**:1626–1632.

101. **Federle MJ, Bassler BL.** 2003. Interspecies communication in bacteria. *J Clin Invest* **112**: 1291–1299.

102. **Schauder S, Bassler BL.** 2001. The languages of bacteria. *Genes Dev* **15**:1468–1480.

103. **Fuqua C, Greenberg EP.** 2002. Listening in on bacteria: acyl-homoserine lactone signalling. *Nat Rev Mol Cell Biol* **3**:685–695.

104. **Parsek MR, Val DL, Hanzelka BL, Cronan JE Jr, Greenberg EP.** 1999. Acyl homoserine-lactone quorum-sensing signal generation. *Proc Natl Acad Sci USA* **96**:4360–4365.

105. **de Kievit TR, Iglewski BH.** 2000. Bacterial quorum sensing in pathogenic relationships. *Infect Immun* **68**:4839–4849.

106. **Dunny GM, Leonard BA.** 1997. Cell-cell communication in Gram-positive bacteria. *Annu Rev Microbiol* **51**:527–564.

107. **Novick RP.** 2003. Autoinduction and signal transduction in the regulation of staphylococcal virulence. *Mol Microbiol* **48**:1429–1449.

108. **Claverys JP, Prudhomme M, Martin B.** 2006. Induction of competence regulons as a general response to stress in Gram-positive bacteria. *Annu Rev Microbiol* **60**:451–475.

109. **Mashburn-Warren L, Morrison DA, Federle MJ.** 2010. A novel double-tryptophan peptide pheromone controls competence in *Streptococcus* spp. via an Rgg regulator. *Mol Microbiol* **78**:589–606.

110. **Fleuchot B, Gitton C, Guillot A, Vidic J, Nicolas P, Besset C, Fontaine L, Hols P, Leblond-Bourget N, Monnet V, Gardan R.** 2011. Rgg proteins associated with internalized small hydrophobic peptides: a new quorum-sensing mechanism in streptococci. *Mol Microbiol* **80**:1102–1119.

111. **Fontaine L, Boutry C, de Frahan MH, Delplace B, Fremaux C, Horvath P, Boyaval P, Hols P.** 2010. A novel pheromone quorum-sensing system controls the development of natural competence in *Streptococcus thermophilus* and *Streptococcus salivarius*. *J Bacteriol* **192**:1444–1454.

112. **Chen X, Schauder S, Potier N, Van Dorsselaer A, Pelczer I, Bassler BL, Hughson FM.** 2002. Structural identification of a bacterial quorum-

sensing signal containing boron. *Nature* **415**: 545–549.

113. **Rezzonico F, Smits TH, Duffy B.** 2012. Detection of AI-2 receptors in genomes of *Enterobacteriaceae* suggests a role of type-2 quorum sensing in closed ecosystems. *Sensors (Basel)* **12**:6645–6665.

114. **Costerton W, Veeh R, Shirtliff M, Pasmore M, Post C, Ehrlich G.** 2003. The application of biofilm science to the study and control of chronic bacterial infections. *J Clin Invest* **112**:1466–1477.

115. **von Rosenvinge EC, O'May GA, Macfarlane S, Macfarlane GT, Shirtliff ME.** 2013. Microbial biofilms and gastrointestinal diseases. *Pathog Dis* **67**:25–38.

116. **Johansson ME, Larsson JM, Hansson GC.** 2011. The two mucus layers of colon are organized by the MUC2 mucin, whereas the outer layer is a legislator of host-microbial interactions. *Proc Natl Acad Sci USA* **108**(Suppl 1):4659–4665.

117. **Pullan RD, Thomas GA, Rhodes M, Newcombe RG, Williams GT, Allen A, Rhodes J.** 1994. Thickness of adherent mucus gel on colonic mucosa in humans and its relevance to colitis. *Gut* **35**:353–359.

118. **Macfarlane S, Woodmansey EJ, Macfarlane GT.** 2005. Colonization of mucin by human intestinal bacteria and establishment of biofilm communities in a two-stage continuous culture system. *Appl Environ Microbiol* **71**:7483–7492.

119. **Holmén Larsson JM, Karlsson H, Sjövall H, Hansson GC.** 2009. A complex, but uniform O-glycosylation of the human MUC2 mucin from colonic biopsies analyzed by nanoLC/MSn. *Glycobiology* **19**:756–766.

120. **Engevik MA, Aihara E, Montrose MH, Shull GE, Hassett DJ, Worrell RT.** 2013. Loss of NHE3 alters gut microbiota composition and influences *Bacteroides thetaiotaomicron* growth. *Am J Physiol Gastrointest Liver Physiol* **305**:G697–G711.

121. **Engevik MA, Hickerson A, Shull GE, Worrell RT.** 2013. Acidic conditions in the NHE2(−/−) mouse intestine result in an altered mucosa-associated bacterial population with changes in mucus oligosaccharides. *Cell Physiol Biochem* **32**:111–128.

122. **Engevik MA, Yacyshyn MB, Engevik KA, Wang J, Darien B, Hassett DJ, Yacyshyn BR, Worrell RT.** 2015. Human *Clostridium difficile* infection: altered mucus production and composition. *Am J Physiol Gastrointest Liver Physiol* **308**:G510–G524.

123. **Marcobal A, Southwick AM, Earle KA, Sonnenburg JL.** 2013. A refined palate: bacterial consumption of host glycans in the gut. *Glycobiology* **23**:1038–1046.

124. **Ahmed FE.** 2003. Genetically modified probiotics in foods. *Trends Biotechnol* **21**:491–497.

125. **Macfarlane S, Furrie E, Cummings JH, Macfarlane GT.** 2004. Chemotaxonomic analysis of bacterial populations colonizing the rectal mucosa in patients with ulcerative colitis. *Clin Infect Dis* **38**:1690–1699.

126. **Lebeer S, Verhoeven TL, Claes IJ, De Hertogh G, Vermeire S, Buyse J, Van Immerseel F, Vanderleyden J, De Keersmaecker SC.** 2011. FISH analysis of *Lactobacillus* biofilms in the gastrointestinal tract of different hosts. *Lett Appl Microbiol* **52**:220–226.

127. **Macfarlane S, Bahrami B, Macfarlane GT.** 2011. Mucosal biofilm communities in the human intestinal tract. *Adv Appl Microbiol* **75**: 111–143.

128. **Nadell CD, Xavier JB, Foster KR.** 2009. The sociobiology of biofilms. *FEMS Microbiol Rev* **33**:206–224.

129. **Rickard AH, Palmer RJ Jr, Blehert DS, Campagna SR, Semmelhack MF, Egland PG, Bassler BL, Kolenbrander PE.** 2006. Autoinducer 2: a concentration-dependent signal for mutualistic bacterial biofilm growth. *Mol Microbiol* **60**:1446–1456.

130. **Merritt J, Qi F, Goodman SD, Anderson MH, Shi W.** 2003. Mutation of luxS affects biofilm formation in *Streptococcus mutans*. *Infect Immun* **71**:1972–1979.

131. **Trappetti C, Potter AJ, Paton AW, Oggioni MR, Paton JC.** 2011. LuxS mediates iron-dependent biofilm formation, competence, and fratricide in *Streptococcus pneumoniae*. *Infect Immun* **79**:4550–4558.

132. **Vidal JE, Ludewick HP, Kunkel RM, Zähner D, Klugman KP.** 2011. The LuxS-dependent quorum-sensing system regulates early biofilm formation by *Streptococcus pneumoniae* strain D39. *Infect Immun* **79**:4050–4060.

133. **Tannock GW, Ghazally S, Walter J, Loach D, Brooks H, Cook G, Surette M, Simmers C, Bremer P, Dal Bello F, Hertel C.** 2005. Ecological behavior of *Lactobacillus reuteri* 100-23 is affected by mutation of the luxS gene. *Appl Environ Microbiol* **71**:8419–8425.

134. **Belenguer A, Duncan SH, Calder AG, Holtrop G, Louis P, Lobley GE, Flint HJ.** 2006. Two routes of metabolic cross-feeding between *Bifidobacterium adolescentis* and butyrate-producing anaerobes from the human gut. *Appl Environ Microbiol* **72**:3593–3599.

135. **Louis P, Duncan SH, McCrae SI, Millar J, Jackson MS, Flint HJ.** 2004. Restricted distribution of the butyrate kinase pathway among butyrate-producing bacteria from the human colon. *J Bacteriol* **186**:2099–2106.

136. Macfarlane GT, Macfarlane S. 2012. Bacteria, colonic fermentation, and gastrointestinal health. *J AOAC Int* **95**:50–60.

137. Ríos-Covián D, Ruas-Madiedo P, Margolles A, Gueimonde M, de Los Reyes-Gavilán CG, Salazar N. 2016. Intestinal short chain fatty acids and their link with diet and human health. *Front Microbiol* **7**:185.

138. Cummings JH, Pomare EW, Branch WJ, Naylor CP, Macfarlane GT. 1987. Short chain fatty acids in human large intestine, portal, hepatic and venous blood. *Gut* **28**:1221–1227.

139. Kim CH, Park J, Kim M. 2014. Gut microbiota-derived short-chain fatty acids, T cells, and inflammation. *Immune Netw* **14**:277–288.

140. Annison G, Illman RJ, Topping DL. 2003. Acetylated, propionylated or butyrylated starches raise large bowel short-chain fatty acids preferentially when fed to rats. *J Nutr* **133**:3523–3528.

141. Gao Z, Yin J, Zhang J, Ward RE, Martin RJ, Lefevre M, Cefalu WT, Ye J. 2009. Butyrate improves insulin sensitivity and increases energy expenditure in mice. *Diabetes* **58**:1509–1517.

142. Cherrington CA, Hinton M, Chopra I. 1990. Effect of short-chain organic acids on macromolecular synthesis in *Escherichia coli*. *J Appl Bacteriol* **68**:69–74.

143. Prohászka L, Jayarao BM, Fábián A, Kovács S. 1990. The role of intestinal volatile fatty acids in the *Salmonella* shedding of pigs. *Zentralbl Veterinarmed B* **37**:570–574.

144. Duncan SH, Barcenilla A, Stewart CS, Pryde SE, Flint HJ. 2002. Acetate utilization and butyryl coenzyme A (CoA):acetate-CoA transferase in butyrate-producing bacteria from the human large intestine. *Appl Environ Microbiol* **68**:5186–5190.

145. Duncan SH, Holtrop G, Lobley GE, Calder AG, Stewart CS, Flint HJ. 2004. Contribution of acetate to butyrate formation by human faecal bacteria. *Br J Nutr* **91**:915–923.

146. den Besten G, Bleeker A, Gerding A, van Eunen K, Havinga R, van Dijk TH, Oosterveer MH, Jonker JW, Groen AK, Reijngoud DJ, Bakker BM. 2015. Short-chain fatty acids protect against high-fat diet-induced obesity via a PPARγ-dependent switch from lipogenesis to fat oxidation. *Diabetes* **64**:2398–2408.

147. Yanase H, Takebe K, Nio-Kobayashi J, Takahashi-Iwanaga H, Iwanaga T. 2008. Cellular expression of a sodium-dependent monocarboxylate transporter (Slc5a8) and the MCT family in the mouse kidney. *Histochem Cell Biol* **130**:957–966.

148. Miyauchi S, Gopal E, Babu E, Srinivas SR, Kubo Y, Umapathy NS, Thakkar SV, Ganapathy V, Prasad PD. 2010. Sodium-coupled electrogenic transport of pyroglutamate (5-oxoproline) via SLC5A8, a monocarboxylate transporter. *Biochim Biophys Acta* **1798**:1164–1171.

149. Halestrap AP, Wilson MC. 2012. The monocarboxylate transporter family: role and regulation. *IUBMB Life* **64**:109–119.

150. Karaki S, Mitsui R, Hayashi H, Kato I, Sugiya H, Iwanaga T, Furness JB, Kuwahara A. 2006. Short-chain fatty acid receptor, GPR43, is expressed by enteroendocrine cells and mucosal mast cells in rat intestine. *Cell Tissue Res* **324**:353–360.

151. Sleeth ML, Thompson EL, Ford HE, Zac-Varghese SE, Frost G. 2010. Free fatty acid receptor 2 and nutrient sensing: a proposed role for fibre, fermentable carbohydrates and short-chain fatty acids in appetite regulation. *Nutr Res Rev* **23**:135–145.

152. Eberle JA, Widmayer P, Breer H. 2014. Receptors for short-chain fatty acids in brush cells at the "gastric groove". *Front Physiol* **5**:152.

153. Tazoe H, Otomo Y, Kaji I, Tanaka R, Karaki SI, Kuwahara A. 2008. Roles of short-chain fatty acids receptors, GPR41 and GPR43 on colonic functions. *J Physiol Pharmacol* **59**(Suppl 2):251–262.

154. Nøhr MK, Pedersen MH, Gille A, Egerod KL, Engelstoft MS, Husted AS, Sichlau RM, Grunddal KV, Poulsen SS, Han S, Jones RM, Offermanns S, Schwartz TW. 2013. GPR41/FFAR3 and GPR43/FFAR2 as cosensors for short-chain fatty acids in enteroendocrine cells vs FFAR3 in enteric neurons and FFAR2 in enteric leukocytes. *Endocrinology* **154**:3552–3564.

155. Xiong Y, Miyamoto N, Shibata K, Valasek MA, Motoike T, Kedzierski RM, Yanagisawa M. 2004. Short-chain fatty acids stimulate leptin production in adipocytes through the G protein-coupled receptor GPR41. *Proc Natl Acad Sci USA* **101**:1045–1050.

156. Zaibi MS, Stocker CJ, O'Dowd J, Davies A, Bellahcene M, Cawthorne MA, Brown AJ, Smith DM, Arch JR. 2010. Roles of GPR41 and GPR43 in leptin secretory responses of murine adipocytes to short chain fatty acids. *FEBS Lett* **584**:2381–2386.

157. Sina C, Gavrilova O, Förster M, Till A, Derer S, Hildebrand F, Raabe B, Chalaris A, Scheller J, Rehmann A, Franke A, Ott S, Häsler R, Nikolaus S, Fölsch UR, Rose-John S, Jiang HP, Li J, Schreiber S, Rosenstiel P. 2009. G protein-coupled receptor 43 is essential for neutrophil recruitment during intestinal inflammation. *J Immunol* **183**:7514–7522.

158. Brown AJ, Goldsworthy SM, Barnes AA, Eilert MM, Tcheang L, Daniels D, Muir AI, Wigglesworth MJ, Kinghorn I, Fraser NJ,

Pike NB, Strum JC, Steplewski KM, Murdock PR, Holder JC, Marshall FH, Szekeres PG, Wilson S, Ignar DM, Foord SM, Wise A, Dowell SJ. 2003. The Orphan G protein-coupled receptors GPR41 and GPR43 are activated by propionate and other short chain carboxylic acids. *J Biol Chem* **278**:11312–11319.

159. Voltolini C, Battersby S, Etherington SL, Petraglia F, Norman JE, Jabbour HN. 2012. A novel antiinflammatory role for the short-chain fatty acids in human labor. *Endocrinology* **153**:395–403.

160. Furusawa Y, Obata Y, Fukuda S, Endo TA, Nakato G, Takahashi D, Nakanishi Y, Uetake C, Kato K, Kato T, Takahashi M, Fukuda NN, Murakami S, Miyauchi E, Hino S, Atarashi K, Onawa S, Fujimura Y, Lockett T, Clarke JM, Topping DL, Tomita M, Hori S, Ohara O, Morita T, Koseki H, Kikuchi J, Honda K, Hase K, Ohno H. 2013. Commensal microbe-derived butyrate induces the differentiation of colonic regulatory T cells. *Nature* **504**:446–450.

161. Ventura M, Turroni F, Motherway MO, MacSharry J, van Sinderen D. 2012. Host-microbe interactions that facilitate gut colonization by commensal bifidobacteria. *Trends Microbiol* **20**:467–476.

162. Singh N, Gurav A, Sivaprakasam S, Brady E, Padia R, Shi H, Thangaraju M, Prasad PD, Manicassamy S, Munn DH, Lee JR, Offermanns S, Ganapathy V. 2014. Activation of Gpr109a, receptor for niacin and the commensal metabolite butyrate, suppresses colonic inflammation and carcinogenesis. *Immunity* **40**:128–139.

163. Fukuda S, Toh H, Hase K, Oshima K, Nakanishi Y, Yoshimura K, Tobe T, Clarke JM, Topping DL, Suzuki T, Taylor TD, Itoh K, Kikuchi J, Morita H, Hattori M, Ohno H. 2011. Bifidobacteria can protect from enteropathogenic infection through production of acetate. *Nature* **469**:543–547.

164. Smith PM, Howitt MR, Panikov N, Michaud M, Gallini CA, Bohlooly-Y M, Glickman JN, Garrett WS. 2013. The microbial metabolites, short-chain fatty acids, regulate colonic Treg cell homeostasis. *Science* **341**:569–573.

165. Arpaia N, Campbell C, Fan X, Dikiy S, van der Veeken J, deRoos P, Liu H, Cross JR, Pfeffer K, Coffer PJ, Rudensky AY. 2013. Metabolites produced by commensal bacteria promote peripheral regulatory T-cell generation. *Nature* **504**:451–455.

166. Arpaia N, Rudensky AY. 2014. Microbial metabolites control gut inflammatory responses. *Proc Natl Acad Sci USA* **111**:2058–2059.

167. Ishiguro K, Ando T, Maeda O, Watanabe O, Goto H. 2011. Cutting edge: tubulin α functions as an adaptor in NFAT-importin β interaction. *J Immunol* **186**:2710–2713.

168. Wrzosek L, Miquel S, Noordine ML, Bouet S, Joncquel Chevalier-Curt M, Robert V, Philippe C, Bridonneau C, Cherbuy C, Robbe-Masselot C, Langella P, Thomas M. 2013. *Bacteroides thetaiotaomicron* and *Faecalibacterium prausnitzii* influence the production of mucus glycans and the development of goblet cells in the colonic epithelium of a gnotobiotic model rodent. *BMC Biol* **11**:61.

169. Levison ME. 1973. Effect of colon flora and short-chain fatty acids on growth *in vitro* of *Pseudomonas aeruginosa* and *Enterobacteriaceae*. *Infect Immun* **8**:30–35.

170. Shin R, Suzuki M, Morishita Y. 2002. Influence of intestinal anaerobes and organic acids on the growth of enterohaemorrhagic *Escherichia coli* O157:H7. *J Med Microbiol* **51**:201–206.

171. Maslowski KM, Vieira AT, Ng A, Kranich J, Sierro F, Yu D, Schilter HC, Rolph MS, Mackay F, Artis D, Xavier RJ, Teixeira MM, Mackay CR. 2009. Regulation of inflammatory responses by gut microbiota and chemoattractant receptor GPR43. *Nature* **461**:1282–1286.

172. De Vuyst L, Leroy F. 2011. Cross-feeding between bifidobacteria and butyrate-producing colon bacteria explains bifidobacterial competitiveness, butyrate production, and gas production. *Int J Food Microbiol* **149**:73–80.

173. Reichardt N, Duncan SH, Young P, Belenguer A, McWilliam Leitch C, Scott KP, Flint HJ, Louis P. 2014. Phylogenetic distribution of three pathways for propionate production within the human gut microbiota. *ISME J* **8**:1323–1335.

174. Lukovac S, Belzer C, Pellis L, Keijser BJ, de Vos WM, Montijn RC, Roeselers G. 2014. Differential modulation by *Akkermansia muciniphila* and *Faecalibacterium prausnitzii* of host peripheral lipid metabolism and histone acetylation in mouse gut organoids. *MBio* **5**:e01438-14.

175. Hung CC, Garner CD, Slauch JM, Dwyer ZW, Lawhon SD, Frye JG, McClelland M, Ahmer BM, Altier C. 2013. The intestinal fatty acid propionate inhibits *Salmonella* invasion through the post-translational control of HilD. *Mol Microbiol* **87**:1045–1060.

176. Lawhon SD, Maurer R, Suyemoto M, Altier C. 2002. Intestinal short-chain fatty acids alter *Salmonella* Typhimurium invasion gene expression and virulence through BarA/SirA. *Mol Microbiol* **46**:1451–1464.

177. Garner CD, Antonopoulos DA, Wagner B, Duhamel GE, Keresztes I, Ross DA, Young VB, Altier C. 2009. Perturbation of the small

intestine microbial ecology by streptomycin alters pathology in a *Salmonella enterica* serovar Typhimurium murine model of infection. *Infect Immun* 77:2691–2702.

178. **Durant JA, Corrier DE, Ricke SC.** 2000. Short-chain volatile fatty acids modulate the expression of the hilA and invF genes of *Salmonella* Typhimurium. *J Food Prot* 63:573–578.

179. **Vinolo MA, Ferguson GJ, Kulkarni S, Damoulakis G, Anderson K, Bohlooly-Y M, Stephens L, Hawkins PT, Curi R.** 2011. SCFAs induce mouse neutrophil chemotaxis through the GPR43 receptor. *PLoS One* 6:e21205.

180. **Vinolo MA, Rodrigues HG, Nachbar RT, Curi R.** 2011. Regulation of inflammation by short chain fatty acids. *Nutrients* 3:858–876.

181. **Anini Y, Fu-Cheng X, Cuber JC, Kervran A, Chariot J, Roz C.** 1999. Comparison of the postprandial release of peptide YY and proglucagon-derived peptides in the rat. *Pflugers Arch* 438:299–306.

182. **Cherbut C, Ferrier L, Rozé C, Anini Y, Blottière H, Lecannu G, Galmiche JP.** 1998. Short-chain fatty acids modify colonic motility through nerves and polypeptide YY release in the rat. *Am J Physiol* 275:G1415–G1422.

183. **Tolhurst G, Heffron H, Lam YS, Parker HE, Habib AM, Diakogiannaki E, Cameron J, Grosse J, Reimann F, Gribble FM.** 2012. Short-chain fatty acids stimulate glucagon-like peptide-1 secretion via the G-protein-coupled receptor FFAR2. *Diabetes* 61:364–371.

184. **Chambers ES, Viardot A, Psichas A, Morrison DJ, Murphy KG, Zac-Varghese SE, MacDougall K, Preston T, Tedford C, Finlayson GS, Blundell JE, Bell JD, Thomas EL, Mt-Isa S, Ashby D, Gibson GR, Kolida S, Dhillo WS, Bloom SR, Morley W, Clegg S, Frost G.** 2015. Effects of targeted delivery of propionate to the human colon on appetite regulation, body weight maintenance and adiposity in overweight adults. *Gut* 64:1744–1754.

185. **Murphy KG, Bloom SR.** 2006. Gut hormones and the regulation of energy homeostasis. *Nature* 444:854–859.

186. **Louis P, Hold GL, Flint HJ.** 2014. The gut microbiota, bacterial metabolites and colorectal cancer. *Nat Rev Microbiol* 12:661–672.

187. **Louis P, Scott KP, Duncan SH, Flint HJ.** 2007. Understanding the effects of diet on bacterial metabolism in the large intestine. *J Appl Microbiol* 102:1197–1208.

188. **Flint HJ, Duncan SH, Scott KP, Louis P.** 2007. Interactions and competition within the microbial community of the human colon: links between diet and health. *Environ Microbiol* 9:1101–1111.

189. **Thangaraju M, Cresci GA, Liu K, Ananth S, Gnanaprakasam JP, Browning DD, Mellinger JD, Smith SB, Digby GJ, Lambert NA, Prasad PD, Ganapathy V.** 2009. GPR109A is a G-protein-coupled receptor for the bacterial fermentation product butyrate and functions as a tumor suppressor in colon. *Cancer Res* 69:2826–2832.

190. **Ganapathy V, Thangaraju M, Prasad PD, Martin PM, Singh N.** 2013. Transporters and receptors for short-chain fatty acids as the molecular link between colonic bacteria and the host. *Curr Opin Pharmacol* 13:869–874.

191. **Fung KY, Cosgrove L, Lockett T, Head R, Topping DL.** 2012. A review of the potential mechanisms for the lowering of colorectal oncogenesis by butyrate. *Br J Nutr* 108:820–831.

192. **Hamer HM, Jonkers D, Venema K, Vanhoutvin S, Troost FJ, Brummer RJ.** 2008. Review article: the role of butyrate on colonic function. *Aliment Pharmacol Ther* 27:104–119.

193. **Buda A, Qualtrough D, Jepson MA, Martines D, Paraskeva C, Pignatelli M.** 2003. Butyrate downregulates alpha2beta1 integrin: a possible role in the induction of apoptosis in colorectal cancer cell lines. *Gut* 52:729–734.

194. **Clarke JM, Topping DL, Bird AR, Young GP, Cobiac L.** 2008. Effects of high-amylose maize starch and butyrylated high-amylose maize starch on azoxymethane-induced intestinal cancer in rats. *Carcinogenesis* 29:2190–2194.

195. **Chang PV, Hao L, Offermanns S, Medzhitov R.** 2014. The microbial metabolite butyrate regulates intestinal macrophage function via histone deacetylase inhibition. *Proc Natl Acad Sci USA* 111:2247–2252.

196. **Wilson AJ, Chueh AC, Tögel L, Corner GA, Ahmed N, Goel S, Byun DS, Nasser S, Houston MA, Jhawer M, Smartt HJ, Murray LB, Nicholas C, Heerdt BG, Arango D, Augenlicht LH, Mariadason JM.** 2010. Apoptotic sensitivity of colon cancer cells to histone deacetylase inhibitors is mediated by an Sp1/Sp3-activated transcriptional program involving immediate-early gene induction. *Cancer Res* 70:609–620.

197. **Shapiro H, Thaiss CA, Levy M, Elinav E.** 2014. The cross talk between microbiota and the immune system: metabolites take center stage. *Curr Opin Immunol* 30:54–62.

198. **Devillard E, McIntosh FM, Duncan SH, Wallace RJ.** 2007. Metabolism of linoleic acid by human gut bacteria: different routes for biosynthesis of conjugated linoleic acid. *J Bacteriol* 189:2566–2570.

199. **McIntosh FM, Shingfield KJ, Devillard E, Russell WR, Wallace RJ.** 2009. Mechanism of conjugated linoleic acid and vaccenic acid

formation in human faecal suspensions and pure cultures of intestinal bacteria. *Microbiology* **155:**285–294.

200. Gorissen L, Raes K, Weckx S, Dannenberger D, Leroy F, De Vuyst L, De Smet S. 2010. Production of conjugated linoleic acid and conjugated linolenic acid isomers by *Bifidobacterium* species. *Appl Microbiol Biotechnol* **87:**2257–2266.

201. Kishino S, Takeuchi M, Park SB, Hirata A, Kitamura N, Kunisawa J, Kiyono H, Iwamoto R, Isobe Y, Arita M, Arai H, Ueda K, Shima J, Takahashi S, Yokozeki K, Shimizu S, Ogawa J. 2013. Polyunsaturated fatty acid saturation by gut lactic acid bacteria affecting host lipid composition. *Proc Natl Acad Sci USA* **110:**17808–17813.

202. Wall R, Ross RP, Shanahan F, O'Mahony L, O'Mahony C, Coakley M, Hart O, Lawlor P, Quigley EM, Kiely B, Fitzgerald GF, Stanton C. 2009. Metabolic activity of the enteric microbiota influences the fatty acid composition of murine and porcine liver and adipose tissues. *Am J Clin Nutr* **89:**1393–1401.

203. Gudbrandsen OA, Rodríguez E, Wergedahl H, Mørk S, Reseland JE, Skorve J, Palou A, Berge RK. 2009. Trans-10, cis-12-conjugated linoleic acid reduces the hepatic triacylglycerol content and the leptin mRNA level in adipose tissue in obese Zucker fa/fa rats. *Br J Nutr* **102:**803–815.

204. Toomey S, Harhen B, Roche HM, Fitzgerald D, Belton O. 2006. Profound resolution of early atherosclerosis with conjugated linoleic acid. *Atherosclerosis* **187:**40–49.

205. Kelly D, Campbell JI, King TP, Grant G, Jansson EA, Coutts AG, Pettersson S, Conway S. 2004. Commensal anaerobic gut bacteria attenuate inflammation by regulating nuclear-cytoplasmic shuttling of PPAR-gamma and RelA. *Nat Immunol* **5:**104–112.

206. Are A, Aronsson L, Wang S, Greicius G, Lee YK, Gustafsson JA, Pettersson S, Arulampalam V. 2008. *Enterococcus faecalis* from newborn babies regulate endogenous PPARγ activity and IL-10 levels in colonic epithelial cells. *Proc Natl Acad Sci USA* **105:**1943–1948.

207. Moya-Camarena SY, Vanden Heuvel JP, Blanchard SG, Leesnitzer LA, Belury MA. 1999. Conjugated linoleic acid is a potent naturally occurring ligand and activator of PPARalpha. *J Lipid Res* **40:**1426–1433.

208. Itoh T, Fairall L, Amin K, Inaba Y, Szanto A, Balint BL, Nagy L, Yamamoto K, Schwabe JW. 2008. Structural basis for the activation of PPARgamma by oxidized fatty acids. *Nat Struct Mol Biol* **15:**924–931.

209. Chen P, Torralba M, Tan J, Embree M, Zengler K, Starkel P, van Pijkeren JP, DePew J, Loomba R, Ho SB, Bajaj JS, Mutlu EA, Keshavarzian A,

Tsukamoto H, Nelson KE, Fouts DE, Schnabl B. 2015. Supplementation of saturated long-chain fatty acids maintains intestinal eubiosis and reduces ethanol-induced liver injury in mice. *Gastroenterology* **148:**203–214.e216.

210. Hill MJ. 1997. Intestinal flora and endogenous vitamin synthesis. *Eur J Cancer Prev* **6**(Suppl 1): S43–S45.

211. Gill SR, Pop M, Deboy RT, Eckburg PB, Turnbaugh PJ, Samuel BS, Gordon JI, Relman DA, Fraser-Liggett CM, Nelson KE. 2006. Metagenomic analysis of the human distal gut microbiome. *Science* **312:**1355–1359.

212. Brestoff JR, Artis D. 2013. Commensal bacteria at the interface of host metabolism and the immune system. *Nat Immunol* **14:**676–684.

213. Said HM, Mohammed ZM. 2006. Intestinal absorption of water-soluble vitamins: an update. *Curr Opin Gastroenterol* **22:**140–146.

214. Ichihashi T, Takagishi Y, Uchida K, Yamada H. 1992. Colonic absorption of menaquinone-4 and menaquinone-9 in rats. *J Nutr* **122:**506–512.

215. Bhaskaram P. 2002. Micronutrient malnutrition, infection, and immunity: an overview. *Nutr Rev* **60**(suppl 5):S40–S45.

216. Cheng CH, Chang SJ, Lee BJ, Lin KL, Huang YC. 2006. Vitamin B_6 supplementation increases immune responses in critically ill patients. *Eur J Clin Nutr* **60:**1207–1213.

217. Meydani SN, Meydani M, Blumberg JB, Leka LS, Siber G, Loszewski R, Thompson C, Pedrosa MC, Diamond RD, Stollar BD. 1997. Vitamin E supplementation and *in vivo* immune response in healthy elderly subjects. A randomized controlled trial. *JAMA* **277:**1380–1386.

218. Tamura J, Kubota K, Murakami H, Sawamura M, Matsushima T, Tamura T, Saitoh T, Kurabayshi H, Naruse T. 1999. Immunomodulation by vitamin B_{12}: augmentation of CD8+ T lymphocytes and natural killer (NK) cell activity in vitamin B_{12}-deficient patients by methyl-B12 treatment. *Clin Exp Immunol* **116:**28–32.

219. LeBlanc JG, Laiño JE, del Valle MJ, Vannini V, van Sinderen D, Taranto MP, de Valdez GF, de Giori GS, Sesma F. 2011. B-group vitamin production by lactic acid bacteria: current knowledge and potential applications. *J Appl Microbiol* **111:**1297–1309.

220. Bacher A, Eberhardt S, Fischer M, Kis K, Richter G. 2000. Biosynthesis of vitamin B_2 (riboflavin). *Annu Rev Nutr* **20:**153–167.

221. Bacher A, Fischer M, Kis K, Kugelbrey K, Mörtl S, Scheuring J, Weinkauf S, Eberhardt S, Schmidt-Bäse K, Huber R, Ritsert K, Cushman M, Ladenstein R. 1996. Biosynthesis of riboflavin: structure and mechanism of lumazine synthase. *Biochem Soc Trans* **24:**89–94.

222. Capozzi V, Menga V, Digesu AM, De Vita P, van Sinderen D, Cattivelli L, Fares C, Spano G. 2011. Biotechnological production of vitamin B_2-enriched bread and pasta. *J Agric Food Chem* **59:**8013–8020.

223. LeBlanc JG, Burgess C, Sesma F, de Giori GS, van Sinderen D. 2005. *Lactococcus lactis* is capable of improving the riboflavin status in deficient rats. *Br J Nutr* **94:**262–267.

224. LeBlanc JG, Burgess C, Sesma F, Savoy de Giori G, van Sinderen D. 2005. Ingestion of milk fermented by genetically modified *Lactococcus lactis* improves the riboflavin status of deficient rats. *J Dairy Sci* **88:**3435–3442.

225. Burgess C, O'Connell-Motherway M, Sybesma W, Hugenholtz J, van Sinderen D. 2004. Riboflavin production in *Lactococcus lactis*: potential for *in situ* production of vitamin-enriched foods. *Appl Environ Microbiol* **70:**5769–5777.

226. Sydenstricker VP. 1941. Clinical manifestations of ariboflavinosis. *Am J Public Health Nations Health* **31:**344–350.

227. Fabian E, Majchrzak D, Dieminger B, Meyer E, Elmadfa I. 2008. Influence of probiotic and conventional yoghurt on the status of vitamins B_1, B_2 and B_6 in young healthy women. *Ann Nutr Metab* **52:**29–36.

228. LeBlanc JG, Sybesma W, Starrenburg M, Sesma F, de Vos WM, de Giori GS, Hugenholtz J. 2010. Supplementation with engineered *Lactococcus lactis* improves the folate status in deficient rats. *Nutrition* **26:**835–841.

229. LeBlanc JG, Aubry C, Cortes-Perez NG, de Moreno de LeBlanc A, Vergnolle N, Langella P, Azevedo V, Chatel JM, Miyoshi A, Bermúdez-Humarán LG. 2013. Mucosal targeting of therapeutic molecules using genetically modified lactic acid bacteria: an update. *FEMS Microbiol Lett* **344:**1–9.

230. Kim TH, Yang J, Darling PB, O'Connor DL. 2004. A large pool of available folate exists in the large intestine of human infants and piglets. *J Nutr* **134:**1389–1394.

231. Thomas CM, Saulnier DM, Spinler JK, Hemarajata P, Gao C, Jones SE, Grimm A, Balderas MA, Burstein MD, Morra C, Roeth D, Kalkum M, Versalovic J. 2016. FolC2-mediated folate metabolism contributes to suppression of inflammation by probiotic *Lactobacillus reuteri*. *MicrobiologyOpen* **5:**802–818.

232. Crittenden RG, Martinez NR, Playne MJ. 2003. Synthesis and utilisation of folate by yoghurt starter cultures and probiotic bacteria. *Int J Food Microbiol* **80:**217–222.

233. Sybesma W, Starrenburg M, Kleerebezem M, Mierau I, de Vos WM, Hugenholtz J. 2003. Increased production of folate by metabolic engineering of *Lactococcus lactis*. *Appl Environ Microbiol* **69:**3069–3076.

234. Sybesma W, Starrenburg M, Tijsseling L, Hoefnagel MH, Hugenholtz J. 2003. Effects of cultivation conditions on folate production by lactic acid bacteria. *Appl Environ Microbiol* **69:**4542–4548.

235. Sybesma W, Van Den Born E, Starrenburg M, Mierau I, Kleerebezem M, De Vos WM, Hugenholtz J. 2003. Controlled modulation of folate polyglutamyl tail length by metabolic engineering of *Lactococcus lactis*. *Appl Environ Microbiol* **69:**7101–7107.

236. Wegkamp A, Starrenburg M, de Vos WM, Hugenholtz J, Sybesma W. 2004. Transformation of folate-consuming *Lactobacillus gasseri* into a folate producer. *Appl Environ Microbiol* **70:**3146–3148.

237. Santos F, Wegkamp A, de Vos WM, Smid EJ, Hugenholtz J. 2008. High-level folate production in fermented foods by the B_{12} producer *Lactobacillus reuteri* JCM1112. *Appl Environ Microbiol* **74:**3291–3294.

238. Claesson MJ, Li Y, Leahy S, Canchaya C, van Pijkeren JP, Cerdeño-Tárraga AM, Parkhill J, Flynn S, O'Sullivan GC, Collins JK, Higgins D, Shanahan F, Fitzgerald GF, van Sinderen D, O'Toole PW. 2006. Multireplicon genome architecture of *Lactobacillus salivarius*. *Proc Natl Acad Sci USA* **103:**6718–6723.

239. van de Guchte M, Penaud S, Grimaldi C, Barbe V, Bryson K, Nicolas P, Robert C, Oztas S, Mangenot S, Couloux A, Loux V, Dervyn R, Bossy R, Bolotin A, Batto JM, Walunas T, Gibrat JF, Bessières P, Weissenbach J, Ehrlich SD, Maguin E. 2006. The complete genome sequence of *Lactobacillus bulgaricus* reveals extensive and ongoing reductive evolution. *Proc Natl Acad Sci USA* **103:**9274–9279.

240. Pompei A, Cordisco L, Amaretti A, Zanoni S, Matteuzzi D, Rossi M. 2007. Folate production by bifidobacteria as a potential probiotic property. *Appl Environ Microbiol* **73:**179–185.

241. Rossi M, Amaretti A, Raimondi S. 2011. Folate production by probiotic bacteria. *Nutrients* **3:**118–134.

242. Wegkamp A, van Oorschot W, de Vos WM, Smid EJ. 2007. Characterization of the role of para-aminobenzoic acid biosynthesis in folate production by *Lactococcus lactis*. *Appl Environ Microbiol* **73:**2673–2681.

243. Quesada-Chanto A, Afschar AS, Wagner F. 1994. Microbial production of propionic acid and vitamin B_{12} using molasses or sugar. *Appl Microbiol Biotechnol* **41:**378–383.

244. Roth LA, Keenan D. 1971. Acid injury of *Escherichia coli*. *Can J Microbiol* **17:**1005–1008.

245. **Martens J-H, Barg H, Warren M, Jahn D.** 2002. Microbial production of vitamin B_{12}. *Appl Microbiol Biotechnol* **58**:275–285.

246. **Smith AD.** 2007. Folic acid fortification: the good, the bad, and the puzzle of vitamin B-12. *Am J Clin Nutr* **85**:3–5.

247. **Roth JR, Lawrence JG, Bobik TA.** 1996. Cobalamin (coenzyme B_{12}): synthesis and biological significance. *Annu Rev Microbiol* **50**:137–181.

248. **Rodionov DA, Vitreschak AG, Mironov AA, Gelfand MS.** 2003. Comparative genomics of the vitamin B_{12} metabolism and regulation in prokaryotes. *J Biol Chem* **278**:41148–41159.

249. **Taranto MP, Vera JL, Hugenholtz J, De Valdez GF, Sesma F.** 2003. *Lactobacillus reuteri* CRL1098 produces cobalamin. *J Bacteriol* **185**:5643–5647.

250. **Vannini V, de Valdez G, Taranto MFS.** 2008. Identification of new lactobacilli able to produce cobalamin (vitamin B_{12}). *Biocell* **32**:72.

251. **Martin R, Olivares M, Marin ML, Fernandez L, Xaus J, Rodriguez JM.** 2005. Probiotic potential of 3 lactobacilli strains isolated from breast milk. *J Hum Lact* **21**:8–17; quiz 18–21, 41.

252. **Santos F, Vera JL, Lamosa P, de Valdez GF, de Vos WM, Santos H, Sesma F, Hugenholtz J.** 2007. Pseudovitamin B(12) is the corrinoid produced by *Lactobacillus reuteri* CRL1098 under anaerobic conditions. *FEBS Lett* **581**:4865–4870.

253. **Hüfner E, Britton RA, Roos S, Jonsson H, Hertel C.** 2008. Global transcriptional response of *Lactobacillus reuteri* to the sourdough environment. *Syst Appl Microbiol* **31**:323–338.

254. **Hunt A, Harrington D, Robinson S.** 2014. Vitamin B_{12} deficiency. *BMJ* **349**(sep04 1):g5226.

255. **Molina VC, Médici M, Taranto MP, Font de Valdez G.** 2009. *Lactobacillus reuteri* CRL 1098 prevents side effects produced by a nutritional vitamin B deficiency. *J Appl Microbiol* **106**:467–473.

256. **Olson RE.** 1984. The function and metabolism of vitamin K. *Annu Rev Nutr* **4**:281–337.

257. **Lippi G, Franchini M.** 2011. Vitamin K in neonates: facts and myths. *Blood Transfus* **9**:4–9.

258. **Conly JM, Stein K.** 1992. Quantitative and qualitative measurements of K vitamins in human intestinal contents. *Am J Gastroenterol* **87**:311–316.

259. **Cooke G, Behan J, Costello M.** 2006. Newly identified vitamin K-producing bacteria isolated from the neonatal faecal flora. *Microb Ecol Health Dis* **18**:133–138.

260. **Morishita T, Tamura N, Makino T, Kudo S.** 1999. Production of menaquinones by lactic acid bacteria. *J Dairy Sci* **82**:1897–1903.

261. **Olsen I, Amano A.** 2015. Outer membrane vesicles: offensive weapons or good Samaritans? *J Oral Microbiol* **7**:27468.

262. **Gurung M, Moon DC, Choi CW, Lee JH, Bae YC, Kim J, Lee YC, Seol SY, Cho DT, Kim SI, Lee JC.** 2011. *Staphylococcus aureus* produces membrane-derived vesicles that induce host cell death. *PLoS One* **6**:e27958.

263. **Berleman J, Auer M.** 2013. The role of bacterial outer membrane vesicles for intra- and interspecies delivery. *Environ Microbiol* **15**:347–354.

264. **Mayrand D, Grenier D.** 1989. Biological activities of outer membrane vesicles. *Can J Microbiol* **35**:607–613.

265. **Kadurugamuwa JL, Beveridge TJ.** 1995. Virulence factors are released from *Pseudomonas aeruginosa* in association with membrane vesicles during normal growth and exposure to gentamicin: a novel mechanism of enzyme secretion. *J Bacteriol* **177**:3998–4008.

266. **Furuta N, Takeuchi H, Amano A.** 2009. Entry of *Porphyromonas gingivalis* outer membrane vesicles into epithelial cells causes cellular functional impairment. *Infect Immun* **77**:4761–4770.

267. **Lee YK, Mazmanian SK.** 2010. Has the microbiota played a critical role in the evolution of the adaptive immune system? *Science* **330**:1768–1773.

268. **Shen Y, Giardino Torchia ML, Lawson GW, Karp CL, Ashwell JD, Mazmanian SK.** 2012. Outer membrane vesicles of a human commensal mediate immune regulation and disease protection. *Cell Host Microbe* **12**:509–520.

269. **Mazmanian SK, Round JL, Kasper DL.** 2008. A microbial symbiosis factor prevents intestinal inflammatory disease. *Nature* **453**:620–625.

270. **Lee YK, Menezes JS, Umesaki Y, Mazmanian SK.** 2011. Proinflammatory T-cell responses to gut microbiota promote experimental autoimmune encephalomyelitis. *Proc Natl Acad Sci USA* **108**(Suppl 1):4615–4622.

271. **Ochoa-Repáraz J, Mielcarz DW, Ditrio LE, Burroughs AR, Begum-Haque S, Dasgupta S, Kasper DL, Kasper LH.** 2010. Central nervous system demyelinating disease protection by the human commensal *Bacteroides fragilis* depends on polysaccharide A expression. *J Immunol* **185**:4101–4108.

272. **Hsiao EY, McBride SW, Hsien S, Sharon G, Hyde ER, McCue T, Codelli JA, Chow J, Reisman SE, Petrosino JF, Patterson PH, Mazmanian SK.** 2013. Microbiota modulate behavioral and physiological abnormalities associated with neurodevelopmental disorders. *Cell* **155**:1451–1463.

273. **Rühlmann A, Kukla D, Schwager P, Bartels K, Huber R.** 1973. Structure of the complex formed by bovine trypsin and bovine pancreatic trypsin inhibitor: crystal structure determination and stereochemistry of the contact region. *J Mol Biol* **77**:417–436.

274. Potempa J, Korzus E, Travis J. 1994. The serpin superfamily of proteinase inhibitors: structure, function, and regulation. *J Biol Chem* 269:15957–15960.

275. Turroni F, Foroni E, O'Connell Motherway M, Bottacini F, Giubellini V, Zomer A, Ferrarini A, Delledonne M, Zhang Z, van Sinderen D, Ventura M. 2010. Characterization of the serpin-encoding gene of *Bifidobacterium breve* 210B. *Appl Environ Microbiol* 76:3206–3219.

276. Schell MA, Karmirantzou M, Snel B, Vilanova D, Berger B, Pessi G, Zwahlen MC, Desiere F, Bork P, Delley M, Pridmore RD, Arigoni F. 2002. The genome sequence of *Bifidobacterium longum* reflects its adaptation to the human gastrointestinal tract. *Proc Natl Acad Sci USA* 99:14422–14427.

277. Ivanov D, Emonet C, Foata F, Affolter M, Delley M, Fisseha M, Blum-Sperisen S, Kochhar S, Arigoni F. 2006. A serpin from the gut bacterium *Bifidobacterium longum* inhibits eukaryotic elastase-like serine proteases. *J Biol Chem* 281:17246–17252.

278. Haandrikman AJ, Kok J, Laan H, Soemitro S, Ledeboer AM, Konings WN, Venema G. 1989. Identification of a gene required for maturation of an extracellular lactococcal serine proteinase. *J Bacteriol* 171:2789–2794.

279. Haandrikman AJ, Kok J, Venema G. 1991. Lactococcal proteinase maturation protein PrtM is a lipoprotein. *J Bacteriol* 173:4517–4525.

280. Holck A, Axelsson L, Birkeland SE, Aukrust T, Blom H. 1992. Purification and amino acid sequence of sakacin A, a bacteriocin from *Lactobacillus sake* Lb706. *J Gen Microbiol* 138:2715–2720.

281. Hoermannsperger G, Clavel T, Hoffmann M, Reiff C, Kelly D, Loh G, Blaut M, Hölzlwimmer G, Laschinger M, Haller D. 2009. Post-translational inhibition of IP-10 secretion in IEC by probiotic bacteria: impact on chronic inflammation. *PLoS One* 4:e4365.

282. von Schillde MA, Hörmannsperger G, Weiher M, Alpert CA, Hahne H, Bäuerl C, van Huynegem K, Steidler L, Hrncir T, Pérez-Martínez G, Kuster B, Haller D. 2012. Lactocepin secreted by *Lactobacillus* exerts anti-inflammatory effects by selectively degrading proinflammatory chemokines. *Cell Host Microbe* 11:387–396.

283. Yan F, Cao H, Cover TL, Whitehead R, Washington MK, Polk DB. 2007. Soluble proteins produced by probiotic bacteria regulate intestinal epithelial cell survival and growth. *Gastroenterology* 132:562–575.

284. Bäuerl C, Pérez-Martínez G, Yan F, Polk DB, Monedero V. 2010. Functional analysis of the p40 and p75 proteins from *Lactobacillus casei* BL23. *J Mol Microbiol Biotechnol* 19:231–241.

285. Yan F, Liu L, Dempsey PJ, Tsai YH, Raines EW, Wilson CL, Cao H, Cao Z, Liu L, Polk DB. 2013. A *Lactobacillus rhamnosus* GG-derived soluble protein, p40, stimulates ligand release from intestinal epithelial cells to transactivate epidermal growth factor receptor. *J Biol Chem* 288:30742–30751.

286. Ganesh BP, Klopfleisch R, Loh G, Blaut M. 2013. Commensal *Akkermansia muciniphila* exacerbates gut inflammation in *Salmonella* Typhimurium-infected gnotobiotic mice. *PLoS One* 8:e74963.

287. Millet YA, Alvarez D, Ringgaard S, von Andrian UH, Davis BM, Waldor MK. 2014. Insights into *Vibrio cholerae* intestinal colonization from monitoring fluorescently labeled bacteria. *PLoS Pathog* 10:e1004405.

288. Bergstrom KS, Kissoon-Singh V, Gibson DL, Ma C, Montero M, Sham HP, Ryz N, Huang T, Velcich A, Finlay BB, Chadee K, Vallance BA. 2010. Muc2 protects against lethal infectious colitis by disassociating pathogenic and commensal bacteria from the colonic mucosa. *PLoS Pathog* 6:e1000902.

289. Quévrain E, Maubert MA, Michon C, Chain F, Marquant R, Tailhades J, Miquel S, Carlier L, Bermúdez-Humarán LG, Pigneur B, Lequin O, Kharrat P, Thomas G, Rainteau D, Aubry C, Breyner N, Afonso C, Lavielle S, Grill JP, Chassaing G, Chatel JM, Trugnan G, Xavier R, Langella P, Sokol H, Seksik P. 2016. Identification of an anti-inflammatory protein from *Faecalibacterium prausnitzii*, a commensal bacterium deficient in Crohn's disease. *Gut* 65:415–425.

290. Quévrain E, Maubert MA, Sokol H, Devreese B, Seksik P. 2016. The presence of the anti-inflammatory protein MAM, from *Faecalibacterium prausnitzii*, in the intestinal ecosystem. *Gut* 65:882.

291. Devi M, Rebecca LJ, Sumathy S. 2013. Bactericidal activity of the lactic acid bacteria *Lactobacillus delbreukii*. *J Chem Pharm Res* 5:176–180.

292. Nikaido H. 2003. Molecular basis of bacterial outer membrane permeability revisited. *Microbiol Mol Biol Rev* 67:593–656.

293. Alakomi HL, Skyttä E, Saarela M, Mattila-Sandholm T, Latva-Kala K, Helander IM. 2000. Lactic acid permeabilizes gram-negative bacteria by disrupting the outer membrane. *Appl Environ Microbiol* 66:2001–2005.

294. Ray B, Sandine WE. 1992. *Acetic, Propionic, and Lactic Acids of Starter Culture Bacteria as Biopreservatives.* CRC Press, Boca Raton, FL.

295. **Kong Y-J, Park B-K, Oh D-H.** 2001. Antimicrobial activity of *Quercus mongolica* leaf ethanol extract and organic acids against food-borne microorganisms. *Korean J Food Sci Technol* **33:**178–183.

296. **Mani-López E, Garcíaa HS, López-Malo A.** 2012. Organic acids as antimicrobials to control *Salmonella* in meat and poultry products. *Food Res Int* **45:**713–721.

297. **Östling CE, Lindgren SE.** 1993. Inhibition of enterobacteria and *Listeria* growth by lactic, acetic and formic acids. *J Appl Bacteriol* **75:**18–24.

298. **Michetti P, Dorta G, Wiesel PH, Brassart D, Verdu E, Herranz M, Felley C, Porta N, Rouvet M, Blum AL, Corthésy-Theulaz I.** 1999. Effect of whey-based culture supernatant of *Lactobacillus acidophilus* (johnsonii) La1 on *Helicobacter pylori* infection in humans. *Digestion* **60:**203–209.

299. **Stanojević-Nikolić S, Dimić G, Mojović L, Pejin J, Djukić-Vuković A, Kocić-Tanackov S.** 2016. Antimicrobial activity of lactic acid against pathogen and spoilage microorganisms. *J Food Process Preserv* **40:**990–998.

300. **De Keersmaecker SC, Verhoeven TL, Desair J, Marchal K, Vanderleyden J, Nagy I.** 2006. Strong antimicrobial activity of *Lactobacillus rhamnosus* GG against *Salmonella typhimurium* is due to accumulation of lactic acid. *FEMS Microbiol Lett* **259:**89–96.

301. **Aiba Y, Suzuki N, Kabir AM, Takagi A, Koga Y.** 1998. Lactic acid-mediated suppression of Helicobacter pylori by the oral administration of Lactobacillus salivarius as a probiotic in a gnotobiotic murine model. *Am J Gastroenterol* **93:**2097–2101.

302. **Lin WH, Lin CK, Sheu SJ, Hwang CF, Ye WT, Hwang WZ, Tsen HY.** 2009. Antagonistic activity of spent culture supernatants of lactic acid bacteria against *Helicobacter pylori* growth and infection in human gastric epithelial AGS cells. *J Food Sci* **74:**M225–M230.

303. **Fayol-Messaoudi D, Berger CN, Coconnier-Polter MH, Liévin-Le Moal V, Servin AL.** 2005. pH-, lactic acid-, and non-lactic acid-dependent activities of probiotic lactobacilli against *Salmonella enterica* serovar Typhimurium. *Appl Environ Microbiol* **71:**6008–6013.

304. **Adeniyi BA, Adetoye A, Ayeni FA.** 2015. Antibacterial activities of lactic acid bacteria isolated from cow faeces against potential enteric pathogens. *Afr Health Sci* **15:**888–895.

305. **Zheng W, Zhang Y, Lu HM, Li DT, Zhang ZL, Tang ZX, Shi LE.** 2015. Antimicrobial activity and safety evaluation of *Enterococcus faecium* KQ 2.6 isolated from peacock feces. *BMC Biotechnol* **15:**30.

306. **Fujimura S, Watanabe A, Kimura K, Kaji M.** 2012. Probiotic mechanism of *Lactobacillus gasseri* OLL2716 strain against *Helicobacter pylori*. *J Clin Microbiol* **50:**1134–1136.

307. **Lau AS, Liong MT.** 2014. Lactic acid bacteria and bifidobacteria-inhibited *Staphylococcus epidermidis*. *Wounds* **26:**121–131.

308. **Watanabe T, Nishio H, Tanigawa T, Yamagami H, Okazaki H, Watanabe K, Tominaga K, Fujiwara Y, Oshitani N, Asahara T, Nomoto K, Higuchi K, Takeuchi K, Arakawa T.** 2009. Probiotic *Lactobacillus casei* strain Shirota prevents indomethacin-induced small intestinal injury: involvement of lactic acid. *Am J Physiol Gastrointest Liver Physiol* **297:**G506–G513.

309. **Engevik MA, Engevik KA, Yacyshyn MB, Wang J, Hassett DJ, Darien B, Yacyshyn BR, Worrell RT.** 2015. Human *Clostridium difficile* infection: inhibition of NHE3 and microbiota profile. *Am J Physiol Gastrointest Liver Physiol* **308:**G497–G509.

310. **Niku-Paavola ML, Laitila A, Mattila-Sandholm T, Haikara A.** 1999. New types of antimicrobial compounds produced by *Lactobacillus plantarum*. *J Appl Microbiol* **86:**29–35.

311. **Ananthaswamy HN, Eisenstark A.** 1977. Repair of hydrogen peroxide-induced single-strand breaks in *Escherichia coli* deoxyribonucleic acid. *J Bacteriol* **130:**187–191.

312. **Freese EB, Gerson J, Taber H, Rhaese HJ, Freese E.** 1967. Inactivating DNA alterations induced by peroxides and peroxide-producing agents. *Mutat Res* **4:**517–531.

313. **Di Mascio P, Wefers H, Do-Thi HP, Lafleur MV, Sies H.** 1989. Singlet molecular oxygen causes loss of biological activity in plasmid and bacteriophage DNA and induces single-strand breaks. *Biochim Biophys Acta* **1007:**151–157.

314. **Florence TM.** 1986. The production of hydroxyl radical from the reaction between hydrogen peroxide and NADH. *J Inorg Biochem* **28:**33–37.

315. **Dahl TA, Midden WR, Hartman PE.** 1989. Comparison of killing of Gram-negative and Gram-positive bacteria by pure singlet oxygen. *J Bacteriol* **171:**2188–2194.

316. **Servin AL.** 2004. Antagonistic activities of lactobacilli and bifidobacteria against microbial pathogens. *FEMS Microbiol Rev* **28:**405–440.

317. **Pridmore RD, Pittet AC, Praplan F, Cavadini C.** 2008. Hydrogen peroxide production by *Lactobacillus johnsonii* NCC 533 and its role in anti-*Salmonella* activity. *FEMS Microbiol Lett* **283:**210–215.

318. **Ito A, Sato Y, Kudo S, Sato S, Nakajima H, Toba T.** 2003. The screening of hydrogen peroxide-producing lactic acid bacteria and their applica-

tion to inactivating psychrotrophic food-borne pathogens. *Curr Microbiol* **47**:231–236.

319. **Siragusa GR, Johnson MG.** 1989. Inhibition Zof *Listeria monocytogenes* growth by the lactoperoxidase-thiocyanate-H2O2 antimicrobial system. *Appl Environ Microbiol* **55**:2802–2805.

320. **Dahiya RS, Speck ML.** 1968. Hydrogen peroxide formation by lactobacilli and its effect on *Staphylococcus aureus*. *J Dairy Sci* **51**:1568–1572.

321. **Watson JA, Schubert J.** 1969. Action of hydrogen peroxide on growth inhibition of *Salmonella typhimurium*. *J Gen Microbiol* **57**:25–34.

322. **Atassi F, Brassart D, Grob P, Graf F, Servin AL.** 2006. *In vitro* antibacterial activity of *Lactobacillus helveticus* strain KS300 against diarrhoeagenic, uropathogenic and vaginosis-associated bacteria. *J Appl Microbiol* **101**:647–654.

323. **Atassi F, Servin AL.** 2010. Individual and cooperative roles of lactic acid and hydrogen peroxide in the killing activity of enteric strain *Lactobacillus johnsonii* NCC933 and vaginal strain *Lactobacillus gasseri* KS120.1 against enteric, uropathogenic and vaginosis-associated pathogens. *FEMS Microbiol Lett* **304**:29–38.

324. **Dubreuil D, Bisaillon JG, Beaudet R.** 1984. Inhibition of *Neisseria gonorrhoeae* growth due to hydrogen peroxide production by urogenital streptococci. *Microbios* **39**:159–167.

325. **Holmberg K, Hallander HO.** 1973. Production of bactericidal concentrations of hydrogen peroxide by *Streptococcus sanguis*. *Arch Oral Biol* **18**:423–434.

326. **Hillman JD, Socransky SS, Shivers M.** 1985. The relationships between streptococcal species and periodontopathic bacteria in human dental plaque. *Arch Oral Biol* **30**:791–795.

327. **Barnard JP, Stinson MW.** 1996. The alphahemolysin of *Streptococcus gordonii* is hydrogen peroxide. *Infect Immun* **64**:3853–3857.

328. **Barnard JP, Stinson MW.** 1999. Influence of environmental conditions on hydrogen peroxide formation by *Streptococcus gordonii*. *Infect Immun* **67**:6558–6564.

329. **Pericone CD, Overweg K, Hermans PW, Weiser JN.** 2000. Inhibitory and bactericidal effects of hydrogen peroxide production by *Streptococcus pneumoniae* on other inhabitants of the upper respiratory tract. *Infect Immun* **68**:3990–3997.

330. **Regev-Yochay G, Trzcinski K, Thompson CM, Malley R, Lipsitch M.** 2006. Interference between *Streptococcus pneumoniae* and *Staphylococcus aureus*: *in vitro* hydrogen peroxide-mediated killing by *Streptococcus pneumoniae*. *J Bacteriol* **188**:4996–5001.

331. **Klaenhammer TR.** 1993. Genetics of bacteriocins produced by lactic acid bacteria. *FEMS Microbiol Rev* **12**:39–85.

332. **Klaenhammer TR.** 1988. Bacteriocins of lactic acid bacteria. *Biochimie* **70**:337–349.

333. **Dobson A, Cotter PD, Ross RP, Hill C.** 2012. Bacteriocin production: a probiotic trait? *Appl Environ Microbiol* **78**:1–6.

334. **Czárán TL, Hoekstra RF, Pagie L.** 2002. Chemical warfare between microbes promotes biodiversity. *Proc Natl Acad Sci USA* **99**:786–790.

335. **Di Cagno R, De Angelis M, Limitone A, Minervini F, Simonetti MC, Buchin S, Gobbetti M.** 2007. Cell-cell communication in sourdough lactic acid bacteria: a proteomic study in *Lactobacillus sanfranciscensis* CB1. *Proteomics* **7**:2430–2446.

336. **Gobbetti M, De Angelis M, Di Cagno R, Minervini F, Limitone A.** 2007. Cell-cell communication in food related bacteria. *Int J Food Microbiol* **120**:34–45.

337. **Majeed H, Gillor O, Kerr B, Riley MA.** 2011. Competitive interactions in *Escherichia coli* populations: the role of bacteriocins. *ISME J* **5**:71–81.

338. **Riley MA, Wertz JE.** 2002. Bacteriocin diversity: ecological and evolutionary perspectives. *Biochimie* **84**:357–364.

339. **Dawid S, Roche AM, Weiser JN.** 2007. The blp bacteriocins of *Streptococcus pneumoniae* mediate intraspecies competition both *in vitro* and *in vivo*. *Infect Immun* **75**:443–451.

340. **Chen Y, Ludescher RD, Montville TJ.** 1997. Electrostatic interactions, but not the YGNGV consensus motif, govern the binding of pediocin PA-1 and its fragments to phospholipid vesicles. *Appl Environ Microbiol* **63**:4770–4777.

341. **Gut IM, Blanke SR, van der Donk WA.** 2011. Mechanism of inhibition of *Bacillus anthracis* spore outgrowth by the lantibiotic nisin. *ACS Chem Biol* **6**:744–752.

342. **Li J, Aroutcheva AA, Faro S, Chikindas ML.** 2005. Mode of action of lactocin 160, a bacteriocin from vaginal *Lactobacillus rhamnosus*. *Infect Dis Obstet Gynecol* **13**:135–140.

343. **Moll GN, Konings WN, Driessen AJ.** 1999. Bacteriocins: mechanism of membrane insertion and pore formation. *Antonie van Leeuwenhoek* **76**:185–198.

344. **van Kraaij C, de Vos WM, Siezen RJ, Kuipers OP, van Kraaij C, de Vos WM, Siezen RJ.** 1999. Lantibiotics: biosynthesis, mode of action and applications. *Nat Prod Rep* **16**:575–587.

345. **Guder A, Wiedemann I, Sahl HG.** 2000. Posttranslationally modified bacteriocins: the lantibiotics. *Biopolymers* **55**:62–73.

346. **Beuchat LR, Clavero MR, Jaquette CB.** 1997. Effects of nisin and temperature on survival, growth, and enterotoxin production characteristics of psychrotrophic *Bacillus cereus* in beef gravy. *Appl Environ Microbiol* **63:**1953–1958.

347. **Ryan MP, Rea MC, Hill C, Ross RP.** 1996. An application in cheddar cheese manufacture for a strain of *Lactococcus lactis* producing a novel broad-spectrum bacteriocin, lacticin 3147. *Appl Environ Microbiol* **62:**612–619.

348. **Thomas LV, Wimpenny JW.** 1996. Investigation of the effect of combined variations in temperature, pH, and NaCl concentration on nisin inhibition of *Listeria monocytogenes* and *Staphylococcus aureus*. *Appl Environ Microbiol* **62:**2006–2012.

349. **Zapico P, Medina M, Gaya P, Nuñez M.** 1998. Synergistic effect of nisin and the lactoperoxidase system on *Listeria monocytogenes* in skim milk. *Int J Food Microbiol* **40:**35–42.

350. **Taylor LY, Cann DD, Welch BJ.** 1990. Antibotulinal properties of nisin in fresh fish packaged in an atmosphere of carbon dioxide. *J Food Prot* **53:**953–957.

351. **Taylor SL, Somers EB, Krueger LA.** 1985. Antibotulinal effectiveness of nisin-nitrite combinations in culture medium and chicken frankfurter emulsions. *J Food Prot* **48:**234–239.

352. **Wijnker JJ, Weerts EA, Breukink EJ, Houben JH, Lipman LJ.** 2011. Reduction of *Clostridium sporogenes* spore outgrowth in natural sausage casings using nisin. *Food Microbiol* **28:**974–979.

353. **Vessoni Penna TC, Moraes DA, Fajardo DN.** 2002. The effect of nisin on growth kinetics from activated *Bacillus cereus* spores in cooked rice and in milk. *J Food Prot* **65:**419–422.

354. **Beasley SS, Saris PE.** 2004. Nisin-producing *Lactococcus lactis* strains isolated from human milk. *Appl Environ Microbiol* **70:**5051–5053.

355. **Ruhr E, Sahl HG.** 1985. Mode of action of the peptide antibiotic nisin and influence on the membrane potential of whole cells and on cytoplasmic and artificial membrane vesicles. *Antimicrob Agents Chemother* **27:**841–845.

356. **Gao FH, Abee T, Konings WN.** 1991. Mechanism of action of the peptide antibiotic nisin in liposomes and cytochrome c oxidase-containing proteoliposomes. *Appl Environ Microbiol* **57:**2164–2170.

357. **McAuliffe O, Ryan MP, Ross RP, Hill C, Breeuwer P, Abee T.** 1998. Lacticin 3147, a broad-spectrum bacteriocin which selectively dissipates the membrane potential. *Appl Environ Microbiol* **64:**439–445.

358. **Piard JC, Kuipers OP, Rollema HS, Desmazeaud MJ, de Vos WM.** 1993. Structure, organization, and expression of the *lct* gene for lacticin 481, a novel lantibiotic produced by *Lactococcus lactis*. *J Biol Chem* **268:**16361–16368.

359. **Mørtvedt CI, Nissen-Meyer J, Sletten K, Nes IF.** 1991. Purification and amino acid sequence of lactocin S, a bacteriocin produced by *Lactobacillus sake* L45. *Appl Environ Microbiol* **57:** 1829–1834.

360. **Allgaier H, Jung G, Werner RG, Schneider U, Zähner H.** 1986. Epidermin: sequencing of a heterodetic tetracyclic 21-peptide amide antibiotic. *Eur J Biochem* **160:**9–22.

361. **Kellner R, Jung G, Hörner T, Zähner H, Schnell N, Entian KD, Götz F.** 1988. Gallidermin: a new lanthionine-containing polypeptide antibiotic. *Eur J Biochem* **177:**53–59.

362. **Choung SY, Kobayashi T, Inoue J, Takemoto K, Ishitsuka H, Inoue K.** 1988. Hemolytic activity of a cyclic peptide Ro09-0198 isolated from *Streptoverticillium*. *Biochim Biophys Acta* **940:**171–179.

363. **McAuliffe O, Ross RP, Hill C.** 2001. Lantibiotics: structure, biosynthesis and mode of action. *FEMS Microbiol Rev* **25:**285–308.

364. **Dunkley EA Jr, Clejan S, Guffanti AA, Krulwich TA.** 1988. Large decreases in membrane phosphatidylethanolamine and diphosphatidylglycerol upon mutation to duramycin resistance do not change the protonophore resistance of *Bacillus subtilis*. *Biochim Biophys Acta* **943:**13–18.

365. **Sahl HG, Jack RW, Bierbaum G.** 1995. Biosynthesis and biological activities of lantibiotics with unique post-translational modifications. *Eur J Biochem* **230:**827–853.

366. **Fredenhagen A, Fendrich G, Märki F, Märki W, Gruner J, Raschdorf F, Peter HH.** 1990. Duramycins B and C, two new lanthionine containing antibiotics as inhibitors of phospholipase A2. Structural revision of duramycin and cinnamycin. *J Antibiot (Tokyo)* **43:**1403–1412.

367. **Ennahar S, Deschamps N, Richard J.** 2000. Natural variation in susceptibility of *Listeria* strains to class IIa bacteriocins. *Curr Microbiol* **41:**1–4.

368. **Ennahar S, Sashihara T, Sonomoto K, Ishizaki A.** 2000. Class IIa bacteriocins: biosynthesis, structure and activity. *FEMS Microbiol Rev* **24:** 85–106.

369. **Rodríguez JM, Martínez MI, Horn N, Dodd HM.** 2003. Heterologous production of bacteriocins by lactic acid bacteria. *Int J Food Microbiol* **80:**101–116.

370. **Tichaczek PS, Nissen-Meyer J, Nes IF, Vogel RF, Hammes WP.** 1992. Characterization of the bacteriocins curvacin A from *Lactobacillus curvatus* LTH1174 and sakacin P from *L. sake* LTH673. *Syst Appl Microbiol* **15:**460–468.

371. **Henderson JT, Chopko AL, van Wassenaar PD.** 1992. Purification and primary structure of pediocin PA-1 produced by *Pediococcus acidilactici* PAC-1.0. *Arch Biochem Biophys* **295**:5–12.

372. **Motlagh AM, Bhunia AK, Szostek F, Hansen TR, Johnson MC, Ray B.** 1992. Nucleotide and amino acid sequence of pap-gene (pediocin AcH production) in *Pediococcus acidilactici* H. *Lett Appl Microbiol* **15**:45–48.

373. **Hastings JW, Sailer M, Johnson K, Roy KL, Vederas JC, Stiles ME.** 1991. Characterization of leucocin A-UAL 187 and cloning of the bacteriocin gene from *Leuconostoc gelidum*. *J Bacteriol* **173**:7491–7500.

374. **Héchard Y, Dérijard B, Letellier F, Cenatiempo Y.** 1992. Characterization and purification of mesentericin Y105, an anti-*Listeria* bacteriocin from *Leuconostoc mesenteroides*. *J Gen Microbiol* **138**:2725–2731.

375. **Métivier A, Pilet MF, Dousset X, Sorokine O, Anglade P, Zagorec M, Piard JC, Marlon D, Cenatiempo Y, Fremaux C.** 1998. Divercin V41, a new bacteriocin with two disulphide bonds produced by *Carnobacterium divergens* V41: primary structure and genomic organization. *Microbiology* **144**:2837–2844.

376. **Aymerich T, Holo H, Håvarstein LS, Hugas M, Garriga M, Nes IF.** 1996. Biochemical and genetic characterization of enterocin A from *Enterococcus faecium*, a new antilisterial bacteriocin in the pediocin family of bacteriocins. *Appl Environ Microbiol* **62**:1676–1682.

377. **Ferchichi M, Frère J, Mabrouk K, Manai M.** 2001. Lactococcin MMFII, a novel class IIa bacteriocin produced by *Lactococcus lactis* MMFII, isolated from a Tunisian dairy product. *FEMS Microbiol Lett* **205**:49–55.

378. **Yildirim Z, Winters DK, Johnson MG.** 1999. Purification, amino acid sequence and mode of action of bifidocin B produced by *Bifidobacterium bifidum* NCFB 1454. *J Appl Microbiol* **86**:45–54.

379. **Shin MS, Han SK, Ryu JS, Kim KS, Lee WK.** 2008. Isolation and partial characterization of a bacteriocin produced by *Pediococcus pentosaceus* K23-2 isolated from kimchi. *J Appl Microbiol* **105**:331–339.

380. **Balla E, Dicks LM, Du Toit M, Van Der Merwe MJ, Holzapfel WH.** 2000. Characterization and cloning of the genes encoding enterocin 1071A and enterocin 1071B, two antimicrobial peptides produced by *Enterococcus faecalis* BFE 1071. *Appl Environ Microbiol* **66**:1298–1304.

381. **Nissen-Meyer J, Håvarstein LS, Holo H, Sletten K, Nes IF.** 1993. Association of the lactococcin A immunity factor with the cell membrane: purification and characterization of the immunity factor. *J Gen Microbiol* **139**:1503–1509.

382. **van Belkum MJ, Kok J, Venema G, Holo H, Nes IF, Konings WN, Abee T.** 1991. The bacteriocin lactococcin A specifically increases permeability of lactococcal cytoplasmic membranes in a voltage-independent, protein-mediated manner. *J Bacteriol* **173**:7934–7941.

383. **Allison GE, Fremaux C, Klaenhammer TR.** 1994. Expansion of bacteriocin activity and host range upon complementation of two peptides encoded within the lactacin F operon. *J Bacteriol* **176**:2235–2241.

384. **Jiménez-Díaz R, Ruiz-Barba JL, Cathcart DP, Holo H, Nes IF, Sletten KH, Warner PJ.** 1995. Purification and partial amino acid sequence of plantaricin S, a bacteriocin produced by *Lactobacillus plantarum* LPCO10, the activity of which depends on the complementary action of two peptides. *Appl Environ Microbiol* **61**:4459–4463.

385. **Anderssen EL, Diep DB, Nes IF, Eijsink VG, Nissen-Meyer J.** 1998. Antagonistic activity of *Lactobacillus plantarum* C11: two new two-peptide bacteriocins, plantaricins EF and JK, and the induction factor plantaricin A. *Appl Environ Microbiol* **64**:2269–2272.

386. **Davey GP, Richardson BC.** 1981. Purification and some properties of diplococcin from *Streptococcus cremoris* 346. *Appl Environ Microbiol* **41**:84–89.

387. **Herranz C, Chen Y, Chung HJ, Cintas LM, Hernández PE, Montville TJ, Chikindas ML.** 2001. Enterocin P selectively dissipates the membrane potential of *Enterococcus faecium* T136. *Appl Environ Microbiol* **67**:1689–1692.

388. **Moll G, Ubbink-Kok T, Hildeng-Hauge H, Nissen-Meyer J, Nes IF, Konings WN, Driessen AJ.** 1996. Lactococcin G is a potassium ion-conducting, two-component bacteriocin. *J Bacteriol* **178**:600–605.

389. **González C, Langdon GM, Bruix M, Gálvez A, Valdivia E, Maqueda M, Rico M.** 2000. Bacteriocin AS-48, a microbial cyclic polypeptide structurally and functionally related to mammalian NK-lysin. *Proc Natl Acad Sci USA* **97**:11221–11226.

390. **Leer RJ, van der Vossen JM, van Giezen M, van Noort JM, Pouwels PH.** 1995. Genetic analysis of acidocin B, a novel bacteriocin produced by *Lactobacillus acidophilus*. *Microbiology* **141**:1629–1635.

391. **Worobo RW, Henkel T, Sailer M, Roy KL, Vederas JC, Stiles ME.** 1994. Characteristics and genetic determinant of a hydrophobic peptide bacteriocin, carnobacteriocin A, pro-

duced by *Carnobacterium piscicola* LV17A. *Microbiology* **140:**517–526.

392. **Cintas LM, Casaus P, Håvarstein LS, Hernández PE, Nes IF.** 1997. Biochemical and genetic characterization of enterocin P, a novel sec-dependent bacteriocin from *Enterococcus faecium* P13 with a broad antimicrobial spectrum. *Appl Environ Microbiol* **63:**4321–4330.

393. **Nes IF, Diep DB, Håvarstein LS, Brurberg MB, Eijsink V, Holo H.** 1996. Biosynthesis of bacteriocins in lactic acid bacteria. *Antonie van Leeuwenhoek* **70:**113–128.

394. **Holo H, Nilssen O, Nes IF.** 1991. Lactococcin A, a new bacteriocin from *Lactococcus lactis* subsp. *cremoris*: isolation and characterization of the protein and its gene. *J Bacteriol* **173:**3879–3887.

395. **Sandiford S, Upton M.** 2012. Identification, characterization, and recombinant expression of epidermicin NI01, a novel unmodified bacteriocin produced by *Staphylococcus epidermidis* that displays potent activity against staphylococci. *Antimicrob Agents Chemother* **56:**1539–1547.

396. **de Lorenzo V.** 1985. Factors affecting microcin E492 production. *J Antibiot (Tokyo)* **38:**340–345.

397. **de Lorenzo V, Pugsley AP.** 1985. Microcin E492, a low-molecular-weight peptide antibiotic which causes depolarization of the *Escherichia coli* cytoplasmic membrane. *Antimicrob Agents Chemother* **27:**666–669.

398. **Wu JA, Kusuma C, Mond JJ, Kokai-Kun JF.** 2003. Lysostaphin disrupts *Staphylococcus aureus* and *Staphylococcus epidermidis* biofilms on artificial surfaces. *Antimicrob Agents Chemother* **47:**3407–3414.

399. **Gründling A, Missiakas DM, Schneewind O.** 2006. *Staphylococcus aureus* mutants with increased lysostaphin resistance. *J Bacteriol* **188:**6286–6297.

400. **Bastos MD, Coutinho BG, Coelho MLV.** 2010. Lysostaphin: a staphylococcal bacteriolysin with potential clinical applications. *Pharmaceuticals (Basel)* **3:**1139–1161.

401. **Nilsen T, Nes IF, Holo H.** 2003. Enterolysin A, a cell wall-degrading bacteriocin from *Enterococcus faecalis* LMG 2333. *Appl Environ Microbiol* **69:**2975–2984.

402. **Vaughan EE, Daly C, Fitzgerald GF.** 1992. Identification and characterization of helveticin V-1829, a bacteriocin produced by *Lactobacillus helveticus* 1829. *J Appl Bacteriol* **73:**299–308.

403. **Ross RP, Morgan S, Hill C.** 2002. Preservation and fermentation: past, present and future. *Int J Food Microbiol* **79:**3–16.

404. **Müller E, Radler F.** 1993. Caseicin, a bacteriocin from *Lactobacillus casei*. *Folia Microbiol (Praha)* **38:**441–446.

405. **Oman TJ, Boettcher JM, Wang H, Okalibe XN, van der Donk WA.** 2011. Sublancin is not a lantibiotic but an S-linked glycopeptide. *Nat Chem Biol* **7:**78–80.

406. **Stepper J, Shastri S, Loo TS, Preston JC, Novak P, Man P, Moore CH, Havlíček V, Patchett ML, Norris GE.** 2011. Cysteine *S*-glycosylation, a new post-translational modification found in glycopeptide bacteriocins. *FEBS Lett* **585:**645–650.

407. **Maqueda M, Gálvez A, Bueno MM, Sanchez-Barrena MJ, González C, Albert A, Rico M, Valdivia E.** 2004. Peptide AS-48: prototype of a new class of cyclic bacteriocins. *Curr Protein Pept Sci* **5:**399–416.

408. **Maky MA, Ishibashi N, Zendo T, Perez RH, Doud JR, Karmi M, Sonomoto K.** 2015. Enterocin F4-9, a novel *O*-linked glycosylated bacteriocin. *Appl Environ Microbiol* **81:**4819–4826.

409. **Paik SH, Chakicherla A, Hansen JN.** 1998. Identification and characterization of the structural and transporter genes for, and the chemical and biological properties of, sublancin 168, a novel lantibiotic produced by *Bacillus subtilis* 168. *J Biol Chem* **273:**23134–23142.

410. **Kelly W, Asmundson R, Huang C.** 1996. Characterization of plantaricin KW30, a bacteriocin produced by *Lactobacillus plantarum*. *J Appl Microbiol* **81:**657–662.

411. **Rebuffat S.** 2012. Microcins in action: amazing defence strategies of *Enterobacteria*. *Biochem Soc Trans* **40:**1456–1462.

412. **Yang SC, Lin CH, Sung CT, Fang JY.** 2014. Antibacterial activities of bacteriocins: application in foods and pharmaceuticals. *Front Microbiol* **5:**241.

413. **Thomas X, Destoumieux-Garzón D, Peduzzi J, Afonso C, Blond A, Birlirakis N, Goulard C, Dubost L, Thai R, Tabet JC, Rebuffat S.** 2004. Siderophore peptide, a new type of post-translationally modified antibacterial peptide with potent activity. *J Biol Chem* **279:**28233–28242.

414. **Severinov K, Semenova E, Kazakov A, Kazakov T, Gelfand MS.** 2007. Low-molecular-weight post-translationally modified microcins. *Mol Microbiol* **65:**1380–1394.

415. **van den Elzen PJ, Walters HH, Veltkamp E, Nijkamp HJ.** 1983. Molecular structure and function of the bacteriocin gene and bacteriocin protein of plasmid Clo DF13. *Nucleic Acids Res* **11:**2465–2477.

416. **Kleanthous C.** 2010. Swimming against the tide: progress and challenges in our understanding of colicin translocation. *Nat Rev Microbiol* **8:**843–848.

417. **Cascales E, Buchanan SK, Duché D, Kleanthous C, Lloubès R, Postle K, Riley M, Slatin S,**

Cavard D. 2007. Colicin biology. *Microbiol Mol Biol Rev* **71:**158–229.

418. **Gillor O, Giladi I, Riley MA.** 2009. Persistence of colicinogenic *Escherichia coli* in the mouse gastrointestinal tract. *BMC Microbiol* **9:**165.

419. **Goldstein BP, Wei J, Greenberg K, Novick R.** 1998. Activity of nisin against *Streptococcus pneumoniae, in vitro,* and in a mouse infection model. *J Antimicrob Chemother* **42:**277–278.

420. **van Staden AD, Brand AM, Dicks LM.** 2012. Nisin F-loaded brushite bone cement prevented the growth of *Staphylococcus aureusin vivo. J Appl Microbiol* **112:**831–840.

421. **Brand AM, de Kwaadsteniet M, Dicks LM.** 2010. The ability of nisin F to control *Staphylococcus aureus* infection in the peritoneal cavity, as studied in mice. *Lett Appl Microbiol* **51:**645–649.

422. **De Kwaadsteniet M, Doeschate KT, Dicks LM.** 2009. Nisin F in the treatment of respiratory tract infections caused by *Staphylococcus aureus. Lett Appl Microbiol* **48:**65–70.

423. **Campion A, Casey PG, Field D, Cotter PD, Hill C, Ross RP.** 2013. *In vivo* activity of nisin A and nisin V against *Listeria monocytogenes* in mice. *BMC Microbiol* **13:**23.

424. **Mota-Meira M, Morency H, Lavoie MC.** 2005. *In vivo* activity of mutacin B-Ny266. *J Antimicrob Chemother* **56:**869–871.

425. **Castiglione F, Cavaletti L, Losi D, Lazzarini A, Carrano L, Feroggio M, Ciciliato I, Corti E, Candiani G, Marinelli F, Selva E.** 2007. A novel lantibiotic acting on bacterial cell wall synthesis produced by the uncommon actinomycete *Planomonospora* sp. *Biochemistry* **46:**5884–5895.

426. **Rihakova J, Cappelier JM, Hue I, Demnerova K, Fédérighi M, Prévost H, Drider D.** 2010. *In vivo* activities of recombinant divercin V41 and its structural variants against *Listeria monocytogenes. Antimicrob Agents Chemother* **54:**563–564.

427. **Salvucci E, Saavedra L, Hebert EM, Haro C, Sesma F.** 2012. Enterocin CRL35 inhibits *Listeria monocytogenes* in a murine model. *Foodborne Pathog Dis* **9:**68–74.

428. **Sosunov V, Mischenko V, Eruslanov B, Svetoch E, Shakina Y, Stern N, Majorov K, Sorokoumova G, Selishcheva A, Apt A.** 2007. Antimycobacterial activity of bacteriocins and their complexes with liposomes. *J Antimicrob Chemother* **59:**919–925.

429. **Lopez FE, Vincent PA, Zenoff AM, Salomón RA, Farías RN.** 2007. Efficacy of microcin J25 in biomatrices and in a mouse model of *Salmonella* infection. *J Antimicrob Chemother* **59:**676–680.

430. **Wang WL, Liu J, Huo YB, Ling JQ.** 2013. Bacteriocin immunity proteins play a role in quorum-sensing system regulated antimicrobial sensitivity of *Streptococcus mutans* UA159. *Arch Oral Biol* **58:**384–390.

431. **Corr SC, Li Y, Riedel CU, O'Toole PW, Hill C, Gahan CG.** 2007. Bacteriocin production as a mechanism for the antiinfective activity of *Lactobacillus salivarius* UCC118. *Proc Natl Acad Sci USA* **104:**7617–7621.

432. **Kuipers OP, de Ruyter PGGA, Kleerebezem M, de Vos WM.** 1998. Quorum sensing-controlled gene expression in lactic acid bacteria. *J Biotechnol* **64:**15–21.

433. **Kleerebezem M.** 2004. Quorum sensing control of lantibiotic production; nisin and subtilin autoregulate their own biosynthesis. *Peptides* **25:**1405–1414.

434. **Kleerebezem M, Kuipers OP, de Vos WM, Stiles ME, Quadri LE.** 2001. A two-component signal-transduction cascade in *Carnobacterium piscicola* LV17B: two signaling peptides and one sensor-transmitter. *Peptides* **22:**1597–1601.

435. **Kleerebezem M, Quadri LE.** 2001. Peptide pheromone-dependent regulation of antimicrobial peptide production in Gram-positive bacteria: a case of multicellular behavior. *Peptides* **22:**1579–1596.

436. **O'Keeffe T, Hill C, Ross RP.** 1999. Characterization and heterologous expression of the genes encoding enterocin a production, immunity, and regulation in *Enterococcus faecium* DPC1146. *Appl Environ Microbiol* **65:**1506–1515.

437. **Cotter PD, Hill C, Ross RP.** 2005. Bacteriocins: developing innate immunity for food. *Nat Rev Microbiol* **3:**777–788.

438. **van der Ploeg JR.** 2005. Regulation of bacteriocin production in *Streptococcus mutans* by the quorum-sensing system required for development of genetic competence. *J Bacteriol* **187:**3980–3989.

439. **Kreth J, Merritt J, Shi W, Qi F.** 2005. Competition and coexistence between *Streptococcus mutans* and *Streptococcus sanguinis* in the dental biofilm. *J Bacteriol* **187:**7193–7203.

440. **Li YH, Hanna MN, Svensäter G, Ellen RP, Cvitkovitch DG.** 2001. Cell density modulates acid adaptation in *Streptococcus mutans*: implications for survival in biofilms. *J Bacteriol* **183:**6875–6884.

441. **Li YH, Lau PC, Lee JH, Ellen RP, Cvitkovitch DG.** 2001. Natural genetic transformation of *Streptococcus mutans* growing in biofilms. *J Bacteriol* **183:**897–908.

442. **Li YH, Tian XL, Layton G, Norgaard C, Sisson G.** 2008. Additive attenuation of virulence and cariogenic potential of *Streptococcus*

mutans by simultaneous inactivation of the ComCDE quorum-sensing system and HK/RR11 two-component regulatory system. *Microbiology* **154**:3256–3265.

443. **Dufour D, Cordova M, Cvitkovitch DG, Lévesque CM.** 2011. Regulation of the competence pathway as a novel role associated with a streptococcal bacteriocin. *J Bacteriol* **193**:6552–6559.

444. **Perry JA, Jones MB, Peterson SN, Cvitkovitch DG, Lévesque CM.** 2009. Peptide alarmone signalling triggers an auto-active bacteriocin necessary for genetic competence. *Mol Microbiol* **72**:905–917.

445. **Kuramitsu HK, He X, Lux R, Anderson MH, Shi W.** 2007. Interspecies interactions within oral microbial communities. *Microbiol Mol Biol Rev* **71**:653–670.

446. **Rodríguez E, Arqués JL, Rodríguez R, Nuñez M, Medina M.** 2003. Reuterin production by lactobacilli isolated from pig faeces and evaluation of probiotic traits. *Lett Appl Microbiol* **37**:259–263.

447. **Talarico TL, Casas IA, Chung TC, Dobrogosz WJ.** 1988. Production and isolation of reuterin, a growth inhibitor produced by *Lactobacillus reuteri*. *Antimicrob Agents Chemother* **32**:1854–1858.

448. **Lüthi-Peng Q, Dileme FB, Puhan Z.** 2002. Effect of glucose on glycerol bioconversion by *Lactobacillus reuteri*. *Appl Microbiol Biotechnol* **59**:289–296.

449. **Schaefer L, Auchtung TA, Hermans KE, Whitehead D, Borhan B, Britton RA.** 2010. The antimicrobial compound reuterin (3-hydroxypropionaldehyde) induces oxidative stress via interaction with thiol groups. *Microbiology* **156**:1589–1599.

450. **Sriramulu DD, Liang M, Hernandez-Romero D, Raux-Deery E, Lünsdorf H, Parsons JB, Warren MJ, Prentice MB.** 2008. *Lactobacillus reuteri* DSM 20016 produces cobalamin-dependent diol dehydratase in metabolosomes and metabolizes 1,2-propanediol by disproportionation. *J Bacteriol* **190**:4559–4567.

451. **Cleusix V, Lacroix C, Vollenweider S, Duboux M, Le Blay G.** 2007. Inhibitory activity spectrum of reuterin produced by *Lactobacillus reuteri* against intestinal bacteria. *BMC Microbiol* **7**:101.

452. **Arqués JL, Rodríguez E, Nuñez M, Medina M.** 2011. Combined effect of reuterin and lactic acid bacteria bacteriocins on the inactivation of food-borne pathogens in milk. *Food Control* **22**:457–461.

453. **Morita H, Toh H, Fukuda S, Horikawa H, Oshima K, Suzuki T, Murakami M, Hisamatsu S, Kato Y, Takizawa T, Fukuoka H, Yoshimura T, Itoh K, O'Sullivan DJ, McKay LL, Ohno H, Kikuchi J, Masaoka T, Hattori M.** 2008. Comparative genome analysis of *Lactobacillus reuteri* and *Lactobacillus fermentum* reveal a genomic island for reuterin and cobalamin production. *DNA Res* **15**:151–161.

454. **Gänzle MG.** 2004. Reutericyclin: biological activity, mode of action, and potential applications. *Appl Microbiol Biotechnol* **64**:326–332.

455. **Gänzle MG, Höltzel A, Walter J, Jung G, Hammes WP.** 2000. Characterization of reutericyclin produced by *Lactobacillus reuteri* LTH2584. *Appl Environ Microbiol* **66**:4325–4333.

456. **Helander IM, Mattila-Sandholm T.** 2000. Permeability barrier of the Gram-negative bacterial outer membrane with special reference to nisin. *Int J Food Microbiol* **60**:153–161.

The Genomic Basis of Lactobacilli as Health-Promoting Organisms

2

ELISA SALVETTI[1] and PAUL W. O'TOOLE[1]

BENEFICIAL EFFECTS ASSOCIATED WITH LACTOBACILLI

The genus *Lactobacillus* includes 177 species (http://www.bacterio.net/lactobacillus.html): they are non-spore-forming, mostly nonmotile, and rod-shaped (although coccobacilli are observed). They generally have a fermentative metabolism (although genome sequence analysis has provided evidence of potential for respiration [1]) with lactic acid as the main fermentation product.

Lactobacilli grow in rich carbohydrate-containing substrates such as food (dairy products, grain products, meat and fish products, beer, wine, fruits and fruit juices, pickled vegetables, mash, sauerkraut, silage, and sourdough), water, soil, and sewage; they are part of the microbiota associated with the mouth and gastrointestinal and genital tracts of humans and many animals (2).

With regard to their beneficial and protechnological properties, 35 *Lactobacillus* species have Qualified Presumption of Safety (QPS) status from the European Food Safety Authority (EFSA) (3) and 12 species are Generally Recognized as Safe (GRAS) by the FDA (http://www.accessdata.fda.gov/scripts/fdcc/?set=GRASNotices). Lactobacilli constitute 43% (84 species) of the total number of microorganisms with certified beneficial use (195 species representing 28 genera of phyla *Actinobacteria*, *Firmicutes*, and *Proteo-*

[1]School of Microbiology and APC Microbiome Institute, University College Cork, Ireland
Bugs as Drugs: Therapeutic Microbes for the Prevention and Treatment of Disease
Edited by Robert A. Britton and Patrice D. Cani
© 2018 American Society for Microbiology, Washington, DC
doi:10.1128/microbiolspec.BAD-0011-2016

bacteria) (4), with 22 of them represented by strains that are patented in Europe due to their potential probiotic properties (E. Salvetti and P. W. O'Toole, under revision).

Given the rising importance of lactobacilli as beneficial microbes, the focus of the present review is the genetic and genomic basis of health promotion by lactobacilli. A comprehensive survey of the discovery research that first identified these features is beyond the scope of this review, and the reader is referred to excellent recent surveys on this topic including Lebeer et al. (5) and Papadimitriou et al. (6).

Beneficial effects associated with lactobacilli, which have been the subject of decades of research, may be classified into three broad categories—*in vivo* survival mechanisms, *in vivo* colonization mechanisms, and direct effects on the host (see Table 1 for representative examples). Arguably, only effects on the host are true "probiotic" traits,

as defined recently by Hill et al. (7), but because surviving intestinal transit is probably required to exert beneficial effects, work aimed at developing probiotic strains and identifying probiotic features has traditionally included survival and colonization analysis, as well as metabolic adaptation to nutritional substrates typically available in the mammalian intestine. A fourth category, effect on the intestinal microbiota, has recently been formalized (8), although exerting a direct effect on other microbes such as pathogens has always been a recognized potential probiotic trait (5).

A preponderance of the literature on probiotic mode of action in lactobacilli is based on studies performed *in vitro* or in preclinical models, as distinct from in humans or in animals. As a consequence, there are many features and gene products whose actual contribution to probiotic function in lactobacilli is unclear. This is reflected in the lack of

TABLE 1 Selected examples of probiotic traits in lactobacilli

Category	Host benefit	Representative examples and effectors	Reference
In vivo survival	Viable bacteria reach site of action in the gut.	Acid resistance in *L. plantarum* by ATPases	93
		Bile resistance in *L. salivarius* by bile salt hydrolases	94
	Bacteria can metabolize dietary ingredients.	Metabolic diversity of intestinal lactobacilli	12
In vivo adherence	Maintaining bacterial numbers and close host cell association	Biofilm formation in *L. reuteri* 100-23	76
		Aggregation of *L. crispatus* cells during murine colonization	95
		Aggregation and adhesion protein allowing colonization by *L. gasseri*	96
		Production of bacterial surface adhesins	31, 97
Direct effects on host	Altered cellular or organ functions	Alteration of signal transduction, apoptosis and barrier function in epithelial cells by *L. rhamnosus* LGG proteins	98, 99
		Alteration of innate immune cell function by *L. acidophilus* S-layer protein	100
		Suppression of inflammation in colitis by histamine produced by *L. reuteri*	101
		Degradation of proinflammatory cytokines by *L. casei*	32
		Altered cytokine production due to *L. rhamnosus* pili	36
Effect on microbiota or pathogens	Restores normal microbiota or excludes pathogens	Anti-*Listeria monocytogenes* activity of *L. salivarius* bacteriocin	88
		Controversial effects of probiotics on the human gut microbiota	102

success in obtaining EFSA approval for probiotics and functional foods, mainly linked to insufficient characterization of the food and poor scientific support for the claimed effect (9), the absence of a beneficial physiological effect based on the scientific evidence assessed (10), and the nonrecognition of the property of preventing, treating, or curing a human disease with food (11).

In reviewing the literature at this juncture (Fig. 1), a clear stalling in investment in *Lactobacillus* probiotic research is apparent, reflected in the large knowledge gap in molecular mechanisms that still needs to be filled.

GENOMIC DIVERSITY OF LACTOBACILLI

The genome sequences of almost all *Lactobacillus* type strains and some historically associated genera were recently determined (12, 13), providing the definitive genomic framework for mining all relevant phylogenetic and functional information and corroborating the genetic basis of what had been described for nearly a century, namely the extreme phenotypic diversity of lactobacilli (2, 14).

Comparative analysis (12, 13) uncovered the extraordinary level of genomic diversity of the lactobacilli: the sizes of the genomes, in fact, range from 1.23 Mb to 4.91 Mb (four times larger) and the DNA GC content range is from 31.93 to 57.02%. The overall level of genome difference among the members of the *Lactobacillus* genus was found to be comparable to that between members of a bacterial family (12). Even more astonishing is consideration of the pairwise average nucleotide identity values that are comparable for those between members of taxonomic orders or classes (12). The genus as currently defined is polyphyletic, meaning it encompasses the descendants of several most recent common ancestors (MRCAs), specifically those of *Pediococcus*, *Weissella*, *Leuconostoc*, *Oenococcus*, and *Fructobacillus*. The overall significance of this unusually complex phylogenomic landscape is that it makes for a challenging research context. In comparison with studies of pathogens, for example, where comparative genomics has led to discovery of pathogenicity islands and converting bacteriophages, such discovery paradigms are less helpful in lactobacilli, with the

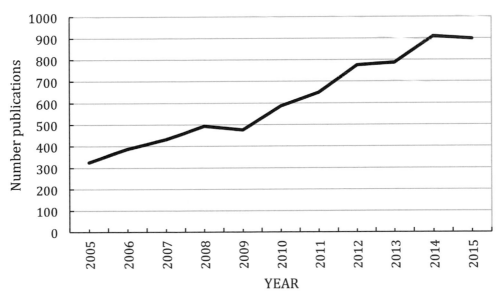

FIGURE 1 Publication numbers by year using search terms (lactobacillus probiotic) in PubMed. Search performed 13 July 2016.

exception of the cobalamin biosynthesis/ propanediol utilization island of *Lactobacillus reuteri* (15, 16). The imminent reallocation of the members of the current genus *Lactobacillus* across a number of smaller, genomically more cohesive new genera (Salvetti et al., in preparation) will provide a more sensible context for genotype-phenotype matching in the lactobacilli.

It is reasonable to expect to be able to understand the interaction of *Lactobacillus* species and their respective environments in the context of their genomic relatedness and genome content. A simple hypothesis is that the MRCAs of all the lactobacilli had a large genome with diverse metabolic capability, and that adaptive radiation to the range of niches occupied by contemporary species was marked by gene loss in those species whose niche is nutrient-rich like the mammalian body or fermented foods, and clade-specific gene acquisition in some clades.

DISTRIBUTION OF PROBIOTIC-RELATED TRAITS IN LACTOBACILLI

Despite these challenges, we and others have been mining the wealth of genomic data for lactobacilli to catalog the number and distribution of traits linked with probiotic function including those in Table 1. These analyses are ongoing (E. Salvetti et al., in preparation), but our initial observations are already instructive. The data provide a framework for testing the well-recognized phenomenon (17) of strain specificity of probiotic effects, and for using comparative genomics and genome annotation mining to uncover probiotic traits in other species. The outcome of analyses based on comparative genomics within species is discussed further below.

Carbohydrate Metabolism

Lactobacilli are saccharolytic but devote a lower proportion of their coding capacity to carbohydrate degradation than, for example,

bifidobacteria (18) or *Bacteroides* spp. (19), even in the larger-genome species such as *L. plantarum* (20). High-throughput annotation of 213 genomes identified glycosyl hydrolases corresponding to 48 of the 133 families of glycoside hydrolases (GHs) in the CAZy database (http://www.cazy.org) (12). Newly identified enzymes included an endo-α-*N*-acetylgalactosaminidase in *L. brantae* and *L. perolens* that may be involved in mucus utilization and could thus be a colonization factor. Glycosyl hydrolase family 95 (GH95) enzymes had not previously been identified in the lactobacilli, but were identified in *L. harbinensis* and *L. perolens* (12), which were isolated from traditional fermented vegetables in China and spoiled soft drinks, respectively. GH95 is a fucosidase, a type of enzyme that is well recognized in bifidobacteria (21), *Bacteroides* spp. (22), and *Akkermansia muciniphila* (23). Although used by bifidobacteria for breaking down human milk oligosaccharides, most of the evidence suggests that these fucosidases are used by gut commensals or pathogens for metabolizing fucose residues on intestinal mucus (reviewed in reference 24). The unusually high proportional gene count encoding glycosyl hydrolases in six *Lactobacillus* clades (12)— *L. (par)alimentarius*, *L. perolens*, *L. plantarum*, *L. rapi*, *L. fructivorans*, and *Carnobacterium* spp.—suggests adaptation of these clades to the selective pressure typically encountered in the gut. Members of these clades have been isolated from the gut of animals (i.e., goat, poultry, and honey bee stomach) and are used as feed additives or probiotics.

Genomics of Surface Carbohydrate Decoration

The major form of surface carbohydrate in Gram-positive bacteria, exopolysaccharide (EPS), contributes to technological features like product viscosity and texture, but also to host interaction (25–27). In *Lactobacillus*, EPS production is strain specific and growth medium dependent, and the EPS can be bound or released by the bacterial cell (e.g., 28, 29), making translation of *in vitro* findings to probiotic effects *in vivo* very challenging. Genus-wide genome comparison identified a number of glycosyltransferases that show restricted presence across species and that may be relevant for probiotic function. For example, the *L. gasseri* genome harbors a gene encoding GT11 (galactoside α-1,2-L-fucosyltransferase), and the *L. delbrueckii* DSM 15996^T encodes GT92 (*N*-glycan core α-1,6-fucoside β-1,4-galactosyltransferase). Production of fucose-containing lipopoly-saccharide is an immune-evasion/antigenic mimicry strategy of pathogens such as *Helicobacter pylori* by virtue of the fucose-containing structures present in Lewis-type blood group antigens (30), and it will be interesting to know if lactobacilli use such a strategy to modulate innate immune interaction. The GT11 enzyme is predicted to be encoded by the *A. muciniphila* genome, so perhaps this trait is present in other gut commensals.

Surface Protein Repertoires

Surface proteins are the next topological interaction layer below EPS on *Lactobacillus* cells, and they thus represent an important interface with the external environment (31). As noted above (Table 1), an extracellular protease of the subtilase type produced by the *L. casei* strain present in the commercial probiotic cocktail called VSL#3 degrades IP-10, an inflammatory mediator involved in colitis (32). This appears to be the only published example of a surface-anchored enzyme contributing to a probiotic trait in lactobacilli (which is distinct from probiotic-derived soluble proteins such as p40 and p75, which have been detected in *L. casei* group members [33]). However, cataloging of the repertoire of this class of protease (lactocepin) in the lactobacilli identified 60 genes among 213 genomes, which were proportionally over-represented in members of the *L. delbrueckii*, *L. casei*, *L. salivarius*, and *L. buchneri* clades,

as well as the carnobacteria. The high level of sequence divergence found between the predicted lactocepin proteins (12) makes it at least plausible that the uncharted specificity of some of these proteases could include human proteins as targets.

A major class of surface proteins in Gram-positives is those that are covalently attached to peptidoglycan by a sortase transpeptidation reaction (34). Searching the translated protein data for the target motifs of the sortase enzyme identified the repertoire of sortase-anchored proteins in the lactobacilli. This identified 1,628 predicted LPXTG-containing proteins and 357 sortase enzymes in the 213 genomes. Species known to contain strains identified as being probiotic did not harbor unusually high numbers of sortase-anchored proteins; in fact, the greatest absolute number or genome-size-normalized number was in the milk isolate *Carnobacterium maltaromaticum*. The fact that sortase-anchored proteins may have almost any biological properties that cannot always be identified from their primary sequence (such as fibrinogen binding, exemplified in reference 35) makes this a difficult bioprospecting approach. A more productive screen identified 67 *pilus* gene clusters in 51 *Lactobacillus* strains, whereby the *pilus* gene search was based on the surface structures identified as mucin binding and immunomodulatory in *L. rhamnosus* GG (36). These clusters were present in clades and species not known to be probiotic, such as *L. thailandensis*, *L. ruminis*, and *L. koreensis*, broadening the avenues of exploration for new beneficial strains.

INTRASPECIFIC DIVERSITY OF *LACTOBACILLUS* SPECIES HARBORING PROBIOTIC STRAINS

Although a number of studies have addressed the similarity and the differences within species of the *Lactobacillus* genus through comparative genomics, knowledge of the evolutionary history and the genomic diversity below the species level is still incomplete. Unraveling the intraspecific diversity of lactobacilli is, in fact, fundamental for the regulatory perspective, for the development of identification tools for tracking isolates during industrial processes, and for the commercial standpoint to differentiate probiotics or starter cultures (37).

The effects of microbial strains that are marketed as established probiotics along with their clinical evidence assessed in clinical studies were recently reviewed by Di Cerbo et al. (38) and Salvetti et al. (39), and they are summarized in Table 2.

Data regarding the evolutionary genomics and population structure of species harboring probiotic strains shown in Table 2 are outlined and reviewed below.

Lactobacillus acidophilus

First described by Moro in 1900, *L. acidophilus* is one of the most commonly used microorganisms for dietary applications and it is available in several foods such as milk, yogurt, formulas, as well as in dietary supplements with reported probiotic effects. The probiotics effects associated with *L. acidophilus* strains are resistance to bile and low pH, adhesion to human colonocytes in cell culture, antimicrobial production, and lactase activity, which contribute to the mediation of host immune response, lowering of serum cholesterol, improving host lactose metabolism, and preventing or treating infection (37).

The first genome sequence published was from strain NCFM (40) which led to the identification of several mucus- and fibronectin-binding proteins, implicated in the adhesion to human intestinal cells, several classes of transporters which were found to be finely regulated by carbohydrate source (induced by their respective substrates but repressed by glucose), likely contributing to the competitive ability of *L. acidophilus* in the human gastrointestinal tract, and nine two-component

TABLE 2 Species for which strains have been ascribed probiotic properties and related applications (according to references 38 and 39)[a]

Trait	*L. acidophilus*	*L. brevis*	*L. casei*	*L. crispatus*	*L. delbrueckii*	*L. fermentum*	*L. gasseri*	*L. johnsonii*	*L. paracasei*	*L. plantarum*	*L. reuteri*	*L. rhamnosus*	*L. sakei*	*L. salivarius*
Gastrointestinal mucosa adhesion	×						×				×	×		
Cancer	×											×		
Vaginal and urinary tract disorders	×	×		×		×	×			×	×	×		×
Hypercholesterolemia	×									×	×			
H. pylori treatment	×	×	×				×	×	×			×		
Oxaluria	×	×								×				
Mastitis							×	×						×
Immunomodulation	×		×			×	×		×	×	×	×	×	×
Gastrointestinal diseases	×		×	×						×				
Survival in the gut	×		×								×	×		
Diarrhea treatment	×		×	×						×	×	×		
Periodontal disease	×									×	×	×		×
Type 2 diabetes mellitus	×		×	×								×		
Muscle, bone, and cartilage diseases											×	×		
Skin disease	×							×	×		×	×	×	×
Ear, nose, and throat diseases	×		×							×				
Respiratory diseases	×		×			×				×	×	×		
Behavior/mental illness	×													
Other	×		×							×	×	×		×

[a]An × means the respective trait has been recorded in that species.

regulatory systems, some of them associated with bacteriocin production and acid tolerance (40, 37).

An updated population structure of *L. acidophilus* based on the comparative analysis of genomic sequences from 34 isolates showed that this species is monophyletic and characterized by a low rate of intraspecific diversity, with the commercial isolates identical at the genome sequence level (41). Although the phenotypic features of the isolates were diverse (i.e., the effects on the immune response following oral vaccination in healthy adults or differences in oxalate depletion), less variation is detected at the genomic level, in accordance with what was unraveled by other genotypic analyses as PCR-fingerprinting assays, randomly amplified polymorphic DNA analysis, and multilocus sequence typing (MLST). This suggests that commercial use has domesticated *L. acidophilus*, with genetically stable, invariant strains being consumed globally by the human population. A limited level of diversity is governed by the variable presence of three prophage remnants, designated as Potentially Autonomic Units (PAU, observed for the first time in *L. acidophilus* NCFM genome [40]), and a region of three contiguous loci with phage-related functions, whose distribution was linked to the isolate history, as commercial or culture collection derived. No active prophages were identified in the panel of strains, according with the absence of the recent description of phages active on *L. acidophilus* strains.

The remarkable genetic stability, supported also by the absence of extrachromosomal DNA, along with their effective phage resistance, has likely contributed to the commercial success of *L. acidophilus* strains, allowing manufacturers to maintain quality control of the cultures for probiotic production and dairy fermentations (41).

Lactobacillus brevis

L. brevis is an obligate heterofermentative Gram-positive organism that produces CO_2

as a side product from glucose metabolism. Strains of this species were isolated from plant materials, fermented beverages, and the human intestinal tract (2).

To date, all genome-based information regarding the intraspecific diversity of probiotic features in *L. brevis* mainly relates to two strains, ATCC 367 and KB290.

L. brevis ATCC 367 was the first *L. brevis* strain studied for probiotic features and its genome, sequenced in 2006 (42), revealed the presence of mucus-binding proteins and other surface layer proteins, which contribute to the adhesion to epithelial cells and extracellular matrices as fibronectin (31, 43).

The probiotic properties of strain KB290, isolated from a traditional Japanese fermented vegetable (*suguki*), include tolerance to gastrointestinal juices, immune system modulation, and gut health improvement (44, 45), and its genome sequence was reported in 2013 (46).

At the genomic level, the main difference between the two strains is the presence of nine plasmids in KB290, which constitute, to date, the highest number of plasmids ever detected among *Lactobacillus* species. The KB290 genome harbors genes for 375 unique proteins, while the ATCC 367 genome harbors genes for 169 unique traits. The majority of unique ATCC 367 genes encode for hypothetical proteins, while, among the unique genes in the KB290 genome, 177 encode proteins of known functions such as putative cell surface proteins, which might enhance the utilization of plant material, and proteins involved in the biosynthesis of cell wall-associated polysaccharides, which could contribute, on one hand, to form a protective shield against host complement factors in the gastrointestinal tract, and, on the other hand, trigger the host differential mucosal responses. The genomic regions harboring these genes in KB290 have a different DNA GC content compared to the genome average, indicating that this strain has undergone events of lateral transfer. This is also supported by the whole-genome alignment between ATCC 367 and KB290, which revealed huge rearrangements generated by homologous recombination between mobile elements, extensively distributed in both genomes.

The nine plasmids in KB290 together carry 191 predicted protein-coding genes (7% of the genome total). Although harboring plasmids constitutes a metabolic/fitness cost for host cells, no strains were found lacking all nine plasmids after plasmid curing attempts, suggesting that the plasmids impart a range of beneficial features to the host. Genes detected on the plasmids were involved in conjugation, presumptive cell wall polysaccharide biosynthesis and stress response (such as multidrug resistance transporters, which possibly confer bile resistance, or DNA protection proteins with ferritin-like domains that could enhance tolerance to oxidative stress and reduce lipid oxidation). Stress-inducible proteins contribute to the survival of probiotic bacteria in the harsh conditions they encounter in the host and they are effectively considered probiotic factors (6).

Based on the data reported by Fukao and colleagues (46), *L. brevis* is considered as a multiniche bacterium which, like other lactobacilli, contains genomic regions of laterally transferred genes; further research is needed to understand the role of *L. brevis* plasmids in the gut (46).

Lactobacillus casei/Lactobacillus paracasei

L. casei and *L. paracasei* are two phylogenetically closely related species, both members of the normal human gut microbiota, used in the food industries as starter cultures for dairy products or beneficial microbes, and reported to improve nutrition and to aid disease prevention and therapy (47).

The high genomic relatedness between these two species is the reason for the ongoing misidentification of strains belonging to *L. casei* and *L. paracasei*: according to the current valid nomenclature, the majority of the sequenced *L. casei* and *L. paracasei* strains would be allotted to *L. paracasei* subsp. *paracasei*, because all of them showed >99% identity with *L. casei* ATCC 334, which is currently the type strain of *L. paracasei* subsp. *paracasei* (48).

Given the interchangeable use of *L. casei* and *L. paracasei* names in many publications, the data presented below will refer to both species.

The evolutionary history of these species has been visualized through MLST, which showed the strains radiating into three distinct lineages (49), and comparative genomic hybridization (CGH), which revealed adaptation of these strains to cheese environment through genome decay of genes involved in carbohydrate utilization and transcriptional regulation (50).

A first comparative genomics analysis of 21 strains representative of the genetic, ecological, and geographical diversity of these species revealed a high level of synteny across the genomes and no major rearrangements (48). Strains of dairy origin had a prevalence of accessory genes with high homology (at protein level) to those detected in *L. fermentum*, another species commonly found in milk, while plant isolates showed the most diverse repertoire of genes coding orthologs with high amino acid identity to species commonly found in other plant isolates. These observations suggested the contribution of niche-associated gene exchange to the composite nature of *L. casei/L. paracasei*, also supported by the detection of a polycistronic region associated with lifestyle adaptation with high nucleotide identity with genomic regions in *L. plantarum* and *L. brevis*, and a polycistronic cluster for L(+)-tartrate catabolism and malate transport in *L. casei/L. paracasei* wine isolates with high identity with the same cluster in *L. plantarum*. Similar to other lactobacilli, horizontal gene transfer has been the dominant force in adaptation of these two species to new habitats and lifestyle in combination with the evolution of genetically distinct clusters shaped by extensive decay of genes associated with carbohydrate utilization (48).

Focusing more on probiotic factors, the analysis of the genomic intraspecific diversity of 34 other strains (dairy, plant, and human isolates) revealed the presence in the *L. casei/L. paracasei* core genome of several factors associated with host-microbe interactions such as cell-envelope proteinase, hydrolases p40 and p75, and the capacity to produce short branched-chain fatty acids (*bkd* operon), which could have an active part in the complex cross talk between bacterial strains and human or animal gut. A particular interest derived from the *bkd* operon, because the branched-chain fatty acids contribute to the preservation of the integrity of the colonic epithelium, inhibition of inflammation, and modulation of energy metabolism; the "fitness advantage" coming from this feature for the strains was provided by the generation of ATP from amino acid metabolism under anaerobic conditions in protein-rich anaerobic environments (51).

Lactobacillus crispatus

Strains belonging to *L. crispatus* have been isolated from the gastrointestinal tract of humans and animals, from the oral cavity, and, above all, from the urovaginal tract, where it counts for more than 80% of all vaginal bacteria (52). As the major component, *L. crispatus* contributes to the maintenance of the healthy vaginal microbiota, and its absence is correlated with several vaginal diseases (i.e., bacterial vaginosis). The beneficial effects described for this species include reduction of recurrent urinary tract infections and bacterial vaginosis in women and the inhibition *in vitro* of the growth, viability, and adhesion of uropathogens, suggesting a role for *L. crispatus* in protecting the vagina from invading pathogens (53, 54).

The intraspecific diversity of *L. crispatus* was investigated by mining the genome sequences of 10 strains (nine vaginal isolates

and one from chicken cecum) (55), which revealed a general collinearity and synteny interrupted only by 5 to 21 genomic islands. These regions were rich in metabolism and EPS biosynthesis genes, prophages, and adaptive immunity traits, pointing to a role for these acquired elements in the adaptation of *L. crispatus* to varying habitats. The genomic fitness related to the adaptation to the vaginal environment was also reflected in the type of CRISPR/Cas systems, which were different between the vaginal isolates and the chicken isolate, and also by the presence of genes encoding enzymatic pathways for the utilization of carbohydrates (such as mannose) available in the vagina (56).

A total of 103 proteins with adhesion- and host colonization-related domains and 30 putative S-layer protein-encoding genes were also identified, along with six strain-specific adhesins, and a sortase-anchored protein with multiple mucus-binding domains.

All the strains under investigation were found to possess genes for antimicrobial substance production, including three to four L-lactate dehydrogenase *loci*, hydrogen peroxide-encoding genes, and sets of putative bacteriocin gene clusters, including two regions coding bacteriolysins. The promotion of the vaginal health may also benefit from the presence in the core genome of components with the same mucin- and fibronectin-binding domains of their counterparts produced by vaginal pathogens such as *Gardnerella vaginalis*, thus actively interfering with the adhesion of these pathogens to the vaginal mucosa.

The comparative genomics analysis of the 10 *L. crispatus* strains provided novel information on their adaptation to the vaginal environment as well as the factors for the competitive exclusion of pathogens, this unveiling the mechanisms at the basis of the role of this species in the maintenance of vaginal health (55).

Lactobacillus delbrueckii

L. delbrueckii is one of the most used lactic acid bacteria related to dairy food production, where, among others, the subspecies *bulgaricus* has been historically applied for yogurt production in protocooperation with *Streptococcus thermophilus*, while the subspecies *lactis* has been traditionally used for cheese making (57).

Yogurt is considered a nutritious, natural, and safe component of a healthy diet and it is at the basis of probiotic concept. Up to now, yogurt is the only functional food product for which a health claim has been validated in Europe, related to the attenuation of lactose intolerance. In addition, both *L. delbrueckii* subsp. *bulgaricus* and *S. thermophilus* were found to be correlated with immune modulation and diarrhea-alleviating effects (58).

The first complete genome sequence of *L. delbrueckii* subsp. *bulgaricus* showed a high number of rRNA and tRNA genes, a signal of a phase of genome size reduction, a higher GC content at codon position 3, supporting an evolution toward high GC content genome, and the loss of superfluous amino acid biosynthesis functions, which could be correlated to the adaptation to the protein-rich milk habitat (58).

The comparative genomics analysis of three strains of *L. delbrueckii* subsp. *bulgaricus* revealed that the three genomes shared a high number of genes encoding putative proteases or peptidases, which are essential for efficient utilization of environmental proteins, along with an aminotransferase, contributing to the transfer of branched-chain amino acids into corresponding α-keto acids, which are known to have cheesy flavors. Among stress tolerance genes, which are essential for industrial fermentation adaptation, a thioredoxin system (composed by two thioredoxin reductases and two thioredoxins) was found, along with a peptide methionine sulfoxide reductase, the genes associated with cell membrane biogenesis and extracellular housekeeping proteases, which confer stability at low pH and are assumed to play an important role in *L. delbrueckii* subsp. *bulgaricus* oxygen tolerance and acid response (59).

The subsp. *lactis* is distinguished from subsp. *bulgaricus* by its more extensive carbohydrate-metabolizing capability, such as sugars of vegetal-origin like maltose, mannose, saccharose, and trehalose.

The comparative genomic analysis of 10 *L. delbrueckii* strains (5 belonging to subsp. *lactis* and 5 to subsp. *bulgaricus*) revealed that *L. delbrueckii* subsp. *bulgaricus* genomes were smaller (1,810 to 1,872 kb) than those of subsp. *lactis* strains (1,844 to 2,125 kb) (57). This difference was linked to the presence of a higher number of IS elements in subsp. *lactis* than in subsp. *bulgaricus*. The genomes of both subspecies showed an aberrant GC content at the third codon position in coding sequences (already observed for subsp. *bulgaricus*), a high number of pseudogenes, and a tendency toward elimination of genes involved in amino acid biosynthesis and carbohydrate metabolism, thus reflecting an ongoing evolution and the adaptation to a protein-rich environment. The analysis of genes related to carbohydrate metabolism revealed that, in contrast to subsp. *lactis*, subsp. *bulgaricus* can only metabolize mannose in addition to the milk sugar lactose, thus showing a more advanced adaptation to the milk medium. A key adaptation to the milk environment is the presence of the major cell wall-bound protease PrtB responsible for the first step in the degradation of milk proteins in both subspecies, while it is not found in closely related lactobacilli.

An acquired lactose-galactose antiporter to import the milk sugar lactose was another important feature in all the strains examined (which is the transport system of choice in a lactose-rich environment), while the ancestral dedicated phosphotransferase system (PTS) (which excels in conditions where the substrate concentration is low) was detected only in *L. delbrueckii* subsp. *lactis* (57). This suggests the evolution of the ancestral organism in the mammalian digestive tract, an environment where both conditions are met. This observation is also consistent with the fact that most of the known closely related lactobacilli are gut isolates and with the presence of genes coding for putative mucus-binding proteins in the majority of *L. delbrueckii* subsp. *lactis* strains under study.

Since subsp. *bulgaricus* is historically faster and more reliable in milk fermentation than the subsp. *lactis,* the similarity of their genomes indicates that the industrially relevant differences between the two subspecies are likely found in gene regulation rather than gene content (57).

Lactobacillus fermentum

L. fermentum is an obligate heterofermentative lactic acid bacterium that is usually isolated in fermented food and in the gastrointestinal tract of humans and animals.

To date, two *L. fermentum* strains are commercially available, namely CECT 5716 and ME-3, which were shown to reduce inflammation and intestinal damage *in vivo,* to improve the effects of influenza vaccination in healthy volunteers, and to have antioxidative properties (60–62).

To date, no extensive analysis of the genomic intraspecific diversity related to the probiotic traits has been performed for this species. However, interesting information can be collected from the study by Archer and colleagues (63) where, in the framework of a project aiming to study the probiotic potential of a panel of acid- and bile-tolerant strains, 12 *L. fermentum* strains (three from infant feces and nine from homemade curd) were found to harbor genes coding for a bile salt hydrolase, a fibronectin-binding protein, a mucin-binding protein, a sortase, and an ATP-binding substrate protein, which also showed 100% similarity both in fecal and dairy strains (63).

In addition, the description of four *L. fermentum* genomes (strains 3872, MTCC 8711, CECT 5716, and F-6) allowed the detection of genes coding for mucus- and collagen-binding proteins, bile salt hydrolases, and proteins involved in EPS production, likely involved in the adhesion mechanisms (64, 65).

A recent picture of the general genomic diversity of this species can be depicted by the MLST derived from 203 *L. fermentum* isolates from different regions and products, which indicated that this species had a clonal population structure and its evolutionary history is not correlated with geography or food type (66).

Lactobacillus gasseri

L. gasseri belongs to the *L. acidophilus* complex and it is usually found in several sites of the human body, such as the mouth, intestines, feces, or vagina. Strains of this species are considered as members of the human intestinal "probiome," which includes commensal intestinal bacteria with beneficial effects on human health (67).

Genome sequencing of strain ATCC 33323[T], of human origin, allowed the detection of a high number of genes coding for proteins predicted to be essential in the gastrointestinal tract, such as bile salt hydrolases, bile transporters and drug resistance traits, cell surface structures, 2CRSs and other transcriptional regulators, *luxS*, bacteriocin and restriction/modification systems and traits involved in sugar transport and metabolism, oxalate degradation (reducing the incidence of disorders related to high levels of oxalic acid in the urine), and stress resistance.

Recently, the genome sequences of four vaginal *L. gasseri* strains were compared, showing a total of 122 protein families shared by all four strains but absent in other vaginal species. Traits reflecting organismal interactions were elucidated, such as an addiction module toxin, a toxin-antitoxin addiction module regulator, and a protein of the toxin-antitoxin system AbrB family; the genomes also harbored a pediocin immunity protein, a signal transduction histidine kinase regulating citrate and malate metabolism, and strain-specific aminotransferases, transcriptional regulators, and inner permeases. The presence of unique proteins not detected in other vaginal lactobacilli suggested that this species has experienced lineage-specific gene gain and loss.

Because this comparative genomics is only based on four vaginal strains, the combined analysis of an increasing number of genome sequences of strains within the same species will help to delineate species-specific genes that influence the ecological and evolutionary dynamics of this species (68).

Lactobacillus johnsonii

L. johnsonii is a natural inhabitant of the gastrointestinal tracts of several hosts, including humans, mice, dogs, poultry, pigs, and honeybees.

The probiotic-associated activities reported for this species are, among others, pathogen inhibition in the chick gut, alleviation of diabetes symptoms, reduction of serum cholesterol levels, immunostimulation, and adhesion to intestinal epithelial cells (69)

The genome sequence of *L. johnsonii* NCC533, a human isolate extensively studied for its probiotic properties, showed that this commensal strain was deficient in biosynthesis of amino acids, purine nucleotides, and cofactors, but it harbored, in compensation, an impressive array of transporters, peptidases, and proteases, along with PTS sugar transporters and β-galactosidases, indicating a reliance on mono-, di-, and trisaccharides for its fermentative metabolism and a major adaptation in the upper gastrointestinal tract, where amino acids, peptides, and lower-order oligosaccharides are abundant. Further metabolic cassettes for saccharide metabolism, cell surface proteins, bile salt hydrolases and bile transporters were identified (69).

Phenotypic analysis and CGH analysis between this strain and the type strain of the species, *L. johnsonii* ATCC 33200[T], showed a lower intestinal persistence in ATCC 33200[T] and allowed the detection of 233 NCC533-specific genes associated with the long-gut-persistence phenotype including

surface proteins and translocases, PTS transporters, bacteriocin, and proteins involved in EPS synthesis (26).

Although an extensive comparative genomic analysis between *L. johnsonii* strains is yet to be reported, a large survey of 39 isolates from fecal-bacterial populations of a few host species was performed with the Simple Sequence Repeats assay and MLST analysis that resolved the isolates into three clusters, according to their hosts (chickens, humans, or mice) (70). These data suggest a phylogenetic separation paralleling host specificity that arose as a result of coevolution of the host and its gastrointestinal tract microbiota.

The bacterial-host specificity identified in *L. johnsonii* constitutes an interesting element to be considered for the selection of health-promoting specific strains based on the microorganisms and host genetics (70).

Lactobacillus plantarum

L. plantarum is one of the most widely known *Lactobacillus* species because of its distribution in a variety of environmental niches (many types of fermented foods, and human body), its versatility, and its metabolic capacity, which facilitates its use in several industrial settlings, either as starter cultures or probiotics. The probiotic properties related to this species are mainly linked to health promotion in humans and animals, and members of this species were found to reduce the concentration of cholesterol and fibrinogen and the risk of cardiovascular diseases and atherosclerosis (71).

L. plantarum WCFS1 was the first sequenced *Lactobacillus* genome (20). It harbored traits for stress response and gastrointestinal tract survival, substrate utilization and respiration, quorum sensing and bacteriocin production, host interaction (with the epithelial barrier as well as with the immune system), modulation of cell shape or surface properties, and interaction with food components and other microorganisms (72).

The comparative genomics analysis based on six strains showed a very high conservation of gene order and sequence identity of orthologs; however, a variety of highly variable regions were detected which mostly included (i) prophages, IS elements and transposases (highly diverse both in gene content and insertion position); (ii) the plantaricin (*L. plantarum*-associated bacteriocin) biosynthesis cluster (composed by highly conserved genes together with less conserved traits); (iii) the CPS/EPS biosynthesis genes; and (iv) the sugar lifestyle cassettes (accumulated within their lifestyle adaptation region). An additional extent of diversity was provided by the presence of numbers of repeated domains, particularly in extracellular proteins (such as adhesins or membrane-anchored protein), which play a role in the interactions between strains and their environment.

These data suggested that the genome diversity of *L. plantarum* is high and explain its flexibility and versatility, which allow this species to succeed in diverse niches and applications. In particular, the presence of genomic islands containing mosaic cassettes of (likely laterally acquired) carbohydrate-metabolism genes indicates the development of a "natural metabolic engineering approach" by *L. plantarum* strains that allows them to optimize their genomes for growth in specific niches (73).

The genome sequences of 54 *L. plantarum* strains isolated from different food sources and natural hosts (as human and insect) (74) revealed a high genetic conservation for orthologous groups involved in energy metabolism, or biosynthesis or degradation of cellular structural components, such as nucleotides, proteins, lipids; however, high variability was shown in regions including genes involved in EPS biosynthesis, restriction modification, sugar-importing PTS and other transport functions, sugar metabolism, and bacteriocin production, as well as elements like prophages, insertion sequences, and transposases. The analysis of the gene content related to the origin of the strain indicated that gene distribution poorly reflected strain origin, different from what was already observed for other lactobacilli such as *L. reuteri* and *L. rhamnosus*.

The absence of niche specialization (74) showed that *L. plantarum* did not undergo the process of bacterial adaptation to specific environments, because it acquired and retained functional capabilities independently of its niche, representing a typical example of a "nomadic" bacterial species.

Lactobacillus reuteri

L. reuteri is autochthonous to several vertebrates because members of this species are isolated from mammalian and avian gastrointestinal tracts, human urogenital tract, and breast milk. It showed several strain-specific beneficial properties relevant to human health including, for example, the production of essential B complex vitamins (folate, cobalamin, thiamin, and riboflavin) and antimicrobial compounds (i.e., reuterin); in addition, *L. reuteri* is considered a model organism for studying host-symbiont interactions as well as microbe-host coevolution. Lineage-specific genomic differences were revealed by the multilocus sequence analysis (MLSA) of more than 100 strains, reflecting the niche characteristics in the gastrointestinal tract of respective hosts. Interestingly, human-derived *L. reuteri* strains clustered in two distinct MLSA clades; one of them (namely clade II) is related specifically to humans, while strains in the other (clade VI) are closely related to isolates from chickens (75).

To gain insight into the distinguishing features of human-derived *L. reuteri* strains, comparative genomic analysis performed on 10 strains from three host origins (human, rat, and pig) unveiled two distinct populations in *L. reuteri* and, among human isolates, the same two clades (clades II and VI) observed with the MLSA. This observation led to the hypothesis that the two human-derived clades had been shaped by different evolutionary forces, since they were as dissimilar to one another as they were to clades that contained rodent- or porcine-derived strains. The two clades, in fact, were characterized by (i) the presence of clade-specific mobile genetic elements (as two complete prophages in clade II genomes and clade-specific transposase families), (ii) distinct metabolic functions and probiotic phenotypes (clade-specific order and composition of genes related to arginine catabolism mechanism and folate production); (iii) diverse rate of production of reuterin, which was enhanced in clade VI strains; (iv) the presence of clade specific of the transcriptional PocR (which gene cluster showed only 80% of identity between clade II and clade VI); (v) the differential effects on cytokine production by human myeloid cells exposed to strain supernatants; (vi) the histamine production by *L. reuteri* clade II strains that corresponded with anti-inflammatory properties.

These differences reflected the distinct ecology of these strains and the symbiotic relations they establish and maintain with their hosts. Clade II strains were all from human fecal samples and they did not cluster with isolates from other hosts, suggesting these members as part of the autochthonous *L. reuteri* population in the human intestinal tract; conversely, strains in clade VI clustered with poultry strains, and thus they might be allochthonous to humans originating from poultry.

As for the non-human isolates, the host specificity of *L. reuteri* in the mouse gut is mediated by specific adhesins and other adaptation factors including the urease cluster, an IgA protease, and genes involved in biofilm formation (76). This specificity was supported by experiments in gnotobiotic mice, which demonstrated that only rodent strains colonized mice efficiently.

These data provided new hints related to host-microbe relationship, and they also highlighted the impact of distinct evolutionary paths within the same species, which determine how microbes act on the fitness of their hosts (77).

Lactobacillus rhamnosus

L. rhamnosus is commonly found in a variety of ecological habitats, including artisanal and industrial dairy products, the oral cavity, the intestinal tract, and the vagina. This species includes the allegedly best-characterized probiotic strain, namely *L. rhamnosus* GG, which displays a wide array of probiotic properties including the reduction of diarrhea, atopic eczema, and respiratory infections (78).

Its genome sequence, released in 2006, showed the presence of genes for three secreted LPXTG-like pilins (*spaCBA*) and a pilin-dedicated sortase that is essential for mucus interaction, likely explaining its ability to persist in the human intestinal tract (79).

An extensive comparative and functional analysis based on 100 strains showed the presence of two geno-phenotypic groups (namely A and B): group A clustered strains which lack of *spaCBA* pili, a different carbohydrate metabolism profile (they could assimilate D-lactose, D-maltose, and L-rhamnose) and a distinct CRISPR system, indicative of the adaptation to a dairy-like environment; conversely, group B included strains characterized by a specific set of traits that confer more competitive fitness to the intestinal tract, such as bile resistance, pilus production, and L-fucose metabolism. Based on these data, strains of group B, which were also very similar to *L. rhamnosus* GG, are likely to be autochthonous in the gastrointestinal tract, and thus actively exert beneficial effects on it (80).

Further information derived from the comparative genomic analysis of two phylogenetically related marketed probiotic strains, *L. casei* BL23 and *L. rhamnosus* GG, unveiled a high degree of synteny, interrupted only by genomic islands with prophages, transposases, and sugar transport systems, confirming again the role of horizontal gene transfer in bacterial evolution. Shared proteins included the identical *spaCBA-srtC* gene cluster, which was also found in other *L. casei* strains. Conversely from *L. rhamnosus* strains, none of *L. casei* strains produced pili, despite the high level of conservation and sequence identity. This could be explained by the transcriptional start site of the *spaCBA* operon, which was characterized by the presence of an IS element in *L. rhamnosus* strains (but absent in *L. casei* strains) that triggers the expression of pili, conferring on *L. rhamnosus* strains a beneficial trait to colonize and persist in mucosa-associated niches (81).

A further comparative genomic analysis based on 40 strains of *L. rhamnosus* from various niches (mostly fermented foods and human-associated niches) provided a better understanding of the variome-associated genes and their distribution in terms of metabolic and regulatory diversity. Furthermore, horizontal gene transfer events were detected in some strains or clades that involved genes related to carbohydrate transport and catabolism functions, EPS biosynthesis, bacteriocin production, restriction modification systems, and bacterial defense systems (CRISP-Cas) together with other elements that reflect niche adaptation such as the diversity of extracellular functions putatively involved in host interactions (i.e., cell adhesion or host immune system modulation) (82).

Lactobacillus sakei

L. sakei is a psychotrophic lactic acid bacterium found naturally on fermented plant material, meat products, and fish. This microorganism is widely known for its biotechnological potential in biopreservation and food safety rather than probiotic properties (which were assessed for strains isolated from the human gut [83]), and it is used as a starter culture for the controlled production of fermented meats.

The analysis of the first genome sequence produced (*L. sakei* 23K) showed a combination of several features used by the organism to adapt and grow in meat products rather than in the gastrointestinal tract, such as the ability to exploit purine nucleosides, abundant in meat, for growth and energy production, and to degrade arginine when carbon sources are lacking; a versatile redox metabolism, combined with iron and heme acquisition and the capability to produce biofilm, allows this microorganism to withstand oxidative stresses and proliferate on meat surfaces (84).

A CGH approach in combination with fermentation profile analysis of 10 and, more recently, 18 strains of *L. sakei* (taking strain 23K as a reference) mainly revealed that the features observed in 23K are distributed also in the other strains of different origin, and they constitute the common gene pool invariant of this species. Interestingly, the clustering based on carbohydrate-fermentation patterns divided the panel of strains into two phenotypic groups that were not consistent with the two genetic groups that emerged with the genome hybridization. In addition, several *rrn* clusters were observed in all strains and they can be related to the ability of an organism to achieve faster doubling times, suggesting the rapid adaptation by this microorganism to changing environmental conditions. No differences were detected between the strains belonging to the two *L. sakei* subspecies, suggesting that niche-specific genes are components of *L. sakei* pangenome (83, 85).

Lactobacillus salivarius

L. salivarius is a natural resident of the oral cavity and the gastrointestinal tract of both humans and animals, and it has been also isolated from human breast milk. The probiotic properties of members of this species include the immunomodulatory effects in cell lines, mice, rats, and humans and the ability to inhibit pathogens, alleviating intestinal disease and promoting host well-being (86).

The first genome sequence available for this species was that from strain UCC118 in 2006, a strain isolated from the terminal ileum of a healthy patient that has been extensively studied for its beneficial properties both in human trials and animal models. The genome comprised a circular chromosome, a megaplasmid, and two plasmids. Genes responsible for the synthesis (*de novo* or by interconversion) of nine amino acids and exopolysaccharides were identified both on the chromosome and on the plasmids, as well as genes related to the central carbohydrate metabolism and transport, including also those of the pentose phosphate pathway. This indicated for the first time that *L. salivarius* should be grouped among the facultatively heterofermentative instead of homofermentative lactobacilli (87), a feature that was also confirmed phenotypically. In addition, the megaplasmid harbored the genes encoding a two-component class IIb bacteriocin, namely Abp118, which is protective against the invasive foodborne pathogen *Listeria monocytogenes* (88). Taken together, all these data indicated how the presence of a multireplicon genome architecture contributed to the metabolic flexibility and adaptation of *L. salivarius* UCC118 to dietary fluctuations and the varying environments encountered in the gastrointestinal tract of different hosts (89).

The genome diversity of *L. salivarius* was explored applying MLST and CGH on a collection of 33 strains derived from different ecological niches, with diverse plasmid content and phenotypic traits. The hybridization signals identified 18 regions characterized by variable traits mainly related to niche adaptation and survival, and they included transposases, bacteriophage genes, CRISPR loci, EPS biosynthesis, and carbohydrate metabolism. Interestingly, the pseudogene number was very different among the panel of strains, suggesting genome decay and an ongoing adaptation within the species. Three major clusters were observed, but they were not consistent with the isolation sources: however, most of the animal-associated isolates clustered together by hierarchical analysis of EPS cluster I and II, whose distribution in

the genomes added an additional extent of diversity among the strains (28).

Data reported by Raftis and colleagues showed that the level of diversity in *L. salivarius* was higher than that in *L. plantarum* and *L. casei*, which was also related to the limited clustering of strains from the same origins, as well as the poor correlation with complex phenotypes (as EPS production) (28).

THE CONTROVERSY IN *LACTOBACILLUS* TAXONOMY

Understanding and ascribing the beneficial effect of particular strains of lactobacilli to the species level is challenging because of the poor correlation between the phylogenetic relationship and the physiological properties of *Lactobacillus* species (13). Since its description by Beijerinck in 1901, the genus *Lactobacillus* has dramatically expanded in membership, often resulting in significant taxonomic changes, causing confusion and leading to the misidentification of lactobacilli (90).

As already mentioned, the most updated phylogenomic analysis based on 73 core proteins of 175 *Lactobacillus* species showed a high molecular diversity that is far too broad to encompass a single well-defined genus, reflected by the DNA GC content and phenotypic diversity (12).

An ongoing multilocus sequence typing and network analysis in our laboratory based on 29 ribosomal proteins and 12 established phylogenetic markers in 238 genomes of *Lactobacillus* and related genera (namely *Pediococcus, Leuconostoc, Weissella, Fructobacillus,* and *Oenococcus*) confirms that genus *Lactobacillus* is polyphyletic, intermixed with the other genera of family *Lactobacillaceae* and *Leuconostocaceae* and characterized by a complex evolutionary history (Salvetti et al., in preparation). The combination of sequence-based (phylogeny) and distance-based methods, namely, the average nucleotide identity (ANI), the average amino acid identity (AAI) and the percentage of conserved proteins (POCP), reveals the presence of 10 consistent subclades whose suitability to be nuclei of novel genera is being substantiated through the ongoing investigation of clade-specific genes and other conventional taxonomic data.

Members of these groups have been shaped by similar evolutionary events and are characterized by patterns of presence/absence of specific sets of genes that may be used as novel tools for their characterization. The absence, in fact, of a discriminative phenotypic feature supports the description of novel genera starting from the genotypic subclusters. This represents the most coherent driving force available to improve the taxonomic description of the genus and to prevent *Lactobacillus* from a never-ending expansion.

The creation of more uniform taxonomic nuclei within the *Lactobacillus* genus will also prevent misidentification issues that are still the major cause of mislabeling of probiotic food products reported worldwide (91). The determination of the genus, the species, and the strain contained in a probiotic product is the first essential requirement for a novel food marketing authorization and a health claim submission (92). Taxonomic characterization provides, in fact, information regarding the main physiological, metabolic, beneficial, and safety properties of the organism.

In addition, unravelling the taxonomic relatedness of health-promoting lactobacilli together with the analysis of the mechanisms by which they adapt to specific environments will provide a new framework for the selection of innovative beneficial microbes.

ACKNOWLEDGMENTS

This project has received funding from the European Union's Horizon 2020 research and innovation program under the Marie Skłodowska-Curie grant agreement No [659801]. Microbiome research in P.W.O'T's laboratory is supported by Science Foundation Ireland through a Centre award to the APC Microbiome Institute, and by FIRM awards to the ELDERFOOD and IMMUNOMET projects from the Dept. Agriculture, Fisheries and Marine of the Government of Ireland.

CITATION

Salvetti E, O'Toole PW. 2017. The genomic basis of lactobacilli as health-promoting organisms. Microbiol Spectrum 5(3):BAD-0011-2016.

REFERENCES

1. **Brooijmans RJ, de Vos WM, Hugenholtz J.** 2009. *Lactobacillus plantarum* WCFS1 electron transport chains. *Appl Environ Microbiol* **75:** 3580–3585.
2. **Salvetti E, Torriani S, Felis GE.** 2012. The genus *Lactobacillus*. a taxonomic update. *Probiotics Antimicrob Proteins* **4:**217–226.
3. **EFSA Panel on Biological Hazards.** 2015. Statement on the update of the list of QPS-recommended biological agents intentionally added to food or feed as notified to EFSA. 2: suitability of taxonomic units notified to EFSA until March 2015. *EFSA J* **13:**4138.
4. **Bourdichon F, Casaregola S, Farrokh C, Frisvad JC, Gerds ML, Hammes WP, Harnett J, Huys G, Laulund S, Ouwehand A, Powell IB, Prajapati JB, Seto Y, Ter Schure E, Van Boven A, Vankerckhoven V, Zgoda A, Tuijtelaars S, Hansen EB.** 2012. Food fermentations: microorganisms with technological beneficial use. *Int J Food Microbiol* **154:**87–97. (Erratum, **156:**301.)
5. **Lebeer S, Vanderleyden J, De Keersmaecker SC.** 2008. Genes and molecules of lactobacilli supporting probiotic action. *Microbiol Mol Biol Rev* **72:** 728–764.
6. **Papadimitriou K, Zoumpopoulou G, Foligné B, Alexandraki V, Kazou M, Pot B, Tsakalidou E.** 2015. Discovering probiotic microorganisms: in vitro, in vivo, genetic and omics approaches. *Front Microbiol* **6:**58.
7. **Hill C, Guarner F, Reid G, Gibson GR, Merenstein DJ, Pot B, Morelli L, Canani RB, Flint HJ, Salminen S, Calder PC, Sanders ME.** 2014. Expert consensus document. The International Scientific Association for Probiotics and Prebiotics consensus statement on the scope and appropriate use of the term probiotic. *Nat Rev Gastroenterol Hepatol* **11:**506–514.

8. **Hemarajata P, Versalovic J.** 2013. Effects of probiotics on gut microbiota: mechanisms of intestinal immunomodulation and neuromodulation. *Therap Adv Gastroenterol* **6:**39–51.

9. **EFSA Panel on Dietetic Products, Nutrition and Allergies (NDA).** 2010. Scientific opinion on the substantiation of health claims related to *Lactobacillus plantarum* 299 (DSM 6595, 67B) (ID 1078) and decreasing potentially pathogenic intestinal microorganisms pursuant to Article 13 (1) of Regulation (EC) No 1924/20061. *EFSA J* **8:**1726.

10. **EFSA Panel on Dietetic Products, Nutrition and Allergies (NDA).** 2011. Scientific opinion on the substantiation of health claims related to various foods/food constituents and "immune function/immune system" (ID 573, 586, 1374, 1566, 1628, 1778, 1793, 1817, 1829, 1939, 2155, 2485, 2486, 2859, 3521, 3774, 3896), "contribution to body defences against external agents" (ID 3635), stimulation of immunological responses (ID 1479, 2064, 2075, 3139), reduction of inflammation (ID 546, 547, 641, 2505, 2862), increase in renal water elimination (ID 2505), treatment of diseases (ID 500), and increasing numbers of gastrointestinal microorganisms (ID 762, 764, 884) pursuant to Article 13(1) of Regulation (EC) No 1924/20061. *EFSA J* **9:**2061.

11. **EFSA Panel on Dietetic Products, Nutrition and Allergies (NDA).** 2012. Scientific opinion on the substantiation of health claims related to *Lactobacillus paracasei* LPC 01 (CNCM I-1390) and treatment of disease (ID 3055, further assessment) pursuant to Article 13(1) of Regulation (EC) No 1924/20061. *EFSA J* **10:**2850.

12. **Sun Z, Harris HM, McCann A, Guo C, Argimón S, Zhang W, Yang X, Jeffery IB, Cooney JC, Kagawa TF, Liu W, Song Y, Salvetti E, Wrobel A, Rasinkangas P, Parkhill J, Rea MC, O'Sullivan O, Ritari J, Douillard FP, Paul Ross R, Yang R, Briner AE, Felis GE, de Vos WM, Barrangou R, Klaenhammer TR, Caufield PW, Cui Y, Zhang H, O'Toole PW.** 2015. Expanding the biotechnology potential of lactobacilli through comparative genomics of 213 strains and associated genera. *Nat Commun* **6:**8322.

13. **Zheng J, Ruan L, Sun M, Gänzle M.** 2015. A genomic view of lactobacilli and pediococci demonstrates that phylogeny matches ecology and physiology. *Appl Environ Microbiol* **81:**7233–7243.

14. **Kant R, Blom J, Palva A, Siezen RJ, de Vos WM.** 2011. Comparative genomics of *Lactobacillus*. *Microb Biotechnol* **4:**323–332.

15. **Morita H, Toh H, Fukuda S, Horikawa H, Oshima K, Suzuki T, Murakami M, Hisamatsu S, Kato Y, Takizawa T, Fukuoka H, Yoshimura T, Itoh K, O'Sullivan DJ, McKay LL, Ohno H, Kikuchi J, Masaoka T, Hattori M.** 2008. Comparative genome analysis of *Lactobacillus reuteri* and *Lactobacillus fermentum* reveal a genomic island for reuterin and cobalamin production. *DNA Res* **15:**151–161.

16. **Santos F, Vera JL, van der Heijden R, Valdez G, de Vos WM, Sesma F, Hugenholtz J.** 2008. The complete coenzyme B12 biosynthesis gene cluster of *Lactobacillus reuteri* CRL1098. *Microbiology* **154:**81–93.

17. **Lee IC, Tomita S, Kleerebezem M, Bron PA.** 2013. The quest for probiotic effector molecules–unraveling strain specificity at the molecular level. *Pharmacol Res* **69:**61–74.

18. **Pokusaeva K, Fitzgerald GF, van Sinderen D.** 2011. Carbohydrate metabolism in Bifidobacteria. *Genes Nutr* **6:**285–306.

19. **Xu J, Bjursell MK, Himrod J, Deng S, Carmichael LK, Chiang HC, Hooper LV, Gordon JI.** 2003. A genomic view of the human-*Bacteroides thetaiotaomicron* symbiosis. *Science* **299:**2074–2076.

20. **Kleerebezem M, Boekhorst J, van Kranenburg R, Molenaar D, Kuipers OP, Leer R, Tarchini R, Peters SA, Sandbrink HM, Fiers MW, Stiekema W, Lankhorst RM, Bron PA, Hoffer SM, Groot MN, Kerkhoven R, de Vries M, Ursing B, de Vos WM, Siezen RJ.** 2003. Complete genome sequence of *Lactobacillus plantarum* WCFS1. *Proc Natl Acad Sci USA* **100:**1990–1995.

21. **Ruas-Madiedo P, Gueimonde M, Fernández-García M, de los Reyes-Gavilán CG, Margolles A.** 2008. Mucin degradation by *Bifidobacterium* strains isolated from the human intestinal microbiota. *Appl Environ Microbiol* **74:**1936–1940.

22. **Berg J-O, Lindqvist L, Nord CE.** 1980. Purification of glycoside hydrolases from *Bacteroides fragilis*. *Appl Environ Microbiol* **40:**40–47.

23. **van Passel MW, Kant R, Zoetendal EG, Plugge CM, Derrien M, Malfatti SA, Chain PS, Woyke T, Palva A, de Vos WM, Smidt H.** 2011. The genome of *Akkermansia muciniphila*, a dedicated intestinal mucin degrader, and its use in exploring intestinal metagenomes. *PLoS One* **6:**e16876.

24. **Tailford LE, Crost EH, Kavanaugh D, Juge N.** 2015. Mucin glycan foraging in the human gut microbiome. *Front Genet* **6:**81.

25. **Fanning S, Hall LJ, Cronin M, Zomer A, MacSharry J, Goulding D, Motherway MO, Shanahan F, Nally K, Dougan G, van Sinderen**

D. 2012. Bifidobacterial surface-exopolysaccharide facilitates commensal-host interaction through immune modulation and pathogen protection. *Proc Natl Acad Sci USA* **109:**2108–2113.

26. **Denou E, Pridmore RD, Berger B, Panoff JM, Arigoni F, Brüssow H.** 2008. Identification of genes associated with the long-gut-persistence phenotype of the probiotic *Lactobacillus johnsonii* strain NCC533 using a combination of genomics and transcriptome analysis. *J Bacteriol* **190:**3161–3168.

27. **Lee IC, Caggianiello G, van Swam II, Taverne N, Meijerink M, Bron PA, Spano G, Kleerebezem M.** 2016. Strain-specific features of extracellular polysaccharides and their impact on *Lactobacillus plantarum*-host interactions. *Appl Environ Microbiol* **82:**3959–3970.

28. **Raftis EJ, Salvetti E, Torriani S, Felis GE, O'Toole PW.** 2011. Genomic diversity of *Lactobacillus salivarius. Appl Environ Microbiol* **77:**954–965.

29. **Sánchez JI, Martínez B, Guillén R, Jiménez-Díaz R, Rodríguez A.** 2006. Culture conditions determine the balance between two different exopolysaccharides produced by *Lactobacillus pentosus* LPS26. *Appl Environ Microbiol* **72:**7495–7502.

30. **Bergman M, Del Prete G, van Kooyk Y, Appelmelk B.** 2006. *Helicobacter pylori* phase variation, immune modulation and gastric autoimmunity. *Nat Rev Microbiol* **4:**151–159.

31. **Kleerebezem M, Hols P, Bernard E, Rolain T, Zhou M, Siezen RJ, Bron PA.** 2010. The extracellular biology of the lactobacilli. *FEMS Microbiol Rev* **34:**199–230.

32. **von Schillde MA, Hörmannsperger G, Weiher M, Alpert CA, Hahne H, Bäuerl C, van Huynegem K, Steidler L, Hrncir T, Pérez-Martínez G, Kuster B, Haller D.** 2012. Lactocepin secreted by *Lactobacillus* exerts anti-inflammatory effects by selectively degrading proinflammatory chemokines. *Cell Host Microbe* **11:**387–396.

33. **Bäuerl C, Pérez-Martínez G, Yan F, Polk DB, Monedero V.** 2010. Functional analysis of the p40 and p75 proteins from *Lactobacillus casei* BL23. *J Mol Microbiol Biotechnol* **19:**231–241.

34. **Dramsi S, Bierne H.** 2016. Spatial organization of cell wall-anchored proteins at the surface of Gram-positive bacteria. *Curr Top Microbiol Immunol.*

35. **Collins J, van Pijkeren JP, Svensson L, Claesson MJ, Sturme M, Li Y, Cooney JC, van Sinderen D, Walker AW, Parkhill J, Shannon O, O'Toole PW.** 2012. Fibrinogen-binding and platelet-aggregation activities of a *Lactobacillus salivarius* septicaemia isolate are mediated by a novel fibrinogen-binding protein. *Mol Microbiol* **85:**862–877.

36. **Vargas García CE, Petrova M, Claes IJ, De Boeck I, Verhoeven TL, Dilissen E, von Ossowski I, Palva A, Bullens DM, Vanderleyden J, Lebeer S.** 2015. Piliation of *Lactobacillus rhamnosus* GG promotes adhesion, phagocytosis, and cytokine modulation in macrophages. *Appl Environ Microbiol* **81:**2050–2062.

37. **Bull M, Plummer S, Marchesi J, Mahenthiralingam E.** 2013. The life history of *Lactobacillus acidophilus* as a probiotic: a tale of revisionary taxonomy, misidentification and commercial success. *FEMS Microbiol Lett* **349:**77–87.

38. **Di Cerbo A, Palmieri B, Aponte M, Morales-Medina JC, Iannitti T.** 2016. Mechanisms and therapeutic effectiveness of lactobacilli. *J Clin Pathol* **69:**187–203.

39. **Salvetti E, Torriani S, Felis GE.** 2015. A survey on established and novel strains for probiotic applications, p 26–44. *In* Foerst P, Santivarangkna C (ed), *Advances in Probiotic Technology.* CRC Press, Boca Raton, FL.

40. **Altermann E, Russell WM, Azcarate-Peril MA, Barrangou R, Buck BL, McAuliffe O, Souther N, Dobson A, Duong T, Callanan M, Lick S, Hamrick A, Cano R, Klaenhammer TR.** 2005. Complete genome sequence of the probiotic lactic acid bacterium *Lactobacillus acidophilus* NCFM. *Proc Natl Acad Sci USA* **102:**3906–3912.

41. **Bull MJ, Jolley KA, Bray JE, Aerts M, Vandamme P, Maiden MC, Marchesi JR, Mahenthiralingam E.** 2014. The domestication of the probiotic bacterium *Lactobacillus acidophilus. Sci Rep* **4:**7202.

42. **Makarova K, Slesarev A, Wolf Y, Sorokin A, Mirkin B, Koonin E, Pavlov A, Pavlova N, Karamychev V, Polouchine N, Shakhova V, Grigoriev I, Lou Y, Rohksar D, Lucas S, Huang K, Goodstein DM, Hawkins T, Plengvidhya V, Welker D, Hughes J, Goh Y, Benson A, Baldwin K, Lee JH, Díaz-Muñiz I, Dosti B, Smeianov V, Wechter W, Barabote R, Lorca G, Altermann E, Barrangou R, Ganesan B, Xie Y, Rawsthorne H, Tamir D, Parker C, Breidt F, Broadbent J, Hutkins R, O'Sullivan D, Steele J, Unlu G, Saier M, Klaenhammer T, Richardson P, Kozyavkin S, Weimer B, Mills D.** 2006. Comparative genomics of the lactic acid bacteria. *Proc Natl Acad Sci USA* **103:**15611–15616.

43. **Boekhorst J, Helmer Q, Kleerebezem M, Siezen RJ.** 2006. Comparative analysis of proteins with a mucus-binding domain found

exclusively in lactic acid bacteria. *Microbiology* 152:273–280.

44. **Yakabe T, Moore EL, Yokota S, Sui H, Nobuta Y, Fukao M, Palmer H, Yajima N.** 2009. Safety assessment of *Lactobacillus brevis* KB290 as a probiotic strain. *Food Chem Toxicol* 47:2450–2453.

45. **Murakami K, Habukawa C, Nobuta Y, Moriguchi N, Takemura T.** 2012. The effect of *Lactobacillus brevis* KB290 against irritable bowel syndrome: a placebo-controlled double-blind crossover trial. *Biopsychosoc Med* 6:16.

46. **Fukao M, Oshima K, Morita H, Toh H, Suda W, Kim SW, Suzuki S, Yakabe T, Hattori M, Yajima N.** 2013. Genomic analysis by deep sequencing of the probiotic *Lactobacillus brevis* KB290 harboring nine plasmids reveals genomic stability. *PLoS One* 8:e60521.

47. **Bao Q, Song Y, Xu H, Yu J, Zhang W, Menghe B, Zhang H, Sun Z.** 2016. Multilocus sequence typing of *Lactobacillus casei* isolates from naturally fermented foods in China and Mongolia. *J Dairy Sci* 99:5202–5213.

48. **Broadbent JR, Neeno-Eckwall EC, Stahl B, Tandee K, Cai H, Morovic W, Horvath P, Heidenreich J, Perna NT, Barrangou R, Steele JL.** 2012. Analysis of the *Lactobacillus casei* supragenome and its influence in species evolution and lifestyle adaptation. *BMC Genomics* 13:533.

49. **Cai H, Rodríguez BT, Zhang W, Broadbent JR, Steele JL.** 2007. Genotypic and phenotypic characterization of *Lactobacillus casei* strains isolated from different ecological niches suggests frequent recombination and niche specificity. *Microbiology* 153:2655–2665.

50. **Cai H, Thompson R, Budinich MF, Broadbent JR, Steele JL.** 2009. Genome sequence and comparative genome analysis of *Lactobacillus casei*: insights into their niche-associated evolution. *Genome Biol Evol* 1:239–257.

51. **Smokvina T, Wels M, Polka J, Chervaux C, Brisse S, Boekhorst J, van Hylckama Vlieg JE, Siezen RJ.** 2013. *Lactobacillus paracasei* comparative genomics: towards species pan-genome definition and exploitation of diversity. *PLoS One* 8:e68731.

52. **Ravel J, Gajer P, Abdo Z, Schneider GM, Koenig SS, McCulle SL, Karlebach S, Gorle R, Russell J, Tacket CO, Brotman RM, Davis CC, Ault K, Peralta L, Forney LJ.** 2011. Vaginal microbiome of reproductive-age women. *Proc Natl Acad Sci USA* 108(Suppl 1):4680–4687.

53. **Zárate G, Nader-Macias ME.** 2006. Influence of probiotic vaginal lactobacilli on *in vitro* adhesion of urogenital pathogens to vaginal epithelial cells. *Lett Appl Microbiol* 43:174–180.

54. **Stapleton AE, Au-Yeung M, Hooton TM, Fredricks DN, Roberts PL, Czaja CA, Yarova-Yarovaya Y, Fiedler T, Cox M, Stamm WE.** 2011. Randomized, placebo-controlled phase 2 trial of a *Lactobacillus crispatus* probiotic given intravaginally for prevention of recurrent urinary tract infection. *Clin Infect Dis* 52:1212–1217.

55. **Ojala T, Kankainen M, Castro J, Cerca N, Edelman S, Westerlund-Wikström B, Paulin L, Holm L, Auvinen P.** 2014. Comparative genomics of *Lactobacillus crispatus* suggests novel mechanisms for the competitive exclusion of *Gardnerella vaginalis*. *BMC Genomics* 15:1070.

56. **Rajan N, Cao Q, Anderson BE, Pruden DL, Sensibar J, Duncan JL, Schaeffer AJ.** 1999. Roles of glycoproteins and oligosaccharides found in human vaginal fluid in bacterial adherence. *Infect Immun* 67:5027–5032.

57. **El Kafsi H, Binesse J, Loux V, Buratti J, Boudebbouze S, Dervyn R, Kennedy S, Galleron N, Quinquis B, Batto JM, Moumen B, Maguin E, van de Guchte M.** 2014. *Lactobacillus delbrueckii* ssp. *lactis* and ssp. *bulgaricus*: a chronicle of evolution in action. *BMC Genomics* 15:407.

58. **van de Guchte M, Penaud S, Grimaldi C, Barbe V, Bryson K, Nicolas P, Robert C, Oztas S, Mangenot S, Couloux A, Loux V, Dervyn R, Bossy R, Bolotin A, Batto JM, Walunas T, Gibrat JF, Bessières P, Weissenbach J, Ehrlich SD, Maguin E.** 2006. The complete genome sequence of *Lactobacillus bulgaricus* reveals extensive and ongoing reductive evolution. *Proc Natl Acad Sci USA* 103:9274–9279.

59. **Hao P, Zheng H, Yu Y, Ding G, Gu W, Chen S, Yu Z, Ren S, Oda M, Konno T, Wang S, Li X, Ji ZS, Zhao G.** 2011. Complete sequencing and pan-genomic analysis of *Lactobacillus delbrueckii* subsp. *bulgaricus* reveal its genetic basis for industrial yogurt production. *PLoS One* 6:e15964.

60. **Mañé J, Lorén V, Pedrosa E, Ojanguren I, Xaus J, Cabré E, Domènech E, Gassull MA.** 2009. *Lactobacillus fermentum* CECT 5716 prevents and reverts intestinal damage on TNBS-induced colitis in mice. *Inflamm Bowel Dis* 15:1155–1163.

61. **Olivares M, Díaz-Ropero MP, Sierra S, Lara-Villoslada F, Fonollá J, Navas M, Rodríguez JM, Xaus J.** 2007. Oral intake of *Lactobacillus fermentum* CECT5716 enhances the effects of influenza vaccination. *Nutrition* 23:254–260.

62. **Mikelsaar M, Zilmer M.** 2009. *Lactobacillus fermentum* ME - 3-an antimicrobial and antioxidative probiotic. *Microb Ecol Health Dis* 21:1–27.

63. **Archer AC, Halami PM.** 2015. Probiotic attributes of *Lactobacillus fermentum* isolated from human feces and dairy products. *Appl Microbiol Biotechnol* **99**:8113–8123.

64. **Jiménez E, Langa S, Martín V, Arroyo R, Martín R, Fernández L, Rodríguez JM.** 2010. Complete genome sequence of *Lactobacillus fermentum* CECT 5716, a probiotic strain isolated from human milk. *J Bacteriol* **192**:4800.

65. **Sun Z, Zhang W, Bilige M, Zhang H.** 2015. Complete genome sequence of the probiotic *Lactobacillus fermentum* F-6 isolated from raw milk. *J Biotechnol* **194**:110–111.

66. **Dan T, Liu W, Song Y, Xu H, Menghe B, Zhang H, Sun Z.** 2015. The evolution and population structure of *Lactobacillus fermentum* from different naturally fermented products as determined by multilocus sequence typing (MLST). *BMC Microbiol* **15**:107. (Erratum, 2016.)

67. **Azcarate-Peril MA, Altermann E, Goh YJ, Tallon R, Sanozky-Dawes RB, Pfeiler EA, O'Flaherty S, Buck BL, Dobson A, Duong T, Miller MJ, Barrangou R, Klaenhammer TR.** 2008. Analysis of the genome sequence of *Lactobacillus gasseri* ATCC 33323 reveals the molecular basis of an autochthonous intestinal organism. *Appl Environ Microbiol* **74**:4610–4625.

68. **Mendes-Soares H, Suzuki H, Hickey RJ, Forney LJ.** 2014. Comparative functional genomics of *Lactobacillus* spp. reveals possible mechanisms for specialization of vaginal lactobacilli to their environment. *J Bacteriol* **196**:1458–1470.

69. **Pridmore RD, Berger B, Desiere F, Vilanova D, Barretto C, Pittet AC, Zwahlen MC, Rouvet M, Altermann E, Barrangou R, Mollet B, Mercenier A, Klaenhammer T, Arigoni F, Schell MA.** 2004. The genome sequence of the probiotic intestinal bacterium *Lactobacillus johnsonii* NCC 533. *Proc Natl Acad Sci USA* **101**:2512–2517.

70. **Buhnik-Rosenblau K, Matsko-Efimov V, Jung M, Shin H, Danin-Poleg Y, Kashi Y.** 2012. Indication for co-evolution of *Lactobacillus johnsonii* with its hosts. *BMC Microbiol* **12**:149.

71. **Liu CJ, Wang R, Gong FM, Liu XF, Zheng HJ, Luo YY, Li XR.** 2015. Complete genome sequences and comparative genome analysis of *Lactobacillus plantarum* strain 5-2 isolated from fermented soybean. *Genomics* **106**:404–411.

72. **van den Nieuwboer M, van Hemert S, Claassen E, de Vos WM.** 2016. *Lactobacillus plantarum* WCFS1 and its host interaction: a dozen years after the genome. *Microb Biotechnol* **9**:452–465.

73. **Siezen RJ, van Hylckama Vlieg JET.** 2011. Genomic diversity and versatility of *Lactobacillus plantarum*, a natural metabolic engineer. *Microb Cell Fact* **10**(Suppl 1):S3.

74. **Martino ME, Bayjanov JR, Caffrey BE, Wels M, Joncour P, Hughes S, Gillet B, Kleerebezem M, van Hijum SA, Leulier F.** 2016. Nomadic lifestyle of *Lactobacillus plantarum* revealed by comparative genomics of 54 strains isolated from different habitats. *Environ Microbiol* **18**:4974–4989.

75. **Oh PL, Benson AK, Peterson DA, Patil PB, Moriyama EN, Roos S, Walter J.** 2010. Diversification of the gut symbiont *Lactobacillus reuteri* as a result of host-driven evolution. *ISME J* **4**:377–387.

76. **Frese SA, Mackenzie DA, Peterson DA, Schmaltz R, Fangman T, Zhou Y, Zhang C, Benson AK, Cody LA, Mulholland F, Juge N, Walter J.** 2013. Molecular characterization of host-specific biofilm formation in a vertebrate gut symbiont. *PLoS Genet* **9**:e1004057.

77. **Spinler JK, Sontakke A, Hollister EB, Venable SF, Oh PL, Balderas MA, Saulnier DM, Mistretta TA, Devaraj S, Walter J, Versalovic J, Highlander SK.** 2014. From prediction to function using evolutionary genomics: human-specific ecotypes of *Lactobacillus reuteri* have diverse probiotic functions. *Genome Biol Evol* **6**:1772–1789.

78. **Douillard FP, Ribbera A, Xiao K, Ritari J, Rasinkangas P, Paulin L, Palva A, Hao Y, de Vos WM.** 2016. Polymorphisms, chromosomal rearrangements, and mutator phenotype development during experimental evolution of *Lactobacillus rhamnosus* GG. *Appl Environ Microbiol* **82**:3783–3792.

79. **Kankainen M, Paulin L, Tynkkynen S, von Ossowski I, Reunanen J, Partanen P, Satokari R, Vesterlund S, Hendrickx AP, Lebeer S, De Keersmaecker SC, Vanderleyden J, Hämäläinen T, Laukkanen S, Salovuori N, Ritari J, Alatalo E, Korpela R, Mattila-Sandholm T, Lassig A, Hatakka K, Kinnunen KT, Karjalainen H, Saxelin M, Laakso K, Surakka A, Palva A, Salusjärvi T, Auvinen P, de Vos WM.** 2009. Comparative genomic analysis of *Lactobacillus rhamnosus* GG reveals pili containing a human-mucus binding protein. *Proc Natl Acad Sci USA* **106**:17193–17198.

80. **Douillard FP, Ribbera A, Kant R, Pietilä TE, Järvinen HM, Messing M, Randazzo CL, Paulin L, Laine P, Ritari J, Caggia C, Lähteinen T, Brouns SJ, Satokari R, von Ossowski I, Reunanen J, Palva A, de Vos WM.** 2013. Comparative genomic and functional analysis of 100 *Lactobacillus rhamnosus* strains and their

comparison with strain GG. *PLoS Genet* **9**: e1003683.

81. **Douillard FP, Ribbera A, Järvinen HM, Kant R, Pietilä TE, Randazzo C, Paulin L, Laine PK, Caggia C, von Ossowski I, Reunanen J, Satokari R, Salminen S, Palva A, de Vos WM.** 2013. Comparative genomic and functional analysis of *Lactobacillus casei* and *Lactobacillus rhamnosus* strains marketed as probiotics. *Appl Environ Microbiol* **79**:1923–1933.

82. **Ceapa C, Davids M, Ritari J, Lambert J, Wels M, Douillard FP, Smokvina T, de Vos WM, Knol J, Kleerebezem M.** 2016. The variable regions of *Lactobacillus rhamnosus* genomes reveal the dynamic evolution of metabolic and host-adaptation repertoires. *Genome Biol Evol* **8**:1889–1905.

83. **Nyquist OL, McLeod A, Brede DA, Snipen L, Aakra Å, Nes IF.** 2011. Comparative genomics of *Lactobacillus sakei* with emphasis on strains from meat. *Mol Genet Genomics* **285**: 297–311.

84. **Chaillou S, Champomier-Vergès MC, Cornet M, Crutz-Le Coq AM, Dudez AM, Martin V, Beaufils S, Darbon-Rongère E, Bossy R, Loux V, Zagorec M.** 2005. The complete genome sequence of the meat-borne lactic acid bacterium *Lactobacillus sakei* 23K. *Nat Biotechnol* **23**:1527–1533.

85. **McLeod A, Nyquist OL, Snipen L, Naterstad K, Axelsson L.** 2008. Diversity of *Lactobacillus sakei* strains investigated by phenotypic and genotypic methods. *Syst Appl Microbiol* **31**: 393–403.

86. **Neville BA, O'Toole PW.** 2010. Probiotic properties of *Lactobacillus salivarius* and closely related *Lactobacillus* species. *Future Microbiol* **5**:759–774.

87. **Li Y, Raftis E, Canchaya C, Fitzgerald GF, van Sinderen D, O'Toole PW.** 2006. Polyphasic analysis indicates that *Lactobacillus salivarius* subsp. *salivarius* and *Lactobacillus salivarius* subsp. *salicinius* do not merit separate subspecies status. *Int J Syst Evol Microbiol* **56**:2397–2403.

88. **Corr SC, Li Y, Riedel CU, O'Toole PW, Hill C, Gahan CG.** 2007. Bacteriocin production as a mechanism for the antiinfective activity of *Lactobacillus salivarius* UCC118. *Proc Natl Acad Sci USA* **104**:7617–7621.

89. **Claesson MJ, Li Y, Leahy S, Canchaya C, van Pijkeren JP, Cerdeño-Tárraga AM, Parkhill J, Flynn S, O'Sullivan GC, Collins JK, Higgins D, Shanahan F, Fitzgerald GF, van Sinderen D, O'Toole PW.** 2006. Multireplicon genome architecture of *Lactobacillus salivarius*. *Proc Natl Acad Sci USA* **103**:6718–6723.

90. **Pot B, Felis GE, De Bruyne K, Tsakalidou E, Papadimitriou K, Leisner J, Vandamme P.** 2014. The genus Lactobacillus, p 249–353. *In* Holzapfel WH, Wood EJB (ed). *Lactic Acid Bacteria: Biodiversity and Taxonomy*. John Wiley & Sons, Hoboken, NJ.

91. **van Loveren H, Sanz Y, Salminen S.** 2012. Health claims in Europe: probiotics and prebiotics as case examples. *Annu Rev Food Sci Technol* **3**:247–261.

92. **EFSA Panel on Dietetic Products, Nutrition and Allergies (NDA).** 2016. General scientific guidance for stakeholders on health and claim applications. *EFSA J* **14**:4367.

93. **Bron PA, Grangette C, Mercenier A, de Vos WM, Kleerebezem M.** 2004. Identification of *Lactobacillus plantarum* genes that are induced in the gastrointestinal tract of mice. *J Bacteriol* **186**:5721–5729.

94. **Fang F, Li Y, Bumann M, Raftis EJ, Casey PG, Cooney JC, Walsh MA, O'Toole PW.** 2009. Allelic variation of bile salt hydrolase genes in *Lactobacillus salivarius* does not determine bile resistance levels. *J Bacteriol* **191**:5743–5757.

95. **Voltan S, Castagliuolo I, Elli M, Longo S, Brun P, D'Incà R, Porzionato A, Macchi V, Palù G, Sturniolo GC, Morelli L, Martines D.** 2007. Aggregating phenotype in *Lactobacillus crispatus* determines intestinal colonization and TLR2 and TLR4 modulation in murine colonic mucosa. *Clin Vaccine Immunol* **14**:1138–1148.

96. **Nishiyama K, Nakazato A, Ueno S, Seto Y, Kakuda T, Takai S, Yamamoto Y, Mukai T.** 2015. Cell surface-associated aggregation-promoting factor from *Lactobacillus gasseri* SBT2055 facilitates host colonization and competitive exclusion of *Campylobacter jejuni*. *Mol Microbiol* **98**:712–726.

97. **Vélez MP, De Keersmaecker SC, Vanderleyden J.** 2007. Adherence factors of *Lactobacillus* in the human gastrointestinal tract. *FEMS Microbiol Lett* **276**:140–148.

98. **Yan F, Cao H, Cover TL, Whitehead R, Washington MK, Polk DB.** 2007. Soluble proteins produced by probiotic bacteria regulate intestinal epithelial cell survival and growth. *Gastroenterology* **132**:562–575.

99. **Seth A, Yan F, Polk DB, Rao RK.** 2008. Probiotics ameliorate the hydrogen peroxide-induced epithelial barrier disruption by a PKC- and MAP kinase-dependent mechanism. *Am J Physiol Gastrointest Liver Physiol* **294**: G1060–G1069.

100. **Konstantinov SR, Smidt H, de Vos WM, Bruijns SC, Singh SK, Valence F, Molle D,**

Lortal S, Altermann E, Klaenhammer TR, van Kooyk Y. 2008. S layer protein A of *Lactobacillus acidophilus* NCFM regulates immature dendritic cell and T cell functions. *Proc Natl Acad Sci USA* **105:**19474–19479.

101. **Gao C, Major A, Rendon D, Lugo M, Jackson V, Shi Z, Mori-Akiyama Y, Versalovic J.** 2015. Histamine H2 receptor-mediated suppression of intestinal inflammation by probiotic *Lactobacillus reuteri*. *MBio* **6:**e01358-15.

102. **Kristensen NB, Bryrup T, Allin KH, Nielsen T, Hansen TH, Pedersen O.** 2016. Alterations in fecal microbiota composition by probiotic supplementation in healthy adults: a systematic review of randomized controlled trials. *Genome Med* **8:**52.

Bifidobacteria and Their Health-Promoting Effects

3

CLAUDIO HIDALGO-CANTABRANA,[1] SUSANA DELGADO,[1]
LORENA RUIZ,[1] PATRICIA RUAS-MADIEDO,[1]
BORJA SÁNCHEZ,[1] and ABELARDO MARGOLLES[1]

THE *BIFIDOBACTERIUM* GENUS

The genus *Bifidobacterium* is included within the phylum *Actinobacteria*, class *Actinobacteria* (high G+C Gram-positive bacteria), order *Bifidobacteriales*, and family *Bifidobacteriaceae*. Currently, this genus contains more than 50 species, including several subspecies; this number rises every year. From a metabolic point of view, the more typical trait of this genus is the catabolism of monosaccharides. Bifidobacteria use a particular route for monosaccharide degradation, the so-called fructose 6-phosphate pathway, or bifid shunt. The fructose 6-phosphate phosphoketolase (Xfp) is the main enzyme of this path. Xfp possesses a dual-substrate specificity on fructose 6-phosphate or xylulose 5-phosphate. The end metabolites of the pathway are acetate, lactate, and ethanol (1). Xfp activity on fructose 6-phosphate is the most common phenotypic test for bifidobacteria, and for many years it has been the main taxonomic test to identify this genus, since this activity is present in members of the family *Bifidobacteriaceae*, but it is not present in other Gram-positive

[1]Department of Microbiology and Biochemistry of Dairy Products, Dairy Research Institute of Asturias, Spanish National Research Council (IPLA-CSIC), Paseo Río Linares s/n 33300, Villaviciosa, Asturias, Spain

Bugs as Drugs: Therapeutic Microbes for the Prevention and Treatment of Disease
Edited by Robert A. Britton and Patrice D. Cani
© 2018 American Society for Microbiology, Washington, DC
doi:10.1128/microbiolspec.BAD-0010-2016

intestinal bacteria. However, currently, DNA-sequencing-based analyses are the standard techniques for identification and typing of bifidobacteria.

The species belonging to the genus *Bifidobacterium* share high rRNA 16S sequence similarity, constituting a coherent phylogenetic unit. During the past few years, genome sequencing has contributed significantly to clarify the phylogenetic relationships among the different *Bifidobacterium* species. In 2002, the first bifidobacterial genome, from a strain of *Bifidobacterium longum*, was published (2). Since then, the number of publicly available bifidobacterial genomes has steadily increased, with more than 50 complete genome sequences available nowadays. In this regard, comparative genomics of the different species has shed light on the phylogeny and the evolutionary adaptation of this genus (3, 4). A recent phylogenetic analysis of bifidobacteria, based on a robust reconstruction of the phylogeny of members of this genus based on 48 genome sequences, has shown that there are seven phylogenetic groups within the genus: *Bifidobacterium adolescentis* group, *Bifidobacterium asteroides* group, *Bifidobacterium boum* group, *Bifidobacterium longum* group, *Bifidobacterium bifidum* group, *Bifidobacterium pseudolongum* group, and *Bifidobacterium pullorum* group (3). These groups partially correlate with the ecological niches from which the representative species were isolated, members of the *B. asteroides* group being the common inhabitants of the microbiota of insects, and those of the *B. pullorum* group being characteristic of birds. In relation to this, members of the *B. pseudolongum* group (especially *Bifidobacterium animalis* subsp. *lactis* strains), *B. longum* group (*Bifidobacterium breve* and *B. longum* strains), *B. bifidum* group (*B. bifidum* strains), and *B. adolescentis* group (*Bi®dobacterium catenulatum*, *Bifidobacterium pseudocatenulatum*, and *B. adolescentis* strains) are often found in the human intestinal microbiota, and most probiotic bifidobacteria belong to these species.

BIFIDOBACTERIA AS MEMBERS OF THE HUMAN INTESTINAL MICROBIOTA

Bifidobacterium Species Evolution with Age, Distribution in the Bowel, and Interindividual Variability

Bifidobacteria are among the dominant bacterial populations in the gastrointestinal tract (GIT) of humans. Among the bifidobacterial species described so far, *B. catenulatum*, *B. pseudocatenulatum*, *B. adolescentis*, *B. longum*, *B. breve*, *B. bifidum*, *B. animalis*, and *Bifidobacterium dentium* are commonly detected in feces of healthy subjects (5, 6). The last two species are not rigorously considered to be autochthonous to the human bowel, being detected in fecal samples but not in mucosa-associated samples. In fact, *B. animalis* subsp. *lactis* is frequently applied in probiotic dairy products and food supplements, and its presence in feces possibly reflects a dietary origin. However, *B. dentium* has been described as residing mainly in the human oral cavity, and several studies link this species to the development of caries (7, 8).

Although bifidobacterial intersubject variability clearly exists, it seems that there are differences between fecal- and mucosa-associated *Bifidobacterium* species, with *B. longum* and *B. pseudocatenulatum* typically being isolated from both mucosa and fecal samples and *B. bifidum* being more related to feces (5, 6). In contrast, a modest diversification of bifidobacterial populations was observed between different intestinal regions within the same individual (6).

Studies of the biodiversity of the human mucosa-associated bifidobacteria by culture-independent techniques have revealed no previously identified bifidobacterial sequences that may represent novel bifidobacterial species (9). By using different approaches and techniques, it has been observed that bifidobacteria numbers and diversity decrease with age, although the fact that particular bifidobacterial types are more related with the elderly still remains obscure (10–12). That bifidobacteria achieve large concentrations during the first few months after birth is more clearly established, as explained in detail below. After weaning, bifidobacterial numbers gradually decrease and other members of the gut microbiota like *Bacteroides* and *Eubacterium* become predominant. Although it has been estimated that the bifidobacterial load in adults is close to 4% of the total fecal microbiota (13), experimental biases in PCR-based culture-independent techniques may be accounting for this modest contribution. A recent work in Japan reported higher abundancies of bifidobacteria for Japanese people (14).

Bifidobacteria Acquisition and Development in Infancy

Although bifidobacteria can be detected in the feces of adults, they form a relatively small proportion of the total bacterial community. However, they are numerous in the feces during the first year of life and are among the pioneers of the bacterial succession that occurs in the large bowel of babies when the gut microbiota begins to be established. Indeed, bifidobacteria are numerically dominant members of the intestinal microbial communities by the age of 3 to 4 months (15, 16). Bifidobacterial members are probably enriched in the bowel of the suckling infants because of the variety of oligosaccharides present in human milk. Additionally, human milk is a source of living bifidobacteria for the infant gut (17, 18). In fact it has been reported that breast-fed infants generally harbor a more complex and numerous *Bifidobacterium* microbiota than formula-fed infants (19, 20). Human colostrum and milk contain high concentrations of human milk oligosaccharides (HMOs). Some of these are recalcitrant to digestion by the infant and thus pass to the large bowel where they can be foraged by gut bacteria. HMOs are structurally diverse and composed of several monosaccharides (glucose, galactose, *N*-acetylglucosamine, fucose, or sialic acid), and

they mainly consist of a lactose core linked to units (n = 0 to 15) of lacto-*N*-biose (type I) or to *N*-acetyl-lactosamine (type II) (21). Bifidobacteria are among the best described gut bacteria with ability to utilize HMOs. Several species possess glycosyl hydrolases that cleave specific linkages within the HMO molecules, the best characterized being those synthesized by *B. bifidum*, which, together with *B. longum* subsp. *infantis* and *B. breve* are the most abundant species in breast-fed neonates (15, 22). Thus the ability of these species to utilize these otherwise indigestible carbohydrates explains their abundance in the breast-fed infant.

Genomic data suggest that bifidobacteria may possess particular adaptation traits to explain this ecological specialization. For example, genome analysis of *B. longum* subsp. *infantis* ATCC15697 has shown that it is an archetypical human milk-utilizing bacterium, because its genome features genes encoding enzymes involved in the breakdown of HMOs (23). *B. bifidum* is predicted to possess lacto-*N*-biosidase activity, which allows an efficient catabolism of HMOs (24). These two species are specialized toward HMO utilization, although they compete for HMOs using different strategies; *B. bifidum* has an array of several membrane-associated glycosyl hydrolases, whereas *B. longum* subsp. *infantis* is more efficient in the import and intracellular breakdown of HMOs (25). Indeed, it seems that strains from the latter species seem to have a similar HMO utilization pattern, while *B. bifidum* strains are more diverse, and some of them are not able to use fucosylated or sialylated HMOs (26). Similarly, the HMO utilization profile of *B. breve* is also variable depending on the strain, but contrary to *B. bifidum*, some strains consume HMOs decorated with fucosyl or sialic acid residues. In any case, the capability of *B. breve* to use these milk oligosaccharides also explains its high presence in the feces of breast-fed babies (27).

In contrast, the genomes of enteric bifidobacteria residing in the intestine of adult humans, such as *B. adolescentis*, do not appear to harbor genes related to the utilization of human milk components, and, instead, they contain a large arsenal of genes dedicated to the metabolism of complex carbohydrates commonly found in the adult-type diet (e.g., starch and starch-derived carbohydrates) (28–31). Until now there have been no clear relationships between type of diet (Western, Asian, Mediterranean) and the enrichment in the gut of particular *Bifidobacterium* species, but differences have been reported between different human groups and countries (14, 32).

A recent bifidobacterial diversity study based on sequence analysis of PCR amplicons of the 16S rRNA gene from infant stools from different geographical origins reinforced the notion of bifidobacteria as being a predominant component of the infant gut microbiota, which may undoubtedly influence the development of the immune system and physiology of the infant (33).

Correlations with Other Members of the Microbiota and Cross Talk Interactions

Bifidobacterium-mediated health benefits are the result of a complex dynamic interplay established among bifidobacteria, other members of the gut microbiota, and the human host. These intricate correlation patterns have not yet been fully deciphered at a molecular level; thus, efforts are currently being pursued to understand the metabolic fluxes within the gut ecosystem discerning the microbiota-host cross talk in health and disease. This will establish the basis for host health modulation through microbiome-targeted approaches, in a more precise, secure, and controlled manner (34).

Some of the first evidence of bifidobacterial capability to interact with other gut bacteria was reported in works pointing toward the existence of a correlation between reduced bifidobacterial presence within the gastrointestinal tract and the overrepresentation of enteropathogens and disease risk

(35, 36). Accordingly, among the bifidobacterial proposed benefits, inhibition of enteropathogens and reduction of rotavirus infection (37) are some of their best established outcomes. Numerous *in vitro* studies have demonstrated that bifidobacteria can inhibit pathogens through the production of organic acids (38), antibacterial peptides (39), quorum-sensing inhibitors (40, 41), or immune stimulation (42) among other mechanisms, providing molecular clues of their capacity to prevent certain infections.

Another fact pointing toward the existence of a critical bifidobacteria-gut microbiota-host cross talk has been provided by the observation that microbiota establishment in early infancy seems to follow an orchestrated and organized pattern of bacterial populations succession (43, 44). The first gut colonizers, among which bifidobacteria represent a dominant group, contribute to reduce the environment and produce metabolites that enable other bacterial populations to stably colonize the gut later on (45). This supports the idea that strong bacterial correlations shape the gut microbiota establishment, stabilization, and evolution (44). Indeed, the fact that HMOs are preferentially metabolized by *B. longum* and *B. bifidum* species, which are the most abundant in the breast-fed infant gut microbiota, supports the existence of critical molecular interaction microbiota-host-dietary components, conditioning bifidobacterial presence in the intestine (46). Furthermore, it is worth mentioning that significant mutualistic effects have been described between bifidobacteria and other intestinal bacteria. In this regard, using colonized germ-free mouse models, it has been shown that *Bacteroides thetaiotaomicron* is able to expand its capacity to utilize polysaccharides in the presence of *B. longum*, suggesting that resident gut symbionts are able to adapt their substrate utilization in response to bifidobacteria (47).

The microbial populations within the gut microbiota coexist in a delicate balance that can be affected by perturbations such as those imposed by antibiotic treatments, enteropathogen challenges, or dietary compounds, e.g., nondigestible carbohydrates (48). Although these perturbations affect the gut microbiota and can have negative consequences on host health, their dependence on environmental factors offers the possibility of modulating gut microbiota composition through various approaches. *In vitro* and *in vivo* studies have shown that modulating bifidobacterial levels through probiotic or prebiotic supplementation can change the overall composition and metabolism of the gut microbiota (49–53). For instance, supplementation with a *B. longum* strain augmented production of pymelate, butyrate, and biotin in a human-gut-derived microbiota mouse model (53). These effects were suggested to be mediated through yet to be deciphered cross talk mechanisms with the human-gut-derived microbiota. However, based on the evidence provided, the authors of this work hypothesized that the increase in biotin production was due to the coexistence of *B. longum* and *Bacteroides caccae*. Moreover, *B. longum* supplementation also correlated with the reduced presence of *Enterobacteriaceae* (54) and augmented representation of *Eubacterium rectale*, supporting a bifidobacterial effect on quantity and functionality of other gut microbiota members (53).

Bifidobacterial molecules, such as the exopolysaccharides present in the outer cell-surface layer, have been proven to be capable of modulating gut microbiota in *in vitro* fecal batch cultures (55) and *in vivo* mice trials (56), thus providing a molecular basis for gut microbiota-bifidobacteria cross talk. In fact, *in vitro* studies have shown that *Bacteroides fragilis* and *Faecalibacterium prausnitzii* modify their metabolism upon growth in the presence of bifidobacterial exopolysaccharides (57–59).

On the other hand, numerous studies have demonstrated the capability of prebiotics to promote bifidobacterial presence within the microbiota, correlating with other changes in the overall microbiota composition and metabolism. Thus, bifidobacterial promotion through prebiotics, including inulin, arabinoxylans, galactooligosaccharides, and fructooligosaccharides, also correlated with greater *Lactobacillus-Bifidobacterium* to *Enterobacteriaceae* ratio, and modulated short-chain fatty acid production (52, 60–62). In fact, most *in vitro* and *in vivo* evidence on bifidobacteria cross talk with other gut microbiota members has been obtained through analysis of prebiotic metabolism. Cross-feeding mechanisms between *B. longum* NCC2705 and *E. rectale* ATCC 33656 were found to be the basis of the bifidogenic and butyrogenic effects of arabinoxylan oligosaccharides (63). Similarly, recent works have provided evidence to understand the cross-feeding mechanisms between *Bifidobacterium* and *Bacteroides* species (59, 64) and *Bifidobacterium* and *F. prausnitzii* (58), respectively, which would help understand butyrogenic activity of coculture fermentations (65). These results also contribute to clarify bacterial interactions within the gut during prebiotic fermentations.

Some other works have also studied the potential cross talk mechanisms between bifidobacterial strains. Ruiz and colleagues analyzed through a proteomic approach the interaction between a *B. longum* and a *B. breve* strain (66), evidencing a significant effect on the production of carbohydrate utilization enzymes. Indeed, a more recent work proved the existence of cross-feeding mechanisms between *B. bifidum* PRL2010, a strain specialized in extracellular breakdown of HMOs, and *B. breve* UCC2003 (67). This latter strain is unable to utilize sialic acid as the sole carbon source *in vitro*, although it can grow at the expense of the residues that *B. bifidum* PRL2010 cleaves from mucins (67). In fact, a detailed analysis on glycoside utilization capabilities within the genus *Bifidobacterium* highlighted that particular species are specialized toward the utilization of specific carbohydrates, therefore suggesting that bifidobacterial species might cooperate for carbohydrate utilization within the gut (48). These facts support the use of mixtures of probiotic strains, which might provide a synergistic effect, improving their capability to exert the desired effects on the gut microbiota and, concomitantly, on host health (68).

It is also worth highlighting that some bifidobacterial colonization traits are modulated by intestinal factors, including the presence of other microorganisms. For instance, Yuan and colleagues (69) found, using an *in vivo* model, that exposure to intestinal environment induces production of a series of proteins which are not expressed upon growth *in vitro* in *B. longum*, like the chologlycine hydrolase. Furthermore, transcription of the bifidobacterial gene clusters required for exopolysaccharide production, a molecule essential for its intestinal colonization ability (42), is strongly upregulated by intestinal factors, as evidenced following growth on fecal-based media (70). Similar observations were made regarding the bifidobacterial pilae structures. The Tad pilus-encoding cluster, which was reported to be essential for *B. breve* UCC2003 colonization of the mouse intestine, was only expressed in the mouse intestine, but not when grown under laboratory conditions (71). Whereas the specific triggering factors of these bifidobacterial traits remain to be determined, it is reasonable to hypothesize that microbial-derived molecules or metabolites, through yet to be deciphered cross talk mechanisms, may be key signaling factors. In fact, in *B. bifidum* PRL2010, pilus expression occurred *in vitro*, but it was strongly upregulated following co-culture with other bifidobacterial and *Lactobacillus* strains (72).

Further evidence of the existence of a bifidobacterial-gut microbiota cross talk has been provided by the fact that individuals with different gut microbiota composition appear to respond differently to *Bifidobacterium* supplementation (73). Although the molecular mechanisms of the cross talk behind this different behavior are far from being understood yet, their comprehension would greatly help to design probiotic-based therapies that can be functional even in those subpopulations currently classified as "nonresponders" on clinical trials (74).

BIFIDOBACTERIA AS PROBIOTICS

In a healthy state of intestinal "eubiosis" there is a population of naturally occurring microbiota that helps to keep our homeostasis by maintaining or adjusting physiological processes to counteract changes. The equilibrium can be broken when internal or external factors alter this microbial community, leading to a state of "dysbiosis," often resulting in a health problem (75). A clear example of an imbalance in the intestinal microbiota is the consequence of the use of antibiotics to treat infections, which are needed to eradicate pathogens, but they also disrupt the symbionts, both mutualists and commensals, inhabiting our gut (76). This fact, together with the increased resistance to antibiotics reported in recent years, leads to the interest in the application of beneficial microorganisms, or probiotics, to help in the recovery of infections through the restoration of the intestinal homeostasis. The first international consensus definition of probiotics was proposed in 2001 by a group of experts, joined by the Food and Agriculture Organization (FAO) and World Health Organization (WHO) (77); it has been recently accepted, with a minor grammatical correction by a Scientific Committee of the International Scientific Association for Probiotics and Prebiotics (ISAAP) (78) as follows: "live microorganisms that, when administered in adequate amounts, confer a health benefit on the host."

The first observations about the occurrence of certain bacteria in "normal" feces in relation to the intestinal physiology and health were established at the beginning of the last century. In 1900, the pediatrician H. Tissier found anaerobic bacteria, with a bifurcated ("bifid") shape, that were abundant in the feces of breast-fed babies and he named them *Bacillus bifidus*; afterward, he proposed the use of this bacterium for the treatment of intestinal infections (79). In the same decade, E. More reported the presence of an acid-tolerant, pleomorphic bacterium, which he named *Bacillus acidophilus*, inhabiting the intestine of infants who subsist entirely on mother's milk (80). Both authors disputed the first assertion that these bacteria constitute the dominant "flora" of the breast-fed infant (81). Simultaneously, at the beginning of the 1900s, E. Metchnikoff postulated that the long life expectancy of Bulgarian peasants was due to the higher consumption of fermented dairy products. These early observations could be considered as the starting point to link the possible benefits of intestinal bacteria and certain foods to human health; later on, after a long evolution of the definition of probiotic based on scientific research (collected in reference 82), the scientific community reached the consensus definition indicated above, which is nowadays widely accepted.

Currently, the genera most commonly used as probiotics to maintain a healthy intestinal function in humans are *Lactobacillus* and *Bifidobacterium*. Some specific species of bifidobacteria, as well as of lactobacilli, have the GRAS (Generally Recognized As Safe) status, given by the FDA. In addition, some of them, based on a long history of safe consumption in different foods, have obtained the QPS (Qualified Presumption of Safety) mark, given by the European Food Safety Authority (EFSA); the last revision of the QPS list maintains the species *B. adolescentis*, *B. animalis*, *B. bifidum*, *B. breve*, and *B. longum* as safe biological agents intentionally added to food or feed (83). However, the probiotic efficacy of bifidobacteria showing positive effects on gastrointestinal functions after human intervention trials has only been studied for a few strains, normally supported by multinational food companies, most of them belonging to the species *B. animalis* subsp. *lactis*, *B. breve*, *B. longum*, and *B. bifidum* (75). In many cases, there is insufficient scientific evidence to support the positive effects reported for the strains, since clear biomarkers for bifidobacterial efficacy are, as yet, not identified (Fig. 1). This is the case of some studies reporting an improvement or alleviation of symptoms related to different inflammatory bowel diseases, such as ulcerative colitis (84, 85) or irritable bowel syndrome (86, 87). In addition, most bifidobacterial strains were tested in combination with other microorganisms, typically lactic acid bacteria (LAB), or with prebiotic carbohydrates, making it difficult to prove the probiotic effect of a single strain (88). Also, the vehicle used for probiotic delivery could play

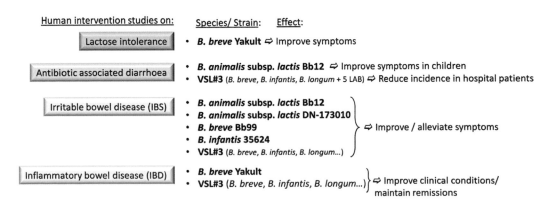

FIGURE 1 Positive effects of some *Bifidobacterium* strains on gastrointestinal functions studied by means of human intervention studies.

a relevant role. In this regard, it has been demonstrated, *in vivo*, that *B. animalis* subsp. *lactis* HN019 changes its effect on the (mice) host when the strain is given in a fermented dairy format in comparison with the unfermented milk (89).

The driving force of the global probiotic market was conducted by dairy companies to launch now well-known products during the past 20 years (90), although other non-dairy-based products have been introduced in the market as well (91). Dairy products, and specifically fermented milks and yogurts, constitute a good matrix for the delivery of bifidobacteria (92). Although (cow) milk is a rich source of nutrients for microbial growth, these are not always bioavailable; in the case of bifidobacteria, some amino acids could be limiting because of the weak proteolytic activity reported for this genus (93), thus limiting the growth in milk and milk-based matrices used to manufacture dairy products. In spite of this, it has been reported that some strains are able to grow in milk and dairy products (94–95); even more, *B. bifidum*, when growing in kefir, increased the expression of genes involved in the host-bacteria interaction, such as pili, thus helping the persistence of the bifidobacteria later on in the gut (96). Besides, it is worth mentioning that breast milk is the most suitable medium to support a high population of bifidobacteria, probably because of the high concentration of human milk oligosaccharides (26). Nevertheless, the dairy matrix is a good environment to improve bifidobacterial survival in food, allowing the delivery of the probiotic in a metabolically active state (97). The preparation of bifidobacterial suspensions in skimmed milk increased significantly their viability under simulated gastrointestinal transit with human stomach and duodenal fluids (98). The protein network of caseins could act as a protectant for the bacteria during the gastrointestinal transit. In this regard, we have visualized, by confocal scanning laser microscopy, strains of *B. animalis* subsp. *lactis* growing inside the pores

enclosed by the casein network formed after fermentation by the bifidobacteria (Fig. 2). In comparison with milk, the use of fermented products containing dairy starters together with bifidobacteria could also lead to an increase in the functional benefit of probiotic foods (89, 99). As an example, the milk fermented by *B. bifidum* MF 20/5 has a strong angiotensin-converting enzyme (ACE) inhibitory activity due to the release of a novel ACE-inhibitory peptide (LVYPFP) from milk protein, thus giving an added functional property to the fermented product (100).

Finally, as previously stated, scientific evidence proving the efficacy of bifidobacteria has been obtained for a few strains/species; given that the beneficial effect, survival, and capability of colonization or persistence in the colon are highly dependent on the strain, the correct identification of the species/strains included in any type of food or food formulation is of pivotal relevance, and is still an issue that must be resolved in the probiotic market. Indeed, in a recent study performed with 16 probiotic products, using DNA-based methods as well as culturing techniques, only one matched its bifidobacterial label; thus, most of them differ from the ingredient list (101). Therefore, to keep the confidence of patients and consumers in probiotic products intended for use in clinical applications, or for specific human populations, more effort must be made in the correct labeling of the strains used to support the proposed claims (77).

BIFIDOBACTERIA FOR PREVENTION AND TREATMENT OF DISEASE

Scientific and medical communities are becoming more conscious about the impact of the composition of the intestinal microbiota in human health. In this sense, there are several publications demonstrating how some imbalanced microbiota populations, or particular dysbiosis, are related to a wide variety of illnesses and abnormal physiolog-

(A) Z-projection of XY field   **(B)** XY field   **(C)** XY-field optical zoom

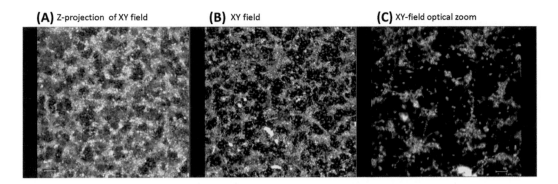

FIGURE 2 Visualization of *B. animalis* subsp. *lactis* growth in skimmed milk by using confocal scanner laser microcopy. The staining method was previously reported by Ruas-Madiedo and Zoon (167); in short, two dyes, rhodamine B (which dyes proteins) and acridine orange (which dyes nucleic acids), were added to the milk at final concentration of 0.001 and 0.002%, respectively. Afterward, stained milk was inoculated (5%) and carefully placed into high-optical-quality plastic μ-Slides (Ibidi GmbH) for direct confocal laser scanning microscopy analysis. The microplates were incubated at 37°C until they reached a pH of ≤4.5, and the confocal microscope Ultra-Spectral Leica TCS AOBS SP2 (Leica Microsystems GmbH, located in the University of Oviedo facilities) was used. Bacteria dyed with acridine orange were visualized with the laser 488 nm ion argon/krypton (green), and proteins (mainly caseins) dyed with rhodamine B were visualized with the laser 543 nm He/Ne (red) but also with the laser 488 nm. Thus, after image treatment, the bacteria are visualized in green and the casein matrix in yellow (combination red and green). The oil immersion objective 63×/1.40 combined with an amplification zoom of 1.58 was directly used (×100 magnification). Microphotographs: (A) a Z-projection (thickness about 10 μm) of 10 slides of an XY-field (bar, 10 μm); (B) a slide of an XY-field (bar, 10 μm); (C) an optical zoom of a region inside the XY-field showed in B (bar, 5 μm).

ical situations, including those associated with intestinal and immunological disorders like allergy, irritable bowel syndrome, inflammatory bowel disease, obesity, metabolic syndrome, systemic lupus erythematosus, etc. (102). Interestingly, alterations in the commensal gut microbiota appear to also be related to some diseases progressing with extraintestinal manifestations, such as psoriasis, rheumatoid arthritis, or mental illnesses (103). In this regard, it has been proposed that the use of bacteriotherapy, mainly through the administration of probiotics, often as an adjuvant to medical treatments, could be helpful for the recovery of a healthy state in the framework of all these pathologies.

Bifidobacterium is one of the main genera of commensal bacteria present in the human GIT and its presence has been related to health benefits in several studies (83). Each *Bifidobacterium* species appeared to elicit different immune effects on the host, noteworthy being the ability of *B. bifidum* to ex-

pand the T-regulatory response, which may be relevant for its use in chronic inflammatory diseases (104). In this regard, supplementation of the gut microbiota obtained from a cohort of systemic lupus erythematosus patients with a *B. bifidum* strain partially corrected the altered immune response characteristic of lupus, using a dendritic cell/naive T-cell model (105). The positive effects that bifidobacteria could exert on human health have been extensively reviewed during the past few years (83, 106, 107). Because of the potential impact on human health and the GRAS, QPS status of some of the species of this genus, several strains have undergone clinical studies and are currently being used as probiotics in human nutrition. Beneficial effects resulting from the consumption of bifidobacteria on human health have mainly been associated with the prevention and treatment of intestinal diseases and immunological disorders (Tables 1 and Table 2). In this section, we will focus on the effectivity of

TABLE 1 *Bifidobacterium* strains used as probiotics with demonstrated effectivity in humans trials

Effect	Strain(s)	Reference(s)
• Improve symptoms in lactose-intolerant patients	• *B. breve* Yakult + *Lb. casei* Shirota	88
• Prevent antibiotic-associated diarrhea	• *B. animalis* subsp. *lactis*	108
	• *B. animalis* subsp. *lactis* BB-12 + *S. thermophilus*	110
• Reduce the incidence of antibiotic-associated diarrhea	• VSL#3 (*B. breve* + *B. infantis* + *B. longum* + *S. thermophilus* + *Lb. acidophilus* + *Lb. paracasei* + *Lb. plantarum* + *Lb. delbrueckii* subsp. *bulgaricus*)	111
• Prevent *C. difficile*-associated diarrhea	• *B. bifidum* + *Lb. acidophilus* (Cultech strains)	112
• Prevent gastrointestinal infections	• *B. animalis* subsp. *lactis* BB-12	109
• Improve functional gastrointestinal symptoms in adults	• *B. animalis* subsp. *lactis* HN019	136
• Improve gastrointestinal symptoms in women	• *B. animalis* subsp. *lactis* CNCM I-2494	168
• Alleviate symptoms of IBS	• *B. animalis* subsp. *lactis* BB-12 + *Lb. rhamnosus* (GG + LC705) + *P. freudenreichii* subsp. *shermanii* JS	86
	• *B. breve* BB99 + *Lb. rhamnosus* (GG + LC705) + *P. freudenreichii* subsp. *shermanii* JS	142
	• *B. infantis* 35624	87, 169
	• *B. longum* 101 + *Lb. acidophilus* 102 + *Lactococcus lactis* 103 + *S. thermophilus* 104	143, 170
• Ameliorate symptoms of IBS in children	• VSL#3	144
• Improve symptoms of IBS	• *B. animalis* DN-173010 + *S. thermophilus* + *Lb. delbrueckii* subsp. *bulgaricus* + *Lc. lactis*	137, 138
• Improve clinical conditions of patients with UC	• *B. breve* Yakult + prebiotic GOS	171
• Reduce symptoms of patients with UC	• VSL#3	140, 141
• Reduce proinflammatory biomarkers in patients with UC	• *B. infantis* 35624	139
• Remission of UC in children	• VSL#3	84
• Maintain remission in recurrent pouchitis	• VSL#3	85, 172
• Reduce the pouchitis activity index	• VSL#3	173

Effect	Strain	Reference
Prevent necrotizing enterocolitis in preterm infants	B. bifidum NCDO 1453 + Lb. acidophilus NCDO1748	147
	Infloran (B. infantis) + Lb. acidophilus	146
Prevent necrotizing enterocolitis in neonate	ABC Dophilus (B. infantis + B. bifidus) + S. thermophilus	148
Reduce levels of Helicobacter pylori	B. bifidum YIT4007	121
Improve immune function in resected CRC patients	B. animalis subsp. lactis BB-12 + Lb. rhamnosus GG	126
Reduce cancer risk, improving epithelial barrier function	B. animalis subsp. lactis BB-12 + Lb. rhamnosus GG + prebiotic	128
Reduce postoperative septicemia in colectomy	Lb. plantarum CGMCC1258 + Lb acidophilus-11 + B. longum-88	129
Reduce postoperative infection complications	B. longum	131
Improve disease score in atopic dermatitis (AD) in children	B. animalis subsp. lactis HN019 + Lb. rhamnosus HN001	153
Improve clinical conditions in children with AD	B. animalis subsp. lactis UABLA-12	154
Improve AD and reduce IgE	B. bifidum + LAB	155
	B. breve M-16V + prebiotics	156
Reduce allergic symptoms, reducing Th2 cytokines	B. animalis subsp. lactis NCC2828	157
Reduce pollinosis symptoms	B. longum BB536	158
Reduce sensitization in infants with mother suffering atopy	B. animalis subsp. lactis BB-12 + Lb. rhamnosus GG	159
Reduce eczema incidence	B. animalis subsp. lactis BB-12	160
	B. animalis subsp. lactis HN019	161
	B. breve BB99 + LAB	162
	B. animalis subsp. lactis AD011 + B. bifidum BGN4	163
Prevent eczema incidence in high-risk children	B. animalis subsp. lactis W52 + B. bifidum W23	164

TABLE 2 Selection of meta-analyses and reviews about the effect of probiotic products containing bifidobacteria on certain diseases

Effect	Reference(s)
• Probiotics effective in prevention of CDAD	113
• Reducing loads or eradicating *H. pylori*	117
• Improve efficacy of antibiotics against *H. pylori* and AAD prevention	118
• Modulate microbiota composition reducing liver disease	134, 135
• Probiotics and gut microbiota role in IBS	145
• Probiotic benefit in eczema prevention	166
• Probiotics and colorectal cancer prevention	133

bifidobacteria in clinical trials, and therefore neither animal models nor *in vitro* or *ex vivo* studies will be considered.

Antibiotic-Associated Diarrhea and Other Intestinal Disorders

Regarding intestinal diseases, administration of bifidobacteria has been used to improve the symptoms of lactose intolerance, mainly using strains of the species *B. animalis* subsp. *lactis* (108), or with the probiotic mixture containing the strain *B. breve* Yakult and *Lactobacillus casei* Shirota (88). The strain *B. animalis* subsp. *lactis* BB-12 has been used in the treatment of intestinal infections; for instance, it has been demonstrated that children fed with an infant formula containing this strain displayed fewer and shorter episodes of diarrhea (109). A commercial probiotic formula containing the same strain of bifidobacteria (BB-12) together with a strain of *Streptococcus thermophilus* was used satisfactorily in a clinical trial focused on the prevention of antibiotic-associated diarrhea (AAD) in infants (110). In this sense, the commercial probiotic mixture VSL#3, which contains several strains, among which are *B. breve*, *B. infantis* (or *B. longum* subsp. *infantis*), and *B. longum*, displayed an ability to reduce the incidence of AAD (111).

Clostridium difficile-Associated Diarrhea

In the case of the *C. difficile*-associated diarrhea (CDAD), a mixture containing a strain of *B. bifidum* and *Lactobacillus acidophilus* was efficient at preventing the proliferation

of this pathogen after antibiotic therapy (112). In this sense, Goldenberg and coworkers (113) concluded, after an exhaustive meta-analysis (23 clinical trials, n = 4,213), that there is moderate evidence suggesting that probiotics are effective in the prevention of CDAD. Regarding *C. difficile* infection, the best methodology to reduce the associated diarrhea and to eradicate this pathogen is the fecal microbiota transplantation, which has shown up to 95.9% success, including recalcitrant and severe cases (114). In this therapy, the complete microbiota of a healthy donor is placed into the patient to modify their intestinal microbiota and to displace *C. difficile* (115). For this purpose, the feces of the healthy donor, in which the intestinal microbiota constitutes a very important part, are homogenized in saline buffer and administered to the patient in different ways, such as colonoscopy, endoscopy, or enema (116). Because it is likely that the feces from a healthy person contain between 1 and 4% bifidobacteria, it remains to be elucidated whether increasing the number of bifidobacteria by appropriate donor selection, or by targeted enrichment of this population before transplantation, could be useful, not only in CDAD, but also in other diseases through fecal microbiota transplantation.

Helicobacter pylori Infection

Regarding the use of bifidobacteria to avoid bacterial infections, it is worth mentioning their application in infections caused by *H. pylori*, a Gram-negative bacterium present in the stomach that is responsible for chronic ulceration, a pathology that has been linked to the development of gastric cancer. Although very successful in the beginning, antibiotic treatments decreased in effectiveness after years of antibiotherapy, which resulted in the emergence of antibiotic resistance in *H. pylori* strains. In this regard, the use of probiotics has been efficient in reducing *H. pylori* loads, or even definitively eradicating the pathogen. Li and coworkers (117) published a meta-analysis that compiled the clinical trial studies involving *H. pylori* treatment, and they showed that the use of probiotics could be as effective as pharmacological approaches. In addition, probiotics were revealed in the same analysis as the best treatment in terms of tolerance for the patient. Recently, Boltin and coworkers (118) reviewed the use of probiotics for *H. pylori*-induced ulcer disease; they concluded that the use of probiotics alone is not enough to eradicate *H. pylori*, but it is suitable to improve the efficacy of antibiotic regimens for *H. pylori* eradication and prevent AAD.

The use of probiotics can be then considered as an adjuvant therapy for the eradication of *H. pylori* thanks to (i) their ability to stimulate mucin production, therefore limiting the adhesion of the pathogen to the gut surface; (ii) production of short-chain fatty acids and other antimicrobial substances that may reduce *H. pylori* density; and (iii) protection against human pathogens due to host receptor competition and immune modulation capabilities (119). On the contrary, and based on other meta-analyses, some authors agree that probiotic supplementation does not improve the eradication rate of *H. pylori* (120). Most probiotics used in these studies are members of the genus *Lactobacillus*, but also some bifidobacteria species were tested as well, such as the strain *B. bifidum* YIT4007. This strain was able to reduce gastric mucosa alterations and other gastrointestinal symptoms due to a reduction in the levels of *H. pylori* (121). Other published works showed that the administration of a pretreatment with yogurt containing mix-

tures of bifidobacteria and lactobacilli improved the eradication of *H. pylori* (122, 123). A recent study reported an *H. pylori* eradication rate of 32.5% in adults after 10 days of administration of the commercial mix of probiotic VSL#3, which includes several probiotic bifidobacteria as mentioned above (118).

Colorectal Cancer

Probiotics have also been used to modify/modulate the microbiota of patients toward a healthy microbiota in those cases in which alterations of microbiota populations are associated with disease. In this context, probiotics have been used to modulate the microbiota in colorectal cancer (CRC). In CRC patients, it is known that the composition of the microbiota is one of the factors favoring the development of carcinogenic lesions, notably by the presence of genotoxic bacteria such as *Fusobacterium nucleatum* or colibactin-producing *Escherichia coli* (124, 125). Only a few clinical trials (involving bifidobacteria administration) have been performed in CRC, although there are promising results in *in vitro* and preclinical studies. As a whole, the main positive effects obtained in the clinical trials are the improvement of the gut environment by reducing the secondary effects of surgery and chemotherapy, notably at the level of the epithelial layer and involving tissue regeneration. In this sense, administration of *B. animalis* subsp. *lactis* BB-12 together with *Lactobacillus rhamnosus* GG and inulin improved the immune functions in resected CRC patients (126). Other works reported on the ability of bifidobacteria to induce fecal microbiota modifications in CRC patients (127) as well as to reduce some cancer risk factors by improving epithelial barrier function and reducing colorectal proliferation by commensal microorganisms (128). Recent studies showed that administration of bifidobacteria as part of a perioperative probiotic treatment reduced the rate of postoperative septicemia in patients undergoing a colectomy (129) and in colorectal liver metastases surgery (130). Moreover, Zhang and coworkers (131) showed that the preoperative administration of bifidobacteria in CRC patients reduced the postoperative infection complications through a mechanism involving maintenance of the intestinal microbiota populations, reduction on the numbers of *E. coli*, and restriction in bacterial translocation from the intestine to the bloodstream.

Chemotherapy Treatments

Chemotherapy treatments cause diarrhea and alter the normal function of the GIT, perturbing the proportions of populations conforming the intestinal microbiota. Alterations in the gut microbiome could be avoided with the use of probiotics before, during, and after the chemotherapy. In this sense, it is estimated that the complex consortia of microorganisms will be more efficient than a single strain when restoring the microbiota. Wada and coworkers (132) showed that the administration of *B. breve* strain Yakult improved the intestinal environment through the production of small-chain fatty acids favoring cross-feeding relationships among the microorganism communities inhabiting the gut of CRC patients receiving chemotherapy. Some of the following works are examples of clinical trials, but many others are indeed preclinical models aimed at analyzing the prevention and treatment ability of bifidobacteria in CRC. To expand this information, the reader is prompted to read an excellent review on the subject by Ambalam and coworkers (133). As has been mentioned, the use of probiotics in CRC is not a direct treatment for the disease, but an adjuvant therapy that would help patients avoid alterations in their gut microbiota. Bifidobacteria-containing probiotics are expected to help recovery from chemotherapy, while reducing the possibilities of septicemia after surgery. Because of the advantages of probiotic consumption, several authors have proposed that

an oral intake of probiotics should be included as a preoperative and postoperative treatment in CRC (133).

Liver Disease

Probiotics, including bifidobacteria, have become part of novel therapeutic approaches in hepatology, mainly because of their beneficial effect modulating the composition of the intestinal microbiota, a factor that can influence liver disease onset (134). The increasing interest in the use of probiotics for prevention and treatment of liver disease is related to the effect of gut microbiota in the pathogenesis of several liver complications including cirrhosis. However, the scientific evidence in this field is still controversial and further studies are required in order to include probiotics in liver treatments with a reasonable guarantee of success (135).

Inflammatory Bowel Disease and Irritable Bowel Syndrome

The positive effects exerted on human health by bifidobacteria and, in general, by probiotics, are related to their ability to modify the composition of the intestinal microbiota and their capability to modulate the immune response. Both parameters are altered in intestinal pathologies like irritable bowel syndrome (IBS), in certain physiological situations such as obesity, autoimmune diseases such as systemic lupus erythematosus, and chronic inflammatory diseases such as inflammatory bowel disease (IBD), including Crohn disease (CD), ulcerative colitis (UC), and pouchitis. Indeed, the prevalence rate of these noncommunicable diseases has increased significantly in developed countries during the past few decades (83). In these pathologies, *B. animalis* subsp. *lactis* HN019 has been able to improve the gastrointestinal function in adults (136), and *B. animalis* subsp. *lactis* DN171010 reduced IBS symptoms (137, 138). The beneficial effect associated with the immune modulation capability of bifidobacteria has been related to their ability to reduce systemic proinflammatory biomarkers. This is the case of the strain *B. infantis* 35624 that was able to reduce pro-inflammatory cytokines at gastrointestinal (mucosal immune system) and nongastrointestinal levels (systemic immune system) (139). The administration of other *Bifidobacterium* strains has also been efficient in alleviating IBS symptoms, such as a probiotic mixture containing *B. breve* BB99 (140) or the strain *B. animalis* subsp. *lactis* BB-12 (86). Another probiotic mixture that reduced IBS symptoms contains the strain *B. longum* 101, together with two strains of the genus *Lactobacillus* (141). Another example was the administration of VSL#3 for 6 weeks, which resulted in the reduction of IBS symptoms and the improvement of the quality of life in children (142). Further reading on the use of probiotics in IBS and the gut microbiota role can be obtained in the review by Distrutti and coworkers (143).

In IBD, the probiotic mixture VSL#3, which contains bifidobacteria of different species, was able to reduce the UC symptoms in adults (144, 145) as well as the remission of the disease in children (84).

Necrotizing Enterocolitis

Regarding prevention of necrotizing enterocolitis (NEC) in newborns, bifidobacteria has also been assayed mainly as part of probiotic mixtures. A commercial product containing a strain of *B. infantis* was able to reduce the incidence and severity of NEC in very-low-birth-weight infants (146) and in very-low-birth-weight preterm infants (147). Moreover, another study showed that a commercial probiotic product containing strains of *B. infantis* and *B. bifidum* reduced the incidence and severity of NEC in a premature neonatal cohort (148). However, some results recently recorded in literature did not support a positive effect of bifidobacteria on NEC. For instance, a phase 3 clinical trial aimed at testing the effectiveness of the probiotic *B. breve*

BBG-001 concluded that there is no evidence of benefit for very preterm infants (149).

Allergic Disease

Probiotic bifidobacteria have also been proposed for the prevention of nonintestinal diseases, such as allergic disease. The prevalence of atopic eczema, food allergy, and asthma has increased during the past decade, becoming a major public health problem, and indeed these allergic disorders are one of the most common causes of chronic illness and hospital admissions (150). Allergic diseases are characterized by an inadequate T-helper immune response balance, involving mainly an overrepresentation of the Th2 response with a concomitant inability to maintain the Th1/Th2 response balance. Moreover, allergic patients usually display a reduced number of T regulatory cells (Treg) (151). During the past 10 years several studies have tried to demonstrate the influence of the intestinal microbiota on allergic processes. It is believed that this influence could be mediated through the interaction of microorganisms with the mucosal immune system. In this sense, several studies aimed to demonstrate the beneficial effects of probiotics on the prevention and treatment of allergic disease through *in vivo* studies with animal models and human trials (152). Regarding human trials for the treatment of allergy, administration of *Lb. rhamnosus* HN001 and *B. animalis* subsp. *lactis* HN019 improved the disease scores of atopic dermatitis (AD) in children suffering from atopic eczema (153). Similar results were obtained with the administration of a probiotic mixture containing *B. animalis* subsp. *lactis* UABLA-12 that significantly improved the clinical conditions in children with AD (154). Improvement in AD scores and reduction of IgE levels associated with eczema have also been observed in children after the administration of *B. bifidum* in combination with other lactic acid bacteria (155), as well as with the strain *B. breve* M-16V combined with a mixture of prebiotics (156). The immune modulatory effect exerted by *B. animalis* subsp. *lactis* NCC2818, which reduced allergic symptoms, was mediated by a reduction in the production of Th2 cytokines (157). Moreover, a human clinical trial performed with the strain *B. longum* BB536 showed that the intake of yogurt supplemented with this strain reduced pollinosis symptoms by modulating the Th1/Th2 balance (158). Use of probiotics to improve atopic eczema needs further investigation and clinical trials to infer recommendations for allergies, especially in adults where no evidence of significant reduction in eczema symptoms has so far been demonstrated.

Regarding the prevention of allergic disease by means of probiotic intake, there are several clinical trials with promising results. In general, the duration of the probiotic intervention, rather than prenatal versus postnatal treatment, seems to be the crucial factor determining the success of probiotics. Administration of *B. animalis* subsp. *lactis* BB-12 and *Lb. rhamnosus* GG during pregnancy and lactation resulted in a reduction of the risk of sensitization of infants whose mothers suffered from atopy (159). Moreover, the strain BB-12 administered during the pre- or postnatal period reduced the incidence of eczema in an atopic dermatitis cohort (160). Another strain able to reduce the atopic eczema incidence was *B. animalis* subsp. *lactis* HN019, administered during the pre- or postnatal periods (161). Another clinical trial combining pre- and postnatal treatments showed a reduction of eczema and IgE-associated eczema when the strain *B. breve* BB99 was administered together with other lactic acid bacteria strains (162). Similar clinical trials, but with longer treatment periods, showed reductions in eczema incidence after the administration of *B. animalis* subsp. *lactis* AD011 and *B. bifidum* BGN4 (163), and a preventive effect of the incidence of eczema in high-risk children after the administration of the strains *B. animalis* subsp. *lactis* W52 and *B. bifidum* W23 (164).

However, not all the clinical trials have been successful and, for instance, no significant differences between the placebo and probiotic groups were found regarding the incidence of atopic eczema when the strain *B. longum* BL999 was administered to Asian infants (165). The World Allergy Organization (WAO) recently published their Guidelines for Allergic Disease Prevention (GLAD-P) based on the use of probiotics (166). The WAO published recommendations about the use of probiotics in the prevention of allergy, based on scientific evidence and from the results of human trials. These guidelines concluded that currently there is no evidence supporting probiotic supplementation for reducing the risk of allergy incidence in children. However, there is likely to be a net benefit using probiotics for eczema prevention, which requires further clinical trials to increase the sample size and the reliability of the results. On the contrary, in case a family history of allergy (eczema) is identified as a risk factor for children, WAO suggests the use of probiotics for pregnant women, women who breastfeed their infants, and in those infants.

CONCLUSIONS

In summary, although positive results of the use of bifidobacteria for the treatment and prevention of different diseases are abundant in scientific literature, further work is needed to improve the solidity of the scientific evidence supporting the beneficial effects of this particular group of intestinal bacteria. It is noteworthy that the health benefits exerted by bifidobacteria seem to be strain dependent, notably at the level of immunomodulation, but they are also dependent on the genetic background of the target population (77). Therefore, and despite the key contribution of probiogenomics efforts in discovering the genetic background of probiotic bacteria (4), investment in basic research is absolutely necessary to clarify the molecular mechanism behind the probiotic action, a key point to be able to define strain-specific effects. Furthermore, it is also necessary to correctly identify not only the strains, but also the pathology and the population to be targeted with probiotic interventions. Finally, for future strain selection, it would be desirable to choose appropriate probiotic strains showing promising results *in vitro* and *in vivo*, and ideally good technological properties, in order to scale up the production of future probiotic bifidobacteria at affordable costs.

ACKNOWLEDGMENTS

Research in our group is supported by grants AGL2015-64901-R, BIO2014-55019-JIN, AGL2013-44761-P, and AGL2013-44039-R from the Spanish Ministry of Economy and Competitiveness.

CITATION

Hidalgo-Cantabrana C, Delgado S, Ruiz L, Ruas-Madiedo P, Sánchez B, Margolles A. 2017. Bifidobacteria and their health-promoting effects. Microbiol Spectrum 5(3):BAD-0010-2016.

REFERENCES

1. **González-Rodríguez I, Gaspar P, Sánchez B, Gueimonde M, Margolles A, Neves AR.** 2013. Catabolism of glucose and lactose in *Bifidobacterium animalis* subsp. *lactis*, studied by ^{13}C Nuclear Magnetic Resonance. *Appl Environ Microbiol* **79:**7628–7638.
2. **Schell MA, Karmirantzou M, Snel B, Vilanova D, Berger B, Pessi G, Zwahlen MC, Desiere F, Bork P, Delley M, Pridmore RD, Arigoni F.** 2002. The genome sequence of *Bifidobacterium longum* reflects its adaptation to the human gastrointestinal tract. *Proc Natl Acad Sci USA* **99:**14422–14427.
3. **Lugli GA, Milani C, Turroni F, Duranti S, Ferrario C, Viappiani A, Mancabelli L, Mangifesta M, Taminiau B, Delcenserie V, van Sinderen D, Ventura M.** 2014. Investigation of the evolutionary development of the genus *Bifidobacterium* by comparative genomics. *Appl Environ Microbiol* **80:**6383–6394.
4. **Milani C, Lugli GA, Duranti S, Turroni F, Bottacini F, Mangifesta M, Sanchez B, Viappiani A, Mancabelli L, Taminiau B, Delcenserie V, Barrangou R, Margolles A, van Sinderen D, Ventura M.** 2014. Genomic encyclopedia of type strains of the genus *Bifidobacterium*. *Appl Environ Microbiol* **80:**6290–6302.
5. **Delgado S, Suárez A, Mayo B.** 2006. Bifidobacterial diversity determined by culturing and by 16S rDNA sequence analysis in feces and mucosa from ten healthy Spanish adults. *Dig Dis Sci* **51:**1878–1885.
6. **Turroni F, Foroni E, Pizzetti P, Giubellini V, Ribbera A, Merusi P, Cagnasso P, Bizzarri B, de'Angelis GL, Shanahan F, van Sinderen D, Ventura M.** 2009. Exploring the diversity of the bifidobacterial population in the human intestinal tract. *Appl Environ Microbiol* **75:**1534–1545.
7. **Aas JA, Griffen AL, Dardis SR, Lee AM, Olsen I, Dewhirst FE, Leys EJ, Paster BJ.** 2008. Bacteria of dental caries in primary and permanent teeth in children and young adults. *J Clin Microbiol* **46:**1407–1417.
8. **Ventura M, Turroni F, Zomer A, Foroni E, Giubellini V, Bottacini F, Canchaya C, Claesson MJ, He F, Mantzourani M, Mulas L, Ferrarini A, Gao B, Delledonne M, Henrissat B, Coutinho P, Oggioni M, Gupta RS, Zhang Z, Beighton D, Fitzgerald GF, O'Toole PW, van Sinderen D.** 2009. The *Bifidobacterium dentium* Bd1 genome sequence reflects its genetic adaptation to the human oral cavity. *PLoS Genet* **5:**e1000785.
9. **Turroni F, Marchesi JR, Foroni E, Gueimonde M, Shanahan F, Margolles A, van Sinderen D, Ventura M.** 2009. Microbiomic analysis of the bifidobacterial population in the human distal gut. *ISME J* **3:**745–751.
10. **Biagi E, Nylund L, Candela M, Ostan R, Bucci L, Pini E, Nikkïla J, Monti D, Satokari R, Franceschi C, Brigidi P, De Vos W.** 2010. Through ageing, and beyond: gut microbiota and inflammatory status in seniors and centenarians. *PLoS One* **5:**e10667. (Erratum, **5:** doi: 10.1371/annotation/df45912f-d15c-44ab-8312-e7ec0607604d)
11. **Drago L, Toscano M, Rodighiero V, De Vecchi E, Mogna G.** 2012. Cultivable and pyrosequenced fecal microflora in centenarians and young subjects. *J Clin Gastroenterol* **46**(Suppl): S81–S84.
12. **Woodmansey EJ, McMurdo ME, Macfarlane GT, Macfarlane S.** 2004. Comparison of compositions and metabolic activities of fecal microbiotas in young adults and in antibiotic-

treated and non-antibiotic-treated elderly subjects. *Appl Environ Microbiol* **70:**6113–6122.

13. **Russell DA, Ross RP, Fitzgerald GF, Stanton C.** 2011. Metabolic activities and probiotic potential of bifidobacteria. *Int J Food Microbiol* **149:** 88–105.

14. **Nishijima S, Suda W, Oshima K, Kim SW, Hirose Y, Morita H, Hattori M.** 2016. The gut microbiome of healthy Japanese and its microbial and functional uniqueness. *DNA Res* **23:**125–133.

15. **Avershina E, Storrø O, Øien T, Johnsen R, Wilson R, Egeland T, Rudi K.** 2013. Bifidobacterial succession and correlation networks in a large unselected cohort of mothers and their children. *Appl Environ Microbiol* **79:**497–507.

16. **Tannock GW.** 2010. Analysis of bifidobacterial populations in bowel ecology studies, p 1–15. *In* Mayo B, van Sinderen D (ed), *Bifidobacteria: Genomics and Molecular Aspects.* Caister Academic Press, Norfolk, England.

17. **Fernández L, Langa S, Martín V, Jiménez E, Martín R, Rodríguez JM.** 2013. The microbiota of human milk in healthy women. *Cell Mol Biol Noisy-le-grand* **59:**31–42.

18. **Martín R, Jiménez E, Heilig H, Fernández L, Marín ML, Zoetendal EG, Rodríguez JM.** 2009. Isolation of bifidobacteria from breast milk and assessment of the bifidobacterial population by PCR-denaturing gradient gel electrophoresis and quantitative real-time PCR. *Appl Environ Microbiol* **75:**965–969.

19. **Mariat D, Firmesse O, Levenez F, Guimarães V, Sokol H, Doré J, Corthier G, Furet JP.** 2009. The Firmicutes/Bacteroidetes ratio of the human microbiota changes with age. *BMC Microbiol* **9:**123.

20. **Roger LC, Costabile A, Holland DT, Hoyles L, McCartney AL.** 2010. Examination of faecal *Bifidobacterium* populations in breast- and formula-fed infants during the first 18 months of life. *Microbiology* **156:**3329–3341.

21. **Smilowitz JT, Lebrilla CB, Mills DA, German JB, Freeman SL.** 2014. Breast milk oligosaccharides: structure-function relationships in the neonate. *Annu Rev Nutr* **34:**143–169.

22. **Zivkovic AM, German JB, Lebrilla CB, Mills DA.** 2011. Human milk glycobiome and its impact on the infant gastrointestinal microbiota. *Proc Natl Acad Sci USA* **108**(Suppl 1):4653–4658.

23. **Sela DA, Chapman J, Adeuya A, Kim JH, Chen F, Whitehead TR, Lapidus A, Rokhsar DS, Lebrilla CB, German JB, Price NP, Richardson PM, Mills DA.** 2008. The genome sequence of *Bifidobacterium longum* subsp. *infantis* reveals adaptations for milk utilization within the infant microbiome. *Proc Natl Acad Sci USA* **105:**18964–18969.

24. **Wada J, Ando T, Kiyohara M, Ashida H, Kitaoka M, Yamaguchi M, Kumagai H, Katayama T, Yamamoto K.** 2008. *Bifidobacterium bifidum* lacto-N-biosidase, a critical enzyme for the degradation of human milk oligosaccharides with a type 1 structure. *Appl Environ Microbiol* **74:**3996–4004.

25. **Garrido D, Dallas DC, Mills DA.** 2013. Consumption of human milk glycoconjugates by infant-associated bifidobacteria: mechanisms and implications. *Microbiology* **159:**649–664.

26. **Garrido D, Ruiz-Moyano S, Lemay DG, Sela DA, German JB, Mills DA.** 2015. Comparative transcriptomics reveals key differences in the response to milk oligosaccharides of infant gut-associated bifidobacteria. *Sci Rep* **5:**13517.

27. **Ruiz-Moyano S, Totten SM, Garrido DA, Smilowitz JT, German JB, Lebrilla CB, Mills DA.** 2013. Variation in consumption of human milk oligosaccharides by infant gut-associated strains of *Bifidobacterium breve*. *Appl Environ Microbiol* **79:**6040–6049.

28. **Duranti S, Turroni F, Lugli GA, Milani C, Viappiani A, Mangifesta M, Gioiosa L, Palanza P, van Sinderen D, Ventura M.** 2014. Genomic characterization and transcriptional studies of the starch-utilizing strain *Bifidobacterium adolescentis* 22L. *Appl Environ Microbiol* **80:** 6080–6090.

29. **Duranti S, Milani C, Lugli GA, Mancabelli L, Turroni F, Ferrario C, Mangifesta M, Viappiani A, Sánchez B, Margolles A, van Sinderen D, Ventura M.** 2016. Evaluation of genetic diversity among strains of the human gut commensal *Bifidobacterium adolescentis*. *Sci Rep* **6:**23971.

30. **Ventura M, Canchaya C, Fitzgerald GF, Gupta RS, van Sinderen D.** 2007. Genomics as a means to understand bacterial phylogeny and ecological adaptation: the case of bifidobacteria. *Antonie van Leeuwenhoek* **91:**351–372. (Erratum, **92:**265)

31. **Ventura M, Canchaya C, Tauch A, Chandra G, Fitzgerald GF, Chater KF, van Sinderen D.** 2007. Genomics of Actinobacteria: tracing the evolutionary history of an ancient phylum. *Microbiol Mol Biol Rev* **71:**495–548.

32. **Ishikawa E, Matsuki T, Kubota H, Makino H, Sakai T, Oishi K, Kushiro A, Fujimoto J, Watanabe K, Watanuki M, Tanaka R.** 2013. Ethnic diversity of gut microbiota: species characterization of *Bacteroides fragilis* group and genus *Bifidobacterium* in healthy Belgian adults, and comparison with data from Japanese subjects. *J Biosci Bioeng* **116:**265–270.

33. **Turroni F, Peano C, Pass DA, Foroni E, Severgnini M, Claesson MJ, Kerr C, Hourihane**

J, Murray D, Fuligni F, Gueimonde M, Margolles A, De Bellis G, O'Toole PW, van Sinderen D, Marchesi JR, Ventura M. 2012. Diversity of bifidobacteria within the infant gut microbiota. *PLoS One* **7**:e36957.

34. Ruiz L, Hevia A, Bernardo D, Margolles A, Sánchez B. 2014. Extracellular molecular effectors mediating probiotic attributes. *FEMS Microbiol Lett* **359**:1–11.

35. Gagnon M, Kheadr EE, Dabour N, Richard D, Fliss I. 2006. Effect of *Bifidobacterium thermacidophilum* probiotic feeding on entero-hemorrhagic *Escherichia coli* O157:H7 infection in BALB/c mice. *Int J Food Microbiol* **111**: 26–33.

36. Henriksson A, Conway PL. 2001. Isolation of human faecal bifidobacteria which reduce signs of *Salmonella* infection when orogastrically dosed to mice. *J Appl Microbiol* **90**:223–228.

37. Muñoz JA, Chenoll E, Casinos B, Bataller E, Ramón D, Genovés S, Montava R, Ribes JM, Buesa J, Fàbrega J, Rivero M. 2011. Novel probiotic *Bifidobacterium longum* subsp. *infantis* CECT 7210 strain active against rotavirus infections. *Appl Environ Microbiol* **77**:8775–8783.

38. Fukuda S, Toh H, Hase K, Oshima K, Nakanishi Y, Yoshimura K, Tobe T, Clarke JM, Topping DL, Taylor TD, Itoh K, Kikuchi J, Morita H, Hattori M, Ohno H. 2011. Bifidobacteria can protect from enteropathogenic infection through production of acetate. *Nature* **469**:543–547.

39. Moroni O, Kheadr E, Boutin Y, Lacroix C, Fliss I. 2006. Inactivation of adhesion and invasion of food-borne *Listeria monocytogenes* by bacteriocin producing *Bifidobacterium* strains of human origin. *Appl Environ Microbiol* **72**:6894–6901.

40. Cotar AI, Chifiriuc MC, Dinu S, Pelinescu D, Banu O, Lazăr V. 2010. Quantitative real-time PCR study of the influence of probiotic culture soluble fraction on the expression of *Pseudomonas aeruginosa* quorum sensing genes. *Roum Arch Microbiol Immunol* **69**:213–223.

41. Kim Y, Lee JW, Kang SG, Oh S, Griffiths MW. 2012. *Bifidobacterium* spp. influences the production of autoinducer-2 and biofilm formation by *Escherichia coli* O157:H7. *Anaerobe* **18**:539–545.

42. Fanning S, Hall LJ, Cronin M, Zomer A, MacSharry J, Goulding D, Motherway MO, Shanahan F, Nally K, Dougan G, van Sinderen D. 2012. Bifidobacterial surface-exopolysaccharide facilitates commensal-host interaction through immune modulation and pathogen protection. *Proc Natl Acad Sci USA* **109**:2108–2113.

43. Koenig JE, Spor A, Scalfone N, Fricker AD, Stombaugh J, Knight R, Angenent LT, Ley RE. 2011. Succession of microbial consortia in the developing infant gut microbiome. *Proc Natl Acad Sci USA* **108**(Suppl 1):4578–4585.

44. Turroni F, Milani C, Duranti S, Mancabelli L, Mangifesta M, Viappiani A, Lugli GA, Ferrario C, Gioiosa L, Ferrarini A, Li J, Palanza P, Delledonne M, van Sinderen D, Ventura M. 2016. Deciphering bifidobacterial-mediated metabolic interactions and their impact on gut microbiota by a multi-omics approach. *ISME J* **10**:1656–1668.

45. Arboleya S, Solís G, Fernández N, de los Reyes-Gavilán CG, Gueimonde M. 2012. Facultative to strict anaerobes ratio in the preterm infant microbiota: a target for intervention? *Gut Microbes* **3**:583–588.

46. Sela DA, Mills DA. 2010. Nursing our microbiota: molecular linkages between bifidobacteria and milk oligosaccharides. *Trends Microbiol* **18**:298–307.

47. Sonnenburg JL, Chen CT, Gordon JI. 2006. Genomic and metabolic studies of the impact of probiotics on a model gut symbiont and host. *PLoS Biol* **4**:e413.

48. Milani C, Lugli GA, Duranti S, Turroni F, Mancabelli L, Ferrario C, Mangifesta M, Hevia A, Viappiani A, Scholz M, Arioli S, Sanchez B, Lane J, Ward DV, Hickey R, Mora D, Segata N, Margolles A, van Sinderen D, Ventura M. 2015. Bifidobacteria exhibit social behavior through carbohydrate resource sharing in the gut. *Sci Rep* **5**:15782.

49. Arboleya S, Salazar N, Solís G, Fernández N, Hernández-Barranco AM, Cuesta I, Gueimonde M, de los Reyes-Gavilán CG. 2013a. Assessment of intestinal microbiota modulation ability of *Bifidobacterium* strains in in vitro fecal batch cultures from preterm neonates. *Anaerobe* **19**: 9–16.

50. Boto-Ordóñez M, Urpi-Sarda M, Queipo-Ortuño MI, Tulipani S, Tinahones FJ, Andres-Lacueva C. 2014. High levels of Bifidobacteria are associated with increased levels of anthocyanin microbial metabolites: a randomized clinical trial. *Food Funct* **5**:1932–1938.

51. Enomoto T, Sowa M, Nishimori K, Shimazu S, Yoshida A, Yamada K, Furukawa F, Nakagawa T, Yanagisawa N, Iwabuchi N, Odamaki T, Abe F, Nakayama J, Xiao JZ. 2014. Effects of bifidobacterial supplementation to pregnant women and infants in the prevention of allergy development in infants and on fecal microbiota. *Allergol Int* **63**:575–585.

52. Monteagudo-Mera A, Arthur JC, Jobin C, Keku T, Bruno-Barcena JM, Azcarate-Peril MA. 2016. High purity galacto-oligosaccharides enhance specific *Bifidobacterium* species and

their metabolic activity in the mouse gut microbiome. *Benef Microbes* **7**:247–264.

53. Sugahara H, Odamaki T, Fukuda S, Kato T, Xiao JZ, Abe F, Kikuchi J, Ohno H. 2015. Probiotic *Bifidobacterium longum* alters gut luminal metabolism through modification of the gut microbial community. *Sci Rep* **5**:13548.

54. **Wu BB, Yang Y, Xu X, Wang WP. 2016.** Effects of *Bifidobacterium* supplementation on intestinal microbiota composition and the immune response in healthy infants. *World J Pediatr* **12**:177–182.

55. **Salazar N, Ruas-Madiedo P, Kolida S, Collins M, Rastall R, Gibson G, de Los Reyes-Gavilán CG. 2009.** Exopolysaccharides produced by *Bifidobacterium longum* IPLA E44 and *Bifidobacterium animalis* subsp. *lactis* IPLA R1 modify the composition and metabolic activity of human faecal microbiota in pH-controlled batch cultures. *Int J Food Microbiol* **135**:260–267.

56. **Salazar N, Binetti A, Gueimonde M, Alonso A, Garrido P, González del Rey C, González C, Ruas-Madiedo P, de los Reyes-Gavilán CG. 2011.** Safety and intestinal microbiota modulation by the exopolysaccharide-producing strains *Bifidobacterium animalis* IPLA R1 and *Bifidobacterium longum* IPLA E44 orally administered to Wistar rats. *Int J Food Microbiol* **144**:342–351.

57. **Rios-Covian D, Arboleya S, Hernandez-Barranco AM, Alvarez-Buylla JR, Ruas-Madiedo P, Gueimonde M, de los Reyes-Gavilan CG. 2013.** Interactions between *Bifidobacterium* and *Bacteroides* species in cofermentations are affected by carbon sources, including exopolysaccharides produced by bifidobacteria. *Appl Environ Microbiol* **79**:7518–7524.

58. **Rios-Covian D, Gueimonde M, Duncan SH, Flint HJ, de los Reyes-Gavilan CG. 2015.** Enhanced butyrate formation by cross-feeding between *Faecalibacterium prausnitzii* and *Bifidobacterium adolescentis*. *FEMS Microbiol Lett* **362**:fnv176.

59. **Rios-Covián D, Sánchez B, Salazar N, Martínez N, Redruello B, Gueimonde M, de Los Reyes-Gavilán CG. 2015.** Different metabolic features of *Bacteroides fragilis* growing in the presence of glucose and exopolysaccharides of bifidobacteria. *Front Microbiol* **6**:825.

60. **Jung TH, Jeon WM, Han KS. 2015.** *In vitro* effects of dietary inulin on human fecal microbiota and butyrate production. *J Microbiol Biotechnol* **25**:1555–1558.

61. **Kato T, Fukuda S, Fujiwara A, Suda W, Hattori M, Kikuchi J, Ohno H. 2014.** Multiple omics uncovers host-gut microbial mutualism during prebiotic fructooligosaccharide supplementation. *DNA Res* **21**:469–480.

62. **Neyrinck AM, Possemiers S, Druart C, Van de Wiele T, De Backer F, Cani PD, Larondelle Y, Delzenne NM. 2011.** Prebiotic effects of wheat arabinoxylan related to the increase in bifidobacteria, *Roseburia* and *Bacteroides/Prevotella* in diet-induced obese mice. *PLoS One* **6**:e20944.

63. **Rivière A, Gagnon M, Weckx S, Roy D, De Vuyst L. 2015.** Mutual cross-feeding interactions between *Bifidobacterium longum* subsp. *longum* NCC2705 and *Eubacterium rectale* ATCC 33656 explain the bifidogenic and butyrogenic effects of arabinoxylan oligosaccharides. *Appl Environ Microbiol* **81**:7767–7781.

64. **Falony G, Calmeyn T, Leroy F, De Vuyst L. 2009.** Coculture fermentations of *Bifidobacterium* species and *Bacteroides thetaiotaomicron* reveal a mechanistic insight into the prebiotic effect of inulin-type fructans. *Appl Environ Microbiol* **75**:2312–2319.

65. **De Vuyst L, Leroy F. 2011.** Cross-feeding between bifidobacteria and butyrate-producing colon bacteria explains bifidobacterial competitiveness, butyrate production, and gas production. *Int J Food Microbiol* **149**:73–80.

66. **Ruiz L, Sánchez B, de Los Reyes-Gavilán CG, Gueimonde M, Margolles A. 2009.** Coculture of *Bifidobacterium longum* and *Bifidobacterium breve* alters their protein expression profiles and enzymatic activities. *Int J Food Microbiol* **133**:148–153.

67. **Egan M, Motherway MO, Kilcoyne M, Kane M, Joshi L, Ventura M, van Sinderen D. 2014.** Cross-feeding by *Bifidobacterium breve* UCC2003 during co-cultivation with *Bifidobacterium bifidum* PRL2010 in a mucin-based medium. *BMC Microbiol* **14**:282.

68. **Tejero-Sariñena S, Barlow J, Costabile A, Gibson GR, Rowland I. 2013.** Antipathogenic activity of probiotics against *Salmonella* Typhimurium and *Clostridium difficile* in anaerobic batch culture systems: is it due to synergies in probiotic mixtures or the specificity of single strains? *Anaerobe* **24**:60–65.

69. **Yuan J, Wang B, Sun Z, Bo X, Yuan X, He X, Zhao H, Du X, Wang F, Jiang Z, Zhang L, Jia L, Wang Y, Wei K, Wang J, Zhang X, Sun Y, Huang L, Zeng M. 2008.** Analysis of host-inducing proteome changes in *bifidobacterium longum* NCC2705 grown *in vivo*. *J Proteome Res* **7**:375–385.

70. **Ferrario C, Milani C, Mancabelli L, Lugli GA, Duranti S, Mangifesta M, Viappiani A, Turroni F, Margolles A, Ruas-Madiedo P, van Sinderen D, Ventura M. 2016.** Modulation of the eps-ome transcription of bifidobacteria through simulation of human intestinal environment. *FEMS Microbiol Ecol* **92**:fiw056.

71. O'Connell Motherway M, Zomer A, Leahy SC, Reunanen J, Bottacini F, Claesson MJ, O'Brien F, Flynn K, Casey PG, Munoz JA, Kearney B, Houston AM, O'Mahony C, Higgins DG, Shanahan F, Palva A, de Vos WM, Fitzgerald GF, Ventura M, O'Toole PW, van Sinderen D. 2011. Functional genome analysis of *Bifidobacterium breve* UCC2003 reveals type IVb tight adherence (Tad) pili as an essential and conserved host-colonization factor. *Proc Natl Acad Sci USA* **108:**11217–11222.

72. Turroni F, Serafini F, Mangifesta M, Arioli S, Mora D, van Sinderen D, Ventura M. 2014. Expression of sortase-dependent pili of *Bifidobacterium bifidum* PRL2010 in response to environmental gut conditions. *FEMS Microbiol Lett* **357:**23–33.

73. Arboleya S, Salazar N, Solís G, Fernández N, Gueimonde M, de los Reyes-Gavilán CG. 2013. *In vitro* evaluation of the impact of human background microbiota on the response to *Bifidobacterium* strains and fructo-oligosaccharides. *Br J Nutr* **110:**2030–2036.

74. Senan S, Prajapati JB, Joshi CG, Sreeja V, Gohel MK, Trivedi S, Patel RM, Pandya H, Singh US, Phatak A, Patel HA. 2015. Geriatric respondents and non-respondents to probiotic intervention can be differentiated by inherent gut microbiome composition. *Front Microbiol* **6:**944.

75. Tojo R, Suárez A, Clemente MG, de los Reyes-Gavilán CG, Margolles A, Gueimonde M, Ruas-Madiedo P. 2014. Intestinal microbiota in health and disease: role of bifidobacteria in gut homeostasis. *World J Gastroenterol* **20:**15163–15176.

76. Reid G, Younes JA, Van der Mei HC, Gloor GB, Knight R, Busscher HJ. 2011. Microbiota restoration: natural and supplemented recovery of human microbial communities. *Nat Rev Microbiol* **9:**27–38.

77. Food and Agriculture Organization. 2006. Probiotics in food: health and nutritional properties and guidelines for evaluation. *FAO Food and Nutrition Paper 85.* ISSN 0254-4725.

78. Hill C, Guarner F, Reid G, Gibson GR, Merenstein DJ, Pot B, Morelli L, Canani RB, Flint HJ, Salminen S, Calder PC, Sanders ME. 2014. Expert consensus document. The International Scientific Association for Probiotics and Prebiotics consensus statement on the scope and appropriate use of the term probiotic. *Nat Rev Gastroenterol Hepatol* **11:**506–514.

79. Tissier H. 1906. Traitement des infections intestinales par la méthode de la flore bactérienne de l'intestin. *Crit Rev Soc Biol* **60:**359–361.

80. Moro E. 1900. Über den *Bacillus acidophilus. Jahrb Kinderheilkunde Physiche Erziehung* **52:**38–55.

81. Rettger LF, Cheplin HA. 1922. *Bacillus acidophilus* and its therapeutic application. *Arch Intern Med (Chic)* **29:**357–367. Chic.

82. Vasiljevic T, Shah NP. 2008. Probiotics—from Metchnikoff to bioactives. *Int Dairy J* **18:**714–728.

83. EFSA, European Food Safety Authority. 2015. Statement on the update of the list of QPS-recommended biological agents intentionally added to food or feed as notified to EFSA. 2: Suitability of taxonomic units notified to EFSA until March 2015. *EFSA J* **13:**4138.

84. Miele E, Pascarella F, Giannetti E, Quaglietta L, Baldassano RN, Staiano A. 2009. Effect of a probiotic preparation (VSL#3) on induction and maintenance of remission in children with ulcerative colitis. *Am J Gastroenterol* **104:**437–443.

85. Mimura T, Rizzello F, Helwig U, Poggioli G, Schreiber S, Talbot IC, Nicholls RJ, Gionchetti P, Campieri M, Kamm MA. 2004. Once daily high dose probiotic therapy (VSL#3) for maintaining remission in recurrent or refractory pouchitis. *Gut* **53:**108–114.

86. Kajander K, Myllyluoma E, Rajilić-Stojanović M, Kyrönpalo S, Rasmussen M, Järvenpää S, Zoetendal EG, de Vos WM, Vapaatalo H, Korpela R. 2008. Clinical trial: multispecies probiotic supplementation alleviates the symptoms of irritable bowel syndrome and stabilizes intestinal microbiota. *Aliment Pharmacol Ther* **27:**48–57.

87. O'Mahony L, McCarthy J, Kelly P, Hurley G, Luo F, Chen K, O'Sullivan GC, Kiely B, Collins JK, Shanahan F, Quigley EM. 2005. *Lactobacillus* and *bifidobacterium* in irritable bowel syndrome: symptom responses and relationship to cytokine profiles. *Gastroenterology* **128:**541–551.

88. Almeida CC, Lorena SL, Pavan CR, Akasaka HM, Mesquita MA. 2012. Beneficial effects of long-term consumption of a probiotic combination of *Lactobacillus casei* Shirota and *Bifidobacterium breve* Yakult may persist after suspension of therapy in lactose-intolerant patients. *Nutr Clin Pract* **27:**247–251.

89. Bogsan CSB, Ferreira L, Maldonado C, Perdigon G, Almeida SR, Oliveira MN. 2014. Fermented or unfermented milk using *Bifidobacterium animalis* subsp. *lactis* HN019: technological approach determines the probiotic modulation of mucosal cellular immunity. *Food Res Int* **64:**283–288.

90. Reid G. 2015. The growth potential for dairy probiotics. *Int Dairy J* **49:**16–22.

91. **Marsh AJ, Hill C, Ross RP, Cotter PD.** 2014. Fermented beverages with health-promoting potential: past and future perspectives. *Trends Food Sci Technol* **38**:113–124.

92. **Prasanna PHP, Grandison AS, Charalampopoulos D.** 2014. Bifidobacteria in milk products: an overview of physiological and biochemical properties, exopolysaccharide production, selection criteria of milk products and health benefits. *Food Res Int* **55**:247–262.

93. **Janer C, Arigoni F, Lee BH, Peláez C, Requena T.** 2005. Enzymatic ability of *Bifidobacterium animalis* subsp. *lactis* to hydrolyze milk proteins: identification and characterization of endopeptidase O. *Appl Environ Microbiol* **71**:8460–8465.

94. **Kehagias C, Csapó J, Konteles S, Kolokitha E, Koulouris S, Csapó-Kiss Z.** 2008. Support of growth and formation of D-amino acids by *Bifidobacterium longum* in cows', ewes', goats' milk and modified whey powder products. *Int Dairy J* **18**:396–402.

95. **Turroni F, Foroni E, Serafini F, Viappiani A, Montanini B, Bottacini F, Ferrarini A, Bacchini PL, Rota C, Delledonne M, Ottonello S, van Sinderen D, Ventura M.** 2011. Ability of *Bifidobacterium breve* to grow on different types of milk: exploring the metabolism of milk through genome analysis. *Appl Environ Microbiol* **77**:7408–7417.

96. **Serafini F, Turroni F, Ruas-Madiedo P, Lugli GA, Milani C, Duranti S, Zamboni N, Bottacini F, van Sinderen D, Margolles A, Ventura M.** 2014. Kefir fermented milk and kefiran promote growth of *Bifidobacterium bifidum* PRL2010 and modulate its gene expression. *Int J Food Microbiol* **178**:50–59.

97. **Hickey CD, Sheehan JJ, Wilkinson MG, Auty MA.** 2015. Growth and location of bacterial colonies within dairy foods using microscopy techniques: a review. *Front Microbiol* **6**:99.

98. **de los Reyes-Gavilán CG, Suárez A, Fernández-García A, Margolles A, Gueimonde M, Ruas-Madiedo P.** 2011. Adhesion of bile-adapted *Bifidobacterium* strains to the HT29-MTX cell line is modified after sequential gastrointestinal challenge simulated *in vitro* using human gastric and duodenal juices. *Res Microbiol* **162**:514–519.

99. **Veiga P, Pons N, Agrawal A, Oozeer R, Guyonnet D, Brazeilles R, Faurie JM, van Hylckama Vlieg JET, Houghton LA, Whorwell PJ, Ehrlich SD, Kennedy SP.** 2014. Changes of the human gut microbiome induced by a fermented milk product. *Sci Rep* **4**:6328.

100. **Gonzalez-Gonzalez C, Gibson T, Jauregi P.** 2013. Novel probiotic-fermented milk with angiotensin I-converting enzyme inhibitory peptides produced by *Bifidobacterium bifidum* MF 20/5. *Int J Food Microbiol* **167**:131–137.

101. **Lewis ZT, Shani G, Masarweh CF, Popovic M, Frese SA, Sela DA, Underwood MA, Mills DA.** 2016. Validating bifidobacterial species and subspecies identity in commercial probiotic products. *Pediatr Res* **79**:445–452.

102. **Hevia A, Milani C, López P, Cuervo A, Arboleya S, Duranti S, Turroni F, González S, Suárez A, Gueimonde M, Ventura M, Sánchez B, Margolles A.** 2014. Intestinal dysbiosis associated with systemic lupus erythematosus. *MBio* **5**:e01548-14.

103. **Dinan TG, Cryan JF.** 2017. Microbes, immunity and behaviour: psychoneuroimmunology meets the microbiome. *Neuropsychopharmacology* **42**:178–192.

104. **López P, González-Rodríguez I, Sánchez B, Gueimonde M, Margolles A, Suárez A.** 2012. Treg-inducing membrane vesicles from *Bifidobacterium bifidum* LMG13195 as potential adjuvants in immunotherapy. *Vaccine* **30**:825–829.

105. **López P, de Paz B, Rodríguez-Carrio J, Hevia A, Sánchez B, Margolles A, Suárez A.** 2016. Th17 responses and natural IgM antibodies are related to gut microbiota composition in systemic lupus erythematosus patients. *Sci Rep* **6**:24072.

106. **Sanders ME, Guarner F, Guerrant R, Holt PR, Quigley EMM, Sartor RB, Sherman PM, Mayer EA.** 2013. An update on the use and investigation of probiotics in health and disease. *Gut* **62**:787–796.

107. **WGO.** 2011. *World Gastroenterology Organisation Global Guidelines: Probiotics and Prebiotics:* http://www.worldgastroenterology.org/probiotics-prebiotics.html

108. **He T, Priebe MG, Zhong Y, Huang C, Harmsen HJM, Raangs GC, Antoine JM, Welling GW, Vonk RJ.** 2008. Effects of yogurt and bifidobacteria supplementation on the colonic microbiota in lactose-intolerant subjects. *J Appl Microbiol* **104**:595–604.

109. **Weizman Z, Asli G, Alsheikh A.** 2005. Effect of a probiotic infant formula on infections in child care centers: comparison of two probiotic agents. *Pediatrics* **115**:5–9.

110. **Corrêa NB, Péret Filho LA, Penna FJ, Lima FM, Nicoli JR.** 2005. A randomized formula controlled trial of *Bifidobacterium lactis* and *Streptococcus thermophilus* for prevention of antibiotic-associated diarrhea in infants. *J Clin Gastroenterol* **39**:385–389.

111. **Selinger CP, Bell A, Cairns A, Lockett M, Sebastian S, Haslam N.** 2013. Probiotic VSL#3 prevents antibiotic-associated diarrhoea in a

double-blind, randomized, placebo-controlled clinical trial. *J Hosp Infect* **84**:159–165.

112. **Plummer S, Weaver MA, Harris JC, Dee P, Hunter J.** 2004. *Clostridium difficile* pilot study: effects of probiotic supplementation on the incidence of *C. difficile* diarrhoea. *Int Microbiol* **7**:59–62.

113. **Goldenberg JZ, Ma SS, Saxton JD, Martzen MR, Vandvik PO, Thorlund K, Guyatt GH, Johnston BC.** 2013. Probiotics for the prevention of *Clostridium difficile*-associated diarrhea in adults and children. *Cochrane Database Syst Rev* **5**:CD006095.

114. **Agrawal M, Aroniadis OC, Brandt LJ, Kelly C, Freeman S, Surawicz C, Broussard E, Stollman N, Giovanelli A, Smith B, Yen E, Trivedi A, Hubble L, Kao D, Borody T, Finlayson S, Ray A, Smith R.** 2016. The long-term efficacy and safety of fecal microbiota transplant for recurrent, severe, and complicated *Clostridium difficile* infection in 146 elderly individuals. *J Clin Gastroenterol* **50**:403–407.

115. **Khoruts A, Sadowsky MJ.** 2016. Understanding the mechanisms of faecal microbiota transplantation. *Nat Rev Gastroenterol Hepatol* **13**:508–516.

116. **Hevia A, Delgado S, Margolles A, Sánchez B.** 2015. Application of density gradient for the isolation of the fecal microbial stool component and the potential use thereof. *Sci Rep* **5**:16807.

117. **Li BZ, Threapleton DE, Wang JY, Xu JM, Yuan JQ, Zhang C, Li P, Ye QL, Guo B, Mao C, Ye DQ.** 2015. Comparative effectiveness and tolerance of treatments for *Helicobacter pylori*: systematic review and network meta-analysis. *BMJ* **351**:h4052.

118. **Boltin D.** 2016. Probiotics in *Helicobacter pylori*-induced peptic ulcer disease. *Best Pract Res Clin Gastroenterol* **30**:99–109.

119. **Talebi Bezmin Abadi A.** 2016. Vaccine against *Helicobacter pylori*: inevitable approach. *World J Gastroenterol* **22**:3150–3157.

120. **Lu C, Sang J, He H, Wan X, Lin Y, Li L, Li Y, Yu C.** 2016. Probiotic supplementation does not improve eradication rate of *Helicobacter pylori* infection compared to placebo based on standard therapy: a meta-analysis. *Sci Rep* **6**:23522.

121. **Miki K, Urita Y, Ishikawa F, Iino T, Shibahara-Sone H, Akahoshi R, Mizusawa S, Nose A, Nozaki D, Hirano K, Nonaka C, Yokokura T.** 2007. Effect of *Bifidobacterium bifidum* fermented milk on *Helicobacter pylori* and serum pepsinogen levels in humans. *J Dairy Sci* **90**:2630–2640.

122. **Sheu BS, Cheng HC, Kao AW, Wang ST, Yang YJ, Yang HB, Wu JJ.** 2006. Pretreatment with *Lactobacillus*- and *Bifidobacterium*-containing yogurt can improve the efficacy of quadruple therapy in eradicating residual *Helicobacter pylori* infection after failed triple therapy. *Am J Clin Nutr* **83**:864–869.

123. **Wang KY, Li SN, Liu CS, Perng DS, Su YC, Wu DC, Jan CM, Lai CH, Wang TN, Wang WM.** 2004. Effects of ingesting *Lactobacillus*- and *Bifidobacterium*-containing yogurt in subjects with colonized *Helicobacter pylori*. *Am J Clin Nutr* **80**:737–741.

124. **Raisch J, Rolhion N, Dubois A, Darfeuille-Michaud A, Bringer MA.** 2015. Intracellular colon cancer-associated *Escherichia coli* promote protumoral activities of human macrophages by inducing sustained COX 2 expression. *Lab Invest* **95**:296–307.

125. **Yu J, Chen Y, Fu X, Zhou X, Peng Y, Shi L, Chen T, Wu Y.** 2016. Invasive *Fusobacterium nucleatum* may play a role in the carcinogenesis of proximal colon cancer through the serrated neoplasia pathway. *Int J Cancer* **139**:1318–1326.

126. **Roller M, Clune Y, Collins K, Rechkemmer G, Watzl B.** 2007. Consumption of prebiotic inulin enriched with oligofructose in combination with the probiotics *Lactobacillus rhamnosus* and *Bifidobacterium lactis* has minor effects on selected immune parameters in polypectomised and colon cancer patients. *Br J Nutr* **97**:676–684.

127. **Worthley DL, Le Leu RK, Whitehall VL, Conlon M, Christophersen C, Belobrajdic D, Mallitt KA, Hu Y, Irahara N, Ogino S, Leggett BA, Young GP.** 2009. A human, double-blind, placebo-controlled, crossover trial of prebiotic, probiotic, and synbiotic supplementation: effects on luminal, inflammatory, epigenetic, and epithelial biomarkers of colorectal cancer. *Am J Clin Nutr* **90**:578–586.

128. **Rafter J, Bennett M, Caderni G, Clune Y, Hughes R, Karlsson PC, Klinder A, O'Riordan M, O'Sullivan GC, Pool-Zobel B, Rechkemmer G, Roller M, Rowland I, Salvadori M, Thijs H, Van Loo J, Watzl B, Collins JK.** 2007. Dietary synbiotics reduce cancer risk factors in polypectomized and colon cancer patients. *Am J Clin Nutr* **85**:488–496.

129. **Liu ZH, Huang MJ, Zhang XW, Wang L, Huang NQ, Peng H, Lan P, Peng JS, Yang Z, Xia Y, Liu WJ, Yang J, Qin HL, Wang JP.** 2013. The effects of perioperative probiotic treatment on serum zonulin concentration and subsequent postoperative infectious complications after colorectal cancer surgery: a double-center and double-blind randomized clinical trial. *Am J Clin Nutr* **97**:117–126.

130. Liu Z, Li C, Huang M, Tong C, Zhang X, Wang L, Peng H, Lan P, Zhang P, Huang N, Peng J, Wu X, Luo Y, Qin H, Kang L, Wang J. 2015. Positive regulatory effects of perioperative probiotic treatment on postoperative liver complications after colorectal liver metastases surgery: a double-center and double-blind randomized clinical trial. *BMC Gastroenterol* **15:**34.

131. Zhang JW, Du P, Gao J, Yang BR, Fang WJ, Ying CM. 2012. Preoperative probiotics decrease postoperative infectious complications of colorectal cancer. *Am J Med Sci* **343:**199–205.

132. Wada M, Nagata S, Saito M, Shimizu T, Yamashiro Y, Matsuki T, Asahara T, Nomoto K. 2010. Effects of the enteral administration of *Bifidobacterium breve* on patients undergoing chemotherapy for pediatric malignancies. *Support Care Cancer* **18:**751–759.

133. Ambalam P, Raman M, Purama RK, Doble M. 2016. Probiotics, prebiotics and colorectal cancer prevention. *Best Pract Res Clin Gastroenterol* **30:**119–131.

134. Ma YY, Li L, Yu CH, Shen Z, Chen LH, Li YM. 2013. Effects of probiotics on nonalcoholic fatty liver disease: a meta-analysis. *World J Gastroenterol* **19:**6911–6918.

135. Lo RS, Austin AS, Freeman JG. 2014. Is there a role for probiotics in liver disease? *Scientific World Journal* **2014:**874768.

136. Waller PA, Gopal PK, Leyer GJ, Ouwehand AC, Reifer C, Stewart ME, Miller LE. 2011. Dose-response effect of *Bifidobacterium lactis* HN019 on whole gut transit time and functional gastrointestinal symptoms in adults. *Scand J Gastroenterol* **46:**1057–1064.

137. Agrawal A, Houghton LA, Morris J, Reilly B, Guyonnet D, Goupil Feuillerat N, Schlumberger A, Jakob S, Whorwell PJ. 2009. Clinical trial: the effects of a fermented milk product containing *Bifidobacterium lactis* DN-173 010 on abdominal distension and gastrointestinal transit in irritable bowel syndrome with constipation. *Aliment Pharmacol Ther* **29:**104–114.

138. Guyonnet D, Chassany O, Ducrotte P, Picard C, Mouret M, Mercier CH, Matuchansky C. 2007. Effect of a fermented milk containing *Bifidobacterium animalis* DN-173 010 on the health-related quality of life and symptoms in irritable bowel syndrome in adults in primary care: a multicentre, randomized, double-blind, controlled trial. *Aliment Pharmacol Ther* **26:**475–486.

139. Groeger D, O'Mahony L, Murphy EF, Bourke JF, Dinan TG, Kiely B, Shanahan F, Quigley EM. 2013. *Bifidobacterium infantis* 35624 modulates host inflammatory processes beyond the gut. *Gut Microbes* **4:**325–339.

140. Kajander K, Hatakka K, Poussa T, Färkkilä M, Korpela R. 2005. A probiotic mixture alleviates symptoms in irritable bowel syndrome patients: a controlled 6-month intervention. *Aliment Pharmacol Ther* **22:**387–394.

141. Moayyedi P, Ford AC, Talley NJ, Cremonini F, Foxx-Orenstein AE, Brandt LJ, Quigley EM. 2010. The efficacy of probiotics in the treatment of irritable bowel syndrome: a systematic review. *Gut* **59:**325–332.

142. Guandalini S, Magazzù G, Chiaro A, La Balestra V, Di Nardo G, Gopalan S, Sibal A, Romano C, Canani RB, Lionetti P, Setty M. 2010. VSL#3 improves symptoms in children with irritable bowel syndrome: a multicenter, randomized, placebo-controlled, double-blind, crossover study. *J Pediatr Gastroenterol Nutr* **51:**24–30.

143. Distrutti E, Monaldi L, Ricci P, Fiorucci S. 2016. Gut microbiota role in irritable bowel syndrome: new therapeutic strategies. *World J Gastroenterol* **22:**2219–2241.

144. Sood A, Midha V, Makharia GK, Ahuja V, Singal D, Goswami P, Tandon RK. 2009. The probiotic preparation, VSL#3 induces remission in patients with mild-to-moderately active ulcerative colitis. *Clin Gastroenterol Hepatol* **7:**1202–1209e1.

145. Tursi A, Brandimarte G, Papa A, Giglio A, Elisei W, Giorgetti GM, Forti G, Morini S, Hassan C, Pistoia MA, Modeo ME, Rodino' S, D'Amico T, Sebkova L, Sacca' N, Di Giulio E, Luzza F, Imeneo M, Larussa T, Di Rosa S, Annese V, Danese S, Gasbarrini A. 2010. Treatment of relapsing mild-to-moderate ulcerative colitis with the probiotic VSL#3 as adjunctive to a standard pharmaceutical treatment: a double-blind, randomized, placebo-controlled study. *Am J Gastroenterol* **105:**2218–2227.

146. Lin HC, Su BH, Chen AC, Lin TW, Tsai CH, Yeh TF, Oh W. 2005. Oral probiotics reduce the incidence and severity of necrotizing enterocolitis in very low birth weight infants. *Pediatrics* **115:**1–4.

147. Lin HC, Hsu CH, Chen HL, Chung MY, Hsu JF, Lien RI, Tsao LY, Chen CH, Su BH. 2008. Oral probiotics prevent necrotizing enterocolitis in very low birth weight preterm infants: a multicenter, randomized, controlled trial. *Pediatrics* **122:**693–700.

148. Bin-Nun A, Bromiker R, Wilschanski M, Kaplan M, Rudensky B, Caplan M, Hammerman C. 2005. Oral probiotics prevent necrotizing enterocolitis in very low birth weight neonates. *J Pediatr* **147:**192–196.

149. Costeloe K, Hardy P, Juszczak E, Wilks M, Millar MR, Probiotics in Preterm Infants

Study Collaborative Group. 2016. *Bifidobacterium breve* BBG-001 in very preterm infants: a randomised controlled phase 3 trial. *Lancet* **387**:649–660.

150. **Zuercher AW, Fritsché R, Corthésy B, Mercenier A.** 2006. Food products and allergy development, prevention and treatment. *Curr Opin Biotechnol* **17**:198–203.

151. **Palomares O, Yaman G, Azkur AK, Akkoc T, Akdis M, Akdis CA.** 2010. Role of Treg in immune regulation of allergic diseases. *Eur J Immunol* **40**:1232–1240.

152. **Toh ZQ, Anzela A, Tang MLK, Licciardi PV.** 2012. Probiotic therapy as a novel approach for allergic disease. *Front Pharmacol* **3**:171.

153. **Sistek D, Kelly R, Wickens K, Stanley T, Fitzharris P, Crane J.** 2006. Is the effect of probiotics on atopic dermatitis confined to food sensitized children? *Clin Exp Allergy* **36**:629–633.

154. **Gerasimov SV, Vasjuta VV, Myhovych OO, Bondarchuk LI.** 2010. Probiotic supplement reduces atopic dermatitis in preschool children: a randomized, double-blind, placebo-controlled, clinical trial. *Am J Clin Dermatol* **11**:351–361.

155. **Yeşilova Y, Çalka Ö, Akdeniz N, Berktaş M.** 2012. Effect of probiotics on the treatment of children with atopic dermatitis. *Ann Dermatol* **24**:189–193.

156. **van der Aa LB, Heymans HS, van Aalderen WM, Sillevis Smitt JH, Knol J, Ben Amor K, Goossens DA, Sprikkelman AB, Synbad Study Group.** 2010. Effect of a new synbiotic mixture on atopic dermatitis in infants: a randomized-controlled trial. *Clin Exp Allergy* **40**:795–804.

157. **Singh A, Hacini-Rachinel F, Gosoniu ML, Bourdeau T, Holvoet S, Doucet-Ladeveze R, Beaumont M, Mercenier A, Nutten S.** 2013. Immune-modulatory effect of probiotic *Bifidobacterium lactis* NCC2818 in individuals suffering from seasonal allergic rhinitis to grass pollen: an exploratory, randomized, placebo-controlled clinical trial. *Eur J Clin Nutr* **67**:161–167.

158. **Xiao JZ, Kondo S, Yanagisawa N, Takahashi N, Odamaki T, Iwabuchi N, Iwatsuki K, Kokubo S, Togashi H, Enomoto K, Enomoto T.** 2006. Effect of probiotic *Bifidobacterium longum* BB536 [corrected] in relieving clinical symptoms and modulating plasma cytokine levels of Japanese cedar pollinosis during the pollen season. A randomized double-blind, placebo-controlled trial. *J Investig Allergol Clin Immunol* **16**:86–93.

159. **Huurre A, Laitinen K, Rautava S, Korkeamari M, Isoulari E.** 2008. Impact of maternal atopy and probiotic supplementation during pregnancy on infant sensibilization: a double-blind placebo-controlled study. *Clin Exp Allergy* **38**:1342–1348.

160. **Dotterud CK, Storrø O, Johnsen R, Oien T.** 2010. Probiotics in pregnant women to prevent allergic disease: a randomized, double-blind trial. *Br J Dermatol* **163**:616–623.

161. **Wickens K, Black PN, Stanley TV, Mitchell E, Fitzharris P, Tannock GW, Purdie G, Crane J, Probiotic Study Group.** 2008. A differential effect of 2 probiotics in the prevention of eczema and atopy: a double-blind, randomized, placebo-controlled trial. *J Allergy Clin Immunol* **122**:788–794.

162. **Kukkonen K, Savilahti E, Haahtela T, Juntunen-Backman K, Korpela R, Poussa T, Tuure T, Kuitunen M.** 2007. Probiotics and prebiotic galacto-oligosaccharides in the prevention of allergic diseases: a randomized, double-blind, placebo-controlled trial. *J Allergy Clin Immunol* **119**:192–198.

163. **Kim JY, Kwon JH, Ahn SH, Lee SI, Han YS, Choi YO, Lee SY, Ahn KM, Ji GE.** 2010. Effect of probiotic mix (*Bifidobacterium bifidum*, *Bifidobacterium lactis*, *Lactobacillus acidophilus*) in the primary prevention of eczema: a double-blind, randomized, placebo-controlled trial. *Pediatr Allergy Immunol* **21**(2p2):e386–e393.

164. **Niers L, Martín R, Rijkers G, Sengers F, Timmerman H, van Uden N, Smidt H, Kimpen J, Hoekstra M.** 2009. The effects of selected probiotic strains on the development of eczema (the PandA study). *Allergy* **64**:1349–1358.

165. **Soh SE, Aw M, Gerez I, Chong YS, Rauff M, Ng YP, Wong HB, Pai N, Lee BW, Shek LP.** 2009. Probiotic supplementation in the first 6 months of life in at risk Asian infants–effects on eczema and atopic sensitization at the age of 1 year. *Clin Exp Allergy* **39**:571–578.

166. **Fiocchi A, Pawankar R, Cuello-Garcia C, Ahn K, Al-Hammadi S, Agarwal A, Beyer K, Burks W, Canonica GW, Ebisawa M, Gandhi S, Kamenwa R, Lee BW, Li H, Prescott S, Riva JJ, Rosenwasser L, Sampson H, Spigler M, Terracciano L, Vereda-Ortiz A, Waserman S, Yepes-Nuñez JJ, Brożek JL, Schünemann HJ.** 2015. World Allergy Organization-McMaster University Guidelines for Allergic Disease Prevention (GLAD-P): probiotics. *World Allergy Organ J* **8**:4.

167. **Ruas-Madiedo P, Zoon P.** 2003. Effect of exopolysaccharide-producing *Lactococcus lactis* strains and temperature on the permeability of skim milk gels. *Colloids Surf A Physicochem Eng Asp* **213**:245–253.

168. **Marteau P, Guyonnet D, Lafaye de Micheaux P, Gelu S.** 2013. A randomized, double-blind,

controlled study and pooled analysis of two identical trials of fermented milk containing probiotic *Bifidobacterium lactis* CNCM I-2494 in healthy women reporting minor digestive symptoms. *Neurogastroenterol Motil* **25:**331–e252.

169. Whorwell PJ, Altringer L, Morel J, Bond Y, Charbonneau D, O'Mahony L, Kiely B, Shanahan F, Quigley EM. 2006. Efficacy of an encapsulated probiotic *Bifidobacterium infantis* 35624 in women with irritable bowel syndrome. *Am J Gastroenterol* **101:**1581–1590.

170. Drouault-Holowacz S, Bieuvelet S, Burckel A, Cazaubiel M, Dray X, Marteau P. 2008. A double blind randomized controlled trial of a probiotic combination in 100 patients with irritable bowel syndrome. *Gastroenterol Clin Biol* **32:**147–152.

171. Ishikawa H, Matsumoto S, Ohashi Y, Imaoka A, Setoyama H, Umesaki Y, Tanaka R, Otani T. 2011. Beneficial effects of probiotic bifidobacterium and galacto-oligosaccharide in patients with ulcerative colitis: a randomized controlled study. *Digestion* **84:**128–133.

172. Gionchetti P, Rizzello F, Helwig U, Venturi A, Lammers KM, Brigidi P, Vitali B, Poggioli G, Miglioli M, Campieri M. 2003. Prophylaxis of pouchitis onset with probiotic therapy: a double-blind, placebo-controlled trial. *Gastroenterology* **124:**1202–1209.

173. Pronio A, Montesani C, Butteroni C, Vecchione S, Mumolo G, Vestri A, Vitolo D, Boirivant M. 2008. Probiotic administration in patients with ileal pouch-anal anastomosis for ulcerative colitis is associated with expansion of mucosal regulatory cells. *Inflamm Bowel Dis* **14:**662–668.

B. NEXT-GENERATION BACTERIOTHERAPY: OPPORTUNITIES IN CHRONIC DISEASES

Microbial Interactions and Interventions in Colorectal Cancer

4

TERENCE VAN RAAY[1] and EMMA ALLEN-VERCOE[1]

INTRODUCTION

Colorectal cancer (CRC), the most common form of gastrointestinal (GI) tract cancer, is globally the third leading cause of cancer and is associated with significant mortality (1). Approximately 90% of CRC cases are sporadic, caused by somatic mutations leading to the progression of invasive carcinomas (2). There are numerous risk factors associated with the development of CRC, and the disease is more common in industrialized countries than it is in the developing world (1). Poor diet (in particular, a diet that is low in fiber and high in fat) appears to be a major influencing factor for disease development and progression, and recently it has been recognized that gut microbes may act as the interface between dietary factors and tumor development (reviewed in reference 3). This chapter will review the pathways that lead to CRC, what is currently known about microbial involvement in these processes, and how these may be manipulated therapeutically.

THE HOST SIDE: PHYSIOLOGY AND DEVELOPMENT IN COLORECTAL CANCER

In order to understand the pathogenesis of CRC and how this is affected by the microbiota, it is important to first understand something of the normal biology

[1]Molecular and Cellular Biology, University of Guelph, 50 Stone Road East, Guelph, Ontario, N1G 2W1, Canada
Bugs as Drugs: Therapeutic Microbes for the Prevention and Treatment of Disease
Edited by Robert A. Britton and Patrice D. Cani
© 2018 American Society for Microbiology, Washington, DC
doi:10.1128/microbiolspec.BAD-0004-2016

of the colon, as well as what is understood about how CRC can arise through mutations and aberrant signaling pathways. The salient points are thus reviewed below, and Fig. 1 is provided as a guide to the physiology and anatomy of the colon to orientate the reader.

COLONIC CRYPT

Makeup of the Colon Epithelium

There are numerous reviews on intestinal crypt stem cells (4–6), and so we mention only the more salient points here. The basic unit of the colon consists of a crypt and the luminal surface. During homeostasis, the colonic crypt contains 14 to 16 multipotent stem cells marked by the transmembrane protein LGR5 (Leu-rich repeat-containing G protein-coupled receptor 5) that are capable of generating all of the differentiated cell types lining the lumen (7, 8). A major difference between the small intestine crypt and the colonic crypt is the absence of Paneth cells in the latter, which intercalate with the LGR5$^+$ cells in the small intestine. The LGR5$^+$ stem cells generate rapidly proliferating transit-amplifying (TA) cells that occupy the approximate top two-thirds of the crypt. These TA cells will differentiate into primarily four differentiated cell types: goblet cells (mucosecreting cells), enteroendocrine cells (hormone-producing cells), absorptive enterocytes, and tuft cells (prostanoid-secreting cells) (4). The majority of these cells are renewed approximately once per week, a rate that provides a sense of the regenerative capacity of the stem cells.

Colonic Crypt Signaling Pathways

There are several signaling pathways that are involved in the proliferation and differentiation of the colonic crypt stem cells (9), but the major players are the Wnt signaling pathway, which maintains the stem cells in the base of the crypt, the Notch-Delta signaling pathway, which aids in specifying progenitors of either the secretory or absorptive fates (10, 11), and the bone morphogenic protein (BMP) signaling pathway, which is involved in differentiation and antagonism of Wnt signaling. For the purposes of this review, the Wnt signaling pathway seems to be the most critical with respect to homeostasis of the intestinal crypt stem cells and its malignant transformation (12). Under normal conditions, the essential signaling pathway involves a Wnt ligand activating the frizzled and LRP5/6 receptors, which in turn activates the scaffolding protein dishevelled, which inhibits the β-catenin destruction complex (Fig. 2A). The main components of this destruction complex consist of the scaffolding proteins adenomatous polyposis coli (APC) and axin and the kinases casein kinase 1 (CK1) and glycogen synthase 3β (GSK3β). In the absence of a Wnt ligand, this destruction complex is charged with seeking out and destroying cytoplasmic β-catenin. Upon its inhibition, β-catenin will accumulate in the nucleus, where it will interact with transcription factors T-cell factor/lymphoid enhancer factor (TCF/Lef) and activate downstream target genes (13).

In addition to cytoplasmic β-catenin involved in Wnt signaling, there is a membrane pool of β-catenin that interacts with the transmembrane protein E-cadherin to form the adherens junction in many differentiated epithelial cells as well as in stem and progenitor cells along the crypt axis. It has been demonstrated that loss of E-cadherin or its substitution with N-cadherin in the intestinal crypt results in increased levels of cytoplasmic and nuclear β-catenin at the expense of the membrane pool (Fig. 2A and B) (14–16).

The major transcriptional targets of the Wnt pathway in the intestinal crypt stem cells are the transmembrane serpentine receptor LGR5, which is a definitive marker of the intestinal stem cell (7), the oncogene Myc, which inhibits differentiation, and the basic helix-loop-helix (bHLH) transcription factor Achaete-Scute Like 2 (ASCL2), which

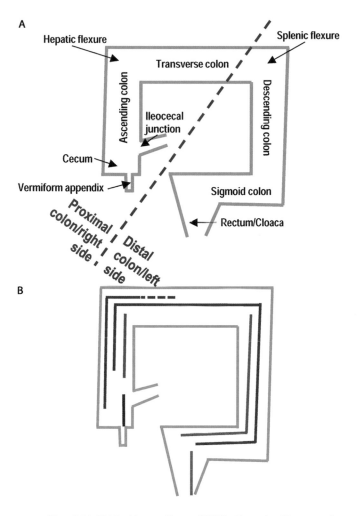

FIGURE 1 (A) Schematic of the anatomy of the human colon, indicating right/proximal and left/distal regions and their designations. (B) Depiction of the overlap between development, innervation, vascularization, and tumorigenesis of the human colon. Abbreviations: superscript c, chick; superscript m, mouse; superscript z, zebrafish; PMF, parasympathetic motor fibers; SMF, sympathetic motor fibers; SF, sensory fibers.

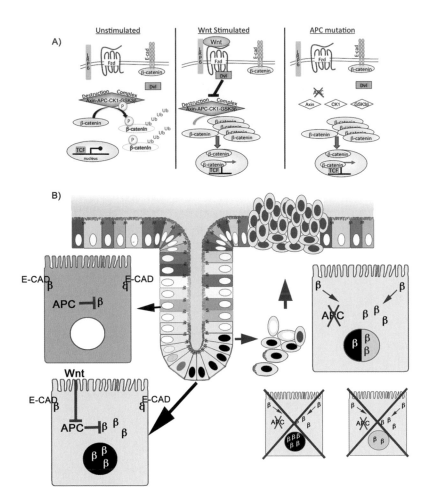

FIGURE 2 Colonic crypt and aberrant Wnt signaling. (A) Model of Wnt signaling. In the absence of Wnt-ligand stimulation, the central signaling molecule β-catenin is degraded and Wnt target genes remain silent (left). In the presence of Wnt ligand-mediated signaling, β-catenin becomes stabilized, resulting in cytoplasmic and nuclear accumulation and active transcription of Wnt target genes (center). APC mutations disrupt the destruction complex resulting in constitutively active Wnt signaling (right). Under normal circumstances, β-catenin-E-cadherin-mediated cell adhesion is not thought to have a role in Wnt signaling. (B) The left side of the crypt depicts normal development. Black nuclei represent β-catenin-positive stem cells, with varying gray scale levels representing decreasing Wnt signaling, which is shut down (white nuclei) as the precursor cells differentiate. Colors represent the four major lineages of the colonic epithelium, with lighter colors representing less differentiated forms in the colonic crypt. On the right side, a mutation in APC renders the Wnt signaling pathway constitutively active, resulting in the proliferation of stem cells that become hyperplastic, eventually forming polyps on the luminal surface. Wnt signaling inhibits mucin-2 synthesis, possibly generating the nonmucinous phenotype characteristic of distal cancers. It is expected that cells in the polyp would consist of a heterogenous mixture of cells, some more differentiated (with less nuclear β-catenin) than others. The selection of APC alleles to generate the just-right amount of Wnt signaling results in the elimination of cells with too much or too little β-catenin signaling. The loss of E-cadherin (E-CAD) could have a role in generating this "just-right" amount of signaling.

is involved in stem cell self-renewal (reviewed in reference 9). In addition to Wnt target gene activation, it is important to remember that one of the main readouts of active Wnt signaling is the nuclear accumulation of β-catenin. As the colonic stem cells migrate into the TA pool of progenitors, they begin to lose their dependence on Wnt signaling and instead become dependent on BMP signaling, which inhibits Wnt signaling to induce differentiation and eventually apoptosis of the luminal epithelial cells (Fig. 2B) (17).

Proximal and Distal Colon

While the Wnt, notch, BMP, hedgehog (HH), and epidermal growth factor (EGF) signaling pathways are the major players in the crypt-villus axis throughout the intestine, there are significant differences in the architecture, cell types, level of signaling, and extracellular matrix between the small and large intestines and between proximal and distal regions within each of these structures. As a prime example, the small intestine contains villi, while the colon has a flat architecture. Also, Paneth cells, which are located at the base of the crypt and secrete antimicrobial agents in the small intestine, are absent in the colon (18). Within the colon, there are also proximal and distal differences at many levels that may influence how the microbiome interacts with the cells and cancers in these different domains. Below, we describe some of the more important differences between the proximal and distal regions of the colon, with a more comprehensive list in Table 1.

Crypt Architecture

The crypt length and cell number per crypt column are significantly larger in the distal colon than in the proximal colon in both humans and rats (19, 20). While overall cell proliferation does not change between proximal and distal colon, there was a difference in the proliferation of cells at the base of

the crypt, with the crypts of the distal colon undergoing higher proliferation rates in rats (20). It is unknown if the same is true in human colonic crypt cells, but the distribution of proliferating cells was similar for the two domains along the crypt axis (19).

Wnt Signaling

As mentioned above, Wnt signaling within the colonic crypt cells gives rise to all of the different cell types of the luminal epithelial cells. However, there are significant differences in the level of Wnt signaling between proximal and distal colon. A comprehensive study by Leedham et al. (21) found significant differences along the entire axis of the small and large intestines. Specific to the colon, they found differences in the levels of Wnt signaling in the proximal-distal axis that were opposite for mouse and human. In mouse, they found an increase in basal Wnt signaling and stem cell number from proximal to distal regions, whereas this was reversed in humans. In humans, the decrease in distal Wnt signaling correlated with the high expression of the Wnt antagonists secreted frizzled related protein (SFRP) and BMP2 and the low expression of the Wnt agonists hepatocyte growth factor (HGF) and Grem1/2 in the distal colon (21).

Goblet Cells and Mucin

Mucin-2 (Muc2) is a highly glycosylated, gel-forming mucin that is the major mucin component in the colon. Two layers of Muc2 exist, with a compact stratified layer forming against the epithelium that is impermeable to bacteria and a looser but thicker layer of Muc2 as an outer layer that is the habitat for the commensal bacteria (22–24). An investigation by Ermund et al. (22) found that the size of the mucus layer differed along the length of the colon, with the distal colon having a thicker and more continuous inner layer than the proximal region. This is consistent with a proteomics screen that found

TABLE 1 Comparison of characteristics across regions[a] of the colon

Study	Class	Category 1	Category 2	Category 3
Glebov et al. (184)	1,000 differentially expressed genes	30% highly expressed	70% highly expressed	
	Chemistry	Genes associated with inorganic chemicals; Genes associated with heterocyclic compounds, polycyclic hydrocarbon, and steroids (protection against procarcinogenic heterocyclic compounds)		Organic chemicals (carboxylic acids and acyclic acids)
	Cell cycle and metabolism		Cell cycle and DNA metabolism groups overexpressed:	
Pekow et al. (185)	miRNAs	miRNA-143, miRNA-145 overexpressed		
	Targets of miRNA-143/145	Low	High	
van der Post and Hansson (25)	Proteins	Metabolism, absorption of nutrients, lipid metabolism; antigen presentation; butyrate transport; amino acid transporters and glucose transporter; organic solute transporter subunit alpha (for bile); chloride secretion proteins; goblet cell-mediated bicarbonate transport	Glycosyltransferases for O-glycosylation, oxidative phosphorylation, carbohydrate metabolism, small molecule transport	
Ermund et al. (22)	Mucin	Partially penetrable to bacterium-sized beads	Impenetrable to bacterium-sized beads	
	Mucin thickness	Inner layer is thinner	Inner layer is thicker and more continuous	
	Mucin	Rich in sialomucin	Rich in sulfomucin	
Filipe and Branfoot (186)	Mucin antigens			
Bara et al. (44)	Mucin antigens			M1, no reactions; M3, stains goblet cells
Lee et al. (39)	Immunology	High	Low	
Noble et al. (187)	Developmental genes		HoxA13, HoxB13 Gli1 Gli3	
MacFarlane et al. (82)	Microbial metabolism	Saccharolytic with production of SCFAs	Proteolytic, with production of nitrogenous compounds	
Aguirre de Cárcer et al. (83)	Abundance of specific bacterial groups	*Streptococcus*, *Enterococcus*, and *Corynebacterium* spp. and *Comamonadaceae*	*Enterobacteriaceae*	

[a]Categories: 1, higher in proximal than distal colon; 2, higher in distal than proximal colon; 3, no change from proximal to distal colon.

higher amounts of O-glycosylation in the distal colon from human biopsies (25) and a higher number of goblet cells in the distal colon in humans (19), although the opposite was found in rat (20).

Development of the Proximal and Distal Colon

Several studies have looked at the molecular and cellular differences between the proximal and distal colon, which clearly identify that these two domains are physiologically different (Table 1). These differences are further supported by and mirror the development of the colon (Fig. 1). At the end of gastrulation, the posterior endoderm that will generate the small and large intestines is a single layer of cells that are patterned by the transcription factor Cdx2. Tubulogenesis is initiated at both ends of the sheet by the formation of ventrally directed pockets termed the anterior and caudal intestinal portals (reviewed in reference 26). The anterior and caudal intestinal portals grow towards each other until tubulogenesis is complete. By embryonic day 14 in the mouse, the endoderm cells have differentiated into columnar epithelium and the gut tube has been subdivided along the anterior-posterior axis, with the cecum being an easily identifiable structure separating the large and small intestines (27, 28). There are many genes and signaling pathways that are involved in patterning the anterior-posterior intestinal axis, including fibroblast growth factor, Wnts, sonic hedgehog, BMPs, and Hox genes (28–30). Most of these signaling pathways are active in the colon crypt of the adult in the proliferation, specification, and differentiation of the stem cells. However, the pattern of Hox gene expression best represents the presence of a future proximal and distal colon (31). The Hox gene expression pattern most likely sets up subsequent developmental processes, such as vascularization and innervation, which physically define the proximal colon and distal colon.

The proximal colon consists of the cecum, ascending colon, and approximately two-thirds of the transverse colon and is supplied by the superior mesenteric artery and innervated by the vagus nerve and superior mesenteric ganglion. The distal colon includes the remainder of the transverse colon, the descending colon, the sigmoid colon, and the rectum and is supplied by the inferior mesenteric artery and innervated by sacral nerves 2 to 4 and inferior mesenteric ganglion. The rectum is separately innervated by the inferior hypogastric plexus (Fig. 1).

COLORECTAL CANCER

Introduction

The initiating event in greater than 90% of all sporadic CRCs is the inactivation of the β-catenin destruction complex, typically by mutations in APC (32–34). These mutations occur within the crypt base stem cells and result in constitutively active Wnt signaling demonstrated by high levels of cytoplasmic and nuclear β-catenin (35). This event establishes the cancer stem cell, which is acted upon by other agents to eventually transform into adenocarcinomas (Fig. 2). For example, there is evidence that the breakdown of membrane E-cadherin releases β-catenin from the membrane to then activate the Wnt pathway, which appears to accelerate the formation of Wnt-induced cancers in mice (15). In addition, the accumulation of these cancer stem cells will form precancerous adenomas that can transform into adenocarcinomas and malignant carcinomas by the accumulation of mutations in KRAS, P53, and transforming growth factor, although these are not universal events in CRCs (36). Similarly, by histology, 80 to 90% of CRCs have a nonmucinous histology, while 10 to 20% have a mucinous histology and most, but not all, have chromosome instability, but only a few have microsatellite instability (MSI) (37). Essentially, not all CRCs are created equal, but until recently all have fallen under the broad umbrella of simply "CRC." While aberrant Wnt signaling is at the root cause of most, if not all, CRCs, there is increasing evidence that there are significant differences in the etiology of cancers on the proximal versus distal parts of the colon. Based on the development, architecture, and physiological differences between the proximal and distal colon, perhaps it should not be unexpected that the cancers located in these regions should be any different.

Proximal versus Distal Colorectal Cancers

There is now substantial evidence that CRC should be clinically divided between proximal and distal based on genetic, epigenetic, morphological, and physiological criteria (Table 2) (38–41). Here, we highlight elements that might be relevant to the gut microbiota. Proximal tumors have an incidence rate of 42% in the United States, but this number is steadily increasing (39). Genetically, proximal tumors consist mostly of microsatellite instable tumors (MSI[+]), in which the mismatch repair genes are mutated (MLH1 and/or MSH2 genes) or inactivated by methylation of the CpG islands in their promoter (positive for CpG island methyla-

tor phenotype [CIMP[+]]). As a result, these tumors are hypermutated, with most containing B-Raf proto-oncogene, serine/threonine kinase (BRAF) mutations (32). Proximal tumors also have a hyperactivated immune response and poor survival compared to distal tumors (42). However, they can also harbor APC mutations, β-catenin-activating mutations, or Axin2 mutations (43). Histologically, proximal tumors are poorly differentiated and have an excess mucinous phenotype and high tumor grade compared to distal tumors (44, 45).

In contrast, distal tumors have a higher incidence (51% of CRCs) than do proximal tumors, but their incidence is decreasing relative to proximal tumors (39). Distal tumors are typically well differentiated; smaller and diagnosed earlier than proximal tumors, their relative numbers are decreasing (reviewed in reference 41). They typically do not have the mucinous phenotype. The vast majority of distal tumors have mutations in APC, which ultimately promotes Wnt/β-catenin signaling (46). Higher levels of Wnt signaling in distal CRC may inhibit the mucinous phenotype, as it has been found that Sox9, a target of the Wnt/β-catenin

TABLE 2 Common elements that distinguish proximal from distal colorectal cancers[a]

Element	Proximal tumors	Distal tumors	Reference(s)
Histology	Mucinous, undifferentiated, larger diameter, exophytic	Nonmucinous, well differentiated, smaller	37, 41, 44
Clinical features	Higher T-stage; higher tumor grade; poorer prognosis; proportion of proximal CRCs is increasing	Lower T-stage; lower tumor grade; better prognosis; present with obstructive symptoms; proportion of distal CRCs is decreasing	37, 39, 41
Genetics	Hypermutated, most with BRAF mutations, many with Wnt pathway mutations and mismatch repair gene mutations, MSI-high; CIMP; diploid genome	Aneuploid genome, MSS; most with mutation in APC, activation of Wnt target genes	32, 37, 41, 42
Immune system	Activation of many immune genes; immune infiltration signature	Not activated	37, 42
APC mutant alleles	Total of 2 or 3 β-catenin binding domains	Total of 0 to 1 β-catenin binding domain	21, 43, 46, 188
Protein expression bias	CD44s; TOPK, E-cadherin, Muc2, p21, CD68	CDX2, β-catenin	37

[a]Abbreviations: MSI, microsatellite instable; MSS, microsatellite stable; CRC, colorectal cancer; CIMP, CpG island methylator phenotype.

pathway, inhibits the expression of Muc2, the major component of the extracellular mucins (47).

Wnt Signaling in Proximal versus Distal CRC

As mentioned above, the Wnt signaling pathway plays a significant role in CRC, with activating mutations in this pathway found in greater than 90% of all CRCs that do not have the MSI, CIMP phenotype (32). As a result, targeting aberrant Wnt signaling in CRC is of prime importance. Mutations in APC cluster around a region that results in a truncated protein with limited ability to bind β-catenin, resulting in its stabilization (46). Further, while it might be expected that any activating mutation in the Wnt pathway within the colorectal stem cells might lead to a cancer phenotype, there is increasing evidence of a "just-right" level of Wnt signaling (21, 43, 46). In this Goldilocks scenario, the authors found that there is a highly significant correlation between the type of APC mutations, the level of Wnt signaling, and the site of CRC. In the proximal colon, APC mutations that select for two or three β-catenin binding sites are selected for, while in the distal colon, APC mutations that select for zero to one β-catenin binding domain are selected for (21, 43, 46). The net result is that there is a lower threshold of Wnt signaling that is selected for in the proximal colon than in the distal colon, which requires a higher activation of the Wnt signaling pathway, but too much Wnt signaling is also not a good thing for CRC (21, 43, 46).

In other studies, the levels of E-cadherin were also found to significantly affect the level of β-catenin available for Wnt signaling (15, 48). In addition to its role in Wnt signaling, a membrane pool of β-catenin binds to E-cadherin to stabilize adherens junctions. Typically, this membrane pool of β-catenin is not accessible to the Wnt pathway. However, loss of E-cadherin in a β-catenin mutant background resulted in an increase in intes-

tinal cancers in mouse and the appearance of more distal tumors than what was seen with β-catenin alone (15, 48). Thus, in addition to the allelic series of APC mutations to create the "just-right" level of Wnt signaling, loss of E-cadherin could also have a role in pushing the Wnt levels over the CRC activation threshold (49).

Conjecture

Combining the distal location of Wnt-high tumors, the role of Wnt signaling in the inhibition of Muc2, the "just-right" hypothesis, and the effect of loss of E-cadherin on enhancement of Wnt signaling, it is easy to conjecture that the gut microbiome would have a significant influence on the development of CRC. In the absence of mucin to protect the distal tumor, gut microbes would have relatively easy access to epithelial cells and may break down barrier integrity, for example, by disrupting adherens junctions, allowing enhanced Wnt signaling. This could potentially drive cells to breach the threshold of Wnt signaling, resulting in a positive-feedback loop to perpetually drive the formation of cancer stem cells and ultimately CRC (Fig. 2). Enhancement of the gut microbiome that promotes the upregulation of E-cadherin may therefore have beneficial effects in reducing the progression of at least the distal CRCs (50).

THE NORMAL COLONIC MICROBIOTA

The human gut microbiota represents a complex community of microbes with representation from bacteria, archaea, fungi, protists, and viruses. Bacteria are the most abundant form of cellular microbe in the gut environment and also the most studied of these microbial residents (51). Thus, the majority of this article will focus on the bacterial components of the gut microbiota and their interactions of relevance to CRC. However, it is important to realize that the study of the human gut microbiota is still in its infancy relative to other fields of importance in CRC, and so the potential effects of non-bacterial microbes in CRC should not be discarded.

The GI tract consists of a chain of connected compartments that can be differentiated from each other by their anatomy, physiology, content (digestion state of consumed food), motility (transit time), pH, oxygen tension, host secretions, and immune system interface. All of these attributes have the potential to modulate the abundance and composition of the resident gut microbiota, and each compartment, in fact, does have distinct microbiota profiles (52). In humans, the colon is the gut compartment with the greatest microbial density (over 10^{11} cells per gram of feces), as well as the greatest species diversity (between 100 and 1,000 bacterial species, although the latter figure differs widely according to methods used for estimation [53–55]). The colon typically maintains a low oxygen tension, which varies from low to extremely low in cross section from the mucosa to the lumen (56, 57). The oxygen gradient through this cross section supports a spectrum of bacterial species, with facultative anaerobes colonizing closer to the mucosa, and strict anaerobes tending to remain within the lumen (56).

The gut microbial ecosystem species composition varies substantially between individuals (58), although metagenomic efforts have revealed that the predicted functional repertoires of the gut microbiomes of different people are similar among individuals, indicating shared gene sets between microbial species repertoires (53). Much of the human gut microbiome consists of genes of unknown function, but metabolomic readouts of the gut microbial ecosystem offer a glimpse into the net outputs of the microbes, and the approach is increasing in popularity as the research community moves from the study of which microbes are present to the study of what such microbes are actually doing.

Diet has been repeatedly demonstrated as a major modulator of gut microbiota functional output. Several studies have indicated, for example, stark differences between the gut microbiota compositions of healthy individuals consuming either a Western-style or a subsistence-associated diet; in general, a Western-style diet is associated with higher ratios of *Firmicutes* as well as *Bacteroides*, whereas a subsistence diet is associated with a higher abundance of *Prevotella* (59–64). A recent, elegant study involved a temporary exchange of diet types between African Americans and rural South Africans such that African Americans consumed a typical rural African low-fat, high-fiber diet, and rural South Africans consumed a typical high-fat, low-fiber diet (59, 60). In this study, only modest shifts in microbial community abundance profiles were seen as a result of dietary switching, and the major effects seemed to be in the overall metabolic profiles generated. As well as variations within the bacterial species compositions between individuals, it has also been reported that there are differences between the gene repertoires of the gut microbiota of individuals; in this case, a high gene count within the microbiota tended to correlate with health, whereas a lower gene count correlated with obesity and associated markers of disease such as insulin resistance (65). Thus, diversity within the gut microbiome seems to be important to health, and diversity is not simply a function of species diversity but of genetic diversity within the microbiome also.

The majority of microbial metabolism within the healthy colon is fermentative, although the presence of a small amount of oxygen acting as an electron acceptor supports energy recovery through both cytochrome- and flavin/thiol-based electron flow in microbes that can respire in this fashion (66). Alternative electron acceptors such as sulfate and hydrogen also support a minority of specialized microbes within the colon (67–69). Saccharolytic fermentation pathways account for the large concentration of short-chain fatty acids (SCFAs) associated with the colon, with acetate, propionate, and butyrate accounting for the bulk of these at a ratio of approximately 3:1:1 (70). Acetate can be utilized in secondary fermentations and is thus particularly important in supporting cross-feeding among microbial species (71, 72). Propionate is produced through several fermentation routes, but the dominant pathway in the human gut appears to be through the conversion of succinate by *Bacteroidetes* members (73); in fact, the relative abundance of *Bacteroidetes* in fecal samples correlates with propionate concentration (74). Butyrate is made using several pathways, but one dominant pathway is utilized by a subset of *Firmicutes* bacteria, including members of the *Lachnospiraceae* and *Ruminococcaceae* families, which are in turn among the most abundant species in the human colon (75, 76). SCFAs are generally considered to be beneficial metabolites in the human gut, and butyrate in particular is known to have anti-inflammatory effects through histone deacetylase inhibition and subsequent down-regulation of proinflammatory cytokines (77), as well as through induction of FOXP3-expressing regulatory T-cells (78, 79). In contrast to saccharolytic fermentation, proteolytic fermentation, carried out for the most part by several *Firmicutes* members and some *Bacteroides* spp., results in the production of less desirable compounds including phenols, indoles, amines, and ammonia (80). Nitrosation reactions, which can be carried out by *Proteobacteria*, lead to the production of *N*-nitroso compounds from dietary proteins in the colon (81). In a small study of sudden-death victims where the colonic metabolite content was measured within a few hours of death, it was found that the cecum and ascending colon were the sites where saccharolytic fermentation predominated, whereas the sigmoid colon and rectum could be characterized by higher proteolytic fermentation (82). This finding correlates with more-recent work that used numeric ecology methods to show evidence of a mi-

crobial species gradient along the GI tract, revealing a higher abundance of *Streptococcus* and *Enterococcus* spp., *Corynebacterium* spp., and *Comamonadaceae* in the proximal part of the colon than in the distal end and a higher abundance of *Enterobacteriaceae* in the sigmoid colon and rectum than in the rest of the colon (83).

The colonic microbiome of the average healthy person develops rapidly during childhood such that by the time a child has weaned onto an adult-type diet at around the age of 3, their fecal microbiota is between 40 and 60% similar to that of a healthy adult (84). However, even through adolescence there appear to be differences in the proportions of species from genera such as *Bacteroides* and *Bifidobacterium* compared to healthy adults (85), suggesting that the development of the gut microbiota may start rapidly in the early years but may then be influenced more subtly by developmental changes through childhood. However, the composition of the gut microbiome tends to remain fairly homeostatic from early adulthood to old age, although the relative proportions of *Proteobacteria* tend to increase with host age, whereas the relative abundance of microbial species associated with production of beneficial metabolites such as butyrate (e.g., *Faecalibacterium prausnitzii* and members of the *Lachnospiraceae* family) tends to decrease over this time. Concomitantly, these age-related microbiome changes are associated with a greater tendency towards a proinflammatory gut phenotype with advancing age (86, 87).

WHEN THINGS GO AWRY: THE GUT MICROBIOTA ASSOCIATED WITH CRC

There is an ever-increasing body of evidence now supporting a role for the gut microbiome in the development of CRC. It is known that, in many cases, specific microbial infections are associated with the development of cancer; however, because the colon houses such a rich diversity of microbes, it can become difficult to tease apart the relative importance of each microbe, as well as microbe-microbe interactions, to the etiology of CRC. A simplified model emerges of the colonic microbiota driving the mucosal immune response, which when activated chronically can have detrimental effects on epithelial cell functions and genetics, leading to oncogenic changes. Several hypotheses have been put forward to try to explain how the colonic microbiota may drive these immune responses that lead to the induction of CRC. These are described below (and summarized in Fig. 3), using examples of specific pathogens and their interactions in CRC to illustrate them. Importantly, these various hypotheses may not be mutually exclusive, since elements of some may be relevant to others.

The Alpha-Bug Hypothesis

The alpha-bug hypothesis, first put forward by Sears and Pardoll (88), suggests that CRC is driven primarily by the actions of certain microbiota members with specific virulence determinants: the "alpha-bugs." These pathogenic species promote oncogenesis via two main activities: the first is through direct interactions with epithelial cells that promote the mucosal immune responses that can eventually lead to cancerous changes; the second is through the selection and remodeling of the local microbiota composition at the site of damage, through either recruitment of other prooncogenic species, thinning out of species that are protective against CRC, or both. To carry out these activities, an alpha-bug needs to have a permanent presence as a colonizer of the affected tissue.

The model organism proposed as an alpha-bug in CRC is enterotoxigenic *Bacteroides fragilis* (ETBF). Although *B. fragilis* itself is a common resident of the human colon, ETBF represents a subset of strains of this species that secrete a 20-kDa metalloprotease toxin,

Bacteroides fragilis toxin (BFT), which has in turn been associated with inflammatory diarrhea (89). The toxin has been shown to indirectly cleave E-cadherin, a host membrane protein that aids in the formation of adherence between colonic epithelial cells. Cleavage of this protein can thus lead to inappropriate exposure of the epithelial cells to luminal antigens, which can thus trigger an inflammatory response. E-cadherin also binds to β-catenin at the plasma membrane, and loss of E-cadherin has been demonstrated to increase the levels of cytoplasmic β-catenin and Wnt signaling in otherwise normal intestinal epithelial cells (15, 16). However, as the majority of CRCs are initiated by activating mutations in this pathway, it is unclear how, or if, the potentially excess β-catenin induced by cleavage of E-cadherin would affect tumor progression. BFT also contributes directly to the inflammatory response by stimulating the production of proinflammatory cytokines such as CXCL-8 and tumor necrosis factor alpha. Promotion of tumorigenesis by ETBF was also found to be due to the induction of signal transducer and activator of transcription 3 (STAT-3), a transcription factor that influences T-cell lineage development pathways. STAT-3 induces a Th17 immune response, and this is suggested, at least in part, to mediate colonic tumor formation in the multiple intestinal neoplasia (Min) mouse model (90).

In addition to ETBF, there are several candidate alpha-bugs that fit the profile for the alpha-bug model of oncogenesis. These include certain *Escherichia coli* serotypes, in particular those associated with the adherent-invasive phenotype (91–94). Adherent-invasive *E. coli* (AIEC), similar to ETBF, can be considered to be part of the normal microbiota; however, these strains have various pathogenic traits that can contribute to the induction of inflammatory pathways. For example, some AIEC strains are able to alter host intestinal permeability by inducing claudin-2 expression and by influencing the rearrangement of apical tight junction

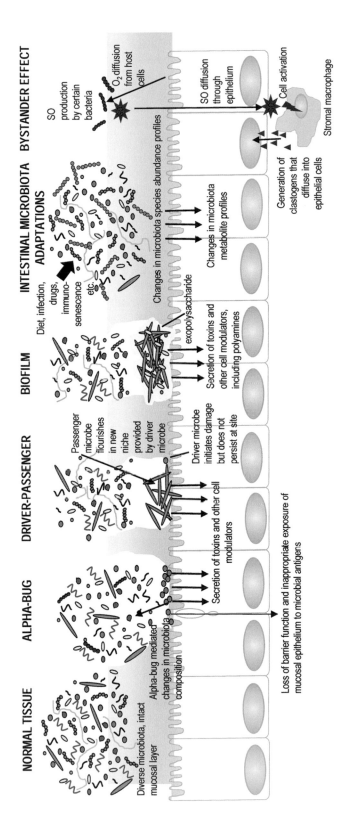

FIGURE 3 Schematic detailing microbiome changes that can lead to the development of CRC. In the normal, healthy state (normal tissue), the gut microbiota is diverse and in balance within the host. The mucosal layer of the gut is intact, and microbes are not found directly in the vicinity of the colonic cells. In the alpha-bug model, certain pathobionts within the microbiome obtain entry to host tissues, e.g., by interfering with mucus secretion or by penetrating the mucus layer, and directly secrete metabolites and/or virulence determinants such as toxins to modulate host cells. Colonization by alpha-bugs in this way can also directly modulate the composition of the local microbiota. The driver-passenger model suggests that the major CRC-promoting factors come from colonization by passenger microbes that can settle within a niche prepared for them by the driver species. The biofilm model indicates that certain colonizing microbes, particularly in the proximal colon, can form aggregates, perhaps with cooperating species, that are able to persist in the niche and to secrete factors (including, in particular, polyamines) that potentiate CRC development. In the intestinal microbiota adaptations model, exogenous factors, such as diet, as well as endogenous factors, such as immune system function, behave as forces that shape the overall balance of cancer-promoting versus cancer-protective microbiota compositions. Finally, the bystander-effect model proposes that certain superoxides produced by the metabolism of certain microbial species can stimulate stromal macrophages to produce clastogens, which in turn have a directly carcinogenic effect on host cells.

proteins, leading to loss of barrier function (92, 95). As for ETBF, the consequence of this loss of barrier integrity is exposure of the mucosa to microbial antigens that can promote a proinflammatory response. AIEC has been particularly associated with pathogenesis in inflammatory bowel disease (IBD) patients, where genetic mutations in innate immune response pathways set the stage for AIEC to cause particular problems with chronic inflammation (94). Chronic intestinal inflammation is a key risk factor for the development of CRC, and suffering from IBD is associated with a 60% higher risk for development of CRC than for healthy individuals (96). A Crohn's disease-associated AIEC isolate was found to be able to attenuate the autophagy response in intestinal epithelial cells by upregulating the expression of microRNAs (miRNAs) 30C and 130A, which have important roles in the regulation of autophagy (97). Some AIEC serotypes are known to make exotoxins, such as cytolethal distending toxin, which can induce direct damage to DNA in host cells (98), and colibactin, which is also genotoxic (99). In summary, alpha-bugs may have a predilection for colonization of the gut mucosa, where they initiate and potentiate inflammatory as well as genotoxic damage by virtue of their virulence determinants. Alpha-bugs may also represent pathogenic strains of otherwise benign commensal species that have become prominent within the colonic environment through unknown selection mechanisms.

The Driver-Passenger Hypothesis

The driver-passenger hypothesis, first proposed by Tjalsma et al. (100), is closely related to the alpha-bug hypothesis in that the alpha-bugs proposed in the latter are likely to represent the driver microbes posited by the former. However, whereas the alpha-bug hypothesis suggests that the alpha-bugs can crowd out microbial species that may be protective against CRC, the driver-passenger hypothesis suggests that the disease progression initiated by the driver/alpha-bug may lead to direct changes in the local environment of infection that can subsequently lead to loss of the initiating driver organisms through outcompetition by other microbes (passengers) that are better suited to the altered tumor microenvironment. Support for the driver-passenger hypothesis can be gained from recent metagenomic and metatranscriptomic studies of the human gut microbiota associated with matched CRC and healthy tissues from the same individuals, which clearly demonstrate the associations of some bacterial species with the microenvironments of tumors and of other species with the microenvironments of healthy tissues. Remarkably, several different studies have independently made an association between CRC tissue and the anaerobic bacterial species *Fusobacterium nucleatum* (101–106); this microbe has also been associated with inflammation in Crohn's disease (107–109) as well as inflammation in appendicitis (110–113), and signatures associated with the *Fusobacterium* genus have additionally been associated with pancreatic cancer tissue specimens (114). The ubiquity of fusobacterial signatures across a range of diseases supports the notion that these microbes may be representative of passenger microbes, able to thrive in the inflamed tissue environment and to perhaps perpetuate inflammation and damage initiated by driver microbes. A recent comparison of the fusobacterial load of clinically distinct CRC phenotypes, i.e., tubular adenoma and sessile serrated adenoma/polyp, revealed that the fusobacterial loads associated with affected tissues were not significantly different, further supporting a role for these bacteria as passengers in the driver-passenger model (115). In addition, the number of *F. nucleatum* organisms present in CRC tissues was found to be associated with disease status; higher loads correlated with poorer outcomes (116) and reduced densities of $CD3^+$ T cells (117). Thus, passenger microbes such as *F. nucleatum*, once established, may perpetuate tumorigenesis through expansion and inappropriate stimulation of the immune system.

F. nucleatum has been investigated for virulence determinants that could be oncogenic, although this is challenging because many of the genes found in fusobacterial genomes code for hypothetical genes with, as yet, no known functions. However, a few of the pathogenic determinants known to be associated with *F. nucleatum* may be important in the development of CRC. These include the FadA adhesin, which has been shown to bind to E-cadherin (118), the capacity for some strains of the species to invade host colonic epithelial cells and potentially upregulate inflammatory pathways while evading host immune responses (109), and the metabolic capability of producing hydrogen sulfide, a potent stimulator of angiogenesis (119). In the Apc^{Min} mouse model, colonization by *F. nucleatum* was shown to increase tumor multiplicity and to selectively recruit tumor infiltrating myeloid cells to potentiate a pro-inflammatory environment (120).

The driver-passenger model of CRC development suggests that there ought to be longitudinal differences in the gut microbiota associated with tissue as it progresses from healthy to hyperproliferative, to adenomatous, and to carcinomatous states, but longitudinal studies of individual human patients (without intervention) would be ethically unsound. Instead, Nakatsu et al. (121) catalogued the associated microbiota of CRC tissues and adjacent healthy tissues in a human cohort, noting the stage of neoplasia for each lesion. As well as the rediscovery of fusobacterial enrichment in CRC tissues, these authors noted distinct bacterial signatures that were enriched in adenomatous tissues, including *E. coli* (associated with genes for colibactin) and *Pseudomonas veronii*. A progressively increasing abundance of *B. fragilis* (associated with *bft* genes) as well as the oral microbe *Granulicatella adiacens* was noted through the advancement of disease state to carcinoma. Intriguingly, a co-occurrence of microbial species associated with the oral cavity, including *Gemella*, *Parvimonas*, and *Peptostreptococcus* spp., were also found to be associated with CRC development (121). This could reflect an ecological niche at gut tumor sites similar to that of the oral cavity (e.g., thickness of mucus layer, oxygen partial pressure). Given that *F. nucleatum* is also an orally associated microbe, there appears to be some future scope to determining the association between oral health and the risk of developing CRC.

The Intestinal Microbiota Adaptations Hypothesis

The gut microbial ecosystem exists in a dynamic state of equilibrium that is influenced directly by its surroundings. The environment of the human colon varies widely, with diet being a major modulating factor (3, 122), but also stressors such as infection, antibiotic exposure, and immunosenescence playing a role (123–125). Consequently, the gut microbiota can be said to live in a constant state of adaptation to its immediate environment. The stability of this ecosystem is a function of its resilience, that is, its ability to continue carrying out fundamental functions in the face of disturbance from stressors. This, in turn, is likely a function of the richness and diversity of the ecosystem, both at the species level and at the gene content level (65, 126). Should stressors act upon an ecosystem in such a way that the underlying balance of the system is damaged, the composition of the ecosystem may change to adapt to the new environment, and as well the members of the ecosystem may change their metabolic strategies to make the most efficient use of the substrates at hand. For example, a stressor that leads to inflammation of the colonic mucosa may alter the oxygen tension of the local area through the induction of an increased blood flow to the tissues. Increased oxygen tension may preferentially benefit facultative anaerobes that can efficiently generate ATP using oxygen as an electron acceptor (e.g., *E. coli*) at the expense of microbes to which even a low oxygen level is toxic and that may be lost from the system.

Support for this hypothesis was given by a recent, elegant study whereby mice were colonized by the microbiota from one of either three healthy or three CRC-affected human hosts. The resulting microbial ecosystems in these mice presented as six compositionally distinct communities according to the source host. The animals were then stressed with a chemical inducer of colitis (dextran sodium sulfate), and susceptibility to subsequent tumorigenesis was demonstrated to correlate with gut microbial profiles, suggesting that some microbiota components may have been protective whereas others may have promoted disease development (127).

Microbiota adaptations are relevant to CRC because they help to explain how the microenvironment of a tumor may drive disease in a positive-feedback loop, and the theory is supportive of the findings that the microbial populations of adenoma, carcinoma, and healthy tissues are distinct. An important point to understand, however, is that adaptations to the microenvironment may also be positive to the host, such that in some cases microbiota shifts may be in the balance of cancer-inhibiting microbes, in which case tumorigenesis will not occur (128). A major goal of current research is to better understand how microbiota adaptations are shaped such that cancer-inhibiting effects might be, to some extent, exploited.

The Biofilm Effect Hypothesis

In nature, microbes tend to exist as biofilm structures: aggregates of cells coated in an exopolymeric matrix that can adhere and remain fixed within a given environment. In some respects, such aggregates can be seen as positive to the function of the ecosystem, as they may foster cell-cell communications and allow for syntrophic interactions that enhance ecosystem stability. However, biofilm production is also a strategy through which different species of pathobionts may interact in order to invade and colonize a given niche while resisting forces that would otherwise remove them.

Recently, Dejea et al. (129) demonstrated that polymicrobial bacterial biofilms are associated with CRCs and, remarkably, most often in right-sided tumors proximal to the hepatic flexure. Such biofilms tended to invade the colonic mucus layer and were associated with prooncogenic changes, for example loss of E-cadherin, activation of STAT3, and increased epithelial cell proliferation. Further work by the same group (130) analyzed the metabolome of colonic tissues associated with biofilms and cancer compared to healthy tissues and revealed that increases in polyamine metabolites, and particularly N^1,N^{12}-diacetylspermine, tended to be associated with cancerous tissues. These metabolites were reduced following antibiotic treatment to clear biofilms, suggesting that biofilm is the driver of these metabolic changes. Polyamines influence both eukaryotic cell proliferation and prokaryotic cell growth and biofilm formation (130–132). Interestingly, polyamine levels tend to decrease from proximal to distal colon (132), which correlates with the predominance of biofilm-associated cancers on the right side of the colon.

The importance of biofilms in CRC is also relevant when considering CRC-associated microbes that have been identified to date. For example, *F. nucleatum* is considered to be a central player in the formation of biofilms in the human mouth (plaque) (133), and the preponderance of oral pathobionts in CRC tissues, as described by Nakutsu et al. and outlined above (121), may reflect a propensity for these species in biofilm formation associated with CRC. Very recent work is starting to uncover further links between particular metabolites associated with CRC with co-occurring microbes, demonstrating that species of *Fusobacterium*, as well as of a further oral biofilm-associated genus, *Porphyromonas*, may be important in CRC development (134).

The Commensal-Driven Bystander Effect Hypothesis

The commensal-driven bystander effect hypothesis is an extension of the bystander effect phenotype that is usually associated with the radiation biology field, whereby ionizing radiation is known to activate the release of diffusible mutagenic agents, or "clastogens," by host cells, which can go on to damage genomic DNA in nonirradiated cells. Clastogens generated by damage through ionizing radiation appear to be small-molecular-weight compounds that are representative of the breakdown products of particular metabolites (with one example being *trans*-4-hydroxy-2-nonenal [4-HNE], a highly reactive aldehyde derived through peroxidation of Ω-6 polyunsaturated fatty acids) (135). Damage to host cell chromosomes that induces changes, such as chromosomal instability, cell cycle arrest, and aneuploidy, can directly contribute to oncogenesis.

Interestingly, extracellular superoxide can behave as an initiator of clastogenesis through polarization of macrophages (136). Certain commensal species of the gut microbiota, most notably *Enterococcus faecalis*, are able to generate extracellular superoxide through reduction of dioxygen by demethylmenaquinones associated with the bacterial cell membrane (137). Gut colonization by *E. faecalis* has been found to be increased in individuals with CRC compared to healthy controls (138), and it is suggested that superoxide produced by this species may ultimately drive DNA damage in colonic epithelial cells, a situation that has been demonstrated in a rodent model (139). The mediators in this situation appear to be stromal macrophages, which respond to superoxide stimulation by inducing cyclooxygenase 2 (COX-2) through NF-κB signaling (140). COX-2 that is upregulated in this way appears to behave as a procarcinogenic enzyme that generates clastogens such as 4-HNE and damages DNA in nearby colonocytes (141).

Under permissive circumstances, such DNA damage may lead to malignant transformation and could contribute to other pathways of microbe-associated CRC etiology discussed here, in an additive fashion.

THE POTENTIAL FOR TREATING CRC WITH MICROBIAL MODULATION THERAPIES

The balance between DNA damage and DNA repair is an important equation for determining the risk of CRC development, but there are many contributors to both factors, and it is difficult to rank how important each of these contributors may be to either promotion or prevention of cancer. However, some of these contributors, for example, diet, have been shown to have particular importance. It has long been understood that dietary choices, for example meat consumption, are associated with higher CRC risk (142). In their study of dietary switching between rural South Africans and African Americans, groups that are highly discordant for CRC risk, Ou et al. found fundamental differences between gut microbiota metabolism, with secondary bile acid production predominating in the Americans and SCFAs predominating in the South Africans (60). This finding could be tightly correlated with dietary differences; for example, the consumption of a typical American high-fat diet may increase hepatic synthesis of bile acids to levels where they can spill over from the enterohepatic circulation and enter the colon. Certain microbes are able to convert these primary bile acids into secondary bile acids, the latter of which can be both proinflammatory and carcinogenic.

If CRC risk is driven at least in part by dietary factors, providing dietary supplementation in the form of probiotics or prebiotics to modulate this risk could represent a useful strategy, particularly for CRC prevention. Considering the clear role of the microbiota in CRC, strategies that modulate microbial communities more directly, such as antibiotics or "microbial ecosystem therapeutics," may also be important, perhaps more so for treatment of early dysplasias. These various strategies are considered below.

Probiotics

Probiotics are live microorganisms that, when administered in adequate amounts, confer a health benefit on the host (143). Most commercial probiotics belong to a very restricted group of bacterial genera, including *Bifidobacterium* and *Lactobacillus*, and may be offered as dietary additives in the form of, e.g., fermented milk products.

Probiotics as CRC-preventative agents may exert their effects through a number of routes. On a simple ecological level, probiotic strains may compete with pathobionts or with microbes that produce prooncolytic compounds, causing a reduction in pathobiont numbers or carcinogen concentrations in the gut (reviewed by Rafter [144]). This premise is supported by a 12-week trial of a combination of two probiotic strains, *Lactobacillus rhamnosus* GG and *Bifidobacterium lactis* Bb12, together with a prebiotic substrate, for the treatment of patients with either adenomatous or cancerous lesions in their colons (145). The authors noted an increase of the numbers of these probiotic strains during treatment that, in adenoma patients in particular, coincided with a reduction in the pathobiont *Clostridium perfringens*. In the same study, a number of key colorectal cancer biomarkers, such as cell proliferation and the ability of fecal water to reduce markers of damage to epithelial cells in tissue culture assays, were noted. Probiotics may also modulate carcinogenic compounds that are either consumed or produced through autochthonous gut microbiota metabolism, to inactivate them. For example, mutagenic compounds found in cooked meat, including derivatives of heterocyclic aromatic amines, can be bound and/or degraded by probiotic strains, rendering them harmless (146–148).

Because the immune system plays a central role in the control of cancer cells through a highly complex antitumor response involving both lymphoid and myeloid cells, and thus both innate and adaptive arms of the immune system, the potential anticancer activities of probiotics have been examined in the context of immune system modulation. Perhaps the most studied probiotic in this respect is *Lactobacillus casei* strain Shirota, which has been tested for antitumor and immunoregulation effects in several rodent models of cancer (149–153) and has been assessed for prophylactic effects against superficial bladder cancer as well as breast cancer in human patients (154, 155). *L. casei* Shirota administered intrapleurally into mice with transplanted fibrosarcoma tumors induced a strong antitumor response through the induction of cytokines such as gamma interferon and tumor necrosis factor alpha, and this response contributed positively to the survival of the animals (156). Matsumoto et al. (157) more recently demonstrated that the activity of *L. casei* Shirota against colitis-associated cancer in mice was dependent upon components of the *L. casei* Shirota cell wall peptidoglycan, which directly inhibited interleukin-6 production (157). Interestingly, lipoteichoic acid (another component of the bacterial cell wall) of *Lactobacillus rhamnosus* strain GG has also been shown to elicit anticancer properties, this time in a UV-induced murine carcinogenesis model, through the production of higher levels of gamma interferon as well as increased numbers of cytotoxic and helper T-cells, as well as activated dendritic cells, compared to control animals (158).

Other probiotic strains have been shown to modify the immune response in a manner that is relevant for CRC. Orally administered *L. casei* strain BL23 was demonstrated to significantly protect mice against 1,2 dimethyl hydrazine-induced CRC through biasing T-cell responses towards Th17, with concomitant increases in the expression of cytokines such as transforming growth factor-β and interleukin-17 (159). A probiotic mixture of eight bacterial strains marketed as VSL#3 was also shown to ameliorate colitis-associated tumor development in a chemically induced colitis model (this time effected with dextran sodium sulfate), through reduction of expression of STAT-3 (160).

Cell proliferation and apoptosis are important components of CRC progression, and the role of probiotics in the modulation of these two mechanisms has been explored using several models. VSL#3 has been shown to suppress COX-2 expression in human colonic epithelial cell lines derived from either adenomatous or cancerous tissues (161). COX-2 expression, which is abnormally elevated in colorectal tumors (162), plays a role in inhibition of apoptosis; thus, VSL#3 may help to overcome this inhibition to reduce tumor cell proliferation. In a rat model of chemically induced colorectal cancer (using azoxymethane), Singh et al. (163) demonstrated that dietary dosing with a milk-derived *Bifidobacterium longum* strain reduced the number and severity of tumors compared to what was seen in control animals, through reduction of ornithine decarboxylase activity, which in turn is a central component of polyamine synthesis. Given that increases in polyamine concentrations have been correlated with biofilms associated with CRC, as described above, there may be scope for probiotic intervention for the specific modulation of colonic biofilm-associated cancers. The antiproliferative effects of probiotics are not limited to the lactic acid bacteria; emerging probiotic strains of species such as *Clostridium butyricum* and *Bacillus subtilis* have been shown to reduce proliferation of, and induce apoptosis in, 1,2 dimethyl hydrazine-induced CRC cells in mice (164), although the mechanisms involved are as yet unexplored.

The antitumor effects of probiotics are not limited to bacterial strains. The probiotic yeast *Saccharomyces cerevisiae* var. *boulardii* strain CNCM I-745 prevented epidermal growth factor-induced proliferation and promoted apoptosis in a human colonic epithelial cell line (HT29) and reduced intestinal tumor growth and dysplasia in *Apc*^{Min} mice (165).

Prebiotics

A prebiotic is defined as a "selectively fermentable non-digestible oligosaccharide or ingredient that brings specific changes, both in the composition and/or activity of the gastrointestinal microflora, conferring health benefits" (166). Generally speaking, the term "prebiotic" is synonymous with fructooligosaccharides (FOS) and galacto-oligosaccharides (GOS) and to a lesser extent xylooligosaccharides (XOS), the most common forms used as dietary supplements in humans (167, 168). Prebiotics may be delivered as a "symbiotic" preparation, with a selected probiotic strain known to ferment the prebiotic with associated production of beneficial metabolites.

The major health-promoting activities of prebiotics lie in their ability to stimulate the growth, and thus metabolism, of microbes, leading to modulation of both the microbial ecosystem and its associated metabonome. Several studies have reported on the inhibitory effects of FOS, GOS, and XOS preparations on the progression of carcinogenesis in chemically induced rodent models of CRC (169–172), and one of these noted the specific stimulation of bifidobacteria (172), suggesting the support of this microbial genus, commonly known as a beneficial microbe, as a major mechanism for the effects seen. However, this early study did not comprehensively analyze the gut microbiotas of the animals in response to, in this case, XOS and FOS, and so while there was a clear bifidogenic effect, it is difficult to know whether this was solely responsible for the modulating effects seen. A study of the effects of GOS on the gut microbiotas of humans fed the substrate as a dietary supplement for a 16-week period showed that *Bifidobacterium* spp. were positively impacted by the substrate, but there were also increases in abundances seen for several other bacterial taxa including *Faecalibacterium prausnitzii* and *Coprococcus comes* (173). An *in vitro* study of GOS fermentation by microbial communities pooled from the stools of eight healthy adult volunteers showed a similar increase of bifidobacteria; however, *F. prausnitzii* abundance in this study was seen to be reduced, and there were also increased amounts of *Enterobacteriaceae* in response to GOS stimulation (174). It is important to remember that the gut microbiotas of different individuals, though functionally similar, can be compositionally different (126), and thus it is likely that studies of prebiotic fermentation patterns need to be normalized to the baseline microbiota makeup in order to fully understand this relationship. However, many studies have clearly shown that prebiotics can increase concentrations of SCFAs in the colon, with associated beneficial effects (as described above and recently reviewed by Bruno-Barcena and Azcarate-Peril [175]).

Through influencing the microbiota, prebiotics can also influence the absorption of dietary minerals, vitamins, and other substrates, which can in turn reduce the risk of cancer development (176, 177). A study by Cloetens et al., in which human volunteers were fed an arabinoxylooligosaccharide prebiotic, indicated a shift from urinary to fecal excretion of ammonia in these volunteers during the trial, suggesting gut microbiota uptake and sequestration of ammonia from the host (thus preventing absorption with subsequent excretion through the kidneys), with expected beneficial effects on health (178). Agaro-oligosaccharides, prebiotics derived from seaweeds, have recently been shown to modulate the detrimental effects of a high-fat diet in mice, for example, by increasing HOX-1 expression (and thus suppressing inflammatory and protumorigenic cytokines) and by reducing polyamine production by certain microbiota members (179–181).

Antibiotics

There is little in the literature to describe the treatment of CRC with antibiotics, although Johnson et al. studied the colonic tissues of CRC patients who had been treated with oral antibiotics 1 day prior to the day of surgical procedure to remove tumors and found that the biofilm and polyamine presence in antibiotic-treated tissues were decreased in these patients compared to findings in control patients who were not exposed to antibiotics (130). The correlation of CRC with the gut microbiome is a relatively recent discovery, which may explain why antibiotic therapy for CRC is somewhat unexplored, but a more likely explanation is that once the process of dysplasia has begun it may be difficult to stop, and since there are large interindividual differences in gut microbiota composition (53), it is not possible to predict the likely efficiency of a given antibiotic in removing problematic microbes. Antibiotic use is generally associated with heavy collateral damage to nontarget members of the gut microbiota (reviewed by Blaser [182]), and this damage can be unpredictable and/or permanent. Considering the intestinal microbiota adaptations hypothesis described above, such an effect may cause a switch between colonization of a niche with protective bacteria to colonization by potentially pathogenic microbes, which could exacerbate CRC progression that might have been otherwise stalled by the presence of tumor-suppressive bacteria. The findings of a nested case-control study that examined the correlation between nonfamilial CRC development and a history of antibiotic use supported this notion, since it was found that previous exposure to multiple courses of penicillins correlated with an increased risk of CRC development (123).

Before the onset of CRC related to gut inflammation, however, could antibiotic therapy be helpful in ameliorating the inflammatory pathways that can lead to oncogenesis? For patients with IBD, a relapsing-remitting condition, the goal is to induce and maintain remission of disease partially to prevent long-term complications such as development of CRC, and it could be perceived that antibiotic therapy might be useful for this purpose. However, because of the rising rates of antibiotic resistance and the potential side effects caused by long-term antibiotic use, these drugs are seldom used in clinical practice for treatment of IBD unless there is a septic complication (reviewed by Sokol [183]). Given these issues, as well as a potential connection between antibiotic use and CRC development, the prospects of using antibiotics as cancer-preventive medicines are poor.

CONCLUSION: CRC TREATMENT OF THE FUTURE—WHERE DO WE GO FROM HERE?

As we continue to study the links between lifestyle, host genetics, and the gut microbiota in the development of CRC, the field is opening up to new hypotheses for prevention and treatment of disease using microbial modulation as a tool. With advances in next-generation sequencing and metabolomics, it may soon be possible to identify risk factors for development of disease or to use stool or blood samples to prescreen for microbial metabolites associated with CRC, thereby identifying individuals who may benefit from more-invasive testing such as colonoscopy and biopsy.

The recent and ongoing identification of specific microbial species associated with the development of CRC perhaps points the way to targeted therapies for removal of these pathobionts. Antibiotics represent too blunt of a tool to carry out such selective work and carry the risk of further damage to the microbiota that may be detrimental to the host. Instead, vaccination strategies against, for example, identified alpha-bugs or microbes that secrete procarcinogenic metabolites may potentially be of benefit. Targeted phage therapy against such microbes may also be a valid tactic (especially for those microbes associated with biofilms in CRC).

However, both of these approaches may be difficult to carry out if, for example, multiple strains of a CRC-associated species exist within a host, only a subset of which are problematic or susceptible to lytic phage.

Perhaps, instead of trying to destroy selected problematic species within a dysbiotic microbial ecosystem, a more durable approach will be to understand the root causes of the dysbiosis and to treat these, thereby restoring balance. The influence of diet on the gut microbiota continues to be uncovered as a major driving force and fits very well with what we understand about CRC rates in the developed world, where dietary habits tend not to be optimal. With the view that prevention is always better than cure, using dietary strategies and interventions to treat dysbioses associated with CRC risk, perhaps incorporating a more personalized view of treatment, given that gut microbiome compositions are unique to individuals, will become a standard of care. And where colonic dysplasia is evident, perhaps replacement or augmentation of dysbiotic microbial ecosystems with microbes known to be protective against disease progression will become an emergent therapeutic avenue.

CITATION

Van Raay T, Allen-Vercoe E. 2017. Microbial interactions and interventions in colorectal cancer. Microbiol Spectrum 5(3):BAD-0004-2016.

REFERENCES

1. **World Health Organization.** 2015. *Fact sheet 297.* http://www.who.int/mediacentre/factsheets/fs297/en/. Accessed April 2016.
2. **Vogelstein B, Fearon ER, Hamilton SR, Kern SE, Preisinger AC, Leppert M, Nakamura Y, White R, Smits AM, Bos JL.** 1988. Genetic alterations during colorectal-tumor development. *N Engl J Med* **319:**525–532.
3. **Vipperla K, O'Keefe SJ.** 2016. Diet, microbiota, and dysbiosis: a "recipe" for colorectal cancer. *Food Funct* **7:**1731–1740.

4. **Barker N.** 2014. Adult intestinal stem cells: critical drivers of epithelial homeostasis and regeneration. *Nat Rev Mol Cell Biol* **15**:19–33.

5. **Biswas S, Davis H, Irshad S, Sandberg T, Worthley D, Leedham S.** 2015. Microenvironmental control of stem cell fate in intestinal homeostasis and disease. *J Pathol* **237**: 135–145.

6. **Clevers H.** 2013. The intestinal crypt, a prototype stem cell compartment. *Cell* **154**:274–284.

7. **Barker N, van Es JH, Kuipers J, Kujala P, van den Born M, Cozijnsen M, Haegebarth A, Korving J, Begthel H, Peters PJ, Clevers H.** 2007. Identification of stem cells in small intestine and colon by marker gene Lgr5. *Nature* **449**:1003–1007.

8. **Sato T, Vries RG, Snippert HJ, van de Wetering M, Barker N, Stange DE, van Es JH, Abo A, Kujala P, Peters PJ, Clevers H.** 2009. Single Lgr5 stem cells build crypt-villus structures in vitro without a mesenchymal niche. *Nature* **459**:262–265.

9. **Clevers H, Batlle E.** 2013. SnapShot: the intestinal crypt. *Cell* **152**:1198–1198e2.

10. **Pellegrinet L, Rodilla V, Liu Z, Chen S, Koch U, Espinosa L, Kaestner KH, Kopan R, Lewis J, Radtke F.** 2011. Dll1- and dll4-mediated notch signaling are required for homeostasis of intestinal stem cells. *Gastroenterology* **140**: 1230–1240e1-7.

11. **van Es JH, van Gijn ME, Riccio O, van den Born M, Vooijs M, Begthel H, Cozijnsen M, Robine S, Winton DJ, Radtke F, Clevers H.** 2005. Notch/gamma-secretase inhibition turns proliferative cells in intestinal crypts and adenomas into goblet cells. *Nature* **435**: 959–963.

12. **van de Wetering M, Sancho E, Verweij C, de Lau W, Oving I, Hurlstone A, van der Horn K, Batlle E, Coudreuse D, Haramis AP, Tjon-Pon-Fong M, Moerer P, van den Born M, Soete G, Pals S, Eilers M, Medema R, Clevers H.** 2002. The beta-catenin/TCF-4 complex imposes a crypt progenitor phenotype on colorectal cancer cells. *Cell* **111**:241–250.

13. **Clevers H, Nusse R.** 2012. Wnt/β-catenin signaling and disease. *Cell* **149**:1192–1205.

14. **Chen YT, Stewart DB, Nelson WJ.** 1999. Coupling assembly of the E-cadherin/beta-catenin complex to efficient endoplasmic reticulum exit and basal-lateral membrane targeting of E-cadherin in polarized MDCK cells. *J Cell Biol* **144**:687–699.

15. **Huels DJ, Ridgway RA, Radulescu S, Leushacke M, Campbell AD, Biswas S, Leedham S, Serra S, Chetty R, Moreaux G, Parry L, Matthews J, Song F, Hedley A, Kalna G, Ceteci F, Reed KR, Meniel VS, Maguire A, Doyle B, Söderberg O, Barker N, Watson A, Larue L, Clarke AR, Sansom OJ.** 2015. E-cadherin can limit the transforming properties of activating β-catenin mutations. *EMBO J* **34**:2321–2333.

16. **Libusova L, Stemmler MP, Hierholzer A, Schwarz H, Kemler R.** 2010. N-cadherin can structurally substitute for E-cadherin during intestinal development but leads to polyp formation. *Development* **137**:2297–2305.

17. **Hardwick JC, Van Den Brink GR, Bleuming SA, Ballester I, Van Den Brande JM, Keller JJ, Offerhaus GJ, Van Deventer SJ, Peppelenbosch MP.** 2004. Bone morphogenetic protein 2 is expressed by, and acts upon, mature epithelial cells in the colon. *Gastroenterology* **126**:111–121.

18. **Rothenberg ME, Nusse Y, Kalisky T, Lee JJ, Dalerba P, Scheeren F, Lobo N, Kulkarni S, Sim S, Qian D, Beachy PA, Pasricha PJ, Quake SR, Clarke MF.** 2012. Identification of a cKit(+) colonic crypt base secretory cell that supports Lgr5(+) stem cells in mice. *Gastroenterology* **142**:1195–1205e6.

19. **Arai T, Kino I.** 1989. Morphometrical and cell kinetic studies of normal human colorectal mucosa. Comparison between the proximal and the distal large intestine. *Acta Pathol Jpn* **39**:725–730.

20. **Hammann A, Arveux P, Martin M.** 1992. Effect of gut-associated lymphoid tissue on cellular proliferation in proximal and distal colon of the rat. *Dig Dis Sci* **37**:1099–1104.

21. **Leedham SJ, Rodenas-Cuadrado P, Howarth K, Lewis A, Mallappa S, Segditsas S, Davis H, Jeffery R, Rodriguez-Justo M, Keshav S, Travis SP, Graham TA, East J, Clark S, Tomlinson IP.** 2013. A basal gradient of Wnt and stem-cell number influences regional tumour distribution in human and mouse intestinal tracts. *Gut* **62**:83–93.

22. **Ermund A, Schütte A, Johansson ME, Gustafsson JK, Hansson GC.** 2013. Studies of mucus in mouse stomach, small intestine, and colon. I. Gastrointestinal mucus layers have different properties depending on location as well as over the Peyer's patches. *Am J Physiol Gastrointest Liver Physiol* **305**:G341–G347.

23. **Johansson ME, Larsson JM, Hansson GC.** 2011. The two mucus layers of colon are organized by the MUC2 mucin, whereas the outer layer is a legislator of host-microbial interactions. *Proc Natl Acad Sci USA* **108**(Suppl 1): 4659–4665.

24. **Pelaseyed T, Bergström JH, Gustafsson JK, Ermund A, Birchenough GM, Schütte A, van der Post S, Svensson F, Rodríguez-Piñeiro AM, Nyström EE, Wising C, Johansson ME,**

Hansson GC. 2014. The mucus and mucins of the goblet cells and enterocytes provide the first defense line of the gastrointestinal tract and interact with the immune system. *Immunol Rev* **260:**8–20.

25. van der Post S, Hansson GC. 2014. Membrane protein profiling of human colon reveals distinct regional differences. *Mol Cell Proteomics* **13:**2277–2287.

26. Noah TK, Donahue B, Shroyer NF. 2011. Intestinal development and differentiation. *Exp Cell Res* **317:**2702–2710.

27. Grapin-Botton A, Melton DA. 2000. Endoderm development: from patterning to organogenesis. *Trends Genet* **16:**124–130.

28. Wells JM, Melton DA. 1999. Vertebrate endoderm development. *Annu Rev Cell Dev Biol* **15:** 393–410.

29. de Santa Barbara P, van den Brink GR, Roberts DJ. 2003. Development and differentiation of the intestinal epithelium. *Cell Mol Life Sci* **60:**1322–1332.

30. Roberts DJ. 2000. Molecular mechanisms of development of the gastrointestinal tract. *Dev Dyn* **219:**109–120.

31. Beck F, Tata F, Chawengsaksophak K. 2000. Homeobox genes and gut development. *BioEssays* **22:**431–441.

32. Cancer Genome Atlas Network. 2012. Comprehensive molecular characterization of human colon and rectal cancer. *Nature* **487:** 330 337.

33. Kinzler KW, Vogelstein B. 1996. Lessons from hereditary colorectal cancer. *Cell* **87:**159–170.

34. Wood LD, Parsons DW, Jones S, Lin J, Sjöblom T, Leary RJ, Shen D, Boca SM, Barber T, Ptak J, Silliman N, Szabo S, Dezso Z, Ustyanksky V, Nikolskaya T, Nikolsky Y, Karchin R, Wilson PA, Kaminker JS, Zhang Z, Croshaw R, Willis J, Dawson D, Shipitsin M, Willson JK, Sukumar S, Polyak K, Park BH, Pethiyagoda CL, Pant PV, Ballinger DG, Sparks AB, Hartigan J, Smith DR, Suh E, Papadopoulos N, Buckhaults P, Markowitz SD, Parmigiani G, Kinzler KW, Velculescu VE, Vogelstein B. 2007. The genomic landscapes of human breast and colorectal cancers. *Science* **318:**1108–1113.

35. Barker N, Ridgway RA, van Es JH, van de Wetering M, Begthel H, van den Born M, Danenberg E, Clarke AR, Sansom OJ, Clevers H. 2009. Crypt stem cells as the cells-of-origin of intestinal cancer. *Nature* **457:**608–611.

36. Terzic J, Grivennikov S, Karin E, Karin M. 2010. Inflammation and colon cancer. *Gastroenterology* **138:**2101–2114e5.

37. Minoo P, Zlobec I, Peterson M, Terracciano L, Lugli A. 2010. Characterization of rectal, proximal and distal colon cancers based on clinicopathological, molecular and protein profiles. *Int J Oncol* **37:**707–718.

38. Gervaz P, Bucher P, Morel P. 2004. Two colons-two cancers: paradigm shift and clinical implications. *J Surg Oncol* **88:**261–266.

39. Lee GH, Malietzis G, Askari A, Bernardo D, Al-Hassi HO, Clark SK. 2015. Is right-sided colon cancer different to left-sided colorectal cancer? - a systematic review. *Eur J Surg Oncol* **41:**300–308.

40. Shen H, Yang J, Huang Q, Jiang MJ, Tan YN, Fu JF, Zhu LZ, Fang XF, Yuan Y. 2015. Different treatment strategies and molecular features between right-sided and left-sided colon cancers. *World J Gastroenterol* **21:**6470–6478.

41. Yahagi M, Okabayashi K, Hasegawa H, Tsuruta M, Kitagawa Y. 2016. The worse prognosis of right-sided compared with left-sided colon cancers: a systematic review and meta-analysis. *J Gastrointest Surg* **20:**648–655.

42. Guinney J, Dienstmann R, Wang X, de Reyniès A, Schlicker A, Soneson C, Marisa L, Roepman P, Nyamundanda G, Angelino P, Bot BM, Morris JS, Simon IM, Gerster S, Fessler E, De Sousa E Melo F, Missiaglia E, Ramay H, Barras D, Homicsko K, Maru D, Manyam GC, Broom B, Boige V, Perez-Villamil B, Laderas T, Salazar R, Gray JW, Hanahan D, Tabernero J, Bernards R, Friend SH, Laurent-Puig P, Medema JP, Sadanandam A, Wessels L, Delorenzi M, Kopetz S, Vermeulen L, Tejpar S. 2015. The consensus molecular subtypes of colorectal cancer. *Nat Med* **21:**1350–1356.

43. Albuquerque C, Baltazar C, Filipe B, Penha F, Pereira T, Smits R, Cravo M, Lage P, Fidalgo P, Claro I, Rodrigues P, Veiga I, Ramos JS, Fonseca I, Leitão CN, Fodde R. 2010. Colorectal cancers show distinct mutation spectra in members of the canonical WNT signaling pathway according to their anatomical location and type of genetic instability. *Genes Chromosomes Cancer* **49:**746–759.

44. Bara J, Nardelli J, Gadenne C, Prade M, Burtin P. 1984. Differences in the expression of mucus-associated antigens between proximal and distal human colon adenocarcinomas. *Br J Cancer* **49:**495–501.

45. Gao P, Song YX, Xu YY, Sun Z, Sun JX, Xu HM, Wang ZN. 2013. Does the prognosis of colorectal mucinous carcinoma depend upon the primary tumour site? Results from two independent databases. *Histopathology* **63:**603–615.

46. Christie M, Jorissen RN, Mouradov D, Sakthianandeswaren A, Li S, Day F, Tsui C, Lipton L, Desai J, Jones IT, McLaughlin S, Ward RL, Hawkins NJ, Ruszkiewicz AR, Moore J, Burgess AW, Busam D, Zhao Q, Strausberg RL, Simpson AJ, Tomlinson IP, Gibbs P, Sieber OM. 2013. Different APC genotypes in proximal and distal sporadic colorectal cancers suggest distinct WNT/β-catenin signalling thresholds for tumourigenesis. *Oncogene* **32**:4675–4682.

47. Pai P, Rachagani S, Dhawan P, Batra SK. 2016. Mucins and Wnt/β-catenin signaling in gastrointestinal cancers: an unholy nexus. *Carcinogenesis* **37**:223–232.

48. Solanas G, Batlle E. 2011. Control of cell adhesion and compartmentalization in the intestinal epithelium. *Exp Cell Res* **317**:2695–2701.

49. Chen GT, Waterman ML. 2015. Cancer: leaping the E-cadherin hurdle. *EMBO J* **34**:2307–2309.

50. Chen L, Brar MS, Leung FC, Hsiao WL. 2016. Triterpenoid herbal saponins enhance beneficial bacteria, decrease sulfate-reducing bacteria, modulate inflammatory intestinal microenvironment and exert cancer preventive effects in ApcMin/+ mice. *Oncotarget* **7**:31226–31242 10.18632/oncotarget.8886.

51. Methé BA, et al, Human Microbiome Project Consortium. 2012. A framework for human microbiome research. *Nature* **486**:215–221.

52. Zilberstein B, Quintanilha AG, Santos MA, Pajecki D, Moura EG, Alves PR, Maluf Filho F, de Souza JA, Gama-Rodrigues J. 2007. Digestive tract microbiota in healthy volunteers. *Clinics (Sao Paulo)* **62**:47–54.

53. Huttenhower C, et al, Human Microbiome Project Consortium. 2012. Structure, function and diversity of the healthy human microbiome. *Nature* **486**:207–214.

54. Zhernakova A, Kurilshikov A, Bonder MJ, Tigchelaar EF, Schirmer M, Vatanen T, Mujagic Z, Vila AV, Falony G, Vieira-Silva S, Wang J, Imhann F, Brandsma E, Jankipersadsing SA, Joossens M, Cenit MC, Deelen P, Swertz MA, Weersma RK, Feskens EJ, Netea MG, Gevers D, Jonkers D, Franke L, Aulchenko YS, Huttenhower C, Raes J, Hofker MH, Xavier RJ, Wijmenga C, Fu J, LifeLines cohort study. 2016. Population-based metagenomics analysis reveals markers for gut microbiome composition and diversity. *Science* **352**:565–569.

55. Avershina E, Rudi K. 2015. Confusion about the species richness of human gut microbiota. *Benef Microbes* **6**:657–659.

56. Albenberg L, Esipova TV, Judge CP, Bittinger K, Chen J, Laughlin A, Grunberg S, Baldassano RN, Lewis JD, Li H, Thom SR, Bushman FD, Vinogradov SA, Wu GD. 2014. Correlation between intraluminal oxygen gradient and radial partitioning of intestinal microbiota. *Gastroenterology* **147**:1055–1063.e8.

57. Espey MG. 2013. Role of oxygen gradients in shaping redox relationships between the human intestine and its microbiota. *Free Radic Biol Med* **55**:130–140.

58. Eckburg PB, Bik EM, Bernstein CN, Purdom E, Dethlefsen L, Sargent M, Gill SR, Nelson KE, Relman DA. 2005. Diversity of the human intestinal microbial flora. *Science* **308**:1635–1638.

59. O'Keefe SJ, Li JV, Lahti L, Ou J, Carbonero F, Mohammed K, Posma JM, Kinross J, Wahl E, Ruder E, Vipperla K, Naidoo V, Mtshali L, Tims S, Puylaert PG, DeLany J, Krasinskas A, Benefiel AC, Kaseb HO, Newton K, Nicholson JK, de Vos WM, Gaskins HR, Zoetendal EG. 2015. Fat, fibre and cancer risk in African Americans and rural Africans. *Nat Commun* **6**:6342.

60. Ou J, Carbonero F, Zoetendal EG, DeLany JP, Wang M, Newton K, Gaskins HR, O'Keefe SJ. 2013. Diet, microbiota, and microbial metabolites in colon cancer risk in rural Africans and African Americans. *Am J Clin Nutr* **98**:111–120.

61. Amato KR, Yeoman CJ, Cerda G, Schmitt CA, Cramer JD, Miller ME, Gomez A, Turner TR, Wilson BA, Stumpf RM, Nelson KE, White BA, Knight R, Leigh SR. 2015. Variable responses of human and non-human primate gut microbiomes to a Western diet. *Microbiome* **3**:53.

62. Greenhill C. 2015. Obesity: gut microbiota, host genetics and diet interact to affect the risk of developing obesity and the metabolic syndrome. *Nat Rev Endocrinol* **11**:630.

63. Schnorr SL, Candela M, Rampelli S, Centanni M, Consolandi C, Basaglia G, Turroni S, Biagi E, Peano C, Severgnini M, Fiori J, Gotti R, De Bellis G, Luiselli D, Brigidi P, Mabulla A, Marlowe F, Henry AG, Crittenden AN. 2014. Gut microbiome of the Hadza hunter-gatherers. *Nat Commun* **5**:3654.

64. De Filippo C, Cavalieri D, Di Paola M, Ramazzotti M, Poullet JB, Massart S, Collini S, Pieraccini G, Lionetti P. 2010. Impact of diet in shaping gut microbiota revealed by a comparative study in children from Europe and rural Africa. *Proc Natl Acad Sci USA* **107**:14691–14696.

65. Le Chatelier E, et al, MetaHIT consortium. 2013. Richness of human gut microbiome correlates with metabolic markers. *Nature* **500**:541–546.

66. **Khan MT, van Dijl JM, Harmsen HJ.** 2014. Antioxidants keep the potentially probiotic but highly oxygen-sensitive human gut bacterium *Faecalibacterium prausnitzii* alive at ambient air. *PLoS One* **9:**e96097.

67. **Rey FE, Faith JJ, Bain J, Muehlbauer MJ, Stevens RD, Newgard CB, Gordon JI.** 2010. Dissecting the in vivo metabolic potential of two human gut acetogens. *J Biol Chem* **285:** 22082–22090.

68. **Rey FE, Gonzalez MD, Cheng J, Wu M, Ahern PP, Gordon JI.** 2013. Metabolic niche of a prominent sulfate-reducing human gut bacterium. *Proc Natl Acad Sci USA* **110:**13582–13587.

69. **Vanderhaeghen S, Lacroix C, Schwab C.** 2015. Methanogen communities in stools of humans of different age and health status and co-occurrence with bacteria. *FEMS Microbiol Lett* **362:**fnv092.

70. **Morrison DJ, Preston T.** 2016. Formation of short chain fatty acids by the gut microbiota and their impact on human metabolism. *Gut Microbes* **7:**189–200.

71. **Kasubuchi M, Hasegawa S, Hiramatsu T, Ichimura A, Kimura I.** 2015. Dietary gut microbial metabolites, short-chain fatty acids, and host metabolic regulation. *Nutrients* **7:** 2839–2849.

72. **Louis P, Hold GL, Flint HJ.** 2014. The gut microbiota, bacterial metabolites and colorectal cancer. *Nat Rev Microbiol* **12:**661–672.

73. **Reichardt N, Duncan SH, Young P, Belenguer A, McWilliam Leitch C, Scott KP, Flint HJ, Louis P.** 2014. Phylogenetic distribution of three pathways for propionate production within the human gut microbiota. *ISME J* **8:**1323–1335.

74. **Salonen A, Lahti L, Salojärvi J, Holtrop G, Korpela K, Duncan SH, Date P, Farquharson F, Johnstone AM, Lobley GE, Louis P, Flint HJ, de Vos WM.** 2014. Impact of diet and individual variation on intestinal microbiota composition and fermentation products in obese men. *ISME J* **8:**2218–2230.

75. **Louis P, Flint HJ.** 2009. Diversity, metabolism and microbial ecology of butyrate-producing bacteria from the human large intestine. *FEMS Microbiol Lett* **294:**1–8.

76. **Louis P, Young P, Holtrop G, Flint HJ.** 2010. Diversity of human colonic butyrate-producing bacteria revealed by analysis of the butyryl-CoA:acetate CoA-transferase gene. *Environ Microbiol* **12:**304–314.

77. **Chang PV, Hao L, Offermanns S, Medzhitov R.** 2014. The microbial metabolite butyrate regulates intestinal macrophage function via histone deacetylase inhibition. *Proc Natl Acad Sci USA* **111:**2247–2252.

78. **Smith PM, Howitt MR, Panikov N, Michaud M, Gallini CA, Bohlooly-Y M, Glickman JN, Garrett WS.** 2013. The microbial metabolites, short-chain fatty acids, regulate colonic Treg cell homeostasis. *Science* **341:**569–573.

79. **Furusawa Y, Obata Y, Fukuda S, Endo TA, Nakato G, Takahashi D, Nakanishi Y, Uetake C, Kato K, Kato T, Takahashi M, Fukuda NN, Murakami S, Miyauchi E, Hino S, Atarashi K, Onawa S, Fujimura Y, Lockett T, Clarke JM, Topping DL, Tomita M, Hori S, Ohara O, Morita T, Koseki H, Kikuchi J, Honda K, Hase K, Ohno H.** 2013. Commensal microbe-derived butyrate induces the differentiation of colonic regulatory T cells. *Nature* **504:**446–450.

80. **Macfarlane GT, Macfarlane S.** 2012. Bacteria, colonic fermentation, and gastrointestinal health. *J AOAC Int* **95:**50–60.

81. **Calmels S, Ohshima H, Vincent P, Gounot AM, Bartsch H.** 1985. Screening of microorganisms for nitrosation catalysis at pH 7 and kinetic studies on nitrosamine formation from secondary amines by *E. coli* strains. *Carcinogenesis* **6:**911–915.

82. **Macfarlane GT, Gibson GR, Cummings JH.** 1992. Comparison of fermentation reactions in different regions of the human colon. *J Appl Bacteriol* **72:**57–64.

83. **Aguirre de Cárcer D, Cuív PO, Wang T, Kang S, Worthley D, Whitehall V, Gordon I, McSweeney C, Leggett B, Morrison M.** 2011. Numerical ecology validates a biogeographical distribution and gender-based effect on mucosa-associated bacteria along the human colon. *ISME J* **5:**801–809.

84. **Yatsunenko T, Rey FE, Manary MJ, Trehan I, Dominguez-Bello MG, Contreras M, Magris M, Hidalgo G, Baldassano RN, Anokhin AP, Heath AC, Warner B, Reeder J, Kuczynski J, Caporaso JG, Lozupone CA, Lauber C, Clemente JC, Knights D, Knight R, Gordon JI.** 2012. Human gut microbiome viewed across age and geography. *Nature* **486:**222–227.

85. **Agans R, Rigsbee L, Kenche H, Michail S, Khamis HJ, Paliy O.** 2011. Distal gut microbiota of adolescent children is different from that of adults. *FEMS Microbiol Ecol* **77:**404–412.

86. **Biagi E, Nylund L, Candela M, Ostan R, Bucci L, Pini E, Nikkïla J, Monti D, Satokari R, Franceschi C, Brigidi P, De Vos W.** 2010. Through ageing, and beyond: gut microbiota and inflammatory status in seniors and centenarians. *PLoS One* **5:**e10667.

87. **Tiihonen K, Ouwehand AC, Rautonen N.** 2010. Human intestinal microbiota and healthy ageing. *Ageing Res Rev* **9:**107–116.

88. **Sears CL, Pardoll DM.** 2011. Perspective: alpha-bugs, their microbial partners, and the link to colon cancer. *J Infect Dis* **203:**306–311.

89. **Sears CL, Islam S, Saha A, Arjumand M, Alam NH, Faruque AS, Salam MA, Shin J, Hecht D, Weintraub A, Sack RB, Qadri F.** 2008. Association of enterotoxigenic *Bacteroides fragilis* infection with inflammatory diarrhea. *Clin Infect Dis* **47:**797–803.

90. **Wu S, Rhee KJ, Albesiano E, Rabizadeh S, Wu X, Yen HR, Huso DL, Brancati FL, Wick E, McAllister F, Housseau F, Pardoll DM, Sears CL.** 2009. A human colonic commensal promotes colon tumorigenesis via activation of T helper type 17 T cell responses. *Nat Med* **15:**1016–1022.

91. **Agus A, Massier S, Darfeuille-Michaud A, Billard E, Barnich N.** 2014. Understanding host-adherent-invasive *Escherichia coli* interaction in Crohn's disease: opening up new therapeutic strategies. *BioMed Res Int* **2014:** 567929.

92. **Denizot J, Sivignon A, Barreau F, Darcha C, Chan HF, Stanners CP, Hofman P, Darfeuille-Michaud A, Barnich N.** 2012. Adherent-invasive *Escherichia coli* induce claudin-2 expression and barrier defect in CEABAC10 mice and Crohn's disease patients. *Inflamm Bowel Dis* **18:**294–304.

93. **Ellermann M, Huh EY, Liu B, Carroll IM, Tamayo R, Sartor RB.** 2015. Adherent-invasive *Escherichia coli* production of cellulose influences iron-induced bacterial aggregation, phagocytosis, and induction of colitis. *Infect Immun* **83:**4068–4080.

94. **Martinez-Medina M, Garcia-Gil LJ.** 2014. *Escherichia coli* in chronic inflammatory bowel diseases: an update on adherent invasive *Escherichia coli* pathogenicity. *World J Gastrointest Pathophysiol* **5:**213–227.

95. **Wine E, Ossa JC, Gray-Owen SD, Sherman PM.** 2009. Adherent-invasive *Escherichia coli*, strain LF82 disrupts apical junctional complexes in polarized epithelia. *BMC Microbiol* **9:**180.

96. **Herrinton LJ, Liu L, Levin TR, Allison JE, Lewis JD, Velayos F.** 2012. Incidence and mortality of colorectal adenocarcinoma in persons with inflammatory bowel disease from 1998 to 2010. *Gastroenterology* **143:**382–389.

97. **Nguyen HT, Dalmasso G, Müller S, Carrière J, Seibold F, Darfeuille-Michaud A.** 2014. Crohn's disease-associated adherent invasive *Escherichia coli* modulate levels of microRNAs in intestinal epithelial cells to reduce autophagy. *Gastroenterology* **146:**508–519.

98. **Nesić D, Hsu Y, Stebbins CE.** 2004. Assembly and function of a bacterial genotoxin. *Nature* **429:**429–433.

99. **Balskus EP.** 2015. Colibactin: understanding an elusive gut bacterial genotoxin. *Nat Prod Rep* **32:**1534–1540.

100. **Tjalsma H, Boleij A, Marchesi JR, Dutilh BE.** 2012. A bacterial driver-passenger model for colorectal cancer: beyond the usual suspects. *Nat Rev Microbiol* **10:**575–582.

101. **Castellarin M, Warren RL, Freeman JD, Dreolini L, Krzywinski M, Strauss J, Barnes R, Watson P, Allen-Vercoe E, Moore RA, Holt RA.** 2012. *Fusobacterium nucleatum* infection is prevalent in human colorectal carcinoma. *Genome Res* **22:**299–306.

102. **Flanagan L, Schmid J, Ebert M, Soucek P, Kunicka T, Liska V, Bruha J, Neary P, Dezeeuw N, Tommasino M, Jenab M, Prehn JH, Hughes DJ.** 2014. *Fusobacterium nucleatum* associates with stages of colorectal neoplasia development, colorectal cancer and disease outcome. *Eur J Clin Microbiol Infect Dis* **33:**1381–1390.

103. **Fukugaiti MH, Ignacio A, Fernandes MR, Ribeiro Júnior U, Nakano V, Avila-Campos MJ.** 2015. High occurrence of *Fusobacterium nucleatum* and *Clostridium difficile* in the intestinal microbiota of colorectal carcinoma patients. *Braz J Microbiol* **46:**1135–1140.

104. **Kostic AD, Gevers D, Pedamallu CS, Michaud M, Duke F, Earl AM, Ojesina AI, Jung J, Bass AJ, Tabernero J, Baselga J, Liu C, Shivdasani RA, Ogino S, Birren BW, Huttenhower C, Garrett WS, Meyerson M.** 2012. Genomic analysis identifies association of *Fusobacterium* with colorectal carcinoma. *Genome Res* **22:**292–298.

105. **McCoy AN, Araújo-Pérez F, Azcárate-Peril A, Yeh JJ, Sandler RS, Keku TO.** 2013. *Fusobacterium* is associated with colorectal adenomas. *PLoS One* **8:**e53653.

106. **Tahara T, Yamamoto E, Suzuki H, Maruyama R, Chung W, Garriga J, Jelinek J, Yamano HO, Sugai T, An B, Shureiqi I, Toyota M, Kondo Y, Estécio MR, Issa JP.** 2014. *Fusobacterium* in colonic flora and molecular features of colorectal carcinoma. *Cancer Res* **74:**1311–1318.

107. **Forbes JD, Van Domselaar G, Bernstein CN.** 2016. Microbiome survey of the inflamed and noninflamed gut at different compartments within the gastrointestinal tract of inflammatory bowel disease patients. *Inflamm Bowel Dis* **22:**817–825.

108. **Naftali T, Reshef L, Kovacs A, Porat R, Amir I, Konikoff FM, Gophna U.** 2016. Distinct microbiotas are associated with ileum-restricted and colon-involving Crohn's disease. *Inflamm Bowel Dis* **22:**293–302.

109. **Strauss J, Kaplan GG, Beck PL, Rioux K, Panaccione R, Devinney R, Lynch T, Allen-Vercoe E.** 2011. Invasive potential of gut

mucosa-derived *Fusobacterium nucleatum* positively correlates with IBD status of the host. *Inflamm Bowel Dis* **17:**1971–1978.

110. **Guinane CM, Tadrous A, Fouhy F, Ryan CA, Dempsey EM, Murphy B, Andrews E, Cotter PD, Stanton C, Ross RP.** 2013. Microbial composition of human appendices from patients following appendectomy. *MBio* **4:**4.

111. **Rogers MB, Brower-Sinning R, Firek B, Zhong D, Morowitz MJ.** 2016. Acute appendicitis in children is associated with a local expansion of *Fusobacteria*. *Clin Infect Dis* **63:**71–78.

112. **Swidsinski A, Dörffel Y, Loening-Baucke V, Tertychnyy A, Biche-Ool S, Stonogin S, Guo Y, Sun ND.** 2012. Mucosal invasion by fusobacteria is a common feature of acute appendicitis in Germany, Russia, and China. *Saudi J Gastroenterol* **18:**55–58.

113. **Zhong D, Brower-Sinning R, Firek B, Morowitz MJ.** 2014. Acute appendicitis in children is associated with an abundance of bacteria from the phylum *Fusobacteria*. *J Pediatr Surg* **49:**441–446.

114. **Mitsuhashi K, Nosho K, Sukawa Y, Matsunaga Y, Ito M, Kurihara H, Kanno S, Igarashi H, Naito T, Adachi Y, Tachibana M, Tanuma T, Maguchi H, Shinohara T, Hasegawa T, Imamura M, Kimura Y, Hirata K, Maruyama R, Suzuki H, Imai K, Yamamoto H, Shinomura Y.** 2015. Association of *Fusobacterium* species in pancreatic cancer tissues with molecular features and prognosis. *Oncotarget* **6:**7209–7220.

115. **Park CH, Han DS, Oh YH, Lee AR, Lee YR, Eun CS.** 2016. Role of *Fusobacteria* in the serrated pathway of colorectal carcinogenesis. *Sci Rep* **6:**25271.

116. **Mima K, Nishihara R, Qian ZR, Cao Y, Sukawa Y, Nowak JA, Yang J, Dou R, Masugi Y, Song M, Kostic AD, Giannakis M, Bullman S, Milner DA, Baba H, Giovannucci EL, Garraway LA, Freeman GJ, Dranoff G, Garrett WS, Huttenhower C, Meyerson M, Meyerhardt JA, Chan AT, Fuchs CS, Ogino S.** 2015. *Fusobacterium nucleatum* in colorectal carcinoma tissue and patient prognosis. *Gut* 10.1136/gutjnl-2015-310101.

117. **Mima K, Sukawa Y, Nishihara R, Qian ZR, Yamauchi M, Inamura K, Kim SA, Masuda A, Nowak JA, Nosho K, Kostic AD, Giannakis M, Watanabe H, Bullman S, Milner DA, Harris CC, Giovannucci E, Garraway LA, Freeman GJ, Dranoff G, Chan AT, Garrett WS, Huttenhower C, Fuchs CS, Ogino S.** 2015. *Fusobacterium nucleatum* and T cells in colorectal carcinoma. *JAMA Oncol* **1:**653–661.

118. **Rubinstein MR, Wang X, Liu W, Hao Y, Cai G, Han YW.** 2013. *Fusobacterium nucleatum* promotes colorectal carcinogenesis by modulating E-cadherin/β-catenin signaling via its FadA adhesin. *Cell Host Microbe* **14:**195–206.

119. **Szabó C, Papapetropoulos A.** 2011. Hydrogen sulphide and angiogenesis: mechanisms and applications. *Br J Pharmacol* **164:**853–865.

120. **Kostic AD, Chun E, Robertson L, Glickman JN, Gallini CA, Michaud M, Clancy TE, Chung DC, Lochhead P, Hold GL, El-Omar EM, Brenner D, Fuchs CS, Meyerson M, Garrett WS.** 2013. *Fusobacterium nucleatum* potentiates intestinal tumorigenesis and modulates the tumor-immune microenvironment. *Cell Host Microbe* **14:**207–215.

121. **Nakatsu G, Li X, Zhou H, Sheng J, Wong SH, Wu WK, Ng SC, Tsoi H, Dong Y, Zhang N, He Y, Kang Q, Cao L, Wang K, Zhang J, Liang Q, Yu J, Sung JJ.** 2015. Gut mucosal microbiome across stages of colorectal carcinogenesis. *Nat Commun* **6:**8727.

122. **Heiman ML, Greenway FL.** 2016. A healthy gastrointestinal microbiome is dependent on dietary diversity. *Mol Metab* **5:**317–320.

123. **Boursi B, Haynes K, Mamtani R, Yang YX.** 2015. Impact of antibiotic exposure on the risk of colorectal cancer. *Pharmacoepidemiol Drug Saf* **24:**534–542.

124. **Duncan SH, Flint HJ.** 2013. Probiotics and prebiotics and health in ageing populations. *Maturitas* **75:**44–50.

125. **Hooper LV, Littman DR, Macpherson AJ.** 2012. Interactions between the microbiota and the immune system. *Science* **336:**1268–1273.

126. **Lozupone CA, Stombaugh JI, Gordon JI, Jansson JK, Knight R.** 2012. Diversity, stability and resilience of the human gut microbiota. *Nature* **489:**220–230.

127. **Baxter NT, Zackular JP, Chen GY, Schloss PD.** 2014. Structure of the gut microbiome following colonization with human feces determines colonic tumor burden. *Microbiome* **2:**20.

128. **Blaut M.** 2013. Ecology and physiology of the intestinal tract. *Curr Top Microbiol Immunol* **358:**247–272.

129. **Dejea CM, Wick EC, Hechenbleikner EM, White JR, Mark Welch JL, Rossetti BJ, Peterson SN, Snesrud EC, Borisy GG, Lazarev M, Stein E, Vadivelu J, Roslani AC, Malik AA, Wanyiri JW, Goh KL, Thevambiga I, Fu K, Wan F, Llosa N, Housseau F, Romans K, Wu X, McAllister FM, Wu S, Vogelstein B, Kinzler KW, Pardoll DM, Sears CL.** 2014. Microbiota organization is a distinct feature of proximal colorectal cancers. *Proc Natl Acad Sci USA* **111:**18321–18326.

130. **Johnson CH, Dejea CM, Edler D, Hoang LT, Santidrian AF, Felding BH, Ivanisevic J, Cho**

K, Wick EC, Hechenbleikner EM, Uritboonthai W, Goetz L, Casero RA Jr, Pardoll DM, White JR, Patti GJ, Sears CL, Siuzdak G. 2015. Metabolism links bacterial biofilms and colon carcinogenesis. *Cell Metab* **21:**891–897.

131. **Canellakis ZN, Marsh LL, Bondy PK.** 1989. Polyamines and their derivatives as modulators in growth and differentiation. *Yale J Biol Med* **62:**481–491.

132. **Fan P, Li L, Rezaei A, Eslamfam S, Che D, Ma X.** 2015. Metabolites of dietary protein and peptides by intestinal microbes and their impacts on gut. *Curr Protein Pept Sci* **16:**646–654.

133. **Kolenbrander PE.** 2011. Multispecies communities: interspecies interactions influence growth on saliva as sole nutritional source. *Int J Oral Sci* **3:**49–54.

134. **Sinha R, Ahn J, Sampson JN, Shi J, Yu G, Xiong X, Hayes RB, Goedert JJ.** 2016. Fecal microbiota, fecal metabolome, and colorectal cancer interrelations. *PLoS One* **11:**e0152126.

135. **Long EK, Picklo MJ Sr.** 2010. Trans-4-hydroxy-2-hexenal, a product of n-3 fatty acid peroxidation: make some room HNE.... *Free Radic Biol Med* **49:**1–8.

136. **Emerit I, Garban F, Vassy J, Levy A, Filipe P, Freitas J.** 1996. Superoxide-mediated clastogenesis and anticlastogenic effects of exogenous superoxide dismutase. *Proc Natl Acad Sci USA* **93:**12799–12804.

137. **Huycke MM, Moore D, Joyce W, Wise P, Shepard L, Kotake Y, Gilmore MS.** 2001. Extracellular superoxide production by *Enterococcus faecalis* requires demethylmenaquinone and is attenuated by functional terminal quinol oxidases. *Mol Microbiol* **42:**729–740.

138. **Balamurugan R, Rajendiran E, George S, Samuel GV, Ramakrishna BS.** 2008. Real-time polymerase chain reaction quantification of specific butyrate-producing bacteria, *Desulfovibrio* and *Enterococcus faecalis* in the feces of patients with colorectal cancer. *J Gastroenterol Hepatol* **23:**1298–1303.

139. **Allen TD, Moore DR, Wang X, Casu V, May R, Lerner MR, Houchen C, Brackett DJ, Huycke MM.** 2008. Dichotomous metabolism of *Enterococcus faecalis* induced by haematin starvation modulates colonic gene expression. *J Med Microbiol* **57:**1193–1204.

140. **Wang X, Huycke MM.** 2015. Colorectal cancer: role of commensal bacteria and bystander effects. *Gut Microbes* **6:**370–376.

141. **Wang X, Allen TD, Yang Y, Moore DR, Huycke MM.** 2013. Cyclooxygenase-2 generates the endogenous mutagen trans-4-hydroxy-2-nonenal in

Enterococcus faecalis-infected macrophages. *Cancer Prev Res (Phila)* **6:**206–216.

142. **Larsson SC, Wolk A.** 2006. Meat consumption and risk of colorectal cancer: a meta-analysis of prospective studies. *Int J Cancer* **119:**2657–2664.

143. **Sanders ME.** 2008. Probiotics: definition, sources, selection, and uses. *Clin Infect Dis* **46**(Suppl 2)**:**S58–S61; discussion S144–S151.

144. **Rafter J.** 2004. The effects of probiotics on colon cancer development. *Nutr Res Rev* **17:**277–284.

145. **Rafter J, Bennett M, Caderni G, Clune Y, Hughes R, Karlsson PC, Klinder A, O'Riordan M, O'Sullivan GC, Pool-Zobel B, Rechkemmer G, Roller M, Rowland I, Salvadori M, Thijs H, Van Loo J, Watzl B, Collins JK.** 2007. Dietary synbiotics reduce cancer risk factors in polypectomized and colon cancer patients. *Am J Clin Nutr* **85:**488–496.

146. **Faridnia F, Hussin AS, Saari N, Mustafa S, Yee LY, Manap MY.** 2010. In vitro binding of mutagenic heterocyclic aromatic amines by *Bifidobacterium pseudocatenulatum* G4. *Benef Microbes* **1:**149–154.

147. **Nowak A, Śliżewska K, Błasiak J, Libudzisz Z.** 2014. The influence of *Lactobacillus casei* DN 114 001 on the activity of faecal enzymes and genotoxicity of faecal water in the presence of heterocyclic aromatic amines. *Anaerobe* **30:**129–136.

148. **Kumar M, Nagpal R, Kumar R, Hemalatha R, Verma V, Kumar A, Chakraborty C, Singh B, Marotta F, Jain S, Yadav H.** 2012. Cholesterol-lowering probiotics as potential biotherapeutics for metabolic diseases. *Exp Diabetes Res* **2012:**902917.

149. **Matsuzaki T, Yokokura T, Azuma I.** 1985. Antitumour activity of *Lactobacillus casei* on Lewis lung carcinoma and line-10 hepatoma in syngeneic mice and guinea pigs. *Cancer Immunol Immunother* **20:**18–22.

150. **Matsuzaki T, Yokokura T, Azuma I.** 1987. Antimetastatic effect of *Lactobacillus casei* YIT9018 (LC 9018) on a highly metastatic variant of B16 melanoma in C57BL/6J mice. *Cancer Immunol Immunother* **24:**99–105.

151. **Matsuzaki T, Yokokura T, Mutai M.** 1988. Antitumor effect of intrapleural administration of *Lactobacillus casei* in mice. *Cancer Immunol Immunother* **26:**209–214.

152. **Takagi A, Matsuzaki T, Sato M, Nomoto K, Morotomi M, Yokokura T.** 1999. Inhibitory effect of oral administration of *Lactobacillus casei* on 3-methylcholanthrene-induced carcinogenesis in mice. *Med Microbiol Immunol (Berl)* **188:**111–116.

153. **Yamazaki K, Tsunoda A, Sibusawa M, Tsunoda Y, Kusano M, Fukuchi K, Yamanaka M, Kushima M, Nomoto K, Morotomi M.** 2000. The effect of an oral administration of *Lactobacillus casei* strain shirota on azoxymethane-induced colonic aberrant crypt foci and colon cancer in the rat. *Oncol Rep* **7**:977–982.

154. **Ohashi Y, Nakai S, Tsukamoto T, Masumori N, Akaza H, Miyanaga N, Kitamura T, Kawabe K, Kotake T, Kuroda M, Naito S, Koga H, Saito Y, Nomata K, Kitagawa M, Aso Y.** 2002. Habitual intake of lactic acid bacteria and risk reduction of bladder cancer. *Urol Int* **68**:273–280.

155. **Toi M, Hirota S, Tomotaki A, Sato N, Hozumi Y, Anan K, Nagashima T, Tokuda Y, Masuda N, Ohsumi S, Ohno S, Takahashi M, Hayashi H, Yamamoto S, Ohashi Y.** 2013. Probiotic beverage with soy isoflavone consumption for breast cancer prevention: a case-control study. *Curr Nutr Food Sci* **9**:194–200.

156. **Yasutake N, Matsuzaki T, Kimura K, Hashimoto S, Yokokura T, Yoshikai Y.** 1999. The role of tumor necrosis factor (TNF)-alpha in the antitumor effect of intrapleural injection of *Lactobacillus casei* strain Shirota in mice. *Med Microbiol Immunol (Berl)* **188**:9–14.

157. **Matsumoto S, Hara T, Nagaoka M, Mike A, Mitsuyama K, Sako T, Yamamoto M, Kado S, Takada T.** 2009. A component of polysaccharide peptidoglycan complex on *Lactobacillus* induced an improvement of murine model of inflammatory bowel disease and colitis-associated cancer. *Immunology* **128**(Suppl):e170–c180.

158. **Weill FS, Cela EM, Paz ML, Ferrari A, Leoni J, González Maglio DH.** 2013. Lipoteichoic acid from *Lactobacillus rhamnosus* GG as an oral photoprotective agent against UV-induced carcinogenesis. *Br J Nutr* **109**:457–466.

159. **Lenoir M, Del Carmen S, Cortes-Perez NG, Lozano-Ojalvo D, Muñoz-Provencio D, Chain F, Langella P, de Moreno de LeBlanc A, LeBlanc JG, Bermúdez-Humarán LG.** 2016. *Lactobacillus casei* BL23 regulates Treg and Th17 T-cell populations and reduces DMH-associated colorectal cancer. *J Gastroenterol* **51**:862–873.

160. **Do EJ, Hwang SW, Kim SY, Ryu YM, Cho EA, Chung EJ, Park S, Lee HJ, Byeon JS, Ye BD, Yang DH, Park SH, Yang SK, Kim JH, Myung SJ.** 2015. Suppression of colitis-associated carcinogenesis through modulation of IL-6/STAT3 pathway by Balsalazide and VSL#3. *J Gastroenterol Hepatol* 10.1111/jgh.13280.

161. **Otte JM, Mahjurian-Namari R, Brand S, Werner I, Schmidt WE, Schmitz F.** 2009. Probiotics regulate the expression of COX-2 in intestinal epithelial cells. *Nutr Cancer* **61**:103–113.

162. **Sano H, Kawahito Y, Wilder RL, Hashiramoto A, Mukai S, Asai K, Kimura S, Kato H, Kondo M, Hla T.** 1995. Expression of cyclooxygenase-1 and -2 in human colorectal cancer. *Cancer Res* **55**:3785–3789.

163. **Singh J, Rivenson A, Tomita M, Shimamura S, Ishibashi N, Reddy BS.** 1997. *Bifidobacterium longum*, a lactic acid-producing intestinal bacterium inhibits colon cancer and modulates the intermediate biomarkers of colon carcinogenesis. *Carcinogenesis* **18**:833–841.

164. **Chen ZF, Ai LY, Wang JL, Ren LL, Yu YN, Xu J, Chen HY, Yu J, Li M, Qin WX, Ma X, Shen N, Chen YX, Hong J, Fang JY.** 2015. Probiotics *Clostridium butyricum* and *Bacillus subtilis* ameliorate intestinal tumorigenesis. *Future Microbiol* **10**:1433–1445.

165. **Chen X, Fruehauf J, Goldsmith JD, Xu H, Katchar KK, Koon HW, Zhao D, Kokkotou EG, Pothoulakis C, Kelly CP.** 2009. *Saccharomyces boulardii* inhibits EGF receptor signaling and intestinal tumor growth in Apc (min) mice. *Gastroenterology* **137**:914–923.

166. **Roberfroid M, Gibson GR, Hoyles L, McCartney AL, Rastall R, Rowland I, Wolvers D, Watzl B, Szajewska H, Stahl B, Guarner F, Respondek F, Whelan K, Coxam V, Davicco MJ, Léotoing L, Wittrant Y, Delzenne NM, Cani PD, Neyrinck AM, Meheust A.** 2010. Prebiotic effects: metabolic and health benefits. *Br J Nutr* **104**(Suppl 2):S1–S63.

167. **Slavin J.** 2013. Fiber and prebiotics: mechanisms and health benefits. *Nutrients* **5**:1417–1435.

168. **Valcheva R, Dieleman LA.** 2016. Prebiotics: definition and protective mechanisms. *Best Pract Res Clin Gastroenterol* **30**:27–37.

169. **Verghese M, Rao DR, Chawan CB, Williams LL, Shackelford L.** 2002. Dietary inulin suppresses azoxymethane-induced aberrant crypt foci and colon tumors at the promotion stage in young Fisher 344 rats. *J Nutr* **132**:2809–2813.

170. **Reddy BS, Hamid R, Rao CV.** 1997. Effect of dietary oligofructose and inulin on colonic preneoplastic aberrant crypt foci inhibition. *Carcinogenesis* **18**:1371–1374.

171. **Rowland IR, Rumney CJ, Coutts JT, Lievense LC.** 1998. Effect of *Bifidobacterium longum* and inulin on gut bacterial metabolism and carcinogen-induced aberrant crypt foci in rats. *Carcinogenesis* **19**:281–285.

172. **Hsu CK, Liao JW, Chung YC, Hsieh CP, Chan YC.** 2004. Xylooligosaccharides and fructooligosaccharides affect the intestinal microbiota and precancerous colonic lesion development in rats. *J Nutr* **134**:1523–1528.

173. **Davis LM, Martínez I, Walter J, Goin C, Hutkins RW.** 2011. Barcoded pyrosequencing reveals that consumption of galactooligosaccharides results in a highly specific bifidogenic response in humans. *PLoS One* **6:**e25200.

174. **Maathuis AJ, van den Heuvel EG, Schoterman MH, Venema K.** 2012. Galacto-oligosaccharides have prebiotic activity in a dynamic in vitro colon model using a (13)C-labeling technique. *J Nutr* **142:**1205–1212.

175. **Bruno-Barcena JM, Azcarate-Peril MA.** 2015. Galacto-oligosaccharides and colorectal cancer: feeding our intestinal probiome. *J Funct Foods* **12:**92–108.

176. **Scholz-Ahrens KE, Ade P, Marten B, Weber P, Timm W, Açil Y, Glüer CC, Schrezenmeir J.** 2007. Prebiotics, probiotics, and synbiotics affect mineral absorption, bone mineral content, and bone structure. *J Nutr* **137**(Suppl 2)**:**838S–846S.

177. **Scholz-Ahrens KE, Schaafsma G, van den Heuvel EG, Schrezenmeir J.** 2001. Effects of prebiotics on mineral metabolism. *Am J Clin Nutr* **73**(Suppl)**:**459S–464S.

178. **Cloetens L, Broekaert WF, Delaedt Y, Ollevier F, Courtin CM, Delcour JA, Rutgeerts P, Verbeke K.** 2010. Tolerance of arabinoxylan-oligosaccharides and their prebiotic activity in healthy subjects: a randomised, placebo-controlled cross-over study. *Br J Nutr* **103:**703–713.

179. **Enoki T, Okuda S, Kudo Y, Takashima F, Sagawa H, Kato I.** 2010. Oligosaccharides from agar inhibit pro-inflammatory mediator release by inducing heme oxygenase 1. *Biosci Biotechnol Biochem* **74:**766–770.

180. **Higashimura Y, Naito Y, Takagi T, Mizushima K, Hirai Y, Harusato A, Ohnogi H, Yamaji R, Inui H, Nakano Y, Yoshikawa T.** 2013. Oligosaccharides from agar inhibit murine intestinal inflammation through the induction of heme oxygenase-1 expression. *J Gastroenterol* **48:**897–909.

181. **Higashimura Y, Naito Y, Takagi T, Uchiyama K, Mizushima K, Ushiroda C, Ohnogi H, Kudo Y, Yasui M, Inui S, Hisada T, Honda A, Matsuzaki Y, Yoshikawa T.** 2016. Protective effect of agaro-oligosaccharides on gut dysbiosis and colon tumorigenesis in high-fat diet-fed mice. *Am J Physiol Gastrointest Liver Physiol* **310:**G367–G375.

182. **Blaser MJ.** 2016. Antibiotic use and its consequences for the normal microbiome. *Science* **352:**544–545.

183. **Sokol H.** 2014. Probiotics and antibiotics in IBD. *Dig Dis* **32**(Suppl 1)**:**10–17.

184. **Glebov OK, Rodriguez LM, Nakahara K, Jenkins J, Cliatt J, Humbyrd CJ, DeNobile J, Soballe P, Simon R, Wright G, Lynch P, Patterson S, Lynch H, Gallinger S, Buchbinder A, Gordon G, Hawk E, Kirsch IR.** 2003. Distinguishing right from left colon by the pattern of gene expression. *Cancer Epidemiol Biomarkers Prev* **12:**755–762.

185. **Pekow J, Meckel K, Dougherty U, Butun F, Mustafi R, Lim J, Crofton C, Chen X, Joseph L, Bissonnette M.** 2015. Tumor suppressors miR-143 and miR-145 and predicted target proteins API5, ERK5, K-RAS, and IRS-1 are differentially expressed in proximal and distal colon. *Am J Physiol Gastrointest Liver Physiol* **308:**G179–G187.

186. **Filipe MI, Branfoot AC.** 1976. Mucin histochemistry of the colon. *Curr Top Pathol* **63:** 143–178.

187. **Noble CL, Abbas AR, Lees CW, Cornelius J, Toy K, Modrusan Z, Clark HF, Arnott ID, Penman ID, Satsangi J, Diehl L.** 2010. Characterization of intestinal gene expression profiles in Crohn's disease by genome-wide microarray analysis. *Inflamm Bowel Dis* **16:**1717–1728.

188. **Albuquerque C, Bakker ER, van Veelen W, Smits R.** 2011. Colorectal cancers choosing sides. *Biochim Biophys Acta* **1816:**219–231.

Microbial Impact on Host Metabolism: Opportunities for Novel Treatments of Nutritional Disorders?

5

HUBERT PLOVIER[1,2] and PATRICE D. CANI[1,2]

INTRODUCTION

Malnutrition, encompassing both excessive and insufficient nutrient intake, is a major public health concern worldwide. On the one hand, overweight and obesity affect more than one-third and one-tenth of the world's population, respectively. Excessive body weight and fat mass gain are classically linked with several metabolic disorders and cardiometabolic risk factors, including insulin resistance, type 2 diabetes, hypertension, low-grade inflammation, and liver diseases (Fig. 1). Over the past 20 years, researchers have gathered evidence showing the involvement of chronic inflammation in the onset of the metabolic syndrome. Among the plethora of factors involved in the etiology of metabolic disorders, our lab and others have shown that the interplay between a too-rich diet and another environmental factor, namely the gut microbiota, plays a major role (for reviews, see references 1 to 5).

On the opposite end of the malnutrition spectrum, undernutrition is the leading cause of death in children under 5 years of age. Arising from dietary deficiencies in either macronutrients, such as proteins, or micronutrients, such as metals (zinc, selenium) and vitamins, undernutrition causes more than 3 million deaths annually (6).

[1]WELBIO—Walloon Excellence in Life Sciences and Biotechnology, Louvain Drug Research Institute, Université catholique de Louvain, Brussels, Belgium; [2]Metabolism and Nutrition Research Group, Louvain Drug Research Institute, Université catholique de Louvain, Brussels, Belgium

Bugs as Drugs: Therapeutic Microbes for the Prevention and Treatment of Disease
Edited by Robert A. Britton and Patrice D. Cani
© 2018 American Society for Microbiology, Washington, DC
doi:10.1128/microbiolspec.BAD-0002-2016

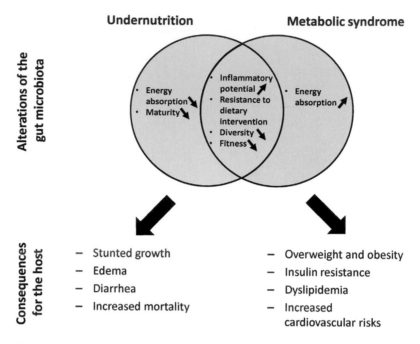

FIGURE 1 Dysbiosis during undernutrition and the metabolic syndrome: two sides of the same coin? Gut microbiota composition is modified in people suffering from undernutrition as well as the metabolic syndrome, the two extremes of malnutrition. Changes in the composition are associated with opposite consequences in terms of energy absorption from the diet, but lead to similar defects in terms of ecological fitness and inflammatory potential.

More than a century ago, two Nobel prizes were awarded for discoveries linking bacteria, immunity, and health (to Robert Koch in 1905 and Ilya Mechnikov in 1908). Since these discoveries, several determinants of host-bacterium interactions have been identified. Microbes are increasingly seen not only as infectious sources but also as symbiotic partners of eukaryotic organisms. The human gut microbiota comprises as many as 10 to 100 trillion microbes. This number is in the same proportion as human cells and goes up to 10 times more microorganisms than human cells when excluding erythrocytes (7). Recent data suggest that each individual houses more than 150 species from a consortium of 1,000 to 1,600 prevalent bacteria (8, 9). As gut microbes provide genetic and metabolic traits that are not encoded by our own genome, they can be seen as a virtual organ involved in the regulation of the host

energy homeostasis, along with glucose and lipid metabolism (10).

The present review will discuss seminal papers and recent data highlighting the influence of the gut microbiota on the host metabolism in overweight and obesity, as well as undernutrition. Data suggesting the therapeutic potential of modulating the gut microbiota composition and activity will also be discussed.

MICROBIAL CONTRIBUTIONS TO ENERGY HOMEOSTASIS—INSIGHTS FROM GERMFREE MICE

The role of the gut microbiota in the regulation of the host energy metabolism has been thoroughly studied using germfree (GF) mice, which are raised without any microorganisms. In a pioneering study in 2004, Bäckhed et al. demonstrated the involvement of the gut microbiota in the host metabolism and growth, showing that GF mice gained significantly less body weight and fat mass than conventionally raised (Conv-R) mice possessing a gut microbiota. This difference was observed despite the increased food consumption and decreased whole-body metabolism of the GF mice. Moreover, the presence of gut microbes increased the levels of serum leptin, insulin, and glucose and increased triglyceride hepatic synthesis and lipid storage in the adipose tissue (11). In another study, insulin-like growth factor 1 (IGF-1) and its downstream effectors IGF-1 binding protein 3 and Akt were also shown to be regulated by the gut microbiota (12). All these components of the somatotropic axis, involved in the postnatal systemic growth, were decreased in GF mice, thereby contributing to the decreased body weight gain observed in the absence of gut microbes.

Another peripheral contribution of the gut microbiota to energy metabolism comes directly from the digestive tract. Indeed, GF mice display markedly lower levels of cecal short-chain fatty acids than Conv-R mice, indicating that the gut microbiota directly contributes to energy absorption by furnishing energy-rich substrates to the host intestinal epithelium (13).

Differences between GF and Conv-R mice also exist at the central level. Indeed, colonization by gut microbes increases the expression of *Pomc* and *Cart* (respectively encoding the anorexigenic peptides proopiomelanocortin and cocain- and amphetamine-regulated transcript) while decreasing the expression of *Npy* and *Agrp* (respectively encoding the orexigenic neuropeptide Y and Agouti-related peptide). This finding might explain the lower food consumption of Conv-R mice (14). However, Conv-R mice are less sensitive to the weight-reducing actions of central leptin, likely contributing to the increased body weight and fat mass gain compared with GF mice (11, 14).

Finally, gut microbes can also modulate the host response to undernutrition. Indeed, in the study of the somatotropic axis, GF and Conv-R mice were exposed to a depleted diet low in proteins, fats, and vitamins. While both groups lost weight compared to mice receiving a normal breeding diet, weight loss and growth defects were more pronounced in the GF mice. Interestingly, colonization of GF mice with strains of *Lactobacillus plantarum* partially compensated these defects through activation of the somatotropic axis (12).

Taken together, these data indicate that gut microbes can act on the host energy homeostasis with consequences on body composition and growth. These effects depend on modulations of nutrient absorption, adipokines, and hormones and central control of food intake.

IMPACT OF THE GUT MICROBIOTA ON MALNUTRITION-ASSOCIATED METABOLIC DISORDERS

A Metabolic Role for Gut Microbes during Obesity

As described at the beginning of this chapter, obesity as a consequence of malnutrition is reaching epidemic proportions around the globe. We recently proposed the concept of MicrObesity (microbes and obesity) (15), devoted to deciphering the impact of alterations in the gut microbiota composition and/or activity on the development of obesity and the metabolic syndrome. Numerous papers have shown that the gut microbiota composition might differ between obese and lean subjects or between prediabetic/type 2 diabetic and normoglycemic subjects (16–28). As these differences have been extensively discussed recently (for reviews, see references 3 and 29 to 32), we highlight the mechanisms underlying the microbial influence on the pathologies associated with obesity as well as the influence of selected bacteria.

Several reports indicate that the gut microbiota contributes to the metabolic syndrome through the modulation of the host energy metabolism. Initial evidence was obtained from experiments in GF mice. Mice lacking gut microbes were protected from the development of obesity, notably through the increased activation of AMP-activated protein kinase (AMPK) in the liver and muscles, leading to higher fatty acid oxidation in peripheral organs (20). The impact of gut microbes on obesity has also been demonstrated using genetically obese *ob/ob* mice. In 2006, Turnbaugh et al. showed that the gut microbiota of these mice is enriched in genes involved in the absorption and conversion of nondigestible polysaccharides into available substrates for the host, leading to increased energy bioavailability. Moreover, colonization of GF mice with the microbiota of *ob/ob* mice provoked a higher fat mass gain than that observed in mice colonized with the gut microbes from lean mice, independently of food intake (18).

Similar results can be observed with the human gut microbiota, as demonstrated by gut microbiota transfer experiments from twins discordant for obesity in GF mice. As observed with *ob/ob* mice, mice colonized with microbes from the obese twin gained more body weight and fat mass than did those receiving the "lean" microbiota, although both groups received a low-fat, high-fiber diet. These results further demonstrate the causative role of gut microbes in the development of obesity. From a metabolic point of view, the microbiota from obese donors presented higher expression of the genes involved in amino acid metabolism, which is associated with the increased abundance of branched-chain amino acids in the serum of colonized mice, similarly to previous observations in obese humans (33). Moreover, mice receiving the "obese" microbiota also displayed an increased concentration of hepatic and muscular acylcarnitines. Interestingly, both branched-chain amino acids and acylcarnitines are linked to the development of insulin resistance (34). These altered levels could therefore further explain the influence of gut microbes on glucose metabolism under conditions of obesity.

Another argument for the role of the gut microbiota in the etiology of obesity comes from studies of antibiotic-treated mice. Indeed, in two recent studies, the group of Martin Blaser has shown that administering mice with subtherapeutic doses of antibiotics in early life moderately increases their body weight, fat mass, and bone density (35). This increase was stronger when antibiotics were given to mice from birth (36). Subtherapeutic antibiotic treatment also tended to increase the effects of a high-fat diet (HFD) on obesity (36). On the host side, antibiotic administration notably caused changes in hormone levels and expression of genes involved in hepatic lipid metabolism. The gut microbiota was also modified by the treatment, with a decreased *Bacteroidetes/Firmicutes* ratio upon antibiotic supplementation and alterations in the metabolism of short-chain fatty acids and bile acids (35, 36). Furthermore, transfer of the microbiota from antibiotic-treated mice to GF mice induced similar effects on body weight and fat mass (36), here again arguing for a causal role of the microbiota during obesity.

The Concept of Metabolic Endotoxemia

Most if not all disorders of the metabolic syndrome have also been associated with a chronic inflammatory tone notably caused by circulating cytokines and macrophage infiltration in the adipose tissue. However, the origin of this inflammation remains a matter of discussion. Several studies have attributed the inflammatory properties of HFDs to specific dietary fatty acids, such as palmitate (C16). In 2004, using culture-independent techniques, we observed that HFD feeding profoundly affects the gut microbiota composition (for a review, see reference 5). We reasoned that a microbial factor might trigger the development of inflammation during HFD exposure. In attempting to identify an eligible candidate, we postulated that the nominee should be continuously produced within the gut, its absorption and/or action should be associated with fatty acid ingestion, and it should be an inflammatory compound of bacterial origin. We hypothesized that lipopolysaccharide (LPS), also known as endotoxin, is a potential culprit. LPS is a constituent of the outer membrane of Gram-negative bacteria, whose abundance is increased in the gut microbiota following HFD feeding. It triggers inflammatory pathways after binding the CD14/Toll-like receptor 4 (TLR-4) complex. Moreover, LPS is physiologically absorbed and carried into the blood through a mechanism involving chylomicron formation, a process stimulated under HFD conditions (37). In 2007, we demonstrated that HFD-fed mice develop a proinflammatory phenotype associated with increased blood LPS levels (19) and that blocking the interaction between LPS and the CD14/TLR-4 complex abolished diet-induced metabolic disorders (19). We further showed that these chronically high LPS levels induce insulin resistance, adipose tissue remodeling, and diabetes (19, 38, 39). We therefore proposed the concept of metabolic endotoxemia as a mechanism associating the gut microbiota with the onset of insulin resistance and low-grade inflammation through this increase in blood LPS levels. Using mice lacking CD14, we showed that metabolic endotoxemia is a key event in the onset of proinflammatory cytokine production. In addition, previous data suggest that metabolic endotoxemia also occurs in *ob/ob* and *db/db* mice (40–42). Furthermore, we demonstrated that the chronic subcutaneous infusion of treatments that quenched LPS *in vivo* (i.e., polymyxin B or a specific endotoxin inhibitor with peptide sequence KTKCKFLKKC) improves glucose metabolism and reduces inflammation and hepatic steatosis (43). The presence of metabolic endotoxemia upon HFD or obesity and diabetes has been extensively confirmed in other studies and in humans (Fig. 1) (44–57). However, we recently demonstrated that the blood of HFD-fed mice activates several TLRs and not only TLR-4, suggesting that other microbe-associated molecular patterns might

be involved in the chronic inflammation observed during obesity (58).

Intestinal Barrier Function and Gut Microbes

While the gut microbiota comprises trillions of microbes, blood and host tissues are nearly devoid of bacteria or bacterial components. This relative sterility reflects the existence of a finely tuned gut barrier function. The intestinal epithelium is notably covered with a mucus layer secreted by goblet cells. This physical barrier contains secreted antimicrobial factors (e.g., primarily regenerating islet-derived 3-gamma [RegIIIγ], α-defensins, lysozyme C, phospholipases) that help maintain microbes at a distance from epithelial cells (59–61). Effectors of the adaptive immune system (e.g., immunoglobulin A [IgA]) are also secreted into the intestinal lumen and restrict bacterial penetration into the host mucus and tissue (62). Epithelial cells themselves also contribute to the regulation of intestinal permeability, and the localization of tight junction proteins strongly influences the efficiency of the gut barrier (41, 63–65).

We and others observed that the gut barrier function is weakened upon HFD feeding and under conditions of obesity, with a decreased mucus layer thickness, lower production of antimicrobial peptides, and a disrupted distribution of tight-junction proteins. Several of these host-derived factors have been shown to shape microbial communities during diet-induced obesity, diabetes, and metabolic inflammation and eventually contribute to the phenotype (41, 67–71). This impairment of the gut barrier leads to the translocation of specific bacterial constituents including LPS in the bloodstream, as well as the presence of bacteria in host tissues during obesity and diabetes (22, 72). Gut permeability can therefore be seen as another mechanism contributing to the chronic inflammation observed during obesity.

Microbial Gene Diversity and Host Metabolism

In 2013, a metagenomic analysis of 292 Danish individuals showed that this cohort could be separated in two distinct groups, namely, high- and low-gene-count groups (HGC and LGC), according to the abundance of the microbial genes present in their microbiomes. Interestingly, HGC individuals notably harbored higher levels of *Akkermansia muciniphila* and the anti-inflammatory bacterium *Faecalibacterium prausnitzii* (27) than did LGC individuals. From a metabolic standpoint, the proportion of obese individuals was higher in the LGC group. The LGC group as a whole also displayed increased adiposity, insulin resistance, dyslipidemia, and inflammatory tone compared with the HGC group (Fig. 1).

In a smaller cohort of 49 overweight and obese subjects, the same bimodal distribution was observed (26). This second cohort was subjected to a weight loss dietary intervention, which partially increased the microbial gene count in LGC individuals and improved clinical parameters, such as adiposity and circulating cholesterol levels. However, this intervention was less efficient in LGC individuals than in the HGC group, suggesting that in addition to increased susceptibility to the development of metabolic syndrome, individuals with a low gene count appear less sensitive to classical dietary therapeutic strategies. The increased efficiency of dietary interventions in HGC individuals requires further investigations. As a more diverse microbiota carries more genes and encodes more potential metabolic pathways, one could argue that it is better suited to adapt to a change in diet. This could in turn allow for a better response of the host to the treatment.

Harnessing the Fitness of the Healthy Microbiota for Therapeutic Purposes

An innovative therapeutic opportunity was suggested in the study of mice colonized with obese and healthy microbiota (33). Indeed, under low-fat, high-fiber diet conditions, cohousing with mice receiving a lean microbiota decreased the fat mass gain in mice originally seeded with an obese microbiota compared with noncohoused mice. However, the opposite was not true, as cohousing did not affect the fat mass gain of mice colonized with lean microbiota. This cohousing-induced protection from obesity reflects the colonization of the obese microbiota by bacteria from the healthy one, reflecting a higher invasive capacity of the healthy microbiota. Notably, the opposite phenomenon was not observed, suggesting that in addition to being more invasive, the healthy microbiota members are also more resistant to colonization, thereby displaying better ecological fitness (33) (Fig. 1). However, it should be noted that under high-fat, low-fiber conditions, colonization of the obese microbiota by bacteria from the lean one was ineffective, highlighting the importance of the interplay between microbes and diet.

Interestingly, these results can at least partially be translated to human medicine. Indeed, a pioneering study used fecal microbial transplantation, a procedure used in antibiotic-resistant *Clostridium difficile* infections (73) to transfer the microbiota from healthy individuals to patients suffering from metabolic syndrome. The procedure improved insulin sensitivity at 6 weeks after treatment compared with patients who received their own microbiota. In addition, the diversity of the microbiota of treated patients increased by 33% (74). As 18 patients were enrolled in this trial, this study should be repeated on a larger scale prior to drawing definite conclusions. Nevertheless, this evidence provides an exciting new strategy for the microbiota-based treatment of metabolic syndrome.

The Role of Classical Probiotic Bacteria

In rodents, various strains of beneficial microbes have been shown to reduce body weight gain, fat mass development, inflammation, and hepatic steatosis or to improve glucose homeostasis. *Lactobacillus* spp. and *Bifidobacterium* spp. are among the most cited genera. The literature published in the last 3 years revealed more than 35 publications reporting the beneficial impact of specific *Lactobacillus* or *Bifidobacterium* strains on obesity and associated disorders in rodents (67, 75–110). However, the magnitude of the metabolic effects might differ according to the strain or species used. In other words, all *Lactobacillus* and *Bifidobacterium* species are not equally potent. This major dissimilarity likely reflects the production of different metabolites and different mechanisms of interactions with other bacteria and the host itself (101, 111). In addition to these "traditional" beneficial microbes, recent research based on metagenomics analyses identified specific gut microbes associated with health that could be used as "next-generation" probiotics (101). In the next section, we describe two of these microorganisms.

Next-Generation Beneficial Microorganisms

Akkermansia muciniphila

Recent research suggests that the relative lower abundance of the bacterium *A. muciniphila* might be linked to obesity and type 2 diabetes (25, 27, 67, 112–114). This bacterium was identified in 2004 and was initially categorized as a mucus degrader residing in the mucus layer (115). In 2011, we published that a prebiotic treatment, such as inulin-type fructans (i.e., oligofructose), dramatically increased the abundance of *A. muciniphila* in obese mice (41). We also positively correlated the presence of *A. muciniphila* with the number of enteroendocrine L cells producing the anorexigenic peptides glucagon-like peptide 1 (GLP-1) and PYY (41). Based on this finding, we examined the impact of *A. muciniphila* on diet-induced obese mice. The results showed that treatment with *A. muciniphila* reduced body weight gain, fat mass, and inflammation. These effects were associated

with a repaired gut lining at different levels (i.e., mucus layer thickness, production of RegIIIγ, and lower metabolic endotoxemia) (67). These results are consistent with those of other studies (116, 117). Remarkably, we observed that the beneficial response to caloric restriction was dependent on the intestinal levels of *A. muciniphila* measured prior to the intervention in obese humans, as higher microbial gene diversity and increased *A. muciniphila* abundance were associated with a better response to dietary restriction. Indeed, HGC patients displayed a higher reduction of fasting glucose, triglycerides, and visceral fat accumulation and increased insulin sensitivity markers and cardiometabolic risk factors (25). These data strengthen the observations in the first cohorts investigating microbial gene diversity (26). Altogether, these observations strongly support the interest of dietary treatments that aim at increasing *A. muciniphila* or direct administration of this microbe in humans.

Saccharomyces cerevisiae var. boulardii

We also recently observed that probiotic yeasts, such as *Saccharomyces cerevisiae* var. *boulardii* CNCM I-745, might improve metabolic parameters associated with obesity and type 2 diabetes. In obese and diabetic *db/db* mice, we observed that *S. cerevisiae* var. *boulardii* CNCM I-745 profoundly changes the microbiota composition associated with reduced fat mass, systemic and hepatic inflammation, and steatosis (118). Interestingly, this yeast has been used primarily in the context of gut inflammation, infections with *C. difficile*, and diarrhea. Whether these effects of *S. cerevisiae* var. *boulardii* are relevant in humans warrants further investigation. Furthermore, a recent study performed in preterm infants showed that the prophylactic supplementation of *S. cerevisiae* var. *boulardii* CNCM I-745 (50 mg/kg of body weight twice a day) improved body weight gain and feeding tolerance, without any adverse effects in these subjects (119). The use of this yeast was thus also beneficial in this specific situation characterized by strong defects in energy storage and intestinal function.

GUT MICROBES IN CHILDHOOD UNDERNUTRITION

The World Health Organization typically defines the clinical forms of childhood undernutrition based on anthropometric parameters: children suffering from severe acute malnutrition (SAM) present a weight-for-height Z score below minus 3 standard deviations from the median of the World Health Organization reference growth standards (6).

One of the most severe forms of SAM is kwashiorkor. Williams initially described this disease in the 1930s (120). Symptoms develop at approximately 2 years of age and include edema, diarrhea, and liver steatosis accompanied by impairments or stunting. Gut barrier function also appears to be dramatically impaired in kwashiorkor patients (120, 121). This form of SAM has been associated with a diet low in protein and micronutrients and impairments in breast-feeding (120). Recently, a ready-to-eat therapeutic food (RUTF) produced from milk powder, oil, peanuts, and sugar and supplemented with micronutrients has been approved as the standard treatment for kwashiorkor (122).

The Gut Microbiota Is Altered in Undernourished Children

The first indications of an association between gut microbes and undernutrition were reported in 1958, when Smythe and collaborators treated children suffering from kwashiorkor with a combination of antibiotics and yogurt containing *Lactobacillus delbrueckii* subsp. *bulgaricus*. This treatment led to a mortality of 9% in treated children, compared to 45% in children admitted the previous years that did not receive this treatment (123). More recently, Trehan and collaborators showed that treatment with either amoxicillin or cefdinir diminished

mortality and increased the efficiency of RUTF treatment in children suffering from undernutrition, regardless of severity (124). A similar trend of increased nutritional recovery in undernourished children receiving similar doses of amoxicillin in addition to RUTF was observed by Isanaka and collaborators, although to a lower extent and without reaching significance (125). However, long-term prophylactic treatment with co-trimoxazole failed to reduce mortality in children with SAM (126), suggesting that different antibiotics might not have the same efficiency.

The involvement of gut microbes in undernutrition is further supported by the results of a comparison of the 16S DNA sequences between healthy and undernourished children (Fig. 1). Most of these studies showed increases in the relative abundance of Proteobacteria in undernourished children, with an enrichment in genera such as *Helicobacter*, *Campylobacter*, *Klebsiella*, and *Escherichia*. Decreases in bacterial diversity and the abundance of several *Firmicutes* were also observed (127–129).

Under normal conditions, the gut microbial community drastically changes during the first 3 years of life prior to reaching an adult-like mature stage. In two distinct cohorts, microbial maturity was greatly impaired in children suffering from kwashiorkor (130, 131). The specific signatures of 220 taxa whose abundance was modified during malnutrition were identified (131). Treatment of the children with either RUTF or a locally produced therapeutic food improved gut microbial maturity associated with recovery, but this change was transient, as the microbial community reverted to an immature state shortly after the end of the treatment.

Priming of the Microbiota: Importance of Milk Oligosaccharides

As previously stated, kwashiorkor is associated with problems during breast-feeding (120). Breast-feeding is a crucial factor in the development of the gut microbiota, as the mother's milk provides the child with specific microbes, human milk oligosaccharides serving as prebiotics, and secreted immunoglobulins, and together these factors converge to modulate the microbiota of the child (132). It was recently demonstrated that the quantity and diversity of human milk oligosaccharides were significantly lower in the milk of mothers with severely stunted children than in the milk of mothers of healthy children (133).

Gnotobiotic experiments confirmed the importance of maternal sialylated milk oligosaccharides in modulating the microbiota and metabolism of the offspring (133). Indeed, GF mice colonized with the microbiota of undernourished children and exposed to a representative Malawian diet gained more weight and lean mass when the diet was supplemented with purified sialylated bovine milk oligosaccharides (S-BMOs) than without this supplement. S-BMOs modulated the microbiota of mice, not through changes in the abundance of some bacterial species but rather through alterations in the transcriptional activity of these microbes. Moreover, S-BMOs impacted the serum and liver metabolomes of mice. In the fed state, the levels of medium- and long-chain acylcarnitines were lower in S-BMO-supplemented mice than in the nonsupplemented mice, reflecting higher anabolic capabilities. During the fasting state, the opposite finding was observed, with increased concentrations of these acylcarnitines, suggesting a higher capability for nutrient mobilization in periods of fasting. Similar results were also obtained in gnotobiotic piglets, whose digestive physiology reflects that of human subjects.

Proof of Causality and Underlying Mechanisms

Microbial transplantation from discordant Malawian twin pairs to GF mice confirmed that gut microbes from children suffering from kwashiorkor are involved in the weight loss observed in this pathology (130). In mice receiving the microbiota from a diseased child, exposure to a representative low-calorie and nutrient-deficient Malawian diet led to severe weight loss, while mice receiving a healthy microbiota did not lose weight. This weight loss did not reflect the transfer of enteric pathogens. Among the most discriminant bacteria, mice with a kwashiorkor microbiota showed an increased proportion of *Bilophila wadsworthia*, associated with inflammatory bowel disease (134). Interestingly, kwashiorkor mice placed on a standard diet did not lose weight, indicating an association between the microbiota and diet in the development of the disease. Switching the mice to RUTF led to body weight normalization, with increases in the abundance of diverse *Bifidobacterium* and *Lactobacillus* species and *F. prausnitzii* and decreases in *Bacteroidales*. Similar to what was seen in human subjects, these changes were transient, as switching the mice back to a Malawian diet reversed these findings, suggesting that RUTF is not entirely sufficient to compensate the disruptions of the gut microbiota linked to undernutrition. Moreover, the metabolomics analyses of mice urinary and cecal samples suggested a disruption of the tricarboxylic acid cycle at the levels of both the host and its microbiota, suggesting that microbial changes associated with kwashiorkor directly impact energy metabolism, thereby impairing energy absorption (130) and worsening the effects of an already low-calorie and nutrient-deficient diet (Fig. 1).

Microbial Species as Prospective Therapeutic Tools against Undernutrition?

In a more recent study, the same group also confirmed the implications of gut microbiota immaturity on the malnourished phenotype. These authors transplanted the immature gut microbiota from diseased children into GF mice fed a representative Malawian diet and showed that body weight and lean mass gain were lower than in mice colonized by a healthy, mature microbiota (135). Moreover, cohousing experiments showed that a healthy microbiota partially compensates for the growth defects observed in mice colonized with an immature community. Similarly to what was observed for obesity, bacteria from the healthy microbiota were able to invade the diseased microbiota. Furthermore, administration of a specific microbial consortium of bacteria selected for their invasive capabilities to mice with an unhealthy microbiota increased the animals' body weight and lean mass gain (135).

In another study, bacteria specifically targeted by IgA were isolated from mice colonized with the microbiota of twins discordant for kwashiorkor (136). In mice colonized with the undernourished microbiota and fed with the Malawian diet, the IgA-positive (kwashiorkor-IgA$^+$) bacteria were significantly enriched in *Enterobacteriaceae*. On the other hand, the most enriched IgA$^+$ bacteria in mice colonized with the healthy microbiota (healthy-IgA$^+$) were *A. muciniphila* organisms, followed by the families *Bacteroidaceae* and *Erysipelotrichaeae*.

Mice on the Malawian diet and colonized by a consortium of kwashiorkor-IgA$^+$ bacteria or healthy-IgA$^+$ bacteria displayed an important difference in terms of survival. Indeed, 50% of the mice receiving the kwashiorkor-IgA$^+$ consortium died 2 weeks after colonization, while no mouse receiving the healthy-IgA$^+$ died in the same period. Interestingly, all mice colonized by a mix of the two consortia also survived, although they experienced greater weight loss than mice receiving only the healthy-IgA$^+$ bacteria. Furthermore, a lower mortality was also observed in mice colonized with the kwashiorkor-IgA$^+$ consortium and treated by receiving live *A. muciniphila* and *Clostridium scindens*, another species specifically enriched in the healthy microbiota. These data reinforce the observations of increased invasive potential from the healthy microbiota compared to the diseased one and

also suggest that specific bacteria such as *A. muciniphila* or *C. scindens* could be used as therapeutic agents in addition to RUTF for the management of undernutrition.

CONCLUSION AND PERSPECTIVES

The gut microbiota can be seen as a virtual organ notably involved in the regulation of several host parameters, including inflammation, immune function, and energy homeostasis (137). Diet exerts a profound influence on the gut microbial composition. In this regard, malnutrition can significantly alter the relative abundance of various gut microbes, with consequences on the functionality of the gut microbiota (Fig. 1). A diet too energy dense or too rich in fat, for example, can increase the energy absorption potential of the gut microbiota, leading to the development of overweight, obesity, and associated metabolic disorders (Fig. 1). Conversely, breast-feeding issues and a diet too poor in energy and nutrients lead to an incomplete priming of the gut microbiota. This can in turn lead to an impaired maturation of the gut microbiota, with profound decreases in its potential for energy absorption, causing stunted growth, edema, and diarrhea. Surprisingly, these seemingly opposite metabolic conditions display similar characteristics, such as an increased inflammatory tone and resistance to classical dietary treatments. On the other hand, the altered microbiota observed under these conditions presents with a decreased ecological fitness characterized by a lower diversity and impaired resistance to colonization.

Interestingly, this lower fitness could be turned into an advantage, as innovative therapeutic strategies aimed at restoring microbial fitness have been shown to cause beneficial effects on the host. The administration of specific microorganisms and fecal transplantation represents a promising tool to restore a healthy microbiota. However, a better characterization of the underlying mechanisms of these strategies is also needed.

In this regard, tools developed for the study of the gut microbiota, such as gnotobiotic models, show tremendous potential for preclinical evaluation. Furthermore, the safety of these procedures requires critical assessment in clinical settings.

ACKNOWLEDGMENTS

P.D.C. is a research associate at FRS-FNRS (Fonds de la Recherche Scientifique), Belgium. H.P. is a research fellow at FRS-FNRS, Belgium. P.D.C. is the recipient of grants from FNRS (convention J.0084.15), PDR (Projet de Recherche, convention: T.0138.14), and ARC (Action de Recherche Concertée—Communauté française de Belgique convention: 12/17-047). This work was financially supported by grants from the Fonds de la Recherche Scientifique—FNRS for the FRFS-WELBIO (grant number WELBIO-CR-2012S-02R). This work was supported in part by the Funds Baillet Latour (Grant for Medical Research 2015). P.D.C. is a recipient of an ERC Starting Grant 2013 (European Research Council, Starting grant 336452-ENIGMO).

CITATION

Plovier H, Cani PD. 2017. Microbial impact on host metabolism: opportunities for novel treatments of nutritional disorders? Microbiol Spectrum 5(2):BAD-0002-2016.

REFERENCES

1. **Nicholson JK, Holmes E, Kinross J, Burcelin R, Gibson G, Jia W, Pettersson S.** 2012. Host-gut microbiota metabolic interactions. *Science* **336:**1262–1267.
2. **Cani PD, Delzenne NM.** 2009. Interplay between obesity and associated metabolic disorders: new insights into the gut microbiota. *Curr Opin Pharmacol* **9:**737–743.
3. **Tremaroli V, Bäckhed F.** 2012. Functional interactions between the gut microbiota and host metabolism. *Nature* **489:**242–249.
4. **Cani PD, Plovier H, Van Hul M, Geurts L, Delzenne NM, Druart C, Everard A.** 2016. Endocannabinoids—at the crossroads between the gut microbiota and host metabolism. *Nat Rev Endocrinol* **12:**133–143.
5. **Cani PD, Everard A.** 2016. Talking microbes: when gut bacteria interact with diet and host organs. *Mol Nutr Food Res* **60:**58–66.
6. **Black RE, Victora CG, Walker SP, Bhutta ZA, Christian P, de Onis M, Ezzati M, Grantham-McGregor S, Katz J, Martorell R, Uauy R, Maternal and Child Nutrition Study Group.** 2013. Maternal and child undernutrition and overweight in low-income and middle-income countries. *Lancet* **382:**427–451.
7. **Sender R, Fuchs S, Milo R.** 2016. Are we really vastly outnumbered? Revisiting the ratio of bacterial to host cells in humans. *Cell* **164:** 337–340.
8. **Qin J, et al, MetaHIT Consortium.** 2010. A human gut microbial gene catalogue established by metagenomic sequencing. *Nature* **464:**59–65.
9. **Li J, Jia H, Cai X, Zhong H, Feng Q, Sunagawa S, Arumugam M, Kultima JR, Prifti E, Nielsen T, Juncker AS, Manichanh C, Chen B, Zhang W, Levenez F, Wang J, Xu X, Xiao L, Liang S, Zhang D, Zhang Z, Chen W, Zhao H, Al-Aama JY, Edris S, Yang H, Wang J, Hansen T, Nielsen HB, Brunak S, Kristiansen K, Guarner F, Pedersen O, Doré J, Ehrlich SD, Bork P, Wang J, MetaHIT Consortium.** 2014. An integrated catalog of reference genes in the human gut microbiome. *Nat Biotechnol* **32:**834–841.
10. **Salazar N, Arboleya S, Valdés L, Stanton C, Ross P, Ruiz L, Gueimonde M, de Los Reyes-Gavilán CG.** 2014. The human intestinal microbiome at extreme ages of life. Dietary intervention as a way to counteract alterations. *Front Genet* **5:**406.
11. **Bäckhed F, Ding H, Wang T, Hooper LV, Koh GY, Nagy A, Semenkovich CF, Gordon JI.** 2004. The gut microbiota as an environmental factor that regulates fat storage. *Proc Natl Acad Sci USA* **101:**15718–15723.
12. **Schwarzer M, Makki K, Storelli G, Machuca-Gayet I, Srutkova D, Hermanova P, Martino ME, Balmand S, Hudcovic T, Heddi A, Rieusset J, Kozakova H, Vidal H, Leulier F.** 2016. *Lactobacillus plantarum* strain maintains growth of infant mice during chronic undernutrition. *Science* **351:**854–857.
13. **Wichmann A, Allahyar A, Greiner TU, Plovier H, Lundén GÖ, Larsson T, Drucker DJ, Delzenne NM, Cani PD, Bäckhed F.** 2013. Microbial modulation of energy availability in the colon regulates intestinal transit. *Cell Host Microbe* **14:**582–590.
14. **Schéle E, Grahnemo L, Anesten F, Hallén A, Bäckhed F, Jansson JO.** 2013. The gut microbiota reduces leptin sensitivity and the expression of the obesity-suppressing neuropeptides

proglucagon (Gcg) and brain-derived neurotrophic factor (Bdnf) in the central nervous system. *Endocrinology* **154**:3643–3651.

15. **Cani PD, Delzenne NM.** 2011. The gut microbiome as therapeutic target. *Pharmacol Ther* **130**:202–212.

16. **Ley RE, Bäckhed F, Turnbaugh P, Lozupone CA, Knight RD, Gordon JI.** 2005. Obesity alters gut microbial ecology. *Proc Natl Acad Sci USA* **102**:11070–11075.

17. **Ley RE, Turnbaugh PJ, Klein S, Gordon JI.** 2006. Microbial ecology: human gut microbes associated with obesity. *Nature* **444**:1022–1023.

18. **Turnbaugh PJ, Ley RE, Mahowald MA, Magrini V, Mardis ER, Gordon JI.** 2006. An obesity-associated gut microbiome with increased capacity for energy harvest. *Nature* **444**:1027–1031.

19. **Cani PD, Amar J, Iglesias MA, Poggi M, Knauf C, Bastelica D, Neyrinck AM, Fava F, Tuohy KM, Chabo C, Waget A, Delmée E, Cousin B, Sulpice T, Chamontin B, Ferrières J, Tanti JF, Gibson GR, Casteilla L, Delzenne NM, Alessi MC, Burcelin R.** 2007. Metabolic endotoxemia initiates obesity and insulin resistance. *Diabetes* **56**:1761–1772.

20. **Bäckhed F, Manchester JK, Semenkovich CF, Gordon JI.** 2007. Mechanisms underlying the resistance to diet-induced obesity in germfree mice. *Proc Natl Acad Sci USA* **104**:979–984.

21. **Larsen N, Vogensen FK, van den Berg FW, Nielsen DS, Andreasen AS, Pedersen BK, Al-Soud WA, Sørensen SJ, Hansen LH, Jakobsen M.** 2010. Gut microbiota in human adults with type 2 diabetes differs from nondiabetic adults. *PLoS One* **5**:e9085.

22. **Amar J, Serino M, Lange C, Chabo C, Iacovoni J, Mondot S, Lepage P, Klopp C, Mariette J, Bouchez O, Perez L, Courtney M, Marre M, Klopp P, Lantieri O, Doré J, Charles M, Balkau B, Burcelin R, DESIR Study Group.** 2011. Involvement of tissue bacteria in the onset of diabetes in humans: evidence for a concept. *Diabetologia* **54**:3055–3061.

23. **Qin J, et al.** 2012. A metagenome-wide association study of gut microbiota in type 2 diabetes. *Nature* **490**:55–60.

24. **Karlsson FH, Tremaroli V, Nookaew I, Bergström G, Behre CJ, Fagerberg B, Nielsen J, Bäckhed F.** 2013. Gut metagenome in European women with normal, impaired and diabetic glucose control. *Nature* **498**:99–103.

25. **Dao MC, Everard A, Aron-Wisnewsky J, Sokolovska N, Prifti E, Verger EO, Kayser BD, Levenez F, Chilloux J, Hoyles L, Dumas ME, Rizkalla SW, Doré J, Cani PD, Clément K, MICRO-Obes Consortium.** 2016. *Akkermansia muciniphila* and improved metabolic health during a dietary intervention in obesity: relationship with gut microbiome richness and ecology. *Gut* **65**:426–436.

26. **Cotillard A, Kennedy SP, Kong LC, Prifti E, Pons N, Le Chatelier E, Almeida M, Quinquis B, Levenez F, Galleron N, Gougis S, Rizkalla S, Batto JM, Renault P, Doré J, Zucker JD, Clément K, Ehrlich SD, ANR MicroObes consortium.** 2013. Dietary intervention impact on gut microbial gene richness. *Nature* **500**:585–588.

27. **Le Chatelier E, et al, MetaHIT consortium.** 2013. Richness of human gut microbiome correlates with metabolic markers. *Nature* **500**:541–546.

28. **Forslund K, Hildebrand F, Nielsen T, Falony G, Le Chatelier E, Sunagawa S, Prifti E, Vieira-Silva S, Gudmundsdottir V, Krogh Pedersen H, Arumugam M, Kristiansen K, Voigt AY, Vestergaard H, Hercog R, Igor Costea P, Kultima JR, Li J, Jørgensen T, Levenez F, Dore J, Nielsen HB, Brunak S, Raes J, Hansen T, Wang J, Ehrlich SD, Bork P, Pedersen O, MetaHIT consortium.** 2015. Disentangling type 2 diabetes and metformin treatment signatures in the human gut microbiota. *Nature* **528**:262–266.

29. **Delzenne NM, Cani PD, Everard A, Neyrinck AM, Bindels LB.** 2015. Gut microorganisms as promising targets for the management of type 2 diabetes. *Diabetologia* **58**:2206–2217.

30. **Tilg H, Kaser A.** 2011. Gut microbiome, obesity, and metabolic dysfunction. *J Clin Invest* **121**:2126–2132.

31. **Tilg H, Moschen AR.** 2014. Microbiota and diabetes: an evolving relationship. *Gut* **63**:1513–1521.

32. **Palau-Rodriguez M, Tulipani S, Isabel Queipo-Ortuño M, Urpi-Sarda M, Tinahones FJ, Andres-Lacueva C.** 2015. Metabolomic insights into the intricate gut microbial-host interaction in the development of obesity and type 2 diabetes. *Front Microbiol* **6**:1151.

33. **Ridaura VK, Faith JJ, Rey FE, Cheng J, Duncan AE, Kau AL, Griffin NW, Lombard V, Henrissat B, Bain JR, Muehlbauer MJ, Ilkayeva O, Semenkovich CF, Funai K, Hayashi DK, Lyle BJ, Martini MC, Ursell LK, Clemente JC, Van Treuren W, Walters WA, Knight R, Newgard CB, Heath AC, Gordon JI.** 2013. Gut microbiota from twins discordant for obesity modulate metabolism in mice. *Science* **341**:1241214.

34. **Koves TR, Ussher JR, Noland RC, Slentz D, Mosedale M, Ilkayeva O, Bain J, Stevens R, Dyck JR, Newgard CB, Lopaschuk GD,**

Muoio DM. 2008. Mitochondrial overload and incomplete fatty acid oxidation contribute to skeletal muscle insulin resistance. *Cell Metab* 7:45–56.

35. Cho I, Yamanishi S, Cox L, Methé BA, Zavadil J, Li K, Gao Z, Mahana D, Raju K, Teitler I, Li H, Alekseyenko AV, Blaser MJ. 2012. Antibiotics in early life alter the murine colonic microbiome and adiposity. *Nature* 488:621–626.

36. Cox LM, Yamanishi S, Sohn J, Alekseyenko AV, Leung JM, Cho I, Kim SG, Li H, Gao Z, Mahana D, Zárate Rodriguez JG, Rogers AB, Robine N, Loke P, Blaser MJ. 2014. Altering the intestinal microbiota during a critical developmental window has lasting metabolic consequences. *Cell* 158:705–721.

37. Vreugdenhil AC, Rousseau CH, Hartung T, Greve JW, van't Veer C, Buurman WA. 2003. Lipopolysaccharide (LPS)-binding protein mediates LPS detoxification by chylomicrons. *J Immunol* 170:1399–1405.

38. Muccioli GG, Naslain D, Bäckhed F, Reigstad CS, Lambert DM, Delzenne NM, Cani PD. 2010. The endocannabinoid system links gut microbiota to adipogenesis. *Mol Syst Biol* 6: 392.

39. Luche E, Cousin B, Garidou L, Serino M, Waget A, Barreau C, André M, Valet P, Courtney M, Casteilla L, Burcelin R. 2013. Metabolic endotoxemia directly increases the proliferation of adipocyte precursors at the onset of metabolic diseases through a CD14-dependent mechanism. *Mol Metab* 2:281–291.

40. Brun P, Castagliuolo I, Di Leo V, Buda A, Pinzani M, Palù G, Martines D. 2007. Increased intestinal permeability in obese mice: new evidence in the pathogenesis of non-alcoholic steatohepatitis. *Am J Physiol Gastrointest Liver Physiol* 292:G518–G525.

41. Everard A, Lazarevic V, Derrien M, Girard M, Muccioli GG, Neyrinck AM, Possemiers S, Van Holle A, François P, de Vos WM, Delzenne NM, Schrenzel J, Cani PD. 2011. Responses of gut microbiota and glucose and lipid metabolism to prebiotics in genetic obese and diet-induced leptin-resistant mice. *Diabetes* 60:2775–2786.

42. Geurts L, Lazarevic V, Derrien M, Everard A, Van Roye M, Knauf C, Valet P, Girard M, Muccioli GG, François P, de Vos WM, Schrenzel J, Delzenne NM, Cani PD. 2011. Altered gut microbiota and endocannabinoid system tone in obese and diabetic leptin-resistant mice: impact on apelin regulation in adipose tissue. *Front Microbiol* 2:149.

43. Cani PD, Bibiloni R, Knauf C, Waget A, Neyrinck AM, Delzenne NM, Burcelin R. 2008. Changes in gut microbiota control metabolic endotoxemia-induced inflammation in high-fat diet-induced obesity and diabetes in mice. *Diabetes* 57:1470–1481.

44. Erridge C, Attina T, Spickett CM, Webb DJ. 2007. A high-fat meal induces low-grade endotoxemia: evidence of a novel mechanism of postprandial inflammation. *Am J Clin Nutr* 86:1286–1292.

45. Amar J, Burcelin R, Ruidavets JB, Cani PD, Fauvel J, Alessi MC, Chamontin B, Ferriéres J. 2008. Energy intake is associated with endotoxemia in apparently healthy men. *Am J Clin Nutr* 87:1219–1223.

46. Pussinen PJ, Havulinna AS, Lehto M, Sundvall J, Salomaa V. 2011. Endotoxemia is associated with an increased risk of incident diabetes. *Diabetes Care* 34:392–397.

47. Lassenius MI, Pietiläinen KH, Kaartinen K, Pussinen PJ, Syrjänen J, Forsblom C, Pörsti I, Rissanen A, Kaprio J, Mustonen J, Groop PH, Lehto M, FinnDiane Study Group. 2011. Bacterial endotoxin activity in human serum is associated with dyslipidemia, insulin resistance, obesity, and chronic inflammation. *Diabetes Care* 34:1809–1815.

48. Laugerette F, Vors C, Géloën A, Chauvin MA, Soulage C, Lambert-Porcheron S, Peretti N, Alligier M, Burcelin R, Laville M, Vidal H, Michalski MC. 2011. Emulsified lipids increase endotoxemia: possible role in early postprandial low-grade inflammation. *J Nutr Biochem* 22:53–59.

49. Serino M, Luche E, Gres S, Baylac A, Bergé M, Cenac C, Waget A, Klopp P, Iacovoni J, Klopp C, Mariette J, Bouchez O, Lluch J, Ouarné F, Monsan P, Valet P, Roques C, Amar J, Bouloumié A, Théodorou V, Burcelin R. 2012. Metabolic adaptation to a high-fat diet is associated with a change in the gut microbiota. *Gut* 61:543–553.

50. Moreno-Navarrete JM, Escoté X, Ortega F, Serino M, Campbell M, Michalski MC, Laville M, Xifra G, Luche E, Domingo P, Sabater M, Pardo G, Waget A, Salvador J, Giralt M, Rodriguez-Hermosa JI, Camps M, Kolditz CI, Viguerie N, Galitzky J, Decaunes P, Ricart W, Frühbeck G, Villarroya F, Mingrone G, Langin D, Zorzano A, Vidal H, Vendrell J, Burcelin R, Vidal-Puig A, Fernández-Real JM. 2013. A role for adipocyte-derived lipopolysaccharide-binding protein in inflammation- and obesity-associated adipose tissue dysfunction. *Diabetologia* 56:2524–2537.

51. Gu Y, Yu S, Park JY, Harvatine K, Lambert JD. 2014. Dietary cocoa reduces metabolic endotoxemia and adipose tissue inflammation

in high-fat fed mice. *J Nutr Biochem* **25**:439–445.

52. **Wang JH, Bose S, Kim GC, Hong SU, Kim JH, Kim JE, Kim H.** 2014. Flos Lonicera ameliorates obesity and associated endotoxemia in rats through modulation of gut permeability and intestinal microbiota. *PLoS One* **9**:e86117.

53. **Kaliannan K, Hamarneh SR, Economopoulos KP, Nasrin Alam S, Moaven O, Patel P, Malo NS, Ray M, Abtahi SM, Muhammad N, Raychowdhury A, Teshager A, Mohamed MM, Moss AK, Ahmed R, Hakimian S, Narisawa S, Millán JL, Hohmann E, Warren HS, Bhan AK, Malo MS, Hodin RA.** 2013. Intestinal alkaline phosphatase prevents metabolic syndrome in mice. *Proc Natl Acad Sci USA* **110**:7003–7008.

54. **Peng X, Nie Y, Wu J, Huang Q, Cheng Y.** 2015. Juglone prevents metabolic endotoxemia-induced hepatitis and neuroinflammation via suppressing TLR4/NF-κB signaling pathway in high-fat diet rats. *Biochem Biophys Res Commun* **462**:245–250.

55. **Luck H, Tsai S, Chung J, Clemente-Casares X, Ghazarian M, Revelo XS, Lei H, Luk CT, Shi SY, Surendra A, Copeland JK, Ahn J, Prescott D, Rasmussen BA, Chng MH, Engleman EG, Girardin SE, Lam TK, Croitoru K, Dunn S, Philpott DJ, Guttman DS, Woo M, Winer S, Winer DA.** 2015. Regulation of obesity-related insulin resistance with gut anti-inflammatory agents. *Cell Metab* **21**:527–542.

56. **Varma MC, Kusminski CM, Azharian S, Gilardini L, Kumar S, Invitti C, McTernan PG.** 2016. Metabolic endotoxaemia in childhood obesity. *BMC Obes* **3**:3.

57. **Radilla-Vázquez RB, Parra-Rojas I, Martínez-Hernández NE, Márquez-Sandoval YF, Illades-Aguiar B, Castro-Alarcón N.** 2016. Gut microbiota and metabolic endotoxemia in young obese Mexican subjects. *Obes Facts* **9**:1–11.

58. **Caesar R, Tremaroli V, Kovatcheva-Datchary P, Cani PD, Bäckhed F.** 2015. Crosstalk between gut microbiota and dietary lipids aggravates WAT inflammation through TLR signaling. *Cell Metab* **22**:658–668.

59. **Bevins CL, Salzman NH.** 2011. Paneth cells, antimicrobial peptides and maintenance of intestinal homeostasis. *Nat Rev Microbiol* **9**:356–368.

60. **Pott J, Hornef M.** 2012. Innate immune signalling at the intestinal epithelium in homeostasis and disease. *EMBO Rep* **13**:684–698.

61. **Hooper LV, Macpherson AJ.** 2010. Immune adaptations that maintain homeostasis with the intestinal microbiota. *Nat Rev Immunol* **10**:159–169.

62. **Macpherson AJ, Geuking MB, Slack E, Hapfelmeier S, McCoy KD.** 2012. The habitat, double life, citizenship, and forgetfulness of IgA. *Immunol Rev* **245**:132–146.

63. **Cani PD, Everard A, Duparc T.** 2013. Gut microbiota, enteroendocrine functions and metabolism. *Curr Opin Pharmacol* **13**:935–940.

64. **Cani PD, Possemiers S, Van de Wiele T, Guiot Y, Everard A, Rottier O, Geurts L, Naslain D, Neyrinck A, Lambert DM, Muccioli GG, Delzenne NM.** 2009. Changes in gut microbiota control inflammation in obese mice through a mechanism involving GLP-2-driven improvement of gut permeability. *Gut* **58**:1091–1103.

65. **Everard A, Lazarevic V, Gaïa N, Johansson M, Ståhlman M, Backhed F, Delzenne NM, Schrenzel J, François P, Cani PD.** 2014. Microbiome of prebiotic-treated mice reveals novel targets involved in host response during obesity. *ISME J* **8**:2116–2130.

66. **Cani PD, Possemiers S, Van de Wiele T, Guiot Y, Everard A, Rottier O, Geurts L, Naslain D, Neyrinck A, Lambert DM, Muccioli GG, Delzenne NM.** 2009. Changes in gut microbiota control inflammation in obese mice through a mechanism involving GLP-2-driven improvement of gut permeability. *Gut* **58**:1091–1103.

67. **Everard A, Belzer C, Geurts L, Ouwerkerk JP, Druart C, Bindels LB, Guiot Y, Derrien M, Muccioli GG, Delzenne NM, de Vos WM, Cani PD.** 2013. Cross-talk between Akkermansia muciniphila and intestinal epithelium controls diet-induced obesity. *Proc Natl Acad Sci USA* **110**:9066–9071.

68. **Everard A, Geurts L, Caesar R, Van Hul M, Matamoros S, Duparc T, Denis RG, Cochez P, Pierard F, Castel J, Bindels LB, Plovier H, Robine S, Muccioli GG, Renauld JC, Dumoutier L, Delzenne NM, Luquet S, Bäckhed F, Cani PD.** 2014. Intestinal epithelial MyD88 is a sensor switching host metabolism towards obesity according to nutritional status. *Nat Commun* **5**:5648.

69. **Vaishnava S, Yamamoto M, Severson KM, Ruhn KA, Yu X, Koren O, Ley R, Wakeland EK, Hooper LV.** 2011. The antibacterial lectin RegIIIgamma promotes the spatial segregation of microbiota and host in the intestine. *Science* **334**:255–258.

70. **Sommer F, Adam N, Johansson ME, Xia L, Hansson GC, Bäckhed F.** 2014. Altered mucus glycosylation in core 1 O-glycan-deficient mice affects microbiota composition and intestinal architecture. *PLoS One* **9**:e85254.

71. **Johansson ME, Larsson JM, Hansson GC.** 2011. The two mucus layers of colon are orga-

nized by the MUC2 mucin, whereas the outer layer is a legislator of host-microbial interactions. *Proc Natl Acad Sci USA* **108**(Suppl 1): 4659–4665.

72. **Lluch J, Servant F, Païssé S, Valle C, Valière S, Kuchly C, Vilchez G, Donnadieu C, Courtney M, Burcelin R, Amar J, Bouchez O, Lelouvier B.** 2015. The characterization of novel tissue microbiota using an optimized 16s metagenomic sequencing pipeline. *PLoS One* **10**:e0142334.

73. **Bowman KA, Broussard EK, Surawicz CM.** 2015. Fecal microbiota transplantation: current clinical efficacy and future prospects. *Clin Exp Gastroenterol* **8**:285–291.

74. **Vrieze A, Van Nood E, Holleman F, Salojärvi J, Kootte RS, Bartelsman JF, Dallinga-Thie GM, Ackermans MT, Serlie MJ, Oozeer R, Derrien M, Druesne A, Van Hylckama Vlieg JE, Bloks VW, Groen AK, Heilig HG, Zoetendal EG, Stroes ES, de Vos WM, Hoekstra JB, Nieuwdorp M.** 2012. Transfer of intestinal microbiota from lean donors increases insulin sensitivity in individuals with metabolic syndrome. *Gastroenterology* **143**:913–6.e7.

75. **Firouzi S, Barakatun-Nisak MY, Ismail A, Majid HA, Nor Azmi K.** 2013. Role of probiotics in modulating glucose homeostasis: evidence from animal and human studies. *Int J Food Sci Nutr* **64**:780–786.

76. **Bernardeau M, Vernoux JP.** 2013. Overview of differences between microbial feed additives and probiotics for food regarding regulation, growth promotion effects and health properties and consequences for extrapolation of farm animal results to humans. *Clin Microbiol Infect* **19**:321–330.

77. **Delzenne NM, Neyrinck AM, Bäckhed F, Cani PD.** 2011. Targeting gut microbiota in obesity: effects of prebiotics and probiotics. *Nat Rev Endocrinol* **7**:639–646.

78. **Ben Salah R, Trabelsi I, Hamden K, Chouayekh H, Bejar S.** 2013. *Lactobacillus plantarum* TN8 exhibits protective effects on lipid, hepatic and renal profiles in obese rat. *Anaerobe* **23**:55–61.

79. **Jung SP, Lee KM, Kang JH, Yun SI, Park HO, Moon Y, Kim JY.** 2013. Effect of *Lactobacillus gasseri* BNR17 on overweight and obese adults: a randomized, double-blind clinical trial. *Korean J Fam Med* **34**:80–89.

80. **Kadooka Y, Sato M, Ogawa A, Miyoshi M, Uenishi H, Ogawa H, Ikuyama K, Kagoshima M, Tsuchida T.** 2013. Effect of *Lactobacillus gasseri* SBT2055 in fermented milk on abdominal adiposity in adults in a randomised controlled trial. *Br J Nutr* **110**:1696–1703.

81. **Kang JH, Yun SI, Park MH, Park JH, Jeong SY, Park HO.** 2013. Anti-obesity effect of *Lactobacillus gasseri* BNR17 in high-sucrose diet-induced obese mice. *PLoS One* **8**:e54617.

82. **Kondo S, Kamei A, Xiao JZ, Iwatsuki K, Abe K.** 2013. *Bifidobacterium breve* B-3 exerts metabolic syndrome-suppressing effects in the liver of diet-induced obese mice: a DNA microarray analysis. *Benef Microbes* **4**:247–251.

83. **Okubo T, Takemura N, Yoshida A, Sonoyama K.** 2013. KK/Ta mice administered *Lactobacillus plantarum* strain no. 14 have lower adiposity and higher insulin sensitivity. *Biosci Microbiota Food Health* **32**:93–100.

84. **Park DY, Ahn YT, Park SH, Huh CS, Yoo SR, Yu R, Sung MK, McGregor RA, Choi MS.** 2013. Supplementation of *Lactobacillus curvatus* HY7601 and *Lactobacillus plantarum* KY1032 in diet-induced obese mice is associated with gut microbial changes and reduction in obesity. *PLoS One* **8**:e59470.

85. **Poutahidis T, Kleinewietfeld M, Smillie C, Levkovich T, Perrotta A, Bhela S, Varian BJ, Ibrahim YM, Lakritz JR, Kearney SM, Chatzigiagkos A, Hafler DA, Alm EJ, Erdman SE.** 2013. Microbial reprogramming inhibits Western diet-associated obesity. *PLoS One* **8**: e68596.

86. **Sakai T, Taki T, Nakamoto A, Shuto E, Tsutsumi R, Toshimitsu T, Makino S, Ikegami S.** 2013. *Lactobacillus plantarum* OLL2712 regulates glucose metabolism in C57BL/6 mice fed a high-fat diet. *J Nutr Sci Vitaminol (Tokyo)* **59**:144–147.

87. **Yadav H, Lee JH, Lloyd J, Walter P, Rane SG.** 2013. Beneficial metabolic effects of a probiotic via butyrate-induced GLP-1 hormone secretion. *J Biol Chem* **288**:25088 25097.

88. **Yoo SR, Kim YJ, Park DY, Jung UJ, Jeon SM, Ahn YT, Huh CS, McGregor R, Choi MS.** 2013. Probiotics *L. plantarum* and *L. curvatus* in combination alter hepatic lipid metabolism and suppress diet-induced obesity. *Obesity (Silver Spring)* **21**:2571–2578.

89. **Karlsson Videhult F, Öhlund I, Stenlund H, Hernell O, West CE.** 2014. Probiotics during weaning: a follow-up study on effects on body composition and metabolic markers at school age. *Eur J Nutr* **54**:355–363.

90. **Lindsay KL, Kennelly M, Culliton M, Smith T, Maguire OC, Shanahan F, Brennan L, McAuliffe FM.** 2014. Probiotics in obese pregnancy do not reduce maternal fasting glucose: a double-blind, placebo-controlled, randomized trial (Probiotics in Pregnancy Study). *Am J Clin Nutr* **99**:1432–1439.

91. **Miyoshi M, Ogawa A, Higurashi S, Kadooka Y.** 2014. Anti-obesity effect of *Lactobacillus gasseri* SBT2055 accompanied by inhibition

of pro-inflammatory gene expression in the visceral adipose tissue in diet-induced obese mice. *Eur J Nutr* **53:**599–606.

92. **Moya-Pérez A, Romo-Vaquero M, Tomás-Barberán F, Sanz Y, García-Conesa MT.** 2014. Hepatic molecular responses to *Bifidobacterium pseudocatenulatum* CECT 7765 in a mouse model of diet-induced obesity. *Nutr Metab Cardiovasc Dis* **24:**57–64.

93. **Ogawa A, Kadooka Y, Kato K, Shirouchi B, Sato M.** 2014. *Lactobacillus gasseri* SBT2055 reduces postprandial and fasting serum non-esterified fatty acid levels in Japanese hypertriacylglycerolemic subjects. *Lipids Health Dis* **13:**36.

94. **Park JE, Oh SH, Cha YS.** 2014. *Lactobacillus plantarum* LG42 isolated from gajami sik-hae decreases body and fat pad weights in diet-induced obese mice. *J Appl Microbiol* **116:**145–156.

95. **Plaza-Diaz J, Gomez-Llorente C, Abadia-Molina F, Saez-Lara MJ, Campaña-Martin L, Muñoz-Quezada S, Romero F, Gil A, Fontana L.** 2014. Effects of *Lactobacillus paracasei* CNCM I-4034, *Bifidobacterium breve* CNCM I-4035 and *Lactobacillus rhamnosus* CNCM I-4036 on hepatic steatosis in Zucker rats. *PLoS One* **9:**e98401.

96. **Reichold A, Brenner SA, Spruss A, Förster-Fromme K, Bergheim I, Bischoff SC.** 2014. *Bifidobacterium adolescentis* protects from the development of nonalcoholic steatohepatitis in a mouse model. *J Nutr Biochem* **25:**118–125.

97. **Ritze Y, Bárdos G, Claus A, Ehrmann V, Bergheim I, Schwiertz A, Bischoff SC.** 2014. *Lactobacillus rhamnosus* GG protects against non-alcoholic fatty liver disease in mice. *PLoS One* **9:**e80169.

98. **Sanchez M, Darimont C, Drapeau V, Emady-Azar S, Lepage M, Rezzonico E, Ngom-Bru C, Berger B, Philippe L, Ammon-Zuffrey C, Leone P, Chevrier G, St-Amand E, Marette A, Doré J, Tremblay A.** 2014. Effect of *Lactobacillus rhamnosus* CGMCC1.3724 supplementation on weight loss and maintenance in obese men and women. *Br J Nutr* **111:**1507–1519.

99. **Toral M, Gómez-Guzmán M, Jiménez R, Romero M, Sánchez M, Utrilla MP, Garrido-Mesa N, Rodríguez-Cabezas ME, Olivares M, Gálvez J, Duarte J.** 2014. The probiotic *Lactobacillus coryniformis* CECT5711 reduces the vascular pro-oxidant and pro-inflammatory status in obese mice. *Clin Sci (Lond)* **127:**33–45.

100. **Wang J, Tang H, Zhang C, Zhao Y, Derrien M, Rocher E, van-Hylckama Vlieg JE, Strissel K, Zhao L, Obin M, Shen J.** 2015. Modulation of gut microbiota during probiotic-mediated attenuation of metabolic syndrome in high fat diet-fed mice. *ISME J* **9:**1–15.

101. **Cani PD, Van Hul M.** 2015. Novel opportunities for next-generation probiotics targeting metabolic syndrome. *Curr Opin Biotechnol* **32:**21–27.

102. **Minami J, Kondo S, Yanagisawa N, Odamaki T, Xiao JZ, Abe F, Nakajima S, Hamamoto Y, Saitoh S, Shimoda T.** 2015. Oral administration of *Bifidobacterium breve* B-3 modifies metabolic functions in adults with obese tendencies in a randomised controlled trial. *J Nutr Sci* **4:**e17.

103. **Moya-Pérez A, Neef A, Sanz Y.** 2015. *Bifidobacterium pseudocatenulatum* CECT 7765 reduces obesity-associated inflammation by restoring the lymphocyte-macrophage balance and gut microbiota structure in high-fat diet-fed mice. *PLoS One* **10:**e0126976.

104. **Pothuraju R, Sharma RK, Kavadi PK, Chagalamarri J, Jangra S, Bhakri G, De S.** 2016. Anti-obesity effect of milk fermented by *Lactobacillus plantarum* NCDC 625 alone and in combination with herbs on high fat diet fed C57BL/6J mice. *Benef Microbes* **7:**375–385.

105. **Park S, Bae JH.** 2015. Probiotics for weight loss: a systematic review and meta-analysis. *Nutr Res* **35:**566–575.

106. **Karimi G, Sabran MR, Jamaluddin R, Parvaneh K, Mohtarrudin N, Ahmad Z, Khazaai H, Khodavandi A.** 2015. The anti-obesity effects of *Lactobacillus casei* strain Shirota versus Orlistat on high fat diet-induced obese rats. *Food Nutr Res* **59:**29273.

107. **Ukibe K, Miyoshi M, Kadooka Y.** 2015. Administration of *Lactobacillus gasseri* SBT2055 suppresses macrophage infiltration into adipose tissue in diet-induced obese mice. *Br J Nutr* **114:**1180–1187.

108. **Novotny Núñez I, Maldonado Galdeano C, de Moreno de LeBlanc A, Perdigón G.** 2015. *Lactobacillus casei* CRL 431 administration decreases inflammatory cytokines in a diet-induced obese mouse model. *Nutrition* **31:**1000–1007.

109. **Wu M, McNulty NP, Rodionov DA, Khoroshkin MS, Griffin NW, Cheng J, Latreille P, Kerstetter RA, Terrapon N, Henrissat B, Osterman AL, Gordon JI.** 2015. Genetic determinants of in vivo fitness and diet responsiveness in multiple human gut Bacteroides. *Science* **350:**aac5992.

110. **Ivanovic N, Minic R, Dimitrijevic L, Radojevic Skodric S, Zivkovic I, Djordjevic B.** 2015. *Lactobacillus rhamnosus* LA68 and *Lactobacillus plantarum* WCFS1 differently influence metabolic and immunological parameters in high fat diet-induced hypercholesterolemia and hepatic steatosis. *Food Funct* **6:**558–565.

111. **Druart C, Alligier M, Salazar N, Neyrinck AM, Delzenne NM.** 2014. Modulation of the gut microbiota by nutrients with prebiotic and probiotic properties. *Adv Nutr* **5:**624S–633S.

112. **Zhang H, DiBaise JK, Zuccolo A, Kudrna D, Braidotti M, Yu Y, Parameswaran P, Crowell MD, Wing R, Rittmann BE, Krajmalnik-Brown R.** 2009. Human gut microbiota in obesity and after gastric bypass. *Proc Natl Acad Sci USA* **106:**2365–2370.

113. **Karlsson CL, Onnerfält J, Xu J, Molin G, Ahrné S, Thorngren-Jerneck K.** 2012. The microbiota of the gut in preschool children with normal and excessive body weight. *Obesity (Silver Spring)* **20:**2257–2261.

114. **Zhang X, Shen D, Fang Z, Jie Z, Qiu X, Zhang C, Chen Y, Ji L.** 2013. Human gut microbiota changes reveal the progression of glucose intolerance. *PLoS One* **8:**e71108.

115. **Derrien M, Vaughan EE, Plugge CM, de Vos WM.** 2004. *Akkermansia muciniphila* gen. nov., sp. nov., a human intestinal mucin-degrading bacterium. *Int J Syst Evol Microbiol* **54:**1469–1476.

116. **Shin NR, Lee JC, Lee HY, Kim MS, Whon TW, Lee MS, Bae JW.** 2014. An increase in the *Akkermansia* spp. population induced by metformin treatment improves glucose homeostasis in diet-induced obese mice. *Gut* **63:**727–735.

117. **Org E, Parks BW, Joo JW, Emert B, Schwartzman W, Kang EY, Mehrabian M, Pan C, Knight R, Gunsalus R, Drake TA, Eskin E, Lusis AJ.** 2015. Genetic and environmental control of host-gut microbiota interactions. *Genome Res* **25:**1558–1569.

118. **Everard A, Matamoros S, Geurts L, Delzenne NM, Cani PD.** 2014. *Saccharomyces boulardii* administration changes gut microbiota and reduces hepatic steatosis, low-grade inflammation, and fat mass in obese and type 2 diabetic db/db mice. *MBio* **5:**e01011–e01014.

119. **Xu L, Wang Y, Wang Y, Fu J, Sun M, Mao Z, Vandenplas Y.** 2016. A double-blinded randomized trial on growth and feeding tolerance with *Saccharomyces boulardii* CNCM I-745 in formula-fed preterm infants. *J Pediatr (Rio J)* **92:**296–301.

120. **Williams CD, Oxon BM, Lond H.** 1973. Kwashiorkor. A nutritional disease of children associated with a maize diet by Cicely D. Williams from the Lancet, Nov. 16, 1935, p. 1151. *Nutr Rev* **31:**350–351.

121. **Brewster DR, Manary MJ, Menzies IS, O'Loughlin EV, Henry RL.** 1997. Intestinal permeability in kwashiorkor. *Arch Dis Child* **76:**236–241.

122. **World Health Organization.** 2007. *Community-based management of severe acute malnutrition: a joint statement of the World Health Organization, World Food Programme, the United Nations System Standing Committee on Nutrition, and the United Nations Children's Fund.* World Health Organization, Geneva, Switzerland.

123. **Smythe PM.** 1958. Changes in intestinal bacterial flora and role of infection in kwashiorkor. *Lancet* **2:**724–727.

124. **Trehan I, Goldbach HS, LaGrone LN, Meuli GJ, Wang RJ, Maleta KM, Manary MJ.** 2013. Antibiotics as part of the management of severe acute malnutrition. *N Engl J Med* **368:**425–435.

125. **Isanaka S, Langendorf C, Berthé F, Gnegne S, Li N, Ousmane N, Harouna S, Hassane H, Schaefer M, Adehossi E, Grais RF.** 2016. Routine amoxicillin for uncomplicated severe acute malnutrition in children. *N Engl J Med* **374:**444–453.

126. **Berkley JA, Ngari M, Thitiri J, Mwalekwa L, Timbwa M, Hamid F, Ali R, Shangala J, Mturi N, Jones KD, Alphan H, Mutai B, Bandika V, Hemed T, Awuondo K, Morpeth S, Kariuki S, Fegan G.** 2016. Daily co-trimoxazole prophylaxis to prevent mortality in children with complicated severe acute malnutrition: a multicentre, double-blind, randomised placebo-controlled trial. *Lancet Glob Health* **4:**e464–e473.

127. **Gupta SS, Mohammed MH, Ghosh TS, Kanungo S, Nair GB, Mande SS.** 2011. Metagenome of the gut of a malnourished child. *Gut Pathog* **3:**7.

128. **Monira S, Nakamura S, Gotoh K, Izutsu K, Watanabe II, Alam NH, Endtz HP, Cravioto A, Ali SI, Nakaya T, Horii T, Iida T, Alam M.** 2011. Gut microbiota of healthy and malnourished children in bangladesh. *Front Microbiol* **2:**228.

129. **Ghosh TS, Gupta SS, Bhattacharya T, Yadav D, Barik A, Chowdhury A, Das B, Mande SS, Nair GB.** 2014. Gut microbiomes of Indian children of varying nutritional status. *PLoS One* **9:**e95547.

130. **Smith MI, Yatsunenko T, Manary MJ, Trehan I, Mkakosya R, Cheng J, Kau AL, Rich SS, Concannon P, Mychaleckyj JC, Liu J, Houpt E, Li JV, Holmes E, Nicholson J, Knights D, Ursell LK, Knight R, Gordon JI.** 2013. Gut microbiomes of Malawian twin pairs discordant for kwashiorkor. *Science* **339:**548–554.

131. **Subramanian S, Huq S, Yatsunenko T, Haque R, Mahfuz M, Alam MA, Benezra A, DeStefano J, Meier MF, Muegge BD, Barratt MJ, VanArendonk LG, Zhang Q, Province MA, Petri WA Jr, Ahmed T, Gordon JI.** 2014. Persistent

gut microbiota immaturity in malnourished Bangladeshi children. *Nature* **510**:417–421.

132. **Walker WA, Iyengar RS.** 2015. Breast milk, microbiota, and intestinal immune homeostasis. *Pediatr Res* **77**:220–228.

133. **Charbonneau MR, O'Donnell D, Blanton LV, Totten SM, Davis JC, Barratt MJ, Cheng J, Guruge J, Talcott M, Bain JR, Muehlbauer MJ, Ilkayeva O, Wu C, Struckmeyer T, Barile D, Mangani C, Jorgensen J, Fan YM, Maleta K, Dewey KG, Ashorn P, Newgard CB, Lebrilla C, Mills DA, Gordon JI.** 2016. Sialylated milk oligosaccharides promote microbiota-dependent growth in models of infant undernutrition. *Cell* **164**:859–871.

134. **Devkota S, Chang EB.** 2015. Interactions between diet, bile acid metabolism, gut microbiota, and inflammatory bowel diseases. *Dig Dis* **33**: 351–356.

135. **Blanton LV, Charbonneau MR, Salih T, Barratt MJ, Venkatesh S, Ilkaveya O, Subramanian S, Manary MJ, Trehan I, Jorgensen JM, Fan YM, Henrissat B, Leyn SA, Rodionov DA, Osterman AL, Maleta KM, Newgard CB, Ashorn P, Dewey KG, Gordon JI.** 2016. Gut bacteria that prevent growth impairments transmitted by microbiota from malnourished children. *Science* **351**:aad3311.

136. **Kau AL, Planer JD, Liu J, Rao S, Yatsunenko T, Trehan I, Manary MJ, Liu TC, Stappenbeck TS, Maleta KM, Ashorn P, Dewey KG, Houpt ER, Hsieh CS, Gordon JI.** 2015. Functional characterization of IgA-targeted bacterial taxa from undernourished Malawian children that produce diet-dependent enteropathy. *Sci Transl Med* **7**:276ra24.

137. **O'Hara AM, Shanahan F.** 2006. The gut flora as a forgotten organ. *EMBO Rep* **7**:688–693.

Therapeutic Opportunities in the Vaginal Microbiome

6

GREGOR REID[1]

SCOPE OF THIS REVIEW

In order to design and apply a therapeutic, there must be a vaginal disease or disorder in need of treatment or a condition influenced by the vaginal microbiota. There must also be a way for a new therapeutic agent to function through the microbiome. Those conditions include bacterial vaginosis (BV), aerobic vaginitis (AV), urinary tract infection, urethritis, cervicitis, vulvovaginal candidiasis, vulvodynia, endometriosis, and chorioamnitis. In addition, sexually transmitted infections are included, as arguably some may be prevented by vaginal microbes. Cancer is included, not only because of the association with viral infection, but also because microbial dysbiosis has been associated with cancers at other sites.

The size of this list demonstrates the enormity of not only the burden of disease among females but also the challenge of reviewing each satisfactorily and suggesting opportunities for novel approaches to prevention and treatment. Rather than provide exhaustive details of these conditions, I will refer the reader to appropriate articles for further insight and try to focus on the elements that offer an opportunity for intervention through microbial manipulation. Much of this will, by necessity, be conjecture, but hopefully reasoned and realistic.

[1]Lawson Health Research Institute and Departments of Microbiology and Immunology and Surgery, University of Western Ontario, London, Ontario, Canada

Bugs as Drugs: Therapeutic Microbes for the Prevention and Treatment of Disease
Edited by Robert A. Britton and Patrice D. Cani
© 2018 American Society for Microbiology, Washington, DC
doi:10.1128/microbiolspec.BAD-0001-2016

THE CERVICOVAGINAL MICROBIOME AND ITS INFLUENCE ON HEALTH

Studies using various molecular methods over the past 15 years have provided insight into the array of microbes that can be detected in the vagina, vulva/labia, cervix, and uterus (1–18). The list is extensive, exceeding 250 bacterial species as well as yeast, *Chlamydia, Archaea*, viruses, and protozoa. Using statistical methodologies, attempts have been made to create groupings of bacterial species or genera into which the status of a given female might fall. In the first use of Illumina next-generation sequencing (NGS), we reported two major clusters (community state types [CSTs]) associated with a normal vaginal microbiota, one dominated by *Lactobacillus iners* and another by *Lactobacillus crispatus* (7). There were four CSTs strongly associated with BV, and these were dominated by *Prevotella bivia, Gardnerella vaginalis, Lachnospiraceae*, or a mixture of different species. This study of 132 subjects was more insightful than the one involving four phylum groups proposed from only 8 subjects (6), but there was still consistency in the findings of dominant lactobacilli or a mixed microbiota with depleted lactobacilli. Another study suggested one *Lactobacillus* grouping and three related to dysbiosis with the order *Lachnospiraceae* and genera *Sneathia* and *Prevotella* being dominant (19). Further studies in pregnant and nonpregnant HIV-negative women (8, 11) proposed five CST groupings: (i) *Lactobacillus crispatus* dominant; (ii) *Lactobacillus gasseri* dominant; (iii) *L. iners* dominant; (iv) *Peptoniphilus, Prevotella*, and *Anaerococcus* species and elevated *Gardnerella* or *Ureaplasma* abundances; and (v) *Lactobacillus jensenii* dominant. Despite issues with sampling, storage, processing, DNA extraction kits' error rates from bias in samples, technical variation with PCR amplification, and the use of different primers and statistical methods (20–22), the creation of subgroups of microbiota is intended to help design better treatment strategies. But is it realistic?

The abject failure of industry to develop novel treatments for vaginal health in 40 or so years surely suggests that creating five to eight new ones is not likely to happen soon. In addition, simply identifying which organisms are present is inadequate information to devise new treatment strategies. Understanding how they got there and what they are doing is critically important. We performed the only transcriptomic study to date and showed that *L. iners* has the ability to adapt to the very different BV environment from that of a healthy vagina (23). Ideally, such a study should examine changes that occur to move the pendulum towards dysbiosis (Fig. 1). Ravel and others have performed such regular sampling over 16 weeks (9), but not using transcriptomics. Nevertheless, their findings and those of others (24–28) have shown that menstruation, sexual activity, spermicides, douching, and antibiotics can dramatically alter the species abundance. Thus, it is impossible to define a single composition associated with health. So, for all the impressive NGS studies that have been undertaken, the basic principle is the same as it was based on culture results 40 years ago, with a high presence of lactobacilli associated with health (29, 30). It remains to be seen whether women with one of the four species (*L. crispatus, L. iners, Lactobacillus jensenii, Lactobacillus gasseri*) are more protected against dysbiosis than women who do not harbor such species. To prove this, one would have to provide *in vivo* evidence that certain factors confer protective functions.

TARGETS FOR THERAPY: MECHANISMS WHEREBY LACTOBACILLI PROTECT THE HOST

One of the features of a microscopic analysis of a vaginal swab from a healthy woman is the number of epithelial cells with few adherent bacteria, mostly presumptive lactobacilli. If so few beneficial bacteria are "protecting" the host, how are they doing it?

The theory that hydrogen peroxide (H_2O_2) produced by lactobacilli is the key defense mechanism (31) makes some sense, as this compound could inhibit the growth of pathogens. However, it has not been verified by a study measuring concentrations of H_2O_2 in the vagina. Therefore, the concentration required per milliliter of vaginal fluid or per surface area of epithelium is not known. Also, if it is protective, why do strains producing it, such as *L. crispatus*, become so apparently easy to displace when BV arises? Arguably, a more plausible protective mechanism, but also one that has not been proven in humans, is that biosurfactants produced by some strains of lactobacilli can cover cell surfaces and interfere with pathogen binding (32, 33) (Fig. 1). This process represents a thermodynamic effect, which has a good theoretical basis (34). Not only do the surface tensions of bacteria and host cells influence bacterial adhesion but so does also the suspending fluid. Thus, biosurfactants can alter the latter and make it less receptive to bacteria. *Lactobacillus* strains vary in the extent of biosurfactant production (35), but no studies have been done to determine if common vaginal isolates produce more than others. Efforts to purify biosurfactants and define their components and associated gene pathways have been limited, as have efforts to enhance their production. Industrialization of yeast-derived biosurfactants is being attempted (36), but not with vaginal applications in mind.

It is possible that bacteriocins or bacteriocin-like compounds are produced and help protect the host against pathogens, thereby leaving a relatively clear epithelial cell (37). But these compounds tend to have quite restricted target organisms, and it seems difficult to imagine that they control the wide range of BV and AV causative agents. Having said that, a recent study identified bacteriocin-like substances produced by vaginal lactobacilli that inhibited the growth of aerobic bacteria *Klebsiella*, *Staphylococcus aureus*, *Escherichia coli*, and *Enterococcus faecalis* and the yeast *Candida parapsilosis* as well as

some *Lactobacillus* species (38). A strain of a somewhat rarer vaginal species, *Lactobacillus pentosus*, isolated from a healthy Nigerian woman, was found to contain a putative cluster of genes for biosynthesis of a cyclic bacteriocin precursor (39). It is not clear if such a strain would be more effective in African women than the four *Lactobacillus* species of the CSTs. No such association has been tested to date. While bacteriocins have been known for many years, few if any, and none for the vagina, have been developed as therapeutic agents. If this approach is to be effective, it may require a more targeted bacteriocin, such as directly against one pathogen. Group B streptococci would be one such target, given their prevalence, their danger to newborns, and the need to administer antibiotics in women at the time of delivery (40). An oral probiotic, *Streptococcus salivarius*, may be one option, given its bacteriocin activity against group B streptococci (41).

The possibility of controlling pathogenesis by coaggregating lactobacilli with pathogens and thereby tying up the latter's ability to spread across surfaces, or by interfering with virulence expression such as production of toxins, has been considered (37) (Fig. 1). The latter concept suggests that a pathogen may not need to direct its energy to producing a toxin, if it can survive and colonize a surface. From a therapeutic point of view, the existence of a pathogen able to infect the host is not ideal, especially one such as *S. aureus* that can produce toxic shock toxin. But if the cocci are bound to lactobacilli, this potentially makes them less able to propagate and infect. In the case of *Lactobacillus reuteri* RC-14, cyclic dipeptides were identified to counter *S. aureus* toxins (42). Compounds such as these and quorum-sensing molecules, including coumarin, a natural plant phenolic compound, are being considered for antivirulence activity against a spectrum of pathogens (43).

The action of lactobacilli on host cell surfaces has been considered for a number of reasons. The most primitive is to simply

Mechanism Illustration	Mechanism Description
	Co-aggregation: This illustrates the concept of non-pathogens binding to pathogens and interfering with their ability to infect the host.
	Biosurfactant Production: Biosurfactants are produced by lactobacilli and their presence on the mucosal surface helps prevent adhesion and infection by the pathogenic organisms.
	Bacteriocin and Hydrogen Peroxide Production: Lactobacilli produce substances that can inhibit the growth or kill pathogens. Illustrated here are hydrogen peroxide and bacteriocins.
	Signalling effects: Bacteria communicate through a number of signalling mechanisms including quorum sensing. In this illustration, the Lactobacillus signalling molecules down-regulate toxin production in the Gram negative pathogen (e.g. *E. coli* 0157:H7 in the gut) and Gram positive pathogen (e.g. *S. aureus* on the vaginal surface).
	Competitive Exclusion: The concept of competitive exclusion is that lactobacilli can physically exclude pathogens from surfaces by competing for nutrients and receptor sites on the surface. This is overly simplistic as pathogens have a number of means to survive in the host. Nevertheless, applying probiotics or fecal transplanted organisms can help to exclude pathogens and prevent infection.

FIGURE 1 Different mechanisms by which beneficial microbes might influence vaginal health.

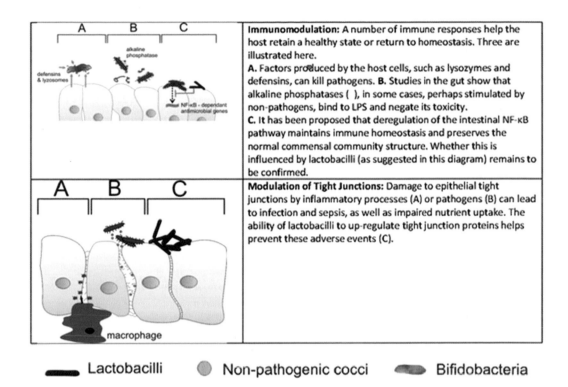

| | Immunomodulation: A number of immune responses help the host retain a healthy state or return to homeostasis. Three are illustrated here.
A. Factors produced by the host cells, such as lysozymes and defensins, can kill pathogens. **B.** Studies in the gut show that alkaline phosphatases ( ), in some cases, perhaps stimulated by non-pathogens, bind to LPS and negate its toxicity.
C. It has been proposed that deregulation of the intestinal NF-κB pathway maintains immune homeostasis and preserves the normal commensal community structure. Whether this is influenced by lactobacilli (as suggested in this diagram) remains to be confirmed. |
| **Modulation of Tight Junctions:** Damage to epithelial tight junctions by inflammatory processes (A) or pathogens (B) can lead to infection and sepsis, as well as impaired nutrient uptake. The ability of lactobacilli to up-regulate tight junction proteins helps prevent these adverse events (C). |

FIGURE 1 *(Continued)*

block the access of pathogens to the surface. Such a competitive-exclusion model would require high inoculum volumes to cover the vaginal epithelium and repeated application, which seem impractical. Rather than blocking access to the host epithelium, this might provide a surface to which pathogens adhere (coaggregate), and if their subsequent growth is not reduced, they might persist. Nevertheless, some groups continue to pursue this competitive-exclusion concept, with genes that aid adherence and inhibit *G. vaginalis* proposed as a means for candidate probiotic *L. crispatus* to improve vaginal health (44). The ability of lactobacilli to improve epithelial integrity by upregulating tight-junction proteins has been shown (45). The question is why this would be advantageous to the lactobacilli. In fact, it may not be important to

lactobacilli but rather may be a by-product of the metabolites that they produce. An interesting study on intestinal cells showed that *Lactobacillus rhamnosus* GG could increase tight-junction proteins Zonula occludens-1, claudin-1, and occludin gene expression by utilizing polyamines (46). Polyamines are found in the vagina and can be used by *Trichomonas* to adhere and infect (47), so the potential exists for lactobacilli to compete for these compounds and improve epithelial integrity.

The nature of the vagina in reproductive-age women is such that different levels of inflammatory processes occur during the menstrual cycle and pregnancy. The ability to maintain immune homeostasis requires more than microbial modulation, but certainly microbes can influence the process.

Alternatively, the process can influence the microbes. For example, during menstruation, the bacterial diversity appears to increase, albeit with variations among individuals (48). The ability to influence mucosal immunity using vaccines, antibodies, and antigens has been successful, but in the urogenital tract, modulation affecting bacterial dysbiosis has not been attempted. One exception has been efforts to create a multisubunit vaccine that elicits antibody against uropathogenic *E. coli* (49). Studies in mice are encouraging, and the concept has great appeal, as this process would stimulate IgG and not eradicate the commensal lactobacilli as antibiotics do. Other vaccine approaches include using flagellin proteins from *Pseudomonas aeruginosa* to passively immunize against pyelonephritis (50). Immune modulation to prevent BV has not been attempted, and one study of patients receiving a quadrivalent human papillomavirus (HPV) vaccine (HPV–6, –11, –16, and –18) surprisingly reported an increase in the management rate of *Gardnerella*/BV in women aged 50 years and older (51). If indeed vaccines increase the risk of BV, this requires closer investigation. A Hungarian vaccine comprising five inactivated strains of lactobacilli administered prophylactically to women was reported to prevent BV, but this approach seems more like a way to circumvent drug regulations requiring to deliver living bacteria than a true vaccine (52). Why would dead or inactivated lactobacilli be better at inducing a protective immune response than live lactobacilli? While one study has shown that heat-treated *Lactobacillus paracasei* NCC 2461 stabilizes interleukin-10 (IL–10) mRNA (53), IL-10 has not been shown to mediate vaginal protection against pathogens.

Aerobic vaginitis is more of an inflammatory disease than BV (54), so it would be interesting to test if vaccines against *E. coli*, streptococci, and staphylococci make an impact on this condition.

Overall, there is no clear path at present to enhance the vaginal mucosal immune parameters over the menstrual cycle, to reduce the recurrence of BV. Stimulation of anti-BV host defenses to the point of being effective without increasing inflammation and discharge will not be simple, but one case study using intravaginally administered *L. rhamnosus* GR-1 (1×10^9 cells in 1 ml once daily for 5 days) suggested that it may potentially work (45).

Can Targets Be Developed from Metabolomics Data?

While the cell surfaces *per se* of bacteria mediate activity in the host and the response can influence outcomes, the metabolic by-products are also important. The compounds that bacteria produce are clearly influenced by the organisms' genomic capabilities, the nutrients available, the microbial milieu in which they live, and environmental factors such as pH, mucins, antimicrobials, hormones, host cells, and immune factors.

Studies of the metabolome of vaginal bacteria are relatively recent, using liquid and gas chromatography with mass spectrometry, nuclear magnetic resonance spectroscopy, and databases that can interpret the resultant spectra (55–57). These studies have identified lactic acid, acetic acid, glycerol, and other metabolites consistent with the known capacities of lactobacilli and other vaginal organisms. Our study (57) was the first to identify and verify metabolites associated with high diversity and clinical BV, specifically 2-hydroxyisovalerate and γ-hydroxybutyrate (GHB), but not succinate as others had previously reported (58). This provides a means to develop a diagnostic system to detect GHB in vaginal swabs. If combined with elevated pH, it would likely be an effective tool to identify patients requiring therapy.

For AV, no such studies have been undertaken, but given the nature of the aerobic organisms and infection, it should be feasible to identify levels of lipopolysaccharide or other inflammatory compounds in vaginal fluid.

Engineered Strains to Deliver Vaccines

The encouraging results from probiotic applications to various areas of the host have stimulated the search for ways to further enhance benefits. One way would be to engineer bacteria either to deliver specific factors that promote health or prevent disease or to increase the production of compounds known to provide benefits.

The first efforts to engineer lactic acid bacteria for this purpose came from the insertion of murine IL-2 into lactococci (59). This was a precursor for the creation of strains engineered with biological containment (60) designed to deliver IL-10 to treat inflammatory bowel disease (61). However, these efforts have so far failed to make a clinical impact.

For vaginal applications, Mercenier et al. (62) were the first to consider using lactobacilli to increase mucosal immunity against pathogens such as *Chlamydia trachomatis*, but these efforts fell by the wayside. With the intent of preventing HIV infection in women, Lee and others (63) engineered an *L. jensenii* strain that secreted 2D CD4, which recognized a conformation-dependent anti-CD4 antibody and bound HIV type 1 gp120. They have continued their research to express single-chain and single-domain antibodies in *L. jensenii* 1153–1128 to passively transfer these antibodies to the mucosa and through colonization of the lactobacilli provide protection at the vaginal site of HIV transmission (64). Using a different approach, we genetically modified *L. reuteri* RC-14 to produce HIV entry or fusion inhibitors fused to the native expression and secretion signals of BspA, Mlp, or Sep proteins capable of blocking the three main steps of HIV entry into human peripheral blood mononuclear cells (65). The expression cassettes were stably inserted into the chromosome, but funding for the project was not forthcoming, so progress was halted. It remains to be seen if these approaches will be sufficiently effective and affordable to warrant large-scale applications, especially to countries where sexual transmission of the virus is most prevalent.

A final recombination strategy is being considered by Israeli researchers following studies that showed that lactobacilli are important for sperm motility and conception (66). The idea is to inhibit this *Lactobacillus* function and presumably then make the sperm less mobile and more apt to not reach the egg (http://nocamels.com/2013/02/the-new-contraceptive-suppository-that-disables-sperm/). The challenges with this approach are many, including overcoming the sheer number and mobility of the sperm, covering the whole area that semen reaches, and taking into account the vaginal microbiota, which if colonized by *Prevotella* or *Pseudomonas* (67) may inhibit fertilization but if colonized by competing lactobacilli may not.

COMMUNITY PROBIOTICS

Given the success of fecal microbiota transplantation in curing *Clostridium difficile* infections (68), the concept of using a full microbiome from one person to reset the aberrant microbiome of another is being considered for niches other than the gut. The use of antibiotics to prepare the gut for entrance of a new microbiota has been important so far, and potentially it could also eradicate many vaginal organisms. On the other hand, if it led to recalcitrant biofilms, persister strains, and invasion of epithelial cells, as in the bladder (69, 70), this could perhaps reduce the ability of the implanted microbiota to fully take over.

Much research is needed to determine the ideal composition of a donor vaginal microbiota. While the proportion of species may be identifiable, it should be appreciated that these organisms were presumably arranged by early life factors, diet, hormones, and metabolic linkages. Some of these will inevitably differ in a recipient. Nevertheless, this approach will no doubt be tested. This may require a sponge to collect the microbiota from the donor or use a synthetically prepared microbial collection, similar to that designed by Allen-Vercoe for the gut (71). The latter has the advantage of being devoid of virulence factors and phage, but the potential disadvantage of not coming from the vagina *per se*, where metabolic interactions had been actively occurring just prior to transplant. Presumably, this real-time functionality is at the core of fecal microbiota transplant success.

It would be particularly interesting to assess whether microbiota transplants could reverse the risk of reproductive tract cancers. One mechanism might be to reduce viral shedding and enhance immune defenses in women with early abnormalities, for example, those associated with HPV infection. Another might be to reduce recurrence of BV and AV, conditions that may be associated with a higher risk of cancer. Further research is required to link dysbiosis with cancer and to assess how lactobacilli influence carcinogenesis of the reproductive tract.

SUMMARY

It does not seem that long ago that our work on beneficial bacteria in the female urogenital tract was met with disdain or disregard. Today, the level of interest in this area is astounding, crossing all parts of life from soil and plants to fish and animals and every part of the human body. A multibillion-dollar industry continues to expand, and consumers the world over, with the exception of Africa, are using probiotics to restore and maintain health.

Likewise, interest in the reproductive tract microbiome has also seen a resurgence, which is long overdue considering the relatively primitive diagnostic and treatment options that have been available to women. Dysbiosis in the tract is frequent and can be debilitating for the woman and influential in the fetus. Our level of understanding of these microbiotas has increased significantly with NGS technology, but it must continue, particularly using functional investigations, if we are to truly improve lifelong reproductive tract health. Therapeutic options will emerge from such research for diagnostics and for treatment and maintenance. The ability to manipulate the microbiome through probiotics, prebiotics, and bacterial metabolites would reduce our reliance on unnatural chemical drugs and empower women if they wish to self-manage their vaginal health. Currently, only the use of urine dipsticks for urinary tract infection and antifungals for vulvovaginal candidiasis are accessible over the counter. This is changing with access to probiotics, but further clinical studies are needed to align which composition is best for which subject. Such personalized care will be feasible, especially since only relatively few CSTs are present, and each woman will presumably fit one of them.

Markers of success will be the extent to which innovations are funded sufficiently to continue through human testing and the extent to which clinicians and regulators embrace this new microbiome paradigm.

ACKNOWLEDGMENTS

Our work is funded by a Vogue Team grant from CIHR.

CITATION

Reid G. 2017. Therapeutic opportunities in the vaginal microbiome. Microbiol Spectrum 5(3):BAD-0001-2016.

REFERENCES

1. **Burton JP, Reid G.** 2002. Evaluation of the bacterial vaginal flora of 20 postmenopausal women by direct (Nugent score) and molecular (polymerase chain reaction and denaturing gradient gel electrophoresis) techniques. *J Infect Dis* **186:**1770–1780.
2. **Heinemann C, Reid G.** 2005. Vaginal microbial diversity among postmenopausal women

with and without hormone replacement therapy. *Can J Microbiol* **51**:777–781.

3. **Thies FL, König W, König B.** 2007. Rapid characterization of the normal and disturbed vaginal microbiota by application of 16S rRNA gene terminal RFLP fingerprinting. *J Med Microbiol* **56**:755–761.

4. **Brown CJ, Wong M, Davis CC, Kanti A, Zhou X, Forney LJ.** 2007. Preliminary characterization of the normal microbiota of the human vulva using cultivation-independent methods. *J Med Microbiol* **56**:271–276.

5. **Schellenberg J, Links MG, Hill JE, Dumonceaux TJ, Peters GA, Tyler S, Ball TB, Severini A, Plummer FA.** 2009. Pyrosequencing of the chaperonin-60 universal target as a tool for determining microbial community composition. *Appl Environ Microbiol* **75**:2889–2898.

6. **Kim TK, Thomas SM, Ho M, Sharma S, Reich CI, Frank JA, Yeater KM, Biggs DR, Nakamura N, Stumpf R, Leigh SR, Tapping RI, Blanke SR, Slauch JM, Gaskins HR, Weisbaum JS, Olsen GJ, Hoyer LL, Wilson BA.** 2009. Heterogeneity of vaginal microbial communities within individuals. *J Clin Microbiol* **47**:1181–1189.

7. **Hummelen R, Fernandes AD, Macklaim JM, Dickson RJ, Changalucha J, Gloor GB, Reid G.** 2010. Deep sequencing of the vaginal microbiota of women with HIV. *PLoS One* **5**:e12078.

8. **Ravel J, Gajer P, Abdo Z, Schneider GM, Koenig SS, McCulle SL, Karlebach S, Gorle R, Russell J, Tacket CO, Brotman RM, Davis CC, Ault K, Peralta L, Forney LJ.** 2011. Vaginal microbiome of reproductive-age women. *Proc Natl Acad Sci USA* **108**(Suppl 1):4680–4687.

9. **Gajer P, Brotman RM, Bai G, Sakamoto J, Schütte UM, Zhong X, Koenig SS, Fu L, Ma ZS, Zhou X, Abdo Z, Forney LJ, Ravel J.** 2012. Temporal dynamics of the human vaginal microbiota. *Sci Transl Med* **4**:132ra52.

10. **Wylie KM, Mihindukulasuriya KA, Zhou Y, Sodergren E, Storch GA, Weinstock GM.** 2014. Metagenomic analysis of double-stranded DNA viruses in healthy adults. *BMC Biol* **12**:71.

11. **DiGiulio DB, Callahan BJ, McMurdie PJ, Costello EK, Lyell DJ, Robaczewska A, Sun CL, Goltsman DS, Wong RJ, Shaw G, Stevenson DK, Holmes SP, Relman DA.** 2015. Temporal and spatial variation of the human microbiota during pregnancy. *Proc Natl Acad Sci USA* **112**:11060–11065.

12. **Tamames J, Abellán JJ, Pignatelli M, Camacho A, Moya A.** 2010. Environmental distribution of prokaryotic taxa. *BMC Microbiol* **10**:85.

13. **Dridi B, Raoult D, Drancourt M.** 2011. Archaea as emerging organisms in complex human microbiomes. *Anaerobe* **17**:56–63.

14. **Hirt RP, Sherrard J.** 2015. *Trichomonas vaginalis* origins, molecular pathobiology and clinical considerations. *Curr Opin Infect Dis* **28**: 72–79.

15. **Borgdorff H, Verwijs MC, Wit FW, Tsivtsivadze E, Ndayisaba GF, Verhelst R, Schuren FH, van de Wijgert JH.** 2015. The impact of hormonal contraception and pregnancy on sexually transmitted infections and on cervicovaginal microbiota in African sex workers. *Sex Transm Dis* **42**:143–152.

16. **Ling Z, Liu X, Chen X, Zhu H, Nelson KE, Xia Y, Li L, Xiang C.** 2011. Diversity of cervicovaginal microbiota associated with female lower genital tract infections. *Microb Ecol* **61**: 704–714.

17. **Zheng NN, Guo XC, Lv W, Chen XX, Feng GF.** 2013. Characterization of the vaginal fungal flora in pregnant diabetic women by 18S rRNA sequencing. *Eur J Clin Microbiol Infect Dis* **32**:1031–1040.

18. **Mitchell CM, Haick A, Nkwopara E, Garcia R, Rendi M, Agnew K, Fredricks DN, Eschenbach D.** 2015. Colonization of the upper genital tract by vaginal bacterial species in nonpregnant women. *Am J Obstet Gynecol* **212**:611e1–611e9.

19. **Muzny CA, Sunesara IR, Kumar R, Mena LA, Griswold ME, Martin DH, Lefkowitz EJ, Schwebke JR, Swiatlo E.** 2013. Characterization of the vaginal microbiota among sexual risk behavior groups of women with bacterial vaginosis. *PLoS One* **8**:e80254.

20. **Di Bella JM, Bao Y, Gloor GB, Burton JP, Reid G.** 2013. High throughput sequencing methods and analysis for microbiome research. *J Microbiol Methods* **95**:401–414.

21. **Fernandes AD, Reid JN, Macklaim JM, McMurrough TA, Edgell DR, Gloor GB.** 2014. Unifying the analysis of high-throughput sequencing datasets: characterizing RNA-seq, 16S rRNA gene sequencing and selective growth experiments by compositional data analysis. *Microbiome* **2**:15.

22. **Brooks JP, Edwards DJ, Harwich MD II, Rivera MC, Fettweis JM, Serrano MG, Reris RA, Sheth NU, Huang B, Girerd P, Vaginal Microbiome Consortium, Strauss JF III, Jefferson KK, Buck GA.** 2015. The truth about metagenomics: quantifying and counteracting bias in 16S rRNA studies. *BMC Microbiol* **15**:66.

23. **Macklaim JM, Fernandes AD, Di Bella JM, Hammond JA, Reid G, Gloor GB.** 2013. Comparative meta-RNA-seq of the vaginal microbiota and differential expression by *Lactobacillus iners* in health and dysbiosis. *Microbiome* **1**:12.

24. **McGroarty JA, Reid G, Bruce AW.** 1994. The influence of nonoxynol-9-containing spermicides on urogenital infection. *J Urol* **152:**831–833.

25. **Reid G, Bruce AW, Cook RL, Llano M.** 1990. Effect on urogenital flora of antibiotic therapy for urinary tract infection. *Scand J Infect Dis* **22:**43–47.

26. **Ravel J, Gajer P, Fu L, Mauck CK, Koenig SS, Sakamoto J, Motsinger-Reif AA, Doncel GF, Zeichner SL.** 2012. Twice-daily application of HIV microbicides alter the vaginal microbiota. *MBio* **3:**e00370-12.

27. **Brown JM, Hess KL, Brown S, Murphy C, Waldman AL, Hezareh M.** 2013. Intravaginal practices and risk of bacterial vaginosis and candidiasis infection among a cohort of women in the United States. *Obstet Gynecol* **121:**773–780.

28. **Mayer BT, Srinivasan S, Fiedler TL, Marrazzo JM, Fredricks DN, Schiffer JT.** 2015. Rapid and profound shifts in the vaginal microbiota following antibiotic treatment for bacterial vaginosis. *J Infect Dis* **212:**793–802.

29. **de Louvois J, Hurley R, Stanley VC.** 1975. Microbial flora of the lower genital tract during pregnancy: relationship to morbidity. *J Clin Pathol* **28:**731–735.

30. **Bruce AW, Chadwick P, Hassan A, VanCott GF.** 1973. Recurrent urethritis in women. *Can Med Assoc J* **108:**973–976.

31. **Schellenberg JJ, Dumonceaux TJ, Hill JE, Kimani J, Jaoko W, Wachihi C, Mungai JN, Lane M, Fowke KR, Ball TB, Plummer FA.** 2012. Selection, phenotyping and identification of acid and hydrogen peroxide producing bacteria from vaginal samples of Canadian and East African women. *PLoS One* **7:**e41217.

32. **Velraeds MM, van der Mei HC, Reid G, Busscher HJ.** 1997. Inhibition of initial adhesion of uropathogenic *Enterococcus faecalis* to solid substrata by an adsorbed biosurfactant layer from *Lactobacillus acidophilus. Urology* **49:**790–794.

33. **Velraeds MM, van de Belt-Gritter B, van der Mei HC, Reid G, Busscher HJ.** 1998. Interference in initial adhesion of uropathogenic bacteria and yeasts to silicone rubber by a *Lactobacillus acidophilus* biosurfactant. *J Med Microbiol* **47:**1081–1085.

34. **Absolom DR, Lamberti FV, Policova Z, Zingg W, van Oss CJ, Neumann AW.** 1983. Surface thermodynamics of bacterial adhesion. *Appl Environ Microbiol* **46:**90–97.

35. **Velraeds MMC, van der Mei HC, Reid G, Busscher HJ.** 1996. Physicochemical and biochemical characterization of biosurfactants released from *Lactobacillus* strains. *Colloids Surf B Biointerfaces* **8:**51–61.

36. **Roelants SL, Ciesielska K, De Maeseneire SL, Moens H, Everaert B, Verweire S, Denon Q, Vanlerberghe B, Van Bogaert IN, Van der Meeren P, Devreese B, Soetaert W.** 2016. Towards the industrialization of new biosurfactants: biotechnological opportunities for the lactone esterase gene from *Starmerella bombicola. Biotechnol Bioeng* **113:**550–559.

37. **Reid G, Younes JA, Van der Mei HC, Gloor GB, Knight R, Busscher HJ.** 2011. Microbiota restoration: natural and supplemented recovery of human microbial communities. *Nat Rev Microbiol* **9:**27–38.

38. **Stoyancheva G, Marzotto M, Dellaglio F, Torriani S.** 2014. Bacteriocin production and gene sequencing analysis from vaginal *Lactobacillus* strains. *Arch Microbiol* **196:**645–653.

39. **Anukam KC, Macklaim JM, Gloor GB, Reid G, Boekhorst J, Renckens B, van Hijum SA, Siezen RJ.** 2013. Genome sequence of *Lactobacillus pentosus* KCA1: vaginal isolate from a healthy premenopausal woman. *PLoS One* **8:**e59239.

40. **Verani JR, McGee L, Schrag SJ, Division of Bacterial Diseases, National Center for Immunization and Respiratory Diseases, Centers for Disease Control and Prevention (CDC).** 2010. Prevention of perinatal group B streptococcal disease–revised guidelines from CDC, 2010. *MMWR Recomm Rep* **59**(RR-10):1–36.

41. **Patras KA, Wescombe PA, Rösler B, Hale JD, Tagg JR, Doran KS.** 2015. *Streptococcus salivarius* K12 limits group B *Streptococcus* vaginal colonization. *Infect Immun* **83:**3438–3444.

42. **Li J, Wang W, Xu SX, Magarvey NA, McCormick JK.** 2011. *Lactobacillus reuteri*-produced cyclic dipeptides quench agr-mediated expression of toxic shock syndrome toxin-1 in staphylococci. *Proc Natl Acad Sci USA* **108:**3360–3365.

43. **Gutiérrez-Barranquero JA, Reen FJ, McCarthy RR, O'Gara F.** 2015. Deciphering the role of coumarin as a novel quorum sensing inhibitor suppressing virulence phenotypes in bacterial pathogens. *Appl Microbiol Biotechnol* **99:**3303–3316.

44. **Ojala T, Kankainen M, Castro J, Cerca N, Edelman S, Westerlund-Wikström B, Paulin L, Holm L, Auvinen P.** 2014. Comparative genomics of *Lactobacillus crispatus* suggests novel mechanisms for the competitive exclusion of *Gardnerella vaginalis. BMC Genomics* **15:**1070.

45. **Kirjavainen PK, Laine RM, Carter D, Hammond J-A, Reid G.** 2008. Expression of anti-microbial

defense factors in vaginal mucosa following exposure to *Lactobacillus rhamnosus* GR-1. *Int J Probiotics* **3**:99–106.

46. **Orlando A, Linsalata M, Notarnicola M, Tutino V, Russo F.** 2014. *Lactobacillus* GG restoration of the gliadin induced epithelial barrier disruption: the role of cellular polyamines. *BMC Microbiol* **14**:19.

47. **Garcia AF, Benchimol M, Alderete JF.** 2005. *Trichomonas vaginalis* polyamine metabolism is linked to host cell adherence and cytotoxicity. *Infect Immun* **73**:2602–2610.

48. **Hickey RJ, Abdo Z, Zhou X, Nemeth K, Hansmann M, Osborn TW III, Wang F, Forney LJ.** 2013. Effects of tampons and menses on the composition and diversity of vaginal microbial communities over time. *BJOG* **120**:695–704, discussion 704–706.

49. **Mobley HL, Alteri CJ.** 2015. Development of a vaccine against *Escherichia coli* urinary tract infections. *Pathogens* **5**(1).pii:E1

50. **Sabharwal N, Chhibber S, Harjai K.** 2016. Divalent flagellin immunotherapy provides homologous and heterologous protection in experimental urinary tract infections in mice. *Int J Med Microbiol* **306**:29–37.

51. **Harrison C, Britt H, Garland S, Conway L, Stein A, Pirotta M, Fairley C.** 2014. Decreased management of genital warts in young women in Australian general practice post introduction of national HPV vaccination program: results from a nationally representative cross-sectional general practice study. *PLoS One* **9**:e105967.

52. **Lazar E, Varga R.** 2011. Gynevac-a vaccine, containing lactobacillus for therapy and prevention of bacterial vaginosis and related diseases. *Akush Ginekol (Sofiia)* **50**:36–42.

53. **Demont A, Hacini-Rachinel F, Doucet-Ladevèze R, Ngom-Bru C, Mercenier A, Prioult G, Blanchard C.** 2016. Live and heat-treated probiotics differently modulate IL10 mRNA stabilization and microRNA expression. *J Allergy Clin Immunol* **137**:1264–7. e1, 10.

54. **Donders GG, Vereecken A, Bosmans E, Dekeersmaecker A, Salembier G, Spitz B.** 2002. Definition of a type of abnormal vaginal flora that is distinct from bacterial vaginosis: aerobic vaginitis. *BJOG* **109**:34–43.

55. **Gajer P, Brotman RM, Bai G, Sakamoto J, Schütte UM, Zhong X, Koenig SS, Fu L, Ma ZS, Zhou X, Abdo Z, Forney LJ, Ravel J.** 2012. Temporal dynamics of the human vaginal microbiota. *Sci Transl Med* **4**:132ra52.

56. **Yeoman CJ, Thomas SM, Miller ME, Ulanov AV, Torralba M, Lucas S, Gillis M, Cregger M, Gomez A, Ho M, Leigh SR, Stumpf R, Creedon DJ, Smith MA, Weisbaum JS, Nelson KE, Wilson BA, White BA.** 2013. A multi-omic systems-based approach reveals metabolic markers of bacterial vaginosis and insight into the disease. *PLoS One* **8**:e56111.

57. **McMillan A, Rulisa S, Sumarah M, Macklaim JM, Renaud J, Bisanz JE, Gloor GB, Reid G.** 2015. A multi-platform metabolomics approach identifies highly specific biomarkers of bacterial diversity in the vagina of pregnant and nonpregnant women. *Sci Rep* **5**:14174.

58. **Srinivasan S, Morgan MT, Fiedler TL, Djukovic D, Hoffman NG, Raftery D, Marrazzo JM, Fredricks DN.** 2015. Metabolic signatures of bacterial vaginosis. *mBio* **6**:e00204–e00215.

59. **Steidler L, Wells JM, Raeymaekers A, Vandekerckhove J, Fiers W, Remaut E.** 1995. Secretion of biologically active murine interleukin-2 by *Lactococcus lactis* subsp. *lactis*. *Appl Environ Microbiol* **61**:1627–1629.

60. **Steidler L, Neirynck S, Huyghebaert N, Snoeck V, Vermeire A, Goddeeris B, Cox E, Remon JP, Remaut E.** 2003. Biological containment of genetically modified *Lactococcus lactis* for intestinal delivery of human interleukin 10. *Nat Biotechnol* **21**:785–789.

61. **Vandenbroucke K, Hans W, Van Huysse J, Neirynck S, Demetter P, Remaut E, Rottiers P, Steidler L.** 2004. Active delivery of trefoil factors by genetically modified *Lactococcus lactis* prevents and heals acute colitis in mice. *Gastroenterology* **127**:502–513.

62. **Mercenier A, Müller-Alouf H, Grangette C.** 2000. Lactic acid bacteria as live vaccines. *Curr Issues Mol Biol* **2**:17–25.

63. **Chang TL, Chang CH, Simpson DA, Xu Q, Martin PK, Lagenaur LA, Schoolnik GK, Ho DD, Hillier SL, Holodniy M, Lewicki JA, Lee PP.** 2003. Inhibition of HIV infectivity by a natural human isolate of *Lactobacillus jensenii* engineered to express functional two-domain CD4. *Proc Natl Acad Sci USA* **100**: 11672–11677.

64. **Marcobal A, Liu X, Zhang W, Dimitrov A, Jia L, Lee PP, Fouts T, Parks TP, Lagenaur LA.** 2016. Expression of human immunodeficiency virus type 1neutralizing antibody fragments using human vaginal *Lactobacillus*. *AIDS Res Hum Retroviruses* **32**:964–971.

65. **Liu JJ, Reid G, Jiang Y, Turner MS, Tsai CC.** 2007. Activity of HIV entry and fusion inhibitors expressed by the human vaginal colonizing probiotic *Lactobacillus reuteri* RC-14. *Cell Microbiol* **9**:120–130.

66. **Barbonetti A, Vassallo MR, Cinque B, Filipponi S, Mastromarino P, Cifone MG, Francavilla S, Francavilla F.** 2013. Soluble

products of *Escherichia coli* induce mitochondrial dysfunction-related sperm membrane lipid peroxidation which is prevented by lactobacilli. *PLoS One* **8:**e83136.

67. **Weng SL, Chiu CM, Lin FM, Huang WC, Liang C, Yang T, Yang TL, Liu CY, Wu WY, Chang YA, Chang TH, Huang HD.** 2014. Bacterial communities in semen from men of infertile couples: metagenomic sequencing reveals relationships of seminal microbiota to semen quality. *PLoS One* **9:**e110152.

68. **Fuentes S, van Nood E, Tims S, Heikamp-de Jong I, ter Braak CJ, Keller JJ, Zoetendal EG, de Vos WM.** 2014. Reset of a critically disturbed microbial ecosystem: faecal transplant in recurrent *Clostridium difficile* infection. *ISME J* **8:**1621–1633.

69. **Anderson GG, Palermo JJ, Schilling JD, Roth R, Heuser J, Hultgren SJ.** 2003. Intracellular bacterial biofilm-like pods in urinary tract infections. *Science* **301:**105–107.

70. **Goneau LW, Hannan TJ, MacPhee RA, Schwartz DJ, Macklaim JM, Gloor GB, Razvi H, Reid G, Hultgren SJ, Burton JP.** 2015. Subinhibitory antibiotic therapy alters recurrent urinary tract infection pathogenesis through modulation of bacterial virulence and host immunity. *mBio* **6:**e00356–e15.

71. **Petrof EO, Gloor GB, Vanner SJ, Weese SJ, Carter D, Daigneault MC, Brown EM, Schroeter K, Allen-Vercoe E.** 2013. Stool substitute transplant therapy for the eradication of *Clostridium difficile* infection: 'RePOOPulating' the gut. *Microbiome* **1:**3.

Lung Microbiota and Its Impact on the Mucosal Immune Phenotype

7

BENJAMIN G. WU[1] and LEOPOLDO N. SEGAL[1]

INTRODUCTION

In 2007, the Human Microbiome Project (HMP) was added to the National Institutes of Health (NIH) Roadmap for Medical Research, and since then, over $200 million has been invested in the exploration of the human microbiome. Several sites on the human body, including the nares, oral cavity, skin, gastrointestinal tract, and urogenital tract, have been studied by the HMP (1). The gastrointestinal tract remains the most thoroughly investigated organ-microbiome interaction studied thus far, and its role in shaping the host immune response is rapidly becoming defined within the context of inflammatory response (2–4). Observations have noted associations of specific microbes and the gut microbiome in obesity (5–8), coronary artery disease (9–12), *Clostridium difficile* colitis (13, 14), type 2 diabetes (15, 16), and inflammatory bowel disease (4, 17, 18). While the nares and oral cavity were included as locations to be studied for the HMP, the lower airway respiratory system was not included as a location of interest. The microbial community of the oropharynx had been well described even before the advances of next-generation sequencing and multiplexed data (19, 20). Microbiome approaches to the upper and lower respiratory systems created a deluge of associations

[1]Department of Medicine, NYU Division of Pulmonary, Critical Care, & Sleep Medicine, New York City, NY 10016
Bugs as Drugs: Therapeutic Microbes for the Prevention and Treatment of Disease
Edited by Robert A. Britton and Patrice D. Cani
© 2018 American Society for Microbiology, Washington, DC
doi:10.1128/microbiolspec.BAD-0005-2016

between host and microbes in health and disease (21–23). Over the past few years, our understanding of the airway microbiome has shifted, upending the old adage of the lungs being a sterile field (24) to a new paradigm of a continuous organ system with a rich and vibrant mucosal surface that embodies complex interactions between the microbiome and its host that can propagate or resist disease (21, 24). Moreover, little is known regarding how the respiratory microbiome interacts with the host immune response. While multiple research projects have focused on the effects of the gut microbiota on the immune response of the gastrointestinal mucosa (25–27), few papers have focused on the effects of the lower airway microbiota on the respiratory mucosa that it inhabits (23, 28–30).

Some of the unique challenges in studying the lower airway microbiome include the technical difficulty of sampling the lower respiratory tract, the extremely low bacterial burden in healthy lung leading to a ratio of low signal to high noise, and the lack of animal models to study the lung microbiome (31, 32). Shifts in gastrointestinal microorganism composition in organ systems that contain high bacterial biomass, such as the gastrointestinal tract, can lead to broad observations resulting in disease states (33). However, the lung microbiome is a low-bacterial-burden organ in which transient perturbations of its microbiome can have dramatic effects on the diversity of its composition and the host inflammatory response to dysbiosis (23). Thus, the upper and lower respiratory tract microbiome is unique, as it represents an organ with a significant biomass gradient, moving from a high-bacterial-burden reservoir in the upper respiratory tract to a very-low-bacterial-burden area in the lung microbiome (32, 34). We will discuss first the microbiomes of the upper and lower respiratory tracts and then the possible mechanisms for microbial migration and colonization, followed by the recent finding of the host immune response to the microbiome and the

inflammatory pathways that the microbiome may impact, and finally we will address possible microbial targets or markers for specific diseases.

The airway microbiome can only be understood as the sum of its individual parts. In the upper airways, the nasal and oral cavities contain a very distinct microbiome. In the nasal cavity, the microbiota is characterized by enrichment with *Streptococcus, Acinetobacter, Lactococcus, Staphylococcus,* and *Corynebacterium*. In the oral cavity, the microbiota is characterized by enrichment with *Prevotella, Streptococcus, Fusobacterium, Neisseria, Leptotrichia,* and *Veillonella* (35). Further defining the qualities of each location, the upper airways are characterized by a constant exposure to airborne microbes and microbes ingested as part of each individual's diet. Although the respiratory system and its mucosa are a continuum, the lower airway microbiota has very distinctive features that set it apart from that of the upper respiratory tract. The boundary between what we define as the upper and the lower airways is classically defined by anatomical structures, with the vocal cords being analogous to a natural "dam" against aspiration (36, 37). Similar to the water held by a dam, the upper airways hold a high bacterial burden, while the lower-airway microbiota has about 100 to 10,000 times less of a bacterial burden than the upper microbiota based on 16S rRNA copies (32, 38). Microaspiration occurs in healthy individuals (39), and its prevalence is higher in several lung diseases, including chronic obstructive pulmonary disease (COPD), asthma, obstructive sleep apnea, cystic fibrosis, and lung infections due to atypical (such as nontuberculous mycobacteria) and typical microorganisms (40–45).

Charlson and colleagues, who in initial studies examined bronchoscopy results from six healthy patients, concluded that the microbiome of the lower respiratory tract resembled that of the upper respiratory tract (32). Further microbiome work studying cell-free bronchoalveolar lavage (BAL) fluids has noted that the bacteria characteristic of the oral cavity are found in about 45% of relatively healthy subjects and that the remaining subjects had a lung microbiome whose members resembled the background taxa (23, 30). Other studies have found bacteria characteristic of the oral cavity at a higher prevalence, although it is unclear if this is related to the sample type utilized (acellular BAL fluid versus whole BAL fluid versus airway brush sample) or differences in cohorts (32, 46–48). Importantly, a dichotomized view of the lower airway microbiota (i.e., enriched with upper airway microbes or not) may be an oversimplification of a more likely physiological continuum of similarity between the lower and upper airway microbiotas. Of note, older studies using radiotracers have found that a similar proportion of healthy individuals microaspirate (39, 49). Using culture-independent techniques, various studies have shown that bacteria commonly found in the upper airways are also frequently found in multiple other disease states, such as asthma (29, 50–58), cystic fibrosis (59–62), HIV infection (47, 63, 64), and advanced COPD (21, 23, 28, 65, 66). Considering the continuity of the airway mucosa, it is no surprise that the upper airway microbiota with its high bacterial burden is the major source of microbes for the lower airways. However, even when the lower airways are enriched with microbes found in the oral cavity, differences can still be noted between the upper and lower airway microbiotas (30, 32). This suggests that there are other important factors that affect the dynamic homeostasis of the lower airway. Several questions remained unanswered regarding (i) what other microbiotas from different mucosae contribute to the "cross pollination" of microbes to the lower airways, (ii) what selection pressures microbes suffer as they enter the lower airways, and (iii) how this selection pressure changes in different compartments of the lower airways.

UNIQUE CHALLENGES IN EVALUATING THE LUNG MICROBIOME

One particular challenge that research in the lung microbiome has yet to resolve is the microbiome signal-to-background noise ratio during health and early disease (Fig. 1) (31). While this might also be important in advanced disease states, the signal-to-noise ratio is highly unfavorable in early stages of disease, when there is low microbial biomass in lower airway samples. Functionally, the lungs have a 100- to 10,000 times-lower bacterial burden than the upper airways (23, 38). Thus, the low-bacterial-burden nature of the pulmonary system poses unique challenges: signal-to-noise ratios that are characterized by high background noise signals (31), lack of standardized methods for background removal, and limited ability to detect signals from low-abundance taxa. These challenges confound researchers and make the lung microbiome difficult to study. One consistent finding in multiple studies is that background environmental samples, such as sterile saline and prebronchoscopic wash through the bronchoscope (prior to the procedure), contain microbial DNA that is characterized as belonging to a diverse environmental background microbiota (30, 31). This is understandable and predictable, since instruments are "clean" but not necessarily DNA free. Furthermore, reagents utilized for DNA isolation and library preparation may also contribute to background DNA (67). A large percentage of healthy subjects have a lower airway microbiota enriched with microbial DNA that is characteristic of background samples (21, 23). Thus, the background microbiome may confound observations in a low-biomass host microbiome in approximately 60% of healthy subjects that will have a microbiome enriched with background predominant taxa (also referred as pneumotype$_{BPT}$) (23, 30). Even in these subjects, bioinformatic approaches that identify the contribution of background taxa (e.g., SourceTracker) to a sample showed

Conceptual Model: Signal to Noise Ratio

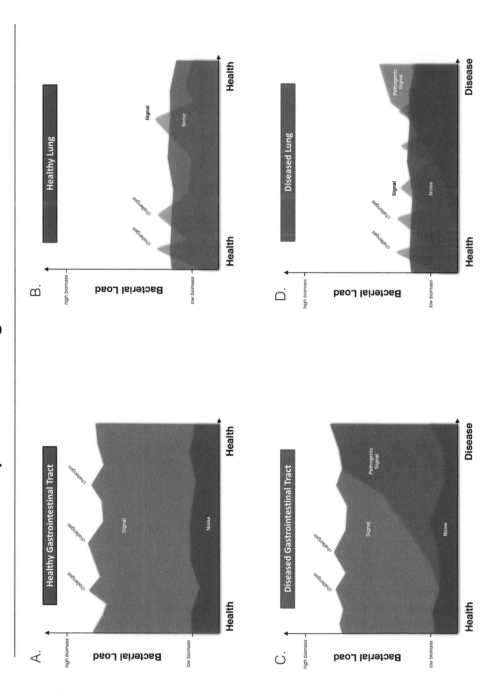

that close to one-half of the composition of a BAL sample was not present in background samples (e.g., bronchoscope) (30). This result suggests that there is still a significant amount of information to be gained from these low-biomass samples. Consider for comparison the microbiome of the gastrointestinal tract. This high-bacterial-burden and diverse microbial community is subjected to multiple microbial challenges (e.g., food intake, medications, etc.). In this setting, the background microbiota is rarely seen as an important source of contamination. However, the background microbiota may influence the recovery of rare or less abundant microorganisms or, in the setting of gross contamination, may play a role in obscuring the bacterial composition. Microbial changes due to different microbial challenges or active disease processes are more likely to be detected in the gastrointestinal tract (Fig. 1A and C). Conversely, the low bacterial burden found in the respiratory tract makes the microbial assessment using culture-independent techniques commonly influenced by the background microbiome. Thus, when microbial challenges that disturb the underlying lung microbiome occur, they may not be apparent due to the low signal that needs to overcome a high background noise (Fig. 1B and D). This model also suggests that the signal can be transient and subjected to the dynamics that dictate the microbial host interaction in the lower airways. The low microbial load of the respiratory system may lead to large shifts in the microbiome when faced with upper airway tract microbial challenges. The microbial challenges caused by microaspiration may then be seen as the enrichment of the lower airway microbiome with upper airway microbes (also referred as pneumotype$_{SPT}$, where SPT stands for supraglottic predominant taxa) (23, 30). The lower microbial biomass and low signal-to-noise ratio present a distinct challenge when studying the lung microbiome. It is therefore important to include the study of the background microbiome in microbiome research involving low-biomass samples.

Questions remain regarding what to do with background taxa when studying the lower airway microbiome. Curation of the sequencing data commonly includes removal of technical contaminating taxa that can be done as part of the upstream processing of the data. Neutral modeling is a technique that can be utilized to identify taxa preferentially enriched in one sample type (68). Taxa that are found but deviate from this model are the most likely to be true inhabitants of the area that was sampled. For example, this technique can then be used to remove taxa found in the bronchoscope to identify microbes that are resident in the lung. SourceTracker is another technique utilized to estimate the degree of microbial contribution that sources of background microbiota (e.g., bronchoscope) may have on a biological sample (69). While these methods have been utilized in lung microbiome research, there is a lack of consensus on how to standardize the analysis. One concern is that in samples with

---

FIGURE 1 Conceptual model: signal-to-noise ratio. (A) Healthy gastrointestinal microbiome, where there is an organ of healthy biomass and background "noise" or signal amplified by background (e.g., background microbiota present in the colonoscope) that does not represent the gut microbiome. This background microbiome is overwhelmed by the large biomass present the sample. (B) Healthy lung microbiome, where there is relatively low biomass and background signals tend to overwhelm the lung microbiome signal. (C) Diseased gastrointestinal microbiome, where the pathogenic signal (dysbiosis) will eventually overcome the high underlying biomass. The pathogenic signal will overpower the background microbiome and be apparent given the high amount of biomass present in the gut. (D) Diseased lung microbiome. Unlike the diseased gut microbiome, the pathogenic signal may be confounded by the background noise and may not be apparent until sufficient progression of disease supports the altered dysbiosis.

a predominance of background taxa (e.g., pneumotype$_{BPT}$), the removal of background taxa may yield low reads and, given the relative-abundance nature of the microbiome data, will inflate the relative proportion of the taxa that were not removed. Also, taxon removal approaches have the potential of excluding taxa existing in both the lung and the possible contamination sources (e.g., bronchoscope) that might be meaningful to comprehend the lower airway microbiota. Finally, bacteria may have a significant pathogenic role in a disease state despite its low abundance in a microbial community, and removal of background taxa may in fact change our understanding of the microbe's role in the lung (70). For example, sequence analysis of experimental diarrhea induced by enterotoxigenic *Escherichia coli* has shown that even low abundance of this organism can cause significant disease (71). Thus, in the lung, the high abundance of background noise represents a major challenge to detect a signal that occurs in microorganisms from low-abundance taxa that may be biologically important to health and disease.

SOURCES OF MICROBIAL CHALLENGE TO THE LOWER AIRWAYS

Predictably, the most straightforward explanation for the source of microbes to the lower airways is the delivery of microbes from the upper respiratory tract through micro-aspiration. Although it is generally accepted that aspiration of oral cavity secretions likely affects the lung microbiota, other possible sources must be considered. The contribution of the airborne microbiome present in ambient air may be a significant contributor to the lower airways. The human body ventilates approximately 7,000 to 20,000 liters of ambient air per day (24, 72), potentially exposing the lower airways to microbes present in the air (airborne microbiota) in conjunction with other well-recognized pollutants, chemicals, dust, allergens, and

other particulate matter from the atmosphere. While there is significant knowledge on pathogens that are aerosolized and can transmit infections, such as mycobacteria (73, 74), much less is known about the presence and relevance of other microorganisms present in the air. It is possible that different airborne microbiota members may also significantly contribute to the lower airway microbiome, a subject that needs further investigation.

There is an increasing understanding of the complex airborne microbiome and its contributions to the lower airway microbiome. Adams and colleagues found differences between indoor and outdoor environments that were dictated by human-associated microorganisms (75). In indoor environments, they found an enrichment of *Corynebacterium*, *Streptococcus*, *Staphylococcus*, *Propionibacterium*, *Lactococcus*, and *Enterobacteriaceae*. In outdoor environments, there was enrichment with *Pseudomonas*, *Acinetobacter*, and *Sphingomonas* (75). Also, Meadow and colleagues identified a distinct "microbial cloud" that supports the notion that in an enclosed space, ambient air can be impacted by its occupants (76). However, the effects of exposure to different airborne microbiotas on the lung microbiome or the effects of the exhaled air microbiota on the airborne ambient microbiome have not been studied. The nasal microbiota is distinct from the oral cavity microbiota (35) and likely represents an important microbial reservoir to the lower airways that is enriched by inhalation of ambient air.

Culture-independent methods in chronic rhinosinusitis have shown enrichment with *Haemophilus influenzae* (77, 78) and other pathogens that are frequently associated with development of pneumonia. Postnasal drip is highly associated with cough and bronchial inflammatory diseases, but its effect on the lower airway microbiota has not been elucidated. The gastrointestinal tract represents another potential source of microbial challenge to the lung microbiome. Gastroesophageal reflux disease (GERD) is frequently present in many disease states. The presence of a distinct microbiome in the gut dominated by *Helicobacter pylori* has been associated with decreased risk for asthma (79, 80). The use of proton pump inhibitors affects the composition of not only the gastric microbiota but also the lung microbiome (81). Further, the lower gastrointestinal tract should be considered a potential source of microbial challenge to the lung. Animal models of sepsis have shown that germ-free animals are protected from lung injury (82) while selective gastrointestinal tract decontamination reduces the development of multiple-organ dysfunction syndrome in 50% of the subjects studied (83).

However, the most frequently observed microorganisms in the lower airways are those characteristically present in the oral cavity. Multiple culture-independent investigations have shown that different subjects have various degrees of enrichment of the lower airway microbiota with oral microbes such as *Prevotella*, *Veillonella*, *Rothia*, *Streptococcus*, and *Porphyromonas* (23, 30, 65, 84, 85). Thus, multiple potential sources may contribute to the lower airway microbiome through different routes of microbial challenge, e.g., aspiration, regurgitation, hematogenous, and aerosolized routes. These microbial challenges will then be subjects of unique selection pressures present in the lower airway environment. Although there is limited understanding of what these selection pressures are at individual levels, it is likely that they have a very significant effect on the structure of the microbial communities that may reside in the lower airways.

UNIQUE SELECTION PRESSURES OF THE LOWER AIRWAY MICROBIOME

Several different theories have been adapted from biology, ecology, and environmental studies to explain the composition of the lung microbiome. One of the most purported has been the "adapted island model" (86–88).

Similar to islands, the lungs are influenced by a balance between immigration of microbes from the "mainland" and their extinction (86, 87). Based on this theory, the lungs can be viewed as conceptual "islands" that receive immigration challenges, most commonly from the upper respiratory tract. Thus, the diversity in the lungs is driven mainly by the diversity from the sources of microbial challenges and the selection pressure on a microorganism's viability.

The proximal airways, including the trachea and the main stem bronchi, may be viewed as large swaths of area that due to their location in relation to the upper airway more closely resemble the upper respiratory tract (32). As one progresses distally in the lower respiratory tract, the conducting airways may represent isolated islands (87, 89), potentially forming a unique microbial niche. Thus, diversity is influenced by three main factors: the rate of immigration, the rate of elimination, and the rate of reproduction of the community members (86–88, 90). In health, the diversity of these islands is dictated mainly by immigration from the upper respiratory tract and elimination by various mechanisms including the mucociliary ladder, bacteriophages, and alveolar macrophages. Frequent episodes of microaspiration observed in healthy individuals are likely to be the most dominant source of microbial airway challenge. In the event of disease, different factors may influence the lung microbiome. For example, in active pneumonia, chronic airway colonization in COPD, or cystic fibrosis, the reproduction rate of the organism in the lower airway will offset the mechanisms of immigration and elimination.

Furthermore, the airway mucosa has several unique features: it is a hollow system of mucosa-lined tubes in constant exposure to ambient air with a role to perform gas exchange; it contains high levels of phospholipids in the form of surfactant (91); and as a result of its gas exchange properties, it contains gradients of oxygen and carbon dioxide tension (92). Thus, microbes, as they enter the lower airways, have to overcome or adapt to the changing environment of the lung. Recent investigations have demonstrated that by evaluating microbial genetic variations within a host, multiple lineages can coexist, providing evidence of selective pressures in the lower airways (93). Several environmental factors present in the lower airways potentially shape the lower airway microbiota. The phospholipid-rich environment not only is important to maintain surface tension and aerated alveoli but also has significant effects on microbial metabolism (94). Multiple antimicrobial peptides such as surfactant protein A, lactoferrin, and defensins are present in the airways (94). Experimental evidence shows that secretory immunoglobulin A (SIgA) has an important role in the airway microbiota and its deficiency leads to increased inflammation in response to the resident lung microbiota and progressive airway remodeling and emphysema (95). Thus, the antimicrobial properties of the pulmonary mucosa represent a significant hurdle for microbial colonization. Microbes have developed and evolved specific mechanisms in order to evade or ameliorate the effects of the host defense. As an example, biofilm constitutes its own microbial niche in which anaerobes can find an optimal anaerobic niche (96). For example, *Pseudomonas aeruginosa* advantageously uses biofilm to create its own microenvironment (97). Biofilms, close proximity to aerobes and anaerobes, and development of oxygen-depleted microenvironments may allow for microbial colonization under anaerobic conditions (98). Thus, although the lung is a highly aerated organ, anaerobes are frequently described in the lower airway microbiome, suggesting that biofilms may have an important role in the co-occurrence of aerobes and anaerobes in the lower airways (96, 98). Microbes with different adhesion properties are also affected differently by mechanical selection pressure such as mucociliary clearance (99, 100). Different bacteria express adhesins, pilin, and flagellin in

order to overcome mucociliary removal from the lower airways (101, 102). These are important virulence factors for bacterial colonization and pathogenesis, and not all bacteria express these advantages. Thus, the microorganisms found in the respiratory system likely reflect highly specialized strains or species that are in constant balance with a highly immune-active mucosa (103, 104). Experimental approaches are needed to study how these factors affect the selection pressures that shape the lower airway microbiome.

The lung environment ecosystem can also be thought of as a series of forward and feedback loops that suppresses or allows the underlying lung bacteria to grow (88). A major risk factor for the development of pneumonia in the hospital setting is the use of antibiotics (105). Evidence suggests that it is likely that the pathogen responsible for the development of pneumonia exists in the lung prior to the onset of disease. In a murine model of this theory, Poroyko and colleagues conducted a study of lipopolysaccharide (LPS)-induced acute lung injury and studied the changes in the murine lung microbiome (106). The mice notably had an increase in bacterial burden without an increase in the number of species. There was also an increase in abundance of the family of *Proteobacteria* and a decrease in *Firmicutes*. These findings suggest that challenge with LPS may overwhelm the feedback mechanisms responsible for equilibrium in the lungs, allowing the resident microorganisms in the lung to proliferate unchecked during times of stress and inflammation. Nutrition availability may also affect the alterations in the lung microbiome (107). Issues such as iron availability and nutritional immunity may select for microorganisms that are able to adapt to the lack of or abundance of certain nutrients. Moreover, coinfection with viruses may affect the equilibrium in the lung as well. Molyneaux and colleagues demonstrated that there are intrinsic changes in the lower respiratory tract microbiome when it is challenged with rhinovirus infection. In this study, healthy subjects and those with a history of COPD were challenged with rhinovirus and monitored longitudinally over a period of 42 days (108). Using induced sputum, the authors showed that rhinovirus challenge led to an increase in *Proteobacteria*, driven mainly by an increase in *Haemophilus influenzae* (108). This may explain why lower airway pneumonia occurs after viral infection.

Changes in the host immune system will affect the selection pressure on the lower airway microbiota. An example of this selection is the enrichment with *Tropheryma whipplei*, the etiological agent of Whipple's disease, in the lungs of treatment-naive HIV subjects and the subsequent decline of the relative abundance of *T. whipplei* following antiretroviral therapy (64). Importantly, since this microbe was not found in the upper airway samples or background controls, it seems to reflect a true inhabitant of the lower airways, where growth is favored or promoted by the host's immunodeficient state. Recently, broader microbial differences were noted in advanced HIV and partially corrected with immune reconstitution (109). Twigg and colleagues identified higher relative abundance of *Streptococcus*, *Prevotella*, and *Veillonella* taxa in the lungs of the HIV-infected patients after 1 year of treatment with antiretroviral therapy as compared to the same patients prior to the start of treatment. Moreover, there is increasing evidence of the effects of immune deficiency on nonbacterial microbes in the lung, such as in the mycobiome, the collection of fungi found in a community (110). The response of the host's respiratory system to this environmental and microorganism challenge is an integral facet to understanding the roles of the upper and lower respiratory microbiomes in health and disease (21, 23, 30).

Specific deficiencies in the host immune response play a significant role in the microbiome. Richmond and colleagues explored changes in mucosal immunity by studying the impact of specific SIgA immunodeficiency

(95). The researchers developed mouse models that were deficient in the polymeric immunoglobulin receptor (pIgR) and were not able to produce SIgA on mucosal surfaces. The pIgR deficiency results in the persistent activation of inflammation signaling due to lung microbiota invasion (95). Mice with a pIgR deficiency contained an increase in taxa (400 versus 194) in the lung. Discriminating taxa found in higher relative abundance in pIgR-deficient mice than in wild-type mice included *Veillonella*, *Prevotella*, *Neisseriaceae*, *Bacillus*, *Actinomycetaceae*, *Tissierellaceae*, and *Ruminococcus* (95). Furthermore, germ-free pIgR-deficient mice did not develop the COPD-like phenotype, in contrast to pIgR-deficient mice raised in a conventional environment. Once the germ-free pIgR mice were removed from their germ-free environment and their microbiotas were conventionalized, similar levels of airway wall remodeling, emphysema, and inflammation were measured and found to be comparable to those of pIgR mice raised under conventional (non-germ-free) conditions for the same duration of exposure (95). Upregulation of NF-κB was found in the lungs of pIgR-deficient mice when compared to wild-type age-matched controls (95). This is important, since structural abnormalities in COPD correlate with decreased expression of pIgR and a disruption of the protective mucosal barrier (111, 112).

The use of medications, especially corticosteroids, may also affect the host response to microorganisms. The host immune response determines host susceptibility to microbes, thereby affecting the distinction between pathogens and commensals. In cases where the immune response is inadequate or altered, microorganisms that may regularly colonize or be cleared by the host may have the potential to cause disease. Mucosa-associated invariant T (MAIT) cells are a prevalent and unique T-cell population in humans with the capacity to detect intracellular infections with bacteria, including *Mycobacterium tuberculosis* (113). MAIT cells recognize early intermediates in bacterial riboflavin synthesis that can be potent antigens for these cells (113). Although they are able to recognize a wide variety of bacterial microorganisms, bacteria that do not express riboflavin synthesis pathways do not stimulate MAIT cells (114). Hinks and colleagues demonstrated that in 11 patients who were exposed to inhaled corticosteroids, peripheral serum and bronchial biopsy specimens contained fewer MAIT cells than did healthy controls (115). In *in vitro* studies, nontypeable *Haemophilus influenzae*-infected macrophages obtained from healthy subjects were exposed to fluticasone or budesonide. In the presence of these corticosteroids, significant impairment of the up-regulation of MR1, a stimulatory receptor on macrophages for MAIT cells, as well as a decrease in nontypeable *H. influenzae*-induced gamma interferon expression from MAIT cells was found in these experiments (115). Therefore, steroid-induced suppression of MAIT cells may be responsible for the increased risk of pneumonia in subjects with airway diseases (115).

Unique selection pressures of the lung may have a profound impact on the lung microbiome. There is increasing evidence that the adapted island model may help model the microbial challenges to the lower airways from microaspiration. Once in the lower airways, the oral microorganisms are likely exposed to multiple selection pressures that dictate their persistence or transient nature in the lungs. Microbes that evolutionarily develop advantages to mitigate and avoid the host immune response are more likely to persist in the lower airway microbiome. Their ability to overcome the innate and adaptive immune systems may serve to guide future studies to address new pathways that are regulated by microbes and particular molecular patterns that may dictate these interactions. Most importantly, host responses and medications deserve particular attention, as these mechanisms remain largely unexplored in the current literature in relation to their effects on the lung microbiome.

THE LUNG MICROBIOME IN DISEASE STATES

Morris and colleagues studied the microbiomes of healthy subjects and healthy smokers in a study of the lung microbiome (85). They found that the most common genera in both oral wash and BAL fluid were microorganisms commonly found in the oral cavity (*Prevotella*, *Streptococcus*, and *Veillonella*). Although the study did detect organisms found to be more abundant in the lung than in the oral cavity, including *Haemophilus*, *Enterobacteriaceae*, and *Tropheryma whipplei*, differences in the lung microbiota between smokers and nonsmokers were not found (85). However, despite no differences found in the lung microbiome, microbiota differences were found in the oropharynx of smokers compared with that of nonsmokers. *Neisseria*, *Porphyromonas*, and *Gemella* were depleted in the oral washes of the former set of subjects (85). Several other studies have shown that smoking alone is sufficient to change the upper airway microbiota (20, 35) but not the lower airway microbiota (23, 85).

The exposure to tobacco smoke may also greatly increase an individual's risk of developing COPD. In contrast to what is seen in individuals with exposure to tobacco smoke, subjects with advanced stages of COPD have significant alterations within the underlying lung microbiome. Erb-Downward and colleagues described these differences in lung microbiome in the lungs of end-stage COPD patients (84). Importantly, different areas of the lung have different microbiotas. Presumably, changes in the underlying lung architecture and decreased mucociliary clearance lead to enrichment with *Pseudomonas* and *Streptococcus* (84). Other studies have also described differences in the lung microbiome of COPD (28, 65, 116). However, most COPD microbiome studies have focused on samples from GOLD stage IV COPD patients and samples collected from explanted lungs, where other confounders, such as use of inhaled steroids and frequent courses of antibiotics, are commonly present and may present confusing results regarding the lung microbiome. Hilty and colleagues also described a disordered lung microbiome in patients with asthma and moderate COPD (58). Notably, 60% of these patients were on inhaled corticosteroid therapy.

Dysbiosis may also play a role in COPD exacerbations. Huang and colleagues studied a group of patients (n = 8) who were admitted to their hospital for COPD exacerbations. All of the patients studied were mechanically ventilated and intubated and received antibiotics (117). The subjects studied showed variations in their interpersonal bacterial richness, with subjects with decreased richness having more *Pseudomonaceae* and *Enterobacteriaceae* and subjects with increased richness possessing higher relative abundance of *Clostridiaceae*, *Lachnospiraceae*, *Bacillaceae*, and *Peptostreptococcaceae* (117). One challenging issue with interpreting some of these results may be that the subjects received different lengths and types of antibiotic treatment at the time of the study. Thus, changes in the lung microbiome that may be related to a subject having a COPD exacerbation may be lost early in the disease and the changes seen may be due to an antibiotic effect on the lung microbiome (117).

Pragman and colleagues examined the lung microbiomes of moderate and severe COPD subjects with relatively stable disease and compared them to healthy subjects. They found that while the moderate and severe COPD groups had more operational taxonomic units in common, very few operational taxonomic units (approximately 13%) were shared among all three groups (116). Notably, the study found several anaerobes within the lung, consisting of *Bacteroidetes*, *Fusobacteria*, and the genus *Clostridium*, extending observations that anaerobic bacteria are found in an aerobic environment; however, it is not known if these anaerobic bacteria are metabolically active (116). In a subanalysis of the study, the authors found that the most

discriminant factor for a distinct lung microbiome was the use of inhaled steroids. Emphasizing the effects of medications on the microbiome, a recent investigation showed that in subjects with early emphysema, the use of azithromycin affected the diversity of the lower airway microbiome and increased stress-related microbial metabolites that might have anti-inflammatory properties (118). These data further support the role of the lower airway microbiome on the immune phenotype of the lower airway mucosa and illustrate the selective pressures of medications.

Using core biopsy specimens from explanted lungs, Sze and colleagues also found differences in advanced COPD, with an increase in the relative abundance of *Firmicutes*, including *Lactobacillus* and *Proteobacteria* (65). However, in a follow-up study, the same researchers found that there was a relative expansion of the phylum *Proteobacteria* and a reduction of the phylum *Firmicutes* when they compared the lung specimens from COPD subjects to lungs from transplant donors (28), reinforcing that it remains difficult to define a consistent "core" COPD microbiota. One important finding of the last study was that there were several taxa that were positively and negatively associated with the host immune response, including neutrophil infiltration, eosinophil infiltration, and B-cell infiltration (28).

Despite studies that have examined the lung microbiome in GOLD stage IV COPD patients, early and moderate COPD patients and active smokers remain difficult to study and represent a knowledge deficit in lung microbiome research. Attention should be given to these populations due to several challenging issues, including a need to study early events in the disease process, a way to control and limit possible confounders such as inhaled corticosteroids, and a focus on longitudinal changes in the lung microbiome.

In asthma, there is evidence of enrichment with *Proteobacteria*, including the *Haemophilus* genus (29, 119). Importantly, distinct immunological phenotypes have been associated with changes in the lower airway microbiome. The respiratory tract of asthmatic patients tends to have a higher bacterial burden than that of subjects without asthma (119). Exposure to diverse allergens and microbes (from animal or environmental exposure) in youth proves to be protective against developing asthma, thus supporting the "hygiene hypothesis" (120, 121). In contrast, several taxa in the lung microbiome, including *Streptococcus pneumoniae* and *Haemophilus influenzae*, have been identified as increasing the susceptibility of developing asthma once colonization is established in a neonatal host (122). Huang and colleagues studied asthmatic patients with a disordered lung microbiome. They identified that a greater airway diversity was strongly associated with increased bronchial hyperresponsiveness (119). Moreover, they found that the taxa that were strongly associated with bronchial hyperresponsiveness belonged primarily to the *Proteobacteria* phylum. The treatment of these patients with clarithromycin showed that those showing improvement in their bronchial reactivity following clarithromycin treatment had an increase in their Shannon diversity index (α diversity) (119).

In severe asthmatics, Huang and colleagues also sought to characterize the microbiome associated with subjects with different phenotypes of asthma. They observed that enrichment with *Bacteroidetes* and the *Firmicutes* phylum (including families *Prevotellaceae, Mycoplasmataceae, Lachnospiraceae,* and *Spirochaetaceae*) was associated with obese subjects who were also asthmatics. They also identified certain taxa associated with worsening asthma symptoms such as the *Proteobacteria* phylum (including families *Pasteurellaceae, Enterobacteriaceae, Neisseriaceae, Burkholderiaceae,* and *Pseudomonadaceae*) (123). The researchers demonstrated that different asthma phenotypes might harbor distinct microbiomes, supporting an important aspect of the lung microbiome on the host immune phenotype (29).

In cystic fibrosis, disordered airway clearance is a result of dysfunction of the sodium

chloride channel, leading to thickened secretions and progressive microbial airway colonization and infection. Culture-based data have identified clinically significant bacteria, including *Pseudomonas aeruginosa* (124), *Burkholderia cepacia* complex (124), methicillin-resistant *Staphylococcus aureus* (125), and *Mycobacterium avium* complex (126), in the airways of cystic fibrosis patients. Early microbiome studies in cystic fibrosis patients identified a possible core microbiome represented by 15 taxa from seven genera including *Catonella, Neisseria, Porphyromonas, Prevotella, Pseudomonas, Streptococcus,* and *Veillonella* (127). The lungs of cystic fibrosis subjects may contain high spatial heterogeneity (128). In a study involving 269 cystic fibrosis patients conducted by Coburn and colleagues, the researchers studied a broad range of ages and disease stages (128, 129). The study reaffirmed particular species as belonging to a possible core microbiome including *Streptococcus, Prevotella, Rothia, Veillonella,* and *Actinomyces* (129). More typical cystic fibrosis-related microorganisms (e.g., *Pseudomonas, Burkholderia, Stenotrophomonas,* and *Achromobacter*) were less prevalent but, when present in sputum specimens, tended to dominate the relative abundance within the samples (129). Furthermore, Coburn and colleagues showed that community diversity and lung function were greatest in patients less than 10 years of age, reaching a plateau at age 25, with a subsequent decreasing community diversity in following years correlated with worsening lung function (129). Bacteria that once were thought to be oral contaminants may be important oral microorganisms in lung ecology (90, 130) and may also represent a potential source of inflammatory response by the host in cystic fibrosis (131).

THE LUNG-GUT AXIS AND ITS ROLE IN DISEASE

The gut is a major reservoir for the microbiome within the human body. Evidence suggests that the gastrointestinal tract plays an important role for the immunological priming of the host. This immunological function is not limited to the gut mucosa or systemic circulation, but there is growing evidence of its relevance to the lung through immunological cross talk between the gut and the lung. Thus, the gastrointestinal tract not only may have direct interaction (e.g., aspiration) with the lower airways but also may serve as an immune-modulating organ with ability to cross talk with other organs, contributing cells related to the innate and adaptive immune systems (dendritic cells and macrophages) and possibly inflammatory cytokines and chemokines in times of disease to the respiratory tract (60, 132, 133).

Microbiome studies of asthma patients have also identified possible lung and gut interactions. The exposure to livestock or canines during youth significantly decreases the risk of developing asthma (134, 135). Until recently, the mechanism that protects the subject from the development of asthma remained elusive. Fujimura and colleagues explored this association with experiments using dust collected from households with canines (25). Mice exposed to dust from canine-inhabited houses exhibited protective responses to allergens. In particular, the mice that received canine household dust had elevated relative abundance of *Lactobacillus johnsonii* in their gastrointestinal tract (25). Oral supplementation of this single species of *Lactobacillus* decreased bronchoresponsiveness to allergens and respiratory syncytial virus challenge. Furthermore, the authors purport that while they were able to detect *L. johnsonii* in cecal samples, they did not detect any in the lung samples, providing evidence that the gastrointestinal microbiome affects the local and systemic inflammatory responses (25).

Cystic fibrosis murine models show that there is an appreciable modulation of the lung microbiome due to changes from the intestinal microbiome in response to antibiotic treatment (136, 137). Bazett and col-

leagues observed that treatment with streptomycin, an antibiotic that is not systemically absorbed from the gut in a murine cystic fibrosis model, was associated with a decrease in pulmonary interleukin-17 (IL-17) and γδ T cells, in contrast to the increase seen when wild-type mice were treated with streptomycin (136). Thus, the gut microbiome also plays an important immune-modulating role in cystic fibrosis (138, 139).

Changes in the gut microbiome have also been associated with pulmonary complications in the setting of allogeneic hematopoietic cell transplantation in humans (140). Domination of the fecal microbiota by *Gammaproteobacteria*, of which *Klebsiella pneumoniae* and *Klebsiella oxytoca* are members, was associated with pulmonary complications and doubling of the risk for mortality (140), suggesting that the gut contributes to the translocation of gut bacteria early in transplantation or is able to contribute to indirect lung injury from microbiota-induced local or systemic inflammatory pathways. The gut microbiome may also attenuate and protect against sepsis (141–143). Eradication of the gastrointestinal microbiota with antibiotics is associated with a dramatic reduction in survival in mice intranasally challenged with a pathogenic strain of *Streptococcus pneumoniae*, as shown in a study in which cytokine production of alveolar macrophages, such as IL-1β, IL-6, and CXCL1, was upregulated while IL-10 and tumor necrosis factor alpha were downregulated (144).

The full extent of gut-lung interactions still requires further clarification. There is clear cross talk between the two organs, and both organs represent large areas of mucosal surfaces that likely share similar immune pathways. Thus, the gut-and-lung interactions expose shortcomings that occur when the immunological effects of the lung or gut microbiome are described in isolation. New evidence is beginning to suggest that the gut-lung axis represents an area of communication and sharing of information between

Host-Microbiota Interaction in the Lung

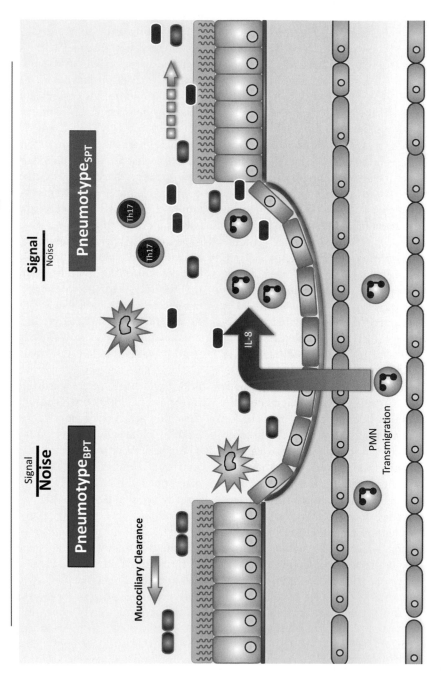

these two organs. The future direction of research is to define and refine these interactions and to take advantage of them to benefit the host.

MICROBIOTA EFFECTS ON THE ACTIVATION OF INFLAMMATORY PATHWAYS OF THE LOWER AIRWAY ENVIRONMENT

The interaction of the host's respiratory system with the environmental and microbiome challenges is an integral component of understanding the role of the upper and lower respiratory microbiomes in health and disease (21, 23, 30). Although examples are currently scant in the pulmonary microbiome literature, several articles have demonstrated the role of the gastrointestinal microbiome in the maturation of the Th17 response in the mucosal immune system (2, 145–147). Within the gastrointestinal literature, there is evidence that the gastrointestinal microbiome plays a significant immune-modulating role in health and disease (2, 146, 147). In particular, the Th17 response on mucosal surfaces is of interest. Ivanov and colleagues demonstrated that segmented filamentous bacilli appear to play a role in the differentiation of Th17 cells in the gastrointestinal tract (2, 147). Furthermore, Suzuki and colleagues demonstrated that in the IgA-deficient mouse model, aberrant and uncontrolled immune responses were associated with the proliferation of segmented filamentous bacilli in these mice (148). In all, the gut microbiome was found to play a necessary role in the maturation of the immune response. However, the lung microbiome may also play a significant role in a mucosa-based immune response.

In the lung mucosa, changes in microbiome in healthy patients are associated with subclinical inflammation (23). In a dichotomized grouping of the lung microbiome, two distinct lung microbiomes (pneumotypes) could be identified: one characterized by enrichment with supraglottic predominant taxa (pneumotype$_{SPT}$) (Fig. 2) and another characterized by enrichment with background predominant taxa (pneumotype$_{BPT}$) (Fig. 2) (23). The degree of similarity with the upper airway microbiome can also be used to characterize the lung microbiome, where lower UniFrac distances (a measurement of dissimilarity based on relative abundance and a phylogenetic tree) occur in BAL samples showing enrichment with supraglottic predominant taxa (pneumotype$_{SPT}$); however, the metabolic activity of these taxa is currently unknown (93, 149). Moreover, the organization of the cohorts into these two pneumotypes (Fig. 2) was supported by contributed phage data (30). The fact that phage data were recovered implies that different phages selected for different taxa in the lungs of our subjects, suggesting that the ecological gradients of the lung may affect the virome as well as the microbiome. The phage data from the cohort also support the existence of an actively replicating phage population; therefore, having an active phage population implies that there also is an actively replicating microbial community (30). Importantly, the lower airway microbiome enriched with oral taxa is associated with a distinct genomic potential and associated with several metabolites of microbial origin.

FIGURE 2 Host-microbiota interaction in the lung. This schema represents the normal lung microbiome and its dysbiosis. In this model, enrichment with background taxa (represented as blue bacteria) in pneumotype$_{BPT}$ occurs in a lung with preserved mucociliary clearance of microorganisms and minimal inflammatory signals within the lung. In the presence of enrichment of the lower airway microbiome with oral taxa (represented as red bacteria) in pneumotype$_{SPT}$, there will be upregulation of the Th17 inflammatory phenotype and recruitment of neutrophils and lymphocytes. PMN, polymorphonuclear leukocyte.

This provides evidence of active microbial metabolism in the lower airways. The host is not merely a bystander in its interaction with the lower respiratory tract microbiome; it can also be affected or benefited by the by-products of bacterial metabolism. A recent investigation has shown that the use of azithromycin in early emphysema promotes the bacterial production of anti-inflammatory metabolites (118), suggesting that some of the anti-inflammatory effects of macrolides might be mediated by their effects on the microbial metabolism in the lower airways.

Further, differences in lung microbiome are associated with a distinct immunological phenotype, demonstrating that the lung microbiome is not a bystander commensal but rather interacts with the host immune system. Specifically, enrichment with supraglottic predominant taxa (pneumotype$_{SPT}$) is associated with the Th17 inflammatory phenotype (Fig. 2). The lower airway microbiome is most likely an active participant in pneumotype$_{SPT}$, and samples that resembled those of the upper respiratory tract were also associated with Th17-chemoattractant cytokines: IL-1α, IL-1β, fractalkine, and IL-7 (30). Furthermore, transcriptome analysis of airway brushes showed that factors important for a Th17 differentiation, such as STAT3 and thymic stromal lymphopoietin, were upregulated in association with pneumotype$_{SPT}$. Given that these microbiome signals were found in both healthy volunteers and those who were exposed to cigarette smoke, enrichment of the lower airways must occur with or without the context of disease (Fig. 2).

Other investigations have also found microbial signatures associated with a Th17 phenotype in severe asthma (29). The mechanism by which this phenotype occurs in the lung is still not clear. Huang and colleagues' study of severe asthmatic patients found that the presence of *Proteobacteria* correlates with Th17-associated gene expression. Members of the *Proteobacteria* taxa include *Pasteurellaceae*, *Enterobacteriaceae*, and *Bacillaceae*. Although both *FKBP5* (a gene

associated with steroid responsiveness in asthma) and genes associated with Th17 inflammation correlated with taxa from the phylum *Proteobacteria*, particular families did not significantly overlap, suggesting that different microorganisms, despite sharing a common phylum, are responsible for different effects on the lower airway (29). Thus, distinct airway microbiotas may promote Th17-associated inflammation but may not be associated with FKBP5-related steroid-induced effects (29). The identification of microorganisms that are associated with Th17 inflammation may represent another pathway of inflammation that is independent of a Th2 and eosinophilic response. The Th17 inflammatory phenotype may represent an important immunomodulatory target in some asthmatics, especially those with a neutrophilic phenotype (29). The Th2 phenotype, however, was not significantly correlated with the microbiome data (29).

Moreover, research by Yadava and colleagues involving an experimental mouse model found that exposure to LPS and elastase leads to a dysbiotic lung microbiome, with an increase of IL-17A expression due to an increase in the γδ$^+$ T cell phenotype (150). This murine inflammatory phenotype is associated with airway abnormalities and emphysematous changes that resembled human COPD. BAL fluids obtained from mice challenged with LPS and elastase demonstrated a decreased α diversity and an increase of relative abundances of *Pseudomonas*, *Lactobacillus*, and *Chryseobacterium* (150). The researchers found that the microbiota enhanced the production of IL-17A by γδ$^+$ T cells by using microbiota-depleted mice. Importantly, researchers recapitulated the upregulated IL-17A immunological phenotype by transfer of enriched microbiotas from LPS- and elastase-treated mice and concurrent challenge with LPS and elastase into antibiotic-treated mice (150). This study demonstrated experimentally that the lung microbiome has a functional role on an immunological phenotype; however, the individual components of this role still need to be clearly elucidated. The use of LPS and elastase in this study raises the question, as does Poroyko and colleagues' study, of whether it is living complex microbial communities or pathogen-associated molecular patterns that are required to induce a Th17 phenotype. Furthermore, LPS may have variable effects depending on the source organism, commonly being *E. coli*, and thus may not be derived from microbes frequently found in the lower airways (106, 150). Given the complexity of the lower airway microbiome, it is likely that other microbial products also play an important role on the host immune phenotype in the lower airways (106, 150).

The presence of the Th17 phenotype and the upregulation of IL-17 have important implications for microbial communities in the lower airway. The lower respiratory tract microbiome, instead of being a nonresponsive passenger, stimulates and attenuates the development of the innate and adaptive immune response. Dysbiosis, here defined by a microbiome that resembles the upper respiratory tract microbiome, is associated with a subclinical proinflammatory phenotype (30). Complex metabolic interactions are present in relationship with this dysbiotic microbiota. Further, there is also evidence of activation of counterregulatory mechanisms being triggered by a distinct lung microbiome. Pulmonary alveolar macrophages collected from subjects who had a lower airway microbiome characterized as pneumotype$_{SPT}$ were associated with a blunted Toll-like receptor 4 response with decreased production of tumor necrosis factor alpha, macrophage-derived chemokine, IL-6, and granulocyte-macrophage colony-stimulating factor in response to LPS stimulation (30). This attenuated innate immune response in this distinct lung microbiome may therefore be an important counterregulatory mechanism present in alveolar macrophages, needed to attenuate the inflammatory immune response in the lung mucosa (3, 30, 145, 147). This is in line with multiple other counter-regulatory mechanisms found in other organ systems, including the gastrointestinal tract (3, 145–147).

The Th17 inflammatory pathway and IL-17 upregulation are not the only pathways that may be upregulated in a host with lung dysbiosis. Richmond and colleagues' study also demonstrated in pIgR-deficient mice that the loss of mucosal immunity resulted in microorganism invasion into the epithelium (95). In contrast, the percentage of bacteria present in the lumen of the airways did not differ between the wild-type mice and pIgR-deficient mice, suggesting that the effects were due to the invasion of microorganisms alone. Mice with pIgR deficiency also demonstrated activation of the NF-κB pathway with associated NF-κB-dependent chemokine keratinocyte chemoattractant in BAL fluid (95). All these results indicate that this mouse model of mucosal immunodeficiency is an example of another pathway that is activated by the interaction between innate microorganisms in the lower airway and represents a target for study.

Metabolites and products of bacterial metabolism will also have immunomodulating properties on the lung microbiome. Chronic inflammation typifies the effects of cystic fibrosis on the pulmonary system. Mechanisms of inflammation revolve around the colonization of typical cystic fibrosis microorganisms but also around the anaerobic metabolism from the facultative anaerobes that make up a smaller portion of the microbiome composition (90). The microorganisms capable of facultative anaerobic metabolism are frequently found in the mouth and have been identified in the lower airway of cystic fibrosis patients. Short-chain fatty acids, a by-product of anaerobic metabolism, have been shown to alter and influence the inflammation in cystic fibrosis (131).

The lung mucosal surface is an important interface with the exterior world, given its roles in the innate and adaptive immune responses that scavenge and respond to microbes and in providing alveolar macrophages that maintain an important function in presenting antigens from opsonized microbes, as well as its ability to regulate signaling cytokines and chemokines (151). The data described above show that there are multiple lines of evidence that support that the lower airway microbiome has an important role in maintaining the immunological tone of the lower airway mucosa. This response may be part of a "healthy" immunological tone required to prime the immune system or may play an important role in the inflammatory process of several inflammatory diseases of the airways.

Microbiome studies have uncovered a complex and diverse microbial community that inhabits within us. With the use of multiomics, we can evaluate the dynamics between the microbes and the host. This new vision of a complex microbial community interacting with the host immune system forces us to reconsider the classical Koch's postulates for our understanding of disease. The great challenge is how to recognize that complex communities of microbes may have a mutualistic and active role in influencing their microenvironment, including the host immune response (152). The effects of communities of microorganisms causing disease represent a challenge to Koch's postulates as they are commonly used, i.e., in positing that a single microbe is the cause of a disease. These postulates have been used to categorize microbes as pathogens (153). In the context of microbial communities interacting with the host and affecting its environment, it is likely that the "pathogenic" role of a microbe and its community will have to be redefined (154, 155). It is then possible that pathogenicity should be viewed in the context of the interaction between the microorganisms and the host, an interface affected by the microorganism's own virulence factors, the associated microbiota, and the host immune response.

Our understanding of many lung diseases is currently limited to association studies, and functional studies have yet to be done in human and mouse models. These different interactions and mechanisms can be further elucidated with the study of the metagenome, metabolomics, metatranscriptomic, metaproteomic, viromics, and other omics studies (22, 23, 30, 155). The use of these approaches will be important to understand how the microbiome communities affect health and disease and to challenge the classical approach to Koch's postulates by addressing the community's role in health and disease as a whole (155).

CONCLUSION

The respiratory mucosa represents a broad and encompassing border between the human host and the environment. The differences between the gastrointestinal tract and the respiratory tract, such as the concentration of microbes, length of organ, ease of sampling, and physiological parameters, represent challenging nuances in the study of the lung microbiome. Attention has shifted from understanding the ecological composition of the respiratory tract microbiome to several key issues, including the colonization and persistence of particular communities of microbes, inflammatory pathways that are upregulated and downregulated in the presence of particular communities, and the functional and mechanistic causes of these inflammatory pathways (23, 30).

The lungs see multiple microbial challenges through different mechanisms such as aerodigestive reflux and microaspiration during the course of the day and night (38). These repetitive microbial challenges may play an important role in the host immune response (23, 30, 156). The effects on the host immunological tone may represent beneficial immunological priming or contribute to a pathogenic immunological process relevant for disease development.

Future directions in the study of the lower respiratory lung microbiome will require focus on dissecting the microbial community function, understanding microbe-microbe interactions, and developing experimental models to uncover causality. Ultimately, the goal is to find potential microbial targets for a more precise manipulation of the lower airway microbiota, such as refined use of antibiotics, phage therapy, or molecules that target specific microbial metabolic pathways, in order to alter the natural course of pulmonary disease processes.

ACKNOWLEDGMENTS

Research support funding was provided by K23 AI102970 (NIH/NIAID), the Flight Attendant Medical Research Institute (FAMRI), a Stony Wold-Herbert Fund Fellowship Award, and 1UL1TR001445 (NIH/NCATS).

CITATION

Wu BG, Segal LN. 2017. Lung microbiota and its impact on the mucosal immune phenotype. Microbiol Spectrum 5(3):BAD-0005-2016.

REFERENCES

1. **Turnbaugh PJ, Ley RE, Hamady M, Fraser-Liggett CM, Knight R, Gordon JI.** 2007. The human microbiome project. *Nature* **449:** 804–810.

2. **Ivanov II, Frutos RL, Manel N, Yoshinaga K, Rifkin DB, Sartor RB, Finlay BB, Littman DR.** 2008. Specific microbiota direct the differentiation of IL-17-producing T-helper cells in the mucosa of the small intestine. *Cell Host Microbe* **4:**337–349.

3. **Atarashi K, Tanoue T, Shima T, Imaoka A, Kuwahara T, Momose Y, Cheng G, Yamasaki S, Saito T, Ohba Y, Taniguchi T, Takeda K, Hori S, Ivanov II, Umesaki Y, Itoh K, Honda K.** 2011. Induction of colonic regulatory T cells by indigenous *Clostridium* species. *Science* **331:** 337–341.

4. **Wright EK, Kamm MA, Teo SM, Inouye M, Wagner J, Kirkwood CD.** 2015. Recent advances in characterizing the gastrointestinal microbiome in Crohn's disease: a systematic review. *Inflamm Bowel Dis* **21:**1219–1228.

5. **Bäckhed F, Ding H, Wang T, Hooper LV, Koh GY, Nagy A, Semenkovich CF, Gordon JI.** 2004. The gut microbiota as an environmental factor that regulates fat storage. *Proc Natl Acad Sci USA* **101:**15718–15723.

6. **Kau AL, Ahern PP, Griffin NW, Goodman AL, Gordon JI.** 2011. Human nutrition, the gut microbiome and the immune system. *Nature* **474:**327–336.

7. **Turnbaugh PJ, Gordon JI.** 2009. The core gut microbiome, energy balance and obesity. *J Physiol* **587:**4153–4158.

8. **Turnbaugh PJ, Hamady M, Yatsunenko T, Cantarel BL, Duncan A, Ley RE, Sogin ML, Jones WJ, Roe BA, Affourtit JP, Egholm M, Henrissat B, Heath AC, Knight R, Gordon JI.** 2009. A core gut microbiome in obese and lean twins. *Nature* **457:**480–484.

9. **Koeth RA, Wang Z, Levison BS, Buffa JA, Org E, Sheehy BT, Britt EB, Fu X, Wu Y, Li L, Smith JD, DiDonato JA, Chen J, Li H, Wu GD, Lewis JD, Warrier M, Brown JM, Krauss RM, Tang WH, Bushman FD, Lusis AJ, Hazen SL.** 2013. Intestinal microbiota metabolism of L-carnitine, a nutrient in red meat, promotes atherosclerosis. *Nat Med* **19:**576–585.

10. **Tang WH, Wang Z, Levison BS, Koeth RA, Britt EB, Fu X, Wu Y, Hazen SL.** 2013. Intestinal microbial metabolism of phosphatidylcholine and cardiovascular risk. *N Engl J Med* **368:** 1575–1584.

11. **Tang WH, Wang Z, Shrestha K, Borowski AG, Wu Y, Troughton RW, Klein AL, Hazen SL.** 2015. Intestinal microbiota-dependent phosphatidylcholine metabolites, diastolic dysfunction, and adverse clinical outcomes in chronic systolic heart failure. *J Card Fail* **21:**91–96.

12. **Wang Z, Klipfell E, Bennett BJ, Koeth R, Levison BS, Dugar B, Feldstein AE, Britt EB, Fu X, Chung YM, Wu Y, Schauer P, Smith JD, Allayee H, Tang WH, DiDonato JA, Lusis AJ, Hazen SL.** 2011. Gut flora metabolism of phosphatidylcholine promotes cardiovascular disease. *Nature* **472:**57–63.

13. **Chang JY, Antonopoulos DA, Kalra A, Tonelli A, Khalife WT, Schmidt TM, Young VB.** 2008. Decreased diversity of the fecal microbiome in recurrent *Clostridium difficile*-associated diarrhea. *J Infect Dis* **197:**435–438.

14. **Lawley TD, Clare S, Walker AW, Stares MD, Connor TR, Raisen C, Goulding D, Rad R, Schreiber F, Brandt C, Deakin LJ, Pickard DJ, Duncan SH, Flint HJ, Clark TG, Parkhill J, Dougan G.** 2012. Targeted restoration of the intestinal microbiota with a simple, defined bacteriotherapy resolves relapsing *Clostridium difficile* disease in mice. *PLoS Pathog* **8:**e1002995.

15. **Qin J, et al.** 2012. A metagenome-wide association study of gut microbiota in type 2 diabetes. *Nature* **490:**55–60.

16. **Forslund K, Hildebrand F, Nielsen T, Falony G, Le Chatelier E, Sunagawa S, Prifti E, Vieira-Silva S, Gudmundsdottir V, Krogh Pedersen H, Arumugam M, Kristiansen K, Voigt AY, Vestergaard H, Hercog R, Igor Costea P, Kultima JR, Li J, Jørgensen T, Levenez F, Dore J, MetaHIT Consortium, Nielsen HB, Brunak S, Raes J, Hansen T, Wang J, Ehrlich SD, Bork P, Pedersen O.** 2015. Disentangling type 2 diabetes and metformin treatment signatures in the human gut microbiota. *Nature* **528:**262–266.

17. **Manichanh C, Rigottier-Gois L, Bonnaud E, Gloux K, Pelletier E, Frangeul L, Nalin R, Jarrin C, Chardon P, Marteau P, Roca J, Dore J.** 2006. Reduced diversity of faecal microbiota in Crohn's disease revealed by a metagenomic approach. *Gut* **55:**205–211.

18. **Morgan XC, Kabakchiev B, Waldron L, Tyler AD, Tickle TL, Milgrom R, Stempak JM, Gevers D, Xavier RJ, Silverberg MS, Huttenhower C.** 2015. Associations between host gene expression, the mucosal microbiome, and clinical outcome in the pelvic pouch of patients with inflammatory bowel disease. *Genome Biol* **16:**67.

19. **Metzker ML.** 2010. Sequencing technologies —the next generation. *Nat Rev Genet* **11:**31–46.

20. **Wu J, Peters BA, Dominianni C, Zhang Y, Pei Z, Yang L, Ma Y, Purdue MP, Jacobs EJ, Gapstur SM, Li H, Alekseyenko AV, Hayes RB, Ahn J.** 2016. Cigarette smoking and the oral microbiome in a large study of American adults. *ISME J* **10:**2435–2446.

21. **Segal LN, Rom WN, Weiden MD.** 2014. Lung microbiome for clinicians. New discoveries about bugs in healthy and diseased lungs. *Ann Am Thorac Soc* **11:**108–116.

22. **Segal LN, Blaser MJ.** 2014. A brave new world: the lung microbiota in an era of change. *Ann Am Thorac Soc* **11**(Suppl 1)**:**S21–S27.

23. **Segal LN, Alekseyenko AV, Clemente JC, Kulkarni R, Wu B, Gao Z, Chen H, Berger KI, Goldring RM, Rom WN, Blaser MJ, Weiden MD.** 2013. Enrichment of lung microbiome with supraglottic taxa is associated with increased pulmonary inflammation. *Microbiome* **1:**19.

24. **Dickson RP, Erb-Downward JR, Martinez FJ, Huffnagle GB.** 2016. The microbiome and the respiratory tract. *Annu Rev Physiol* **78:**481–504.

25. **Fujimura KE, Demoor T, Rauch M, Faruqi AA, Jang S, Johnson CC, Boushey HA, Zoratti E, Ownby D, Lukacs NW, Lynch SV.** 2014. House dust exposure mediates gut microbiome *Lactobacillus* enrichment and airway immune defense against allergens and virus infection. *Proc Natl Acad Sci USA* **111:**805–810.

26. **Noverr MC, Falkowski NR, McDonald RA, McKenzie AN, Huffnagle GB.** 2005. Development of allergic airway disease in mice following antibiotic therapy and fungal microbiota increase: role of host genetics, antigen, and interleukin-13. *Infect Immun* **73:**30–38.

27. **Noverr MC, Noggle RM, Toews GB, Huffnagle GB.** 2004. Role of antibiotics and fungal microbiota in driving pulmonary allergic responses. *Infect Immun* **72:**4996–5003.

28. **Sze MA, Dimitriu PA, Suzuki M, McDonough JE, Campbell JD, Brothers JF, Erb-Downward JR, Huffnagle GB, Hayashi S, Elliott WM, Cooper J, Sin DD, Lenburg ME, Spira A, Mohn WW, Hogg JC.** 2015. Host response to the lung microbiome in chronic obstructive pulmonary disease. *Am J Respir Crit Care Med* **192:**438–445.

29. **Huang YJ, Nariya S, Harris JM, Lynch SV, Choy DF, Arron JR, Boushey H.** 2015. The airway microbiome in patients with severe asthma: associations with disease features and severity. *J Allergy Clin Immunol* **136:**874–884.

30. **Segal LN, Clemente JC, Tsay JCJ, Koralov SB, Keller BC, Wu BG, Li Y, Shen N, Ghedin E, Morris A, Diaz P, Huang L, Wikoff WR, Ubeda C, Artacho A, Rom WN, Sterman DH, Collman RG, Blaser MJ, Weiden MD.** 2016. Enrichment of the lung microbiome with oral taxa is associated with lung inflammation of a Th17 phenotype. *Nat Microbiol* **1:**16031.

31. **Twigg HL III, Morris A, Ghedin E, Curtis JL, Huffnagle GB, Crothers K, Campbell TB, Flores SC, Fontenot AP, Beck JM, Huang L, Lynch S, Knox KS, Weinstock G, Lung HIV Microbiome Project.** 2013. Use of bronchoalveolar lavage to assess the respiratory microbiome: signal in the noise. *Lancet Respir Med* **1:**354–356.

32. **Charlson ES, Bittinger K, Haas AR, Fitzgerald AS, Frank I, Yadav A, Bushman FD, Collman RG.** 2011. Topographical continuity of bacterial populations in the healthy human respiratory tract. *Am J Respir Crit Care Med* **184:**957–963.

33. **Buffie CG, Bucci V, Stein RR, McKenney PT, Ling L, Gobourne A, No D, Liu H, Kinnebrew M, Viale A, Littmann E, van den Brink MR, Jenq RR, Taur Y, Sander C, Cross JR, Toussaint NC, Xavier JB, Pamer EG.** 2015. Precision microbiome reconstitution restores bile acid mediated resistance to *Clostridium difficile*. *Nature* **517:**205–208.

34. **Charlson ES, Bittinger K, Chen J, Diamond JM, Li H, Collman RG, Bushman FD.** 2012. Assessing bacterial populations in the lung by replicate analysis of samples from the upper and lower respiratory tracts. *PLoS One* **7:**e42786.

35. **Charlson ES, Chen J, Custers-Allen R, Bittinger K, Li H, Sinha R, Hwang J, Bushman FD, Collman RG.** 2010. Disordered microbial

communities in the upper respiratory tract of cigarette smokers. *PLoS One* **5:**e15216.

36. **Shaker R, Hogan WJ.** 2000. Reflex-mediated enhancement of airway protective mechanisms. *Am J Med* **108**(Suppl 4a):8S–14S.

37. **Kronenberger MB, Meyers AD.** 1994. Dysphagia following head and neck cancer surgery. *Dysphagia* **9:**236–244.

38. **Bassis CM, Erb-Downward JR, Dickson RP, Freeman CM, Schmidt TM, Young VB, Beck JM, Curtis JL, Huffnagle GB.** 2015. Analysis of the upper respiratory tract microbiotas as the source of the lung and gastric microbiotas in healthy individuals. *MBio* **6:**e00037.

39. **Gleeson K, Eggli DF, Maxwell SL.** 1997. Quantitative aspiration during sleep in normal subjects. *Chest* **111:**1266–1272.

40. **Cvejic L, Harding R, Churchward T, Turton A, Finlay P, Massey D, Bardin PG, Guy P.** 2011. Laryngeal penetration and aspiration in individuals with stable COPD. *Respirology* **16:**269–275.

41. **Morse CA, Quan SF, Mays MZ, Green C, Stephen G, Fass R.** 2004. Is there a relationship between obstructive sleep apnea and gastroesophageal reflux disease? *Clin Gastroenterol Hepatol* **2:**761–768.

42. **Teramoto S, Ohga E, Matsui H, Ishii T, Matsuse T, Ouchi Y.** 1999. Obstructive sleep apnea syndrome may be a significant cause of gastroesophageal reflux disease in older people. *J Am Geriatr Soc* **47:**1273–1274.

43. **Field SK, Underwood M, Brant R, Cowie RL.** 1996. Prevalence of gastroesophageal reflux symptoms in asthma. *Chest* **109:**316–322.

44. **Scott RB, O'Loughlin EV, Gall DG.** 1985. Gastroesophageal reflux in patients with cystic fibrosis. *J Pediatr* **106:**223–227.

45. **Koh WJ, Lee JH, Kwon YS, Lee KS, Suh GY, Chung MP, Kim H, Kwon OJ.** 2007. Prevalence of gastroesophageal reflux disease in patients with nontuberculous mycobacterial lung disease. *Chest* **131:**1825–1830.

46. **Dickson RP, Erb-Downward JR, Prescott HC, Martinez FJ, Curtis JL, Lama VN, Huffnagle GB.** 2014. Cell-associated bacteria in the human lung microbiome. *Microbiome* **2:**28.

47. **Beck JM, Schloss PD, Venkataraman A, Twigg H III, Jablonski KA, Bushman FD, Campbell TB, Charlson ES, Collman RG, Crothers K, Curtis JL, Drews KL, Flores SC, Fontenot AP, Foulkes MA, Frank I, Ghedin E, Huang L, Lynch SV, Morris A, Palmer BE, Schmidt TM, Sodergren E, Weinstock GM, Young VB, Lung HIV Microbiome Project.** 2015. Multicenter comparison of lung and oral microbiomes of HIV-infected and HIV-uninfected individuals. *Am J Respir Crit Care Med* **192:**1335–1344.

48. **Segal LN, Dickson RP.** 2016. The lung microbiome in HIV. Getting to the HAART of the host-microbe interface. *Am J Respir Crit Care Med* **194:**136–137.

49. **Huxley EJ, Viroslav J, Gray WR, Pierce AK.** 1978. Pharyngeal aspiration in normal adults and patients with depressed consciousness. *Am J Med* **64:**564–568.

50. **Simpson JL, Daly J, Baines KJ, Yang IA, Upham JW, Reynolds PN, Hodge S, James AL, Hugenholtz P, Willner D, Gibson PG.** 2016. Airway dysbiosis: *Haemophilus influenzae* and *Tropheryma* in poorly controlled asthma. *Eur Respir J* **47:**792–800.

51. **Smits HH, Hiemstra PS, Prazeres da Costa C, Ege M, Edwards M, Garn H, Howarth PH, Jartti T, de Jong EC, Maizels RM, Marsland BJ, McSorley HJ, Müller A, Pfefferle PI, Savelkoul H, Schwarze J, Unger WW, von Mutius E, Yazdanbakhsh M, Taube C.** 2016. Microbes and asthma: opportunities for intervention. *J Allergy Clin Immunol* **137:**690–697.

52. **Huang YJ.** 2015. The respiratory microbiome and innate immunity in asthma. *Curr Opin Pulm Med* **21:**27–32.

53. **Huang YJ.** 2013. Asthma microbiome studies and the potential for new therapeutic strategies. *Curr Allergy Asthma Rep* **13:**453–461.

54. **Huang YJ, Boushey HA.** 2015. The microbiome in asthma. *J Allergy Clin Immunol* **135:** 25–30.

55. **Huang YJ, Boushey HA.** 2014. The microbiome and asthma. *Ann Am Thorac Soc* **11** (Suppl 1):S48–S51.

56. **Huang YJ, Boushey HA.** 2013. The bronchial microbiome and asthma phenotypes. *Am J Respir Crit Care Med* **188:**1178–1180.

57. **Huang YJ, Charlson ES, Collman RG, Colombini-Hatch S, Martinez FD, Senior RM.** 2013. The role of the lung microbiome in health and disease. A National Heart, Lung, and Blood Institute workshop report. *Am J Respir Crit Care Med* **187:**1382–1387.

58. **Hilty M, Burke C, Pedro H, Cardenas P, Bush A, Bossley C, Davies J, Ervine A, Poulter L, Pachter L, Moffatt MF, Cookson WO.** 2010. Disordered microbial communities in asthmatic airways. *PLoS One* **5:**e8578.

59. **Lynch SV, Bruce KD.** 2013. The cystic fibrosis airway microbiome. *Cold Spring Harb Perspect Med* **3:**a009738.

60. **Huang YJ, LiPuma JJ.** 2016. The microbiome in cystic fibrosis. *Clin Chest Med* **37:**59–67.

61. **Whelan FJ, Surette MG.** 2015. Clinical insights into pulmonary exacerbations in cystic fibrosis from the microbiome. What are we missing? *Ann Am Thorac Soc* **12**(Suppl 2):S207–S211.

62. **Caverly LJ, Zhao J, LiPuma JJ.** 2015. Cystic fibrosis lung microbiome: opportunities to reconsider management of airway infection. *Pediatr Pulmonol* **50**(Suppl 40):S31–S38.

63. **Twigg HL III, Knox KS, Zhou J, Crothers KA, Nelson DE, Toh E, Day RB, Lin H, Gao X, Dong Q, Mi D, Katz BP, Sodergren E, Weinstock GM.** 2016. Effect of advanced HIV infection on the respiratory microbiome. *Am J Respir Crit Care Med* **194**:226–235.

64. **Lozupone C, Cota-Gomez A, Palmer BE, Linderman DJ, Charlson ES, Sodergren E, Mitreva M, Abubucker S, Martin J, Yao G, Campbell TB, Flores SC, Ackerman G, Stombaugh J, Ursell L, Beck JM, Curtis JL, Young VB, Lynch SV, Huang L, Weinstock GM, Knox KS, Twigg H, Morris A, Ghedin E, Bushman FD, Collman RG, Knight R, Fontenot AP, Lung HIV Microbiome Project.** 2013. Widespread colonization of the lung by *Tropheryma whipplei* in HIV infection. *Am J Respir Crit Care Med* **187**:1110–1117.

65. **Sze MA, Dimitriu PA, Hayashi S, Elliott WM, McDonough JE, Gosselink JV, Cooper J, Sin DD, Mohn WW, Hogg JC.** 2012. The lung tissue microbiome in chronic obstructive pulmonary disease. *Am J Respir Crit Care Med* **185**:1073–1080.

66. **Sze MA, Hogg JC, Sin DD.** 2014. Bacterial microbiome of lungs in COPD. *Int J Chron Obstruct Pulmon Dis* **9**:229–238.

67. **Salter SJ, Cox MJ, Turek EM, Calus ST, Cookson WO, Moffatt MF, Turner P, Parkhill J, Loman NJ, Walker AW.** 2014. Reagent and laboratory contamination can critically impact sequence-based microbiome analyses. *BMC Biol* **12**:87.

68. **Venkataraman A, Bassis CM, Beck JM, Young VB, Curtis JL, Huffnagle GB, Schmidt TM.** 2015. Application of a neutral community model to assess structuring of the human lung microbiome. *mBio* **6**:e02284-14.

69. **Knights D, Kuczynski J, Charlson ES, Zaneveld J, Mozer MC, Collman RG, Bushman FD, Knight R, Kelley ST.** 2011. Bayesian community-wide culture-independent microbial source tracking. *Nat Methods* **8**:761–763.

70. **Hajishengallis G, Liang S, Payne MA, Hashim A, Jotwani R, Eskan MA, McIntosh ML, Alsam A, Kirkwood KL, Lambris JD, Darveau RP, Curtis MA.** 2011. Low-abundance biofilm species orchestrates inflammatory periodontal disease through the commensal microbiota and complement. *Cell Host Microbe* **10**:497–506.

71. **Pop M, Paulson JN, Chakraborty S, Astrovskaya I, Lindsay BR, Li S, Bravo HC, Harro C, Parkhill J, Walker AW, Walker RI,** Sack DA, Stine OC. 2016. Individual-specific changes in the human gut microbiota after challenge with enterotoxigenic *Escherichia coli* and subsequent ciprofloxacin treatment. *BMC Genomics* **17**:440.

72. **Schwartz DA, Quinn TJ, Thorne PS, Sayeed S, Yi AK, Krieg AM.** 1997. CpG motifs in bacterial DNA cause inflammation in the lower respiratory tract. *J Clin Invest* **100**:68–73.

73. **Riley RL.** 1957. Aerial dissemination of pulmonary tuberculosis. *Am Rev Tuberc* **76**:931–941.

74. **Riley RL, Mills CC, O'Grady F, Sultan LU, Wittstadt F, Shivpuri DN.** 1962. Infectiousness of air from a tuberculosis ward. Ultraviolet irradiation of infected air: comparative infectiousness of different patients. *Am Rev Respir Dis* **85**:511–525.

75. **Adams RI, Bateman AC, Bik HM, Meadow JF.** 2015. Microbiota of the indoor environment: a meta-analysis. *Microbiome* **3**:49.

76. **Meadow JF, Altrichter AE, Bateman AC, Stenson J, Brown GZ, Green JL, Bohannan BJ.** 2015. Humans differ in their personal microbial cloud. *PeerJ* **3**:e1258.

77. **Stephenson MF, Mfuna L, Dowd SE, Wolcott RD, Barbeau J, Poisson M, James G, Desrosiers M.** 2010. Molecular characterization of the polymicrobial flora in chronic rhinosinusitis. *J Otolaryngol Head Neck Surg* **39**:182–187.

78. **Boase S, Foreman A, Cleland E, Tan L, Melton-Kreft R, Pant H, Hu FZ, Ehrlich GD, Wormald PJ.** 2013. The microbiome of chronic rhinosinusitis: culture, molecular diagnostics and biofilm detection. *BMC Infect Dis* **13**:210.

79. **Blaser MJ, Chen Y, Reibman J.** 2008. Does *Helicobacter pylori* protect against asthma and allergy? *Gut* **57**:561–567.

80. **Reibman J, Marmor M, Filner J, Fernandez-Beros ME, Rogers L, Perez-Perez GI, Blaser MJ.** 2008. Asthma is inversely associated with *Helicobacter pylori* status in an urban population. *PLoS One* **3**:e4060.

81. **Rosen R, Hu L, Amirault J, Khatwa U, Ward DV, Onderdonk A.** 2015. 16S community profiling identifies proton pump inhibitor related differences in gastric, lung, and oropharyngeal microflora. *J Pediatr* **166**:917–923.

82. **Souza DG, Vieira AT, Soares AC, Pinho V, Nicoli JR, Vieira LQ, Teixeira MM.** 2004. The essential role of the intestinal microbiota in facilitating acute inflammatory responses. *J Immunol* **173**:4137–4146.

83. **Silvestri L, van Saene HK, Zandstra DF, Marshall JC, Gregori D, Gullo A.** 2010. Impact of selective decontamination of the digestive

tract on multiple organ dysfunction syndrome: systematic review of randomized controlled trials. *Crit Care Med* 38:1370–1376.

84. **Erb-Downward JR, Thompson DL, Han MK, Freeman CM, McCloskey L, Schmidt LA, Young VB, Toews GB, Curtis JL, Sundaram B, Martinez FJ, Huffnagle GB.** 2011. Analysis of the lung microbiome in the "healthy" smoker and in COPD. *PLoS One* 6:e16384.

85. **Morris A, Beck JM, Schloss PD, Campbell TB, Crothers K, Curtis JL, Flores SC, Fontenot AP, Ghedin E, Huang L, Jablonski K, Kleerup E, Lynch SV, Sodergren E, Twigg H, Young VB, Bassis CM, Venkataraman A, Schmidt TM, Weinstock GM, Lung HIV Microbiome Project.** 2013. Comparison of the respiratory microbiome in healthy non-smokers and smokers. *Am J Respir Crit Care Med* 187:1067–1075.

86. **Lomolino MV, Brown JH.** 2009. The reticulating phylogeny of island biogeography theory. *Q Rev Biol* 84:357–390.

87. **Dickson RP, Erb-Downward JR, Freeman CM, McCloskey L, Beck JM, Huffnagle GB, Curtis JL.** 2015. Spatial variation in the healthy human lung microbiome and the adapted island model of lung biogeography. *Ann Am Thorac Soc* 12:821–830.

88. **Dickson RP, Erb-Downward JR, Huffnagle GB.** 2014. Towards an ecology of the lung: new conceptual models of pulmonary microbiology and pneumonia pathogenesis. *Lancet Respir Med* 2:238–246.

89. **Dickson RP, Martinez FJ, Huffnagle GB.** 2014. The role of the microbiome in exacerbations of chronic lung diseases. *Lancet* 384:691–702.

90. **Whiteson KL, Bailey B, Bergkessel M, Conrad D, Delhaes L, Felts B, Harris JK, Hunter R, Lim YW, Maughan H, Quinn R, Salamon P, Sullivan J, Wagner BD, Rainey PB.** 2014. The upper respiratory tract as a microbial source for pulmonary infections in cystic fibrosis. Parallels from island biogeography. *Am J Respir Crit Care Med* 189:1309–1315.

91. **Veldhuizen R, Nag K, Orgeig S, Possmayer F.** 1998. The role of lipids in pulmonary surfactant. *Biochim Biophys Acta* 1408:90–108.

92. **West JB.** 2012. *Respiratory Physiology: The Essentials*, 9th ed. Wolters Kluwer Health/Lippincott Williams & Wilkins, Philadelphia, PA.

93. **Lieberman TD, Flett KB, Yelin I, Martin TR, McAdam AJ, Priebe GP, Kishony R.** 2014. Genetic variation of a bacterial pathogen within individuals with cystic fibrosis provides a record of selective pressures. *Nat Genet* 46:82–87.

94. **Rogan MP, Geraghty P, Greene CM, O'Neill SJ, Taggart CC, McElvaney NG.** 2006. Antimicrobial proteins and polypeptides in pulmonary innate defence. *Respir Res* 7:29.

95. **Richmond BW, Brucker RM, Han W, Du RH, Zhang Y, Cheng DS, Gleaves L, Abdolrasulnia R, Polosukhina D, Clark PE, Bordenstein SR, Blackwell TS, Polosukhin VV.** 2016. Airway bacteria drive a progressive COPD-like phenotype in mice with polymeric immunoglobulin receptor deficiency. *Nat Commun* 7:11240.

96. **Costerton JW, Lewandowski Z, DeBeer D, Caldwell D, Korber D, James G.** 1994. Biofilms, the customized microniche. *J Bacteriol* 176:2137–2142.

97. **Whitchurch CB, Tolker-Nielsen T, Ragas PC, Mattick JS.** 2002. Extracellular DNA required for bacterial biofilm formation. *Science* 295:1487.

98. **Costerton JW, Stewart PS, Greenberg EP.** 1999. Bacterial biofilms: a common cause of persistent infections. *Science* 284:1318–1322.

99. **Twigg HL III.** 1998. Pulmonary host defenses. *J Thorac Imaging* 13:221–233.

100. **Renshaw SA, Parmar JS, Singleton V, Rowe SJ, Dockrell DH, Dower SK, Bingle CD, Chilvers ER, Whyte MK.** 2003. Acceleration of human neutrophil apoptosis by TRAIL. *J Immunol* 170:1027–1033.

101. **Chmiel JF, Davis PB.** 2003. State of the art: why do the lungs of patients with cystic fibrosis become infected and why can't they clear the infection? *Respir Res* 4:8.

102. **Klemm P, Schembri MA.** 2000. Bacterial adhesins: function and structure. *Int J Med Microbiol* 290:27–35.

103. **Deslée G, Mal H, Dutau H, Bourdin A, Vergnon JM, Pison C, Kessler R, Jounieaux V, Thiberville L, Leroy S, Marceau A, Laroumagne S, Mallet JP, Dukic S, Barbe C, Bulsei J, Jolly D, Durand-Zaleski I, Marquette CH, REVOLENS Study Group.** 2016. Lung volume reduction coil treatment vs usual care in patients with severe emphysema: the REVOLENS randomized clinical trial. *JAMA* 315:175–184.

104. **Oliver A, Cantón R, Campo P, Baquero F, Blázquez J.** 2000. High frequency of hypermutable *Pseudomonas aeruginosa* in cystic fibrosis lung infection. *Science* 288:1251–1254.

105. **Rello J, Ausina V, Ricart M, Castella J, Prats G.** 1993. Impact of previous antimicrobial therapy on the etiology and outcome of ventilator-associated pneumonia. *Chest* 104:1230–1235.

106. **Poroyko V, Meng F, Meliton A, Afonyushkin T, Ulanov A, Semenyuk E, Latif O, Tesic V, Birukova AA, Birukov KG.** 2015. Alterations of lung microbiota in a mouse model of LPS-

induced lung injury. *Am J Physiol Lung Cell Mol Physiol* **309**:L76–L83.

107. **Dickson RP, Erb-Downward JR, Huffnagle GB.** 2015. Homeostasis and its disruption in the lung microbiome. *Am J Physiol Lung Cell Mol Physiol* **309**:L1047–L1055.

108. **Molyneaux PL, Mallia P, Cox MJ, Footitt J, Willis-Owen SA, Homola D, Trujillo-Torralbo MB, Elkin S, Kon OM, Cookson WO, Moffatt MF, Johnston SL.** 2013. Outgrowth of the bacterial airway microbiome after rhinovirus exacerbation of chronic obstructive pulmonary disease. *Am J Respir Crit Care Med* **188**:1224–1231.

109. **Twigg H, Knox KS, Zhou J, Crothers K, Nelson D, Toh E, Day RB, Lin H, Gao X, Dong Q, Mi D, Katz BP, Sodergren E, Weinstock G.** 2016. Effect of advanced HIV infection on the respiratory microbiome. *Am J Respir Crit Care Med* **194**:226–235.

110. **Cui L, Lucht L, Tipton L, Rogers MB, Fitch A, Kessinger C, Camp D, Kingsley L, Leo N, Greenblatt RM, Fong S, Stone S, Dermand JC, Kleerup EC, Huang L, Morris A, Ghedin E.** 2015. Topographic diversity of the respiratory tract mycobiome and alteration in HIV and lung disease. *Am J Respir Crit Care Med* **191**:932–942.

111. **Gohy ST, Detry BR, Lecocq M, Bouzin C, Weynand BA, Amatngalim GD, Sibille YM, Pilette C.** 2014. Polymeric immunoglobulin receptor down-regulation in chronic obstructive pulmonary disease. Persistence in the cultured epithelium and role of transforming growth factor-β. *Am J Respir Crit Care Med* **190**:509–521.

112. **Polosukhin VV, Cates JM, Lawson WE, Zaynagetdinov R, Milstone AP, Massion PP, Ocak S, Ware LB, Lee JW, Bowler RP, Kononov AV, Randell SH, Blackwell TS.** 2011. Bronchial secretory immunoglobulin a deficiency correlates with airway inflammation and progression of chronic obstructive pulmonary disease. *Am J Respir Crit Care Med* **184**:317–327.

113. **Corbett AJ, Eckle SB, Birkinshaw RW, Liu L, Patel O, Mahony J, Chen Z, Reantragoon R, Meehan B, Cao H, Williamson NA, Strugnell RA, Van Sinderen D, Mak JY, Fairlie DP, Kjer-Nielsen L, Rossjohn J, McCluskey J.** 2014. T-cell activation by transitory neo-antigens derived from distinct microbial pathways. *Nature* **509**:361–365.

114. **Gapin L.** 2014. Check MAIT. *J Immunol* **192**:4475–4480.

115. **Hinks TS, Wallington JC, Williams AP, Djukanovič R, Staples KJ, Wilkinson TM.** 2016. Steroid-induced deficiency of mucosal-associated invariant T cells in the COPD lung: implications for NTHi infection. *Am J Respir Crit Care Med* **194**:1208–1218.

116. **Pragman AA, Kim HB, Reilly CS, Wendt C, Isaacson RE.** 2012. The lung microbiome in moderate and severe chronic obstructive pulmonary disease. *PLoS One* **7**:e47305.

117. **Huang YJ, Kim E, Cox MJ, Brodie EL, Brown R, Wiener-Kronish JP, Lynch SV.** 2010. A persistent and diverse airway microbiota present during chronic obstructive pulmonary disease exacerbations. *OMICS* **14**:9–59.

118. **Segal LN, Clemente JC, Wu BG, Wikoff WR, Gao Z, Li Y, Ko JP, Rom WN, Blaser MJ, Weiden MD.** 2016. Randomised, double-blind, placebo-controlled trial with azithromycin selects for anti-inflammatory microbial metabolites in the emphysematous lung. *Thorax* **72**:13–22. 10.1136/thoraxjnl-2016-208599.

119. **Huang YJ, Nelson CE, Brodie EL, Desantis TZ, Baek MS, Liu J, Woyke T, Allgaier M, Bristow J, Wiener-Kronish JP, Sutherland ER, King TS, Icitovic N, Martin RJ, Calhoun WJ, Castro M, Denlinger LC, Dimango E, Kraft M, Peters SP, Wasserman SI, Wechsler ME, Boushey HA, Lynch SV, National Heart, Lung, and Blood Institute's Asthma Clinical Research Network.** 2011. Airway microbiota and bronchial hyperresponsiveness in patients with suboptimally controlled asthma. *J Allergy Clin Immunol* **127**:372–381.e1-3.

120. **Fujimura KE, Johnson CC, Ownby DR, Cox MJ, Brodie EL, Havstad SL, Zoratti EM, Woodcroft KJ, Bobbitt KR, Wegienka G, Boushey HA, Lynch SV.** 2010. Man's best friend? The effect of pet ownership on house dust microbial communities. *J Allergy Clin Immunol* **126**:410–412.e1-3.

121. **Ege MJ, Mayer M, Normand AC, Genuneit J, Cookson WO, Braun-Fahrländer C, Heederik D, Piarroux R, von Mutius E, GABRIELA Transregio 22 Study Group.** 2011. Exposure to environmental microorganisms and childhood asthma. *N Engl J Med* **364**:701–709.

122. **Bisgaard H, Hermansen MN, Buchvald F, Loland L, Halkjaer LB, Bønnelykke K, Brasholt M, Heltberg A, Vissing NH, Thorsen SV, Stage M, Pipper CB.** 2007. Childhood asthma after bacterial colonization of the airway in neonates. *N Engl J Med* **357**:1487–1495.

123. **Huang EY, Inoue T, Leone VA, Dalal S, Touw K, Wang Y, Musch MW, Theriault B, Higuchi K, Donovan S, Gilbert J, Chang EB.** 2015. Using corticosteroids to reshape the gut microbiome: implications for inflammatory bowel diseases. *Inflamm Bowel Dis* **21**:963–972.

124. **Gilligan PH.** 2014. Infections in patients with cystic fibrosis: diagnostic microbiology update. *Clin Lab Med* **34:**197–217.

125. **Dasenbrook EC, Checkley W, Merlo CA, Konstan MW, Lechtzin N, Boyle MP.** 2010. Association between respiratory tract methicillin-resistant *Staphylococcus aureus* and survival in cystic fibrosis. *JAMA* **303:**2386–2392.

126. **Martiniano SL, Nick JA.** 2015. Nontuberculous mycobacterial infections in cystic fibrosis. *Clin Chest Med* **36:**101–115.

127. **van der Gast CJ, Walker AW, Stressmann FA, Rogers GB, Scott P, Daniels TW, Carroll MP, Parkhill J, Bruce KD.** 2011. Partitioning core and satellite taxa from within cystic fibrosis lung bacterial communities. *ISME J* **5:**780–791.

128. **Willner D, Haynes MR, Furlan M, Schmieder R, Lim YW, Rainey PB, Rohwer F, Conrad D.** 2012. Spatial distribution of microbial communities in the cystic fibrosis lung. *ISME J* **6:**471–474.

129. **Coburn B, Wang PW, Diaz Caballero J, Clark ST, Brahma V, Donaldson S, Zhang Y, Surendra A, Gong Y, Elizabeth Tullis D, Yau YC, Waters VJ, Hwang DM, Guttman DS.** 2015. Lung microbiota across age and disease stage in cystic fibrosis. *Sci Rep* **5:**10241.

130. **Goddard AF, Staudinger BJ, Dowd SE, Joshi-Datar A, Wolcott RD, Aitken ML, Fligner CL, Singh PK.** 2012. Direct sampling of cystic fibrosis lungs indicates that DNA-based analyses of upper-airway specimens can misrepresent lung microbiota. *Proc Natl Acad Sci USA* **109:**13769–13774.

131. **Ghorbani P, Santhakumar P, Hu Q, Djiadeu P, Wolever TM, Palaniyar N, Grasemann H.** 2015. Short-chain fatty acids affect cystic fibrosis airway inflammation and bacterial growth. *Eur Respir J* **46:**1033–1045.

132. **Clark JA, Coopersmith CM.** 2007. Intestinal crosstalk: a new paradigm for understanding the gut as the "motor" of critical illness. *Shock* **28:**384–393.

133. **Klingensmith NJ, Coopersmith CM.** 2016. The gut as the motor of multiple organ dysfunction in critical illness. *Crit Care Clin* **32:**203–212.

134. **Ownby DR, Johnson CC, Peterson EL.** 2002. Exposure to dogs and cats in the first year of life and risk of allergic sensitization at 6 to 7 years of age. *JAMA* **288:**963–972.

135. **von Mutius E, Vercelli D.** 2010. Farm living: effects on childhood asthma and allergy. *Nat Rev Immunol* **10:**861–868.

136. **Bazett M, Bergeron ME, Haston CK.** 2016. Streptomycin treatment alters the intestinal microbiome, pulmonary T cell profile and airway hyperresponsiveness in a cystic fibrosis mouse model. *Sci Rep* **6:**19189.

137. **Bazett M, Honeyman L, Stefanov AN, Pope CE, Hoffman LR, Haston CK.** 2015. Cystic fibrosis mouse model-dependent intestinal structure and gut microbiome. *Mamm Genome* **26:**222–234.

138. **Segal LN, Blaser MJ.** 2015. Harnessing the early-life microbiota to protect children with cystic fibrosis. *J Pediatr* **167:**16–18.e11.

139. **Hoen AG, Li J, Moulton LA, O'Toole GA, Housman ML, Koestler DC, Guill MF, Moore JH, Hibberd PL, Morrison HG, Sogin ML, Karagas MR, Madan JC.** 2015. Associations between gut microbial colonization in early life and respiratory outcomes in cystic fibrosis. *J Pediatr* **167:**138–147.e1-3.

140. **Harris B, Morjaria SM, Littmann ER, Geyer AI, Stover DE, Barker JN, Giralt SA, Taur Y, Pamer EG.** 2016. Gut microbiota predict pulmonary infiltrates after allogeneic hematopoietic cell transplantation. *Am J Respir Crit Care Med* **194:**450–463.

141. **Deshmukh HS, Liu Y, Menkiti OR, Mei J, Dai N, O'Leary CE, Oliver PM, Kolls JK, Weiser JN, Worthen GS.** 2014. The microbiota regulates neutrophil homeostasis and host resistance to *Escherichia coli* K1 sepsis in neonatal mice. *Nat Med* **20:**524–530.

142. **Caballero S, Pamer EG.** 2015. Microbiota-mediated inflammation and antimicrobial defense in the intestine. *Annu Rev Immunol* **33:**227–256.

143. **Schuijt TJ, van der Poll T, de Vos WM, Wiersinga WJ.** 2013. The intestinal microbiota and host immune interactions in the critically ill. *Trends Microbiol* **21:**221–229.

144. **Schuijt TJ, Lankelma JM, Scicluna BP, de Sousa e Melo F, Roelofs JJ, de Boer JD, Hoogendijk AJ, de Beer R, de Vos A, Belzer C, de Vos WM, van der Poll T, Wiersinga WJ.** 2016. The gut microbiota plays a protective role in the host defence against pneumococcal pneumonia. *Gut* **65:**575–583.

145. **Kumar P, Monin L, Castillo P, Elsegeiny W, Horne W, Eddens T, Vikram A, Good M, Schoenborn AA, Bibby K, Montelaro RC, Metzger DW, Gulati AS, Kolls JK.** 2016. Intestinal interleukin-17 receptor signaling mediates reciprocal control of the gut microbiota and autoimmune inflammation. *Immunity* **44:**659–671.

146. **Tanabe S.** 2013. The effect of probiotics and gut microbiota on Th17 cells. *Int Rev Immunol* **32:**511–525.

147. **Ivanov II, Atarashi K, Manel N, Brodie EL, Shima T, Karaoz U, Wei D, Goldfarb KC,**

Santee CA, Lynch SV, Tanoue T, Imaoka A, Itoh K, Takeda K, Umesaki Y, Honda K, Littman DR. 2009. Induction of intestinal Th17 cells by segmented filamentous bacteria. *Cell* **139**:485–498.

148. Suzuki K, Meek B, Doi Y, Muramatsu M, Chiba T, Honjo T, Fagarasan S. 2004. Aberrant expansion of segmented filamentous bacteria in IgA-deficient gut. *Proc Natl Acad Sci USA* **101**:1981–1986.

149. Lozupone C, Lladser ME, Knights D, Stombaugh J, Knight R. 2011. UniFrac: an effective distance metric for microbial community comparison. *ISME J* **5**:169–172.

150. Yadava K, Pattaroni C, Sichelstiel AK, Trompette A, Gollwitzer ES, Salami O, von Garnier C, Nicod LP, Marsland BJ. 2016. Microbiota promotes chronic pulmonary inflammation by enhancing IL-17A and auto-antibodies. *Am J Respir Crit Care Med* **193**:975–987.

151. McDermott AJ, Huffnagle GB. 2014. The microbiome and regulation of mucosal immunity. *Immunology* **142**:24–31.

152. Byrd AL, Segre JA. 2016. Infectious disease. Adapting Koch's postulates. *Science* **351**:224–226.

153. Koch R. 1952. Tuberculosis etiology. *Dtsch Gesundheitsw* **7**:457–465. (In German.)

154. Fredricks DN, Relman DA. 1996. Sequence-based identification of microbial pathogens: a reconsideration of Koch's postulates. *Clin Microbiol Rev* **9**:18–33.

155. Wommack KE, Ravel J. 2013. Microbiome, demystifying the role of microbial communities in the biosphere. *Microbiome* **1**:1.

156. Dickson RP. 2016. The microbiome and critical illness. *Lancet Respir Med* **4**:59–72.

Microbiota, Liver Diseases, and Alcohol

8

ANNE-MARIE CASSARD,[1] PHILIPPE GÉRARD,[2] and
GABRIEL PERLEMUTER[1,3]

METABOLIC LIVER DISEASES: FROM DIAGNOSIS TO CURRENT TREATMENTS

Pathogenesis of NAFLD and ALD

Excessive alcohol consumption and being obese/overweight are the leading causes of chronic liver disease in Western countries. Nonalcoholic fatty liver disease (NAFLD) encompasses all liver lesions that can be observed in overweight/obese patients, ranging from pure steatosis to steatohepatitis (nonalcoholic steatohepatitis [NASH]), fibrosis, cirrhosis, and even hepatocellular carcinoma (HCC). Alcoholic liver disease (ALD) defines liver lesions observed in patients with alcohol abuse and includes steatosis, hepatitis, fibrosis, cirrhosis, and HCC. It usually occurs when alcohol consumption is higher than 70 g/day in men and 60 g/day in women. However, only some chronic alcohol consumers develop liver injury, suggesting that factors other than excessive alcohol consumption play a role in ALD. Moreover, some patients with other liver diseases, such as chronic hepatitis C or NAFLD, also

[1]INSERM U996 Inflammation, Chemokines and Immunopathology, DHU Hepatinov, Univ Paris-Sud, Université Paris-Saclay, 92140 Clamart, France; [2]Micalis Institute, INRA, AgroParisTech, Université Paris-Saclay, 78350 Jouy-en-Josas, France; [3]AP-HP, Hepatogastroenterology and Nutrition, Hôpital Antoine-Béclère, Clamart, France

Bugs as Drugs: Therapeutic Microbes for the Prevention and Treatment of Disease
Edited by Robert A. Britton and Patrice D. Cani
© 2018 American Society for Microbiology, Washington, DC
doi:10.1128/microbiolspec.BAD-0007-2016

consume alcohol. Alcohol may lead to liver injury at a lower level of consumption in these patients with another underlying liver disease.

NAFLD usually occurs in patients with a metabolic syndrome. Such patients are overweight and may have hypertension, dyslipidemia, high blood glucose, or diabetes. However, as with chronic alcohol consumers, overweight or obese patients do not systematically develop NAFLD.

NAFLD and ALD encompass a wide spectrum of pathological lesions. Liver lesions in both diseases include a combination of steatosis, inflammation, hepatocyte necrosis, and fibrosis. Thus, NASH is merely a stage of NAFLD. Although the lesions are similar, the mechanisms of the two diseases share similarities, but there are also differences (1, 2).

Steatosis is an accumulation of triglycerides in the cytoplasm of hepatocytes. Steatosis is reversible after withdrawal of its cause (alcohol intake, being overweight), but if its cause remains, it may progress towards inflammation (Fig. 1). The presence of an inflammatory process in alcoholic patients with simple steatosis suggests that they will progress towards alcoholic hepatitis in the absence of alcohol withdrawal (3), whereas the transition from simple steatosis to steatohepatitis in overweight patients is less well understood (4). Another difference between the two diseases is the degree of the liver inflammation. The inflammatory infiltrate in both alcoholic and overweight patients may contain lymphocytes and polymorphonuclear neutrophils along with ballooning and necrosis of hepatocytes. Nevertheless, the intensity

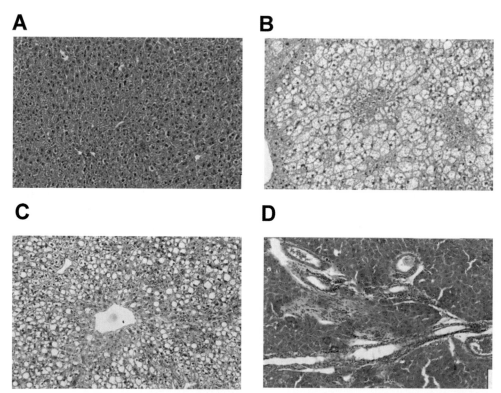

FIGURE 1 Histology of the liver. Paraffin sections (4 μm thick) were stained with hematoxylin and eosin. Images were obtained using a Hamamatsu scanning module (Hamamatsu LX2000) and appropriate software (magnification, ×100). (A) Healthy tissue; (B) steatosis; (C) steatosis with inflammation; (D) fibrosis.

of this process is generally much higher in alcoholic than overweight patients. Mega-mitochondria is often observed in both diseases. The distinction of simple steatosis from true NASH may be difficult. The lesion is considered to be NASH when lobular inflammation and liver cell clarification/ballooning are present (5). The inflammatory process progresses towards fibrosis and cirrhosis in approximately 20% of alcoholic patients. The natural incidence of cirrhosis in overweight patients is less clear, possibly due to death from other diseases associated with being overweight, such as cardiovascular diseases. The incidence of HCC in cirrhotic livers is approximately 3 to 5% each year (6). HCC may occur without cirrhosis in overweight patients, whereas cirrhosis is an obligatory step in alcoholic patients (7). Severe alcoholic hepatitis is a particular form of ALD, characterized by acute hepatocellular insufficiency, severe histological liver injury, and a high mortality rate, as the 1-month survival of such patients is between 50 and 65%. Among patients who survive beyond 1 month, 50% die within the following year (8).

NAFLD and ALD: Clinical Aspects and Diagnosis

A diagnosis of NAFLD is clinically suspected in asymptomatic patients with elevated transaminases or radiological evidence of steatosis. Diagnosis of NAFLD may be associated with other components of metabolic syndrome, such as being overweight/obese, type 2 diabe-

tes mellitus, hypertension, or dyslipidemia. When symptoms occur, they are nonspecific, consisting of fatigue and/or vague right-upper-quadrant abdominal pain. ALD should be suspected in all patients with excessive alcohol intake. The WHO safety threshold for alcohol consumption is approximately 20 g/day for women and 30 g/day for men, with 1 day of abstinence from alcohol each week. Higher consumption may lead to complications, but individual susceptibility to alcohol varies widely. For example, we have shown that overweight patients are more sensitive to alcohol-dependent liver toxicity, due to alcohol-induced inflammation in adipose tissue (9).

Elevated transaminases and gamma-glutamyltransferase are often the only abnormalities detected in overweight and alcoholic patients. A ratio of ALT to aspartate aminotransferase (AST) of <1 is suggestive of ALD in most cases, whereas an ALT/AST ratio of >1 suggests the presence of NAFLD. An ALT/AST ratio of <1 may also be observed when NAFLD progresses towards advanced fibrosis/cirrhosis. Transaminase values do not reflect the extent of liver injury, and a normal transaminase level does not guarantee the absence of underlying steatohepatitis or fibrosis. Conversely, increased transaminase levels are often associated with inflammation. The level of transaminases in ASH and NASH is rarely higher than twice the upper limit of the normal value (Table 1), and prothrombin time and bilirubin and albumin levels remain normal in the absence of

TABLE 1 Main differences between ALD and NAFLD

	ALD	NAFLD
Clinical characteristic	Alcohol intake	Overweight Metabolic syndrome Hypertension
Biology	ALT/AST < 1	ALT/AST > 1 in 66% of cases ALT/AST < 1 usually in patients with advanced fibrosis Dyslipidemia Increased blood glucose
Liver biopsy	Steatosis In patients with alcoholic hepatitis, high inflammatory process	Steatosis In patients with NASH, usually low inflammatory process

hepatocellular insufficiency. Abdominal imaging aids in diagnosing steatosis. Abdominal ultrasound is noninvasive and can detect a steatosis involving more than 30% of hepatocytes (10). Computed tomography scan lacks sensitivity and introduces a radiation hazard. Magnetic resonance imaging (MRI) is expensive but provides the highest precision for quantifying steatosis. Nevertheless, liver imaging cannot distinguish between simple steatosis and NASH in the absence of liver dysmorphy due to cirrhosis (reviewed in reference 1).

Liver biopsy remains the gold standard to assess liver injury because of the lack of good correlations between simple blood tests and histological liver lesions. Noninvasive biological and physical tests, such as transient elastography, are often used for initial screening to limit the use of liver biopsy.

The mortality rate is higher in patients with NAFLD than in the general population (11). NAFLD is associated with an increased risk of cardiovascular disease and liver-related mortality.

Nevertheless, most patients with NAFLD display only simple steatosis, without inflammation. Their risk of progression from steatosis to steatohepatitis (i.e., NASH) is very low. These patients do not generally show a progression of liver injury and increased mortality risk after 20 years of follow-up. Conversely, patients with NASH may progress after several years towards fibrosis, cirrhosis, and HCC, with increased mortality. The three major causes of NASH-related mortality are cardiovascular diseases, all-cause malignancy, and liver-related death. NASH is associated with a >10-fold-increased risk of liver-related death (2.8% versus 0.2%) and a 2-fold-increased risk of death from cardiovascular disease (15.5% versus 7.5%) (12, 13). The presence and severity of fibrosis are the strongest determinants of long-term prognosis (14). The progression of fibrosis is generally slow, taking approximately 8 years to progress from no fibrosis to low-stage fibrosis. However, some patients progress

more rapidly (15), similar to what is seen with those with chronic hepatitis C. Factors leading to more-rapid progression are a body mass index (BMI) of >30 kg/m^2, persistently abnormal liver enzyme levels with an AST/ALT ratio of >1, type 2 diabetes mellitus, hypertension, high triglycerides, low high-density lipoprotein (HDL) cholesterol levels, and a family history of diabetes mellitus (13, 16).

Of note, 30 to 60% of patients with NASH who develop HCC harbor advanced fibrosis without cirrhotic features (7, 17).

NAFLD: Current Treatments

Metabolic syndrome and its components are the primary cause of NAFLD. The management of NAFLD includes treatment of the risk factors that are commonly associated with metabolic syndrome through lifestyle modifications. No treatment is needed for simple steatosis, as it is not associated with increased morbidity. Thus, treatment should be considered in patients with NASH.

Dietary modifications leading to a weight loss of 7% or more may improve liver histology. A hypocaloric diet leading to a weight loss of 0.5 to 1.0 kg/week is generally recommended (18). Nevertheless, most patients do not achieve this weight loss goal.

Exercise, independent of weight loss, may also improve liver histology, decreasing liver fat content and increasing muscle mass (19). Lasting weight loss can be achieved in patients with NAFLD by combining diet and exercise for longer than 12 months (20). No specific treatment is recommended for NASH, despite several clinical trials. The best-studied treatments are insulin sensitizers, such as metformin, thiazolidinediones, and glucagon-like peptide 1 agonists (liraglutide); antioxidants, such as vitamin E; and cytoprotective agents, such as ursodeoxycholic acid (UDCA) and obeticholic acid (OCA) (21). Thiazolidinediones are peroxisome-proliferator-activated receptor gamma agonists. In addition to increasing insulin sensitivity, they promote peripheral fatty acid uptake and thus divert them from the liver towards adipose tissue. They improve steatosis, inflammation, and ballooning degeneration. No significant effect on liver fibrosis has been found. These drugs are no longer used in Europe due to their side effects: weight gain, increased risk of heart failure, and possible increased risk of bladder cancer (22). Metformin led to encouraging results in animal models, but no improvement of NASH has been observed in human clinical trials. However, metformin may decrease the risk of liver cancer and modulate the intestinal microbiota (IM), which may contribute to its beneficial effects. Metformin increases the abundance of the mucin-degrading bacterium *Akkermansia*, which may result in an improved metabolic profile in patients with type 2 diabetes (23). Vitamin E has shown a benefit in steatosis and inflammation, but not fibrosis, in nondiabetic patients with NAFLD (24). However, vitamin E does not improve insulin resistance in these nondiabetic patients and may increase all-cause mortality (24). UDCA may prevent hepatocyte apoptosis and downregulate inflammatory pathways. Improvement of liver transaminases following treatment with UDCA was shown in one clinical trial but not another, and there was only mild improvement of liver lesions, if any. OCA activates the farnesoid X receptor (FXR), whereas UDCA is a weak agonist of FXR. In a clinical trial, OCA improved liver transaminase levels and pathological lesions, fibrosis, hepatocellular ballooning, steatosis, and lobular inflammation. The safety of OCA must be tested, as it also increases alkaline phosphatase and low-density lipoprotein cholesterol (25). Bariatric surgery may be recommended in obese patients with a BMI of >40 kg/m^2 or >35 kg/m^2 with a comorbidity (26). Bariatric surgery improves liver histology and reduces mortality from both NASH-related complications and all-cause mortality in the 7 to 10 years that follow the bariatric procedure.

Overall, lifestyle modifications can provide a strong benefit to patients but are difficult to follow in the long term. Some treatments may be beneficial for patients, but the magnitude of the effects is small, in particular on liver fibrosis.

ALD: Current Treatments

Treatment of ALD relies principally on alcohol withdrawal. Nevertheless, patients with severe alcoholic hepatitis, defined by a Maddrey discriminant function of >32, must also be treated with corticosteroids, which is the reference treatment. Corticosteroids decrease liver inflammation and improve 1-month and possibly 6-month survival. In one of the largest trials to date, mortality after 28 days was 17% (45 of 269 patients) in the placebo group versus 14% (38 of 266 patients) in the prednisolone group (27). However, survival curves converged after 28 days, such that prednisolone therapy provided no benefit to patients after 90 days or 1 year. Pentoxifylline, a phosphodiesterase inhibitor, may reduce tumor necrosis factor alpha production. Its efficacy, alone or in association with corticosteroids, is controversial (28). It may increase survival relative to placebo but does not do so relative to prednisolone (29). N-Acetylcysteine is a glutathione precursor. In one trial, its addition to prednisolone increased survival of patients, but its efficacy needs to be confirmed (30). Enteral or parenteral nutritional supplementation may improve the prognosis, as ALD is often associated with protein, vitamin, and mineral deficiencies, but its impact on survival remains unclear (31). Nevertheless, nutritional support should be considered in patients with severe alcoholic hepatitis. Liver transplantation is generally proposed to patients with severe liver insufficiency after at least 6 months of abstinence. However, the mortality rate of patients with severe alcoholic hepatitis is very high (more than 50% during the first 3 months). Thus, it has been proposed to proceed rapidly to liver transplantation for patients with severe alcoholic hepatitis who do not respond to corticosteroids. In a clinical trial of 26 patients undergoing liver transplantation, the 6-month survival rate was 77%, similar to that of patients who respond to corticosteroids. After 2 years, 71% were still alive and only 3 patients resumed the consumption of alcohol (32).

Therapeutic resources for metabolic liver diseases are scarce, and the recent discovery of the involvement of the IM in NAFLD and ALD opens new therapeutic perspectives.

NAFLD AND THE GUT MICROBIOTA

NASH and Dysbiosis

Dysbiosis is defined as a microbial imbalance associated with a disease. Dysbiosis in NAFLD was first described in animal studies. For example, the severity of steatosis was associated with an increase in the *Lactobacillus* population in mice fed a high-fat diet (HFD) for 10 weeks (33). Since then, an increasing number of studies have investigated the gut microbiota in relation to human NAFLD, using culture-independent techniques, such as quantitative PCR (qPCR) or sequencing (Table 2). Children and adolescents (with or without NASH) were found to have a higher abundance of *Bacteroidetes* and a lower abundance of *Firmicutes* than healthy controls. *Proteobacteria, Enterobacteriaceae,* and *Escherichia* were the only phylum, family, and genus, respectively, exhibiting a significant difference between microbiomes from obese and NASH individuals and were found to be more abundant in patients with NASH (34). In adults, the comparison of 30 obese patients with clinically defined NAFLD and 30 nonobese controls revealed an overrepresentation of *Lactobacillus* species and selected members of the phylum *Firmicutes* (*Lachnospiraceae, Dorea, Robinsoniella,* and *Roseburia*) in NAFLD patients (35). Another study comprising 53 NAFLD patients and 32 healthy subjects found that *Escherichia, Anaerobacter, Lactobacillus,* and *Clostridium* cluster XI were more abundant in the gut microbiotas of NAFLD patients, whereas

Alistipes, Odoribacter, Oscillibacter, and *Flavonifractor* were less abundant (36).

In a prospective, cross-sectional study, the gut microbiota composition (analyzed using qPCR) was compared between adults with biopsy-proven NAFLD (simple steatosis or NASH) and healthy controls. Patients with NASH had a lower proportion of *Bacteroidetes* than individuals with simple steatosis and healthy controls, even after adjusting for body mass index (37). Wong et al. investigated the microbiome composition using 16S rRNA gene sequencing in 16 biopsy-proven NASH patients and 22 healthy controls. The order *Aeromonadales,* the families *Succinivibrionaceae* and *Porphyromonadaceae,* and the genera *Parabacteroides* and *Allisonella* were found to be more abundant in NASH patients. Conversely, the class *Clostridia,* the order *Clostridiales,* and the genera *Anaerosporobacter* and *Faecalibacterium* were less abundant in NASH patients (38). Differences in fecal microbiota between nonobese adults with and without NAFLD have also been found, characterized by a higher abundance of *Bacteroidetes* and a lower abundance of *Firmicutes* in nonobese patients with NAFLD (39).

The effect of a choline-deficient diet on the composition of the human gut microbiome and the development of fatty liver has been studied by Spencer et al. They found that a baseline microbial composition correlated with the development of fatty liver in response to choline deficiency. The abundance of *Gammaproteobacteria* negatively correlated with the development of steatosis, whereas the abundance of *Erysipelotrichia* was positively associated, suggesting that baseline levels of these populations may predict susceptibility to fatty liver due to choline deficiency (40).

Altogether, these human studies revealed taxonomic differences between the gut microbiotas of healthy controls and patients with NASH. However, the results were heterogeneous, even contradictory, despite the identification of dysbiosis at the phylum or genus levels. Factors that may explain these differences include differences in the study design and methods of gut microbiota analysis, the variety of clinical endpoints, or changes of the gut microbiota due to diet or medications. The specific phyla or genera that are the causative agents in NASH development remain unclear.

A Causative Role for the Gut Microbiota in NAFLD

Patients suffering from NAFLD harbor a gut microbiota different from that of healthy controls, but the previously described association studies do not indicate whether this dysbiosis is a cause or a consequence of liver disease. Strategies have been developed in animal models to prove the causality of the gut microbiota in disease development. These strategies aim to transmit a phenotype from one mouse to another by a microbiota transfer that can be performed via cohousing of conventional mice or fecal transplant to germ-free or antibiotic-treated mice. These microbiota transfer strategies have already proven the causative role of the gut bacteria in several diseases including obesity and inflammatory bowel disease (41, 42). It was first demonstrated that cohousing germ-free mice with their conventional counterparts leads to increased glycogenesis in the liver of ex-germ-free mice prior to triggering increases in hepatic triglyceride synthesis. Colonization was also associated with altered hepatic Cyp8b1 expression and changes in bile acid (BA) composition. The hepatic triglyceride, glucose, and glycogen levels were strongly associated with the *Coriobacteriaceae* family (phylum *Actinobacteria*) (43). Henao-Mejia et al. further established the causative role of the gut microbiota in the development of liver disease using mouse models deficient in the proinflammatory multiprotein complex called the inflammasome (44). These inflammasome-deficient mice exhibited exacerbated NAFLD phenotypes when fed a methionine choline-deficient diet or HFD. This was associated with changes in the composition of the gut microbiota, especially an increase in the proportion of bacteria belonging to the *Porphyromonadaceae* family. Strikingly, cohousing of wild-type mice with these inflammasome-deficient mice resulted in increased glucose intolerance and obesity, as well as hepatic steatosis and liver inflammation, in the wild-type mice, indicating that dysbiosis itself can induce NAFLD progression. Another study conducted in mouse models demonstrated that the susceptibility to develop NAFLD can be transmitted by fecal transplant to recipient germ-free mice (45). They first observed that conventionally raised mice displayed various levels of weight gain, glucose intolerance, and steatosis when given an HFD for 16 weeks. They selected two donor mice for microbiota transplant based on their opposite responses to the HFD. Although the mice were the same weight, one displayed low fasting glycemia and slight steatosis ("nonresponder"), and the other displayed insulin resistance and marked steatosis ("responder"). Two groups of germ-free mice were transplanted with the gut microbiota of the two selected mice by oral gavage of donor cecal content. Only the mice transplanted with the responder microbiota developed fasting hyperglycemia, hyperinsulinemia, and liver steatosis after being fed an HFD and showed increased expression of genes involved in lipogenesis. This suggests that differences in susceptibility to develop NAFLD may be controlled primarily by the gut microbiota. *Lachnospiraceae* and *Barnesiella* were found to be overrepresented in the gut microbiotas of mice with glucose intolerance and steatosis, whereas the group of mice that did not develop features of NAFLD had a higher population of *Bacteroides vulgatus* (45).

Mechanisms Linking the Gut Microbiota to NAFLD

Several mechanisms have been proposed to link the gut microbiota to NAFLD, including small intestinal bowel overgrowth (SIBO),

TABLE 2 Microbiotas associated with different stages of NAFLD[a]

Condition	Phylum	Family	Genus	Reference
NAFLD versus healthy controls	[Bacteroidetes] [Firmicutes]	Porphyromonadaceae ⇩ Veillonellaceae ⇧ Lactobacillaceae ⇧ Ruminococcaceae ⇩ Lachnospiraceae ⇧	*Lactobacillus* ⇧ *Oscillibacter* ⇩ *Robinsoniella* ⇧ *Roseburia* ⇧ *Dorea* ⇧	Healthy (*n* = 30, BMI = 22) NAFLD (*n* = 30, BMI = 33) Raman et al., 2013 (35)
	[Proteobacteria] [Bacteroidetes] [Firmicutes]	Kiloniellaceae ⇧ Pasteurellaceae ⇧ [Rikenellaceae] [Porphyromonadaceae] [Lactobacillaceae] [Oscillospiraceae] [Clostridiaceae] [Lachnospiraceae] [Streptococcaceae]	*Alistipes* ⇩ *Odoribacter* ⇩ *Lactobacillus* ⇧ *Oscillibacter* ⇩ *Anaerobacter* ⇧ *Clostridium* XI ⇧ *Streptococcus* ⇧ *Flavonifractor* ⇩	Healthy (*n* = 32, BMI = 22) NAFLD (*n* = 53, BMI = 26) Jiang et al, 2015 (36)
NASH versus healthy controls	[Proteobacteria] *Lentisphaerae* ⇩ *Bacteroidetes* ⇩	[Enterobacteriaceae]	*Escherichia* ⇧	Healthy (*n* = 17, BMI = 26) NASH (*n* = 22, BMI = 32) Mouzaki et al., 2013 (37)
	Bacteroidetes ⇧	Prevotellaceae ⇧ Rikenellaceae ⇩	*Prevotella* ⇧ *Allistipes* ⇩	Healthy (*n* = 16, BMI = 20) NASH (*n* = 22, BMI = 34)

Comparison	Phylum	Family	Genus/species	Population/Study
	Firmicutes ⇩	*Ruminococcaceae* ⇩	*Oscillospira* ⇩	Children
		Lachnospiraceae ⇩	*Ruminococcus* ⇩	Zhu et al., 2013 (34)
			Blautia ⇩	
			Coprococcus ⇩	
			Eubacterium ⇩	
			Roseburia ⇩	
	Proteobacteria ⇧	*Enterobacteriaceae* ⇧	**Escherichia coli** ⇧	Healthy (*n* = 22, BMI = 22)
	Actinobacteria	*Bifidobacteriaceae* ⇩	*Bifidobacterium* ⇩	NASH (*n* = 16, BMI = 29)
	Firmicutes ⇩	Unclassified *Clostridiales* ⇩	*Faecalibacterium* ⇩	Wong et al., 2013 (38)
		[*Ruminococcaceae*]	*Anaerosporobacter* ⇩	
		[*Lachnospiraceae*]	*Allisonella* ⇧	
		[*Veillonellaceae*]		
	[*Bacteroidetes*]	*Porphyromonadaceae* ⇧	*Parabacteroides* ⇧	
	[*Proteobacteria*]	*Succinivibrionaceae* ⇧		
NASH versus obese	*Bacteroidetes* ⇩	[*Lachnospiraceae*]	*Clostridium coccoides* ⇧	Obese (*n* = 11, BMI = 28)
				NASH (*n* = 22, BMI = 32)
				Mouzaki et al., 2013 (37)
	[*Firmicutes*]			Obese (*n* = 25, BMI = 33)
	Proteobacteria ⇧	*Enterobacteriaceae* ⇧	**Escherichia coli** ⇧	NASH (*n* = 22, BMI = 34)
				Zhu et al., 2013 (34)
NAFLD patients NASH versus no NASH	[*Bacteroidetes*]	*Bacteroidaceae* ⇧	*Bacteroides* ⇧	No NASH (*n* = 22, BMI = 30)
				NASH (*n* = 35, BMI = 32)
				Boursier et al., 2016 (122)

aMicrobiota were analyzed using 16S deep sequencing, except in the study by Mouzaki et al., in which qPCR was used. Additional taxonomic information for discriminating taxa is in brackets. Taxa in boldface are those identified in more than one study.

gut leakiness and resulting endotoxemia and inflammation, endogenous ethanol production, or BA and choline metabolism.

SIBO is a condition in which colonic bacteria colonize the small bowel due to altered intestinal motility. The diagnosis of bacterial overgrowth is performed using various techniques including breath testing and the culture of an aspirate from the jejunum, whereas culture-independent techniques, such as qPCR and sequencing, have been rarely applied. Most controlled trials using breath testing revealed a higher prevalence of SIBO in NAFLD patients than in healthy subjects (reviewed in reference 46). Moreover, SIBO correlated with the severity of steatosis but not NASH (47). However, no difference was found in bacterial numbers between patients suffering from NAFLD or NASH and healthy controls in a study using qPCR (37), suggesting that the use of molecular techniques may revise the current view on the role of SIBO in NAFLD.

Numerous studies have shown that the IM tunes the homeostasis of the gut barrier. A disruption of gut barrier integrity, characterized by the disruption of tight junctions and increased permeability, has been found in biopsy-proven NAFLD patients (47). Similarly, increased gut permeability has been observed in children with NAFLD and was found to correlate with the severity of the disease (48). This loss of barrier function leads to increased amounts of microbial products reaching the liver via portal circulation (49). Among these microbial products, lipopolysaccharide (LPS), a component of the bacterial cell wall of Gram-negative bacteria, binds to Toll-like receptor 4 (TLR4), triggering not only inflammation but also production of the extracellular matrix by hepatic stellate cells, leading to fibrosis (Fig. 2) (50, 51). In addition to TLR4, TLR2 and TLR9 may also be involved in NAFLD development, as TLR2- and TLR9-deficient mice display less steatosis and inflammation than their wild-type counterparts. In addition to increased gut permeability, HFD results in increased intestinal LPS absorption through high chylomicron production by intestinal epithelial cells, leading to low-grade endotoxemia (52). Animal studies suggest that endotoxemia alone may induce NASH, and higher endotoxin levels have been observed in NASH patients than in subjects with steatosis (53, 54). However, endotoxemia is not always higher in NASH (55), suggesting that LPS is not the only component that triggers the cascade of increased proinflammatory cytokines, insulin resistance, and fibrosis.

Endogenous ethanol production has also been proposed as a mechanism linking the gut microbiota to NAFLD (56). Indeed, gut bacteria, including the *Enterobacteriaceae* family, carry out mixed-acid fermentation, a major product of which is ethanol. This microbially produced ethanol reaches the liver via the portal vein and is converted to acetate and acetaldehyde. Acetate is a fatty acid substrate, whereas acetaldehyde triggers the production of reactive oxygen species. Moreover, ethanol alters gut permeability, leading to increased endotoxemia. Thus, endogenous ethanol production may be another component that triggers the proinflammatory cascade. Higher ethanol levels have been detected in patients with histology-proven NAFLD than in healthy controls (57) and in non-alcohol-consuming adolescents with NASH than in obese or healthy controls (34). This was associated with an increased abundance of *Escherichia* bacteria, ethanol-producing members of the *Enterobacteriaceae* family.

Choline, a phospholipid component of the cell membrane, is an essential nutrient required for lipid metabolism and neurotransmitter synthesis. Diets deficient in choline lead to triglyceride accumulation in the liver and reduced hepatic secretion of very-low-density lipoproteins, resulting in liver steatosis, which is reversed after choline supplementation (58). The gut microbiota can reduce choline bioavailability, thus mimicking a choline-deficient diet. Different gut bacteria can convert choline to

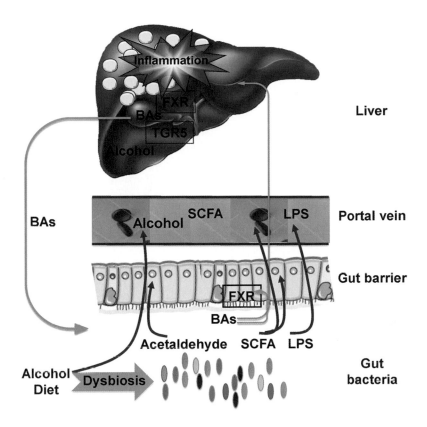

FIGURE 2 Intestinal microbiota in liver disease. Diet and alcohol influence the composition of the gut bacteria. Dysbiosis is associated with changes in bacterial metabolites such as SCFA and BAs. The gut barrier is also altered, leading to increased endotoxemia (LPS). Acetaldehyde is specifically produced by the gut bacteria in ALD. Modifications of BAs and activation of their receptors, FXR and TGR5, participate in the development of liver lesions.

methylamines, which may further induce inflammation when absorbed by the liver. Indeed, the high capacity of the gut microbiota to metabolize choline into methylamines explains the high susceptibility to develop NAFLD in response to an HFD in mouse strain 129S6 (59). However, it is not currently known whether bacterial choline metabolism contributes to NAFLD susceptibility in humans.

Primary BAs (in humans, cholic acid [CA] and chenodeoxycholic acid [CDCA]) are synthesized from cholesterol in the liver and conjugated to either taurine or glycine (60). They are then excreted into the small intestine, where their deconjugation and dehydro-

xylation are dependent on the gut bacterial species and are therefore modified when dysbiosis occurs (61). More than 95% of the BAs secreted in bile are reabsorbed in the distal ileum and return to the liver, taking part in the enterohepatic cycle. The main function of BAs is to assist the absorption of dietary lipids and lipid-soluble nutrients. However, they are also signaling molecules through the activation of receptors, such as the FXR or Takeda G protein-coupled receptor 5 (TGR5). Thus, they may modulate the inflammatory response and lipid, glucose, energy, and drug metabolisms, as well as their own biosynthesis (62). FXR-deficient mice develop features of NAFLD, including increased steatosis and inflammation. Beneficial effects of BAs on glucose and lipid metabolism, as well as on NAFLD, have been recently reported. OCA, a synthetic FXR ligand, improves liver injuries in biopsy-proven NASH patients (25). However, less than 50% of the patients receiving OCA showed histological improvement, whereas transaminases and glucose intolerance returned to baseline levels when the treatment ceased. Dyslipidemia was a side effect of OCA administration, preventing its use as an adjuvant treatment for NAFLD. The fraction of BAs that escape enterohepatic circulation, approximately 5% (i.e., 200 to 800 mg daily in humans), pass into the colon, where they undergo bacterial metabolism leading to the production of over 20 different secondary BAs in adult human feces (63). The capacity to activate the FXR and TGR5 depends on the type of BA. The primary BA, CDCA, is the most potent, whereas secondary BAs activate the FXR and TGR5 to a much lesser extent. The metabolism of the gut microbiota may thus modulate FXR and TGR5 activation, and subsequently NAFLD susceptibility, by altering the composition of the BA pool.

Specific BAs produced by the gut microbiota can also directly affect liver health. For example, the dehydroxylation of CDCA leads to formation of lithocholic acid, which is toxic to liver cells (64), and high levels of deoxycholic acid (DCA) are associated with an increased risk of liver cancer (65). Some studies also showed that DCA can impair gut barrier function (66). Conversely, UDCA, produced by few intestinal bacteria through the epimerization of the 7α-hydroxyl group of CDCA (67), is thought to be chemopreventive and is used to treat cholesterol gallstones and primary biliary cirrhosis. UDCA is also able to reverse the effect of DCA on the gut barrier (66). Finally, the gut microbiota may also modulate host lipid metabolism and NAFLD development through the metabolism of BAs by changing their emulsification and absorption properties, which may affect fatty acid storage in the liver.

Probiotics, Prebiotics, and Symbiotics as Therapeutic Approaches

Prebiotics and probiotics are known modulators of the gut microbiota and have demonstrated beneficial effects in both animal models of NAFLD and humans. Several probiotic strains have been found to be effective in different experimental rodent models of NAFLD. For example, supplementation with *Lactobacillus rhamnosus* GG reduced steatosis in fructose-induced NAFLD (68). This was associated with restored gut barrier function and decreased expression of proinflammatory cytokines in the liver. Similarly, *Bacteroides uniformis* CECT 7771 and *Bifidobacterium pseudocatenulatum* CECT 7765 improved steatosis and immune defense mechanisms in HFD-fed mice (69, 70), whereas *Lactobacillus casei* strain Shirota was shown to protect against NASH induced by a methionine- and choline-deficient diet (71). Also, *Lactobacillus paracasei* F19 reduced steatosis and inflammation in a rat model of ischemia-reperfusion (72). Finally, administration of VSL#3, a preparation composed of eight bacterial strains, improved liver steatosis and insulin resistance in HFD-fed mice (73) and reduced liver inflammation and serum ALT in leptin-deficient (ob/ob) mice (74). Few randomized, prospective clinical trials have been performed in humans to assess the effect of probiotic administration on NAFLD. However, a meta-analysis of four trials involving 134 NAFLD/NASH patients provided evidence that probiotic therapies may be effective in improving NAFLD markers, despite the use of different bacterial strains and administration protocols (75). In particular, the use of probiotics was associated with lower plasma aminotransferase and total cholesterol levels, lower systemic inflammation, and improved insulin resistance.

Prebiotics, which can promote the growth of beneficial bacteria, may also improve markers of NAFLD. For example, fructooligosaccharide (FOS) administration reduced endotoxemia and steatosis in HFD-fed mice, probably via the restoration of *Bifidobacteria* and *Akkermansia muciniphila* populations (76, 77). Similarly, an HFD supplemented with fungal chitin-glucan was found to decrease steatosis as well as fat mass development and hyperglycemia in mice. These beneficial effects correlated with the abundance of *Roseburia* spp., which was decreased by the HFD and restored by the prebiotics. These changes in gut microbiota composition, due to prebiotic treatment, are thought to improve gut barrier integrity through mechanisms including the production of endogenous glucagon-like peptide 2 and endocannabinoids.

Finally, symbiotics, which consist of a mix of probiotics and prebiotics, have been recently used in patients with NAFLD. A 24-week treatment with *Bifidobacterium longum* and FOS (78), together with lifestyle modifications, reduced endotoxemia and serum transaminase and tumor necrosis factor alpha levels, as well as steatosis and liver inflammation (79). However, these parameters also improved in the placebo group. Similarly, a 28-week treatment with a mixture of seven bacterial strains associated with FOS had beneficial effects on hepatic inflammation and overall liver function (80).

These encouraging results strongly suggest that the use of pro-, pre-, and symbiotics may be an effective addition in the treatment of NAFLD.

ALCOHOL LIVER DISEASE

Microbiota, a Key Player in ALD

In 1995, Adachi et al. reported that antibiotics protected rats against alcohol-induced liver injury by lowering Kupffer cell activation, without linking antibiotic use to gut bacteria (81). ALD is also associated with elevated plasma endotoxin levels in alcoholic patients and rodent models of alcohol consumption (82–84), which is further explained by increased intestinal permeability (85). The disruption of the gut barrier is now largely understood (86–88) and is explained by the lower expression of several proteins of the tight junctions (89). Moreover, ethanol consumption modulates the glycosylation of mucin, which modifies the protective mucus layer and, potentially, the adherent bacterial species (90). Using germ-free mice, it was shown that the alcohol-associated increase of intestinal permeability is not induced by alcohol, *per se*, but at least in part by acetaldehyde produced by bacterial ethanol metabolism (91). These data do not exclude that other bacterial metabolites may be involved in the disruption of tight junctions (92). Thus, the IM participates in the disruption of the gut barrier, which may impair liver homeostasis by increasing the level of bacterial products or bacterial translocation into the blood and lymph nodes. This translocation may be particularly deleterious in the case of dysbiosis. Indeed, dysbiosis has already been described in alcohol-fed rodents (93–95). Alcohol intake in rats was associated with a decrease in the abundance of lactic acid bacteria, especially those of the genera *Lactobacillus, Pediococcus, Leuconostoc*, and *Lactococcus* (95). An increase in the abundance of *Proteobacteria* and *Actinobacteria* and decreases in *Bacteroidetes* and *Firmicutes* were described in alcohol-fed mice. Moreover, these modifications were accompanied by a decrease in the bacterial diversity (93). In alcoholic patients, dysbiosis of the colon IM was associated with a decrease in the abundance of *Bacteroidetes* and an increase in *Enterobacteriaceae* and *Proteobacteria* (96). These studies show that dysbiosis is associated with alcohol-induced liver lesions, but the causal role of the IM has only recently been demonstrated.

Patients with severe alcoholic hepatitis (sAH) harbor an IM different from that of alcoholic patients without liver lesions (noAH) (97). The propensity of alcohol-induced inflammation was shown to be transmissible from patients to mice via the transplantation of the IM. Germ-free mice that received the IM of an alcoholic patient with sAH developed more-severe liver lesions than mice that received the IM of an alcoholic patient without AH. They also developed more-pronounced disruption of the intestinal barrier, associated with visceral inflammation. In conventional mice, efficient IM transplantation of a human stool sample from an alcoholic patient with noAH reverted the development of liver lesions in alcohol-fed mice that initially received the IM of an alcoholic patient with sAH (97). Altogether, these findings show that individual susceptibility to ALD is dependent on the IM and provide strong evidence for a causal role of the IM in ALD.

The connections between the microbiota and their host in the development of ALD have been established, but the mechanisms that are involved in the deleterious role mediated by the IM remain unclear (98). However, metabolites produced by bacteria, such as short-chain fatty acids (SCFA) and, more importantly, volatile organic compounds (VOC) or BAs seem to be key players in ALD.

Alcohol consumption is associated with a specific mixture of VOC in stools (99). Among these VOC, SCFA propionate and isobutyrate, involved in intestinal epithelial cell homeostasis and gut barrier integrity, are less abundant in the stools of alcoholics than in those of nonalcoholic healthy individuals. BA profiles are also altered by alcohol intake in rats (100). In humans, alcohol intake induces an increase in total stool BA levels, specifically lithocholic acid and DCA, and more generally an increase in the secondary/primary BA ratio (101). However, these studies compared alcoholic and nonalcoholic individuals, and alcohol as a specific carbohydrate substrate could itself induce marked changes.

Analysis of the fecal metabolome from alcohol-fed mice has highlighted the involvement of BAs in ALD (97). Mice transplanted with the IM of a patient with severe alcoholic hepatitis developed more-severe liver lesions than those transplanted with the IM of an alcoholic patient without liver disease. Comparison of the fecal metabolites allowed

the identification of 13 biomarkers related to alcohol-induced liver toxicity. The most discriminating molecules were BA derivatives and hydroxygenated/oxygenated fatty acids. Higher amounts of the primary BA, CDCA, were found in fecal samples of mice without liver lesions than in those of mice with alcohol-induced liver lesions. The secondary BA, UDCA, was more abundant in the fecal metabolome of mice that received the MI of the alcoholic patient without liver disease than of those that received the MI of the patient with ALD.

The synthesis of BAs is dependent on a negative-feedback loop following FXR activation (102, 103). This cycle also involves several transporters that take part in the secretion of BAs from the liver to the gallbladder and BA reabsorption from the ileum. Specific BAs play a role in gut barrier disruption. UDCA and tauroursodeoxycholic acid attenuate alcohol-induced liver lesions by preventing liver damage (104). UDCA has hepatoprotective properties and was a discriminant metabolite between patients with and without alcohol-induced liver lesions (97). DCA impairs the gut barrier function in the jejunum and colon, and UDCA has a protective effect on the colon against DCA-induced barrier dysfunction (66). Moreover, mice deficient for the BA receptor FXR showed an increase of liver lesions, suggesting that the disruption of BA homeostasis was involved in alcohol-induced liver lesions (105). Thus, the dysregulation of the enterohepatic cycle by IM dysbiosis may be involved in alcohol-induced liver lesions, but further studies are needed to better understand this relationship (Fig. 2).

Disruption of the gut barrier is a prerequisite for ALD, resulting in bacterial translocation (106). The mucus layer and antimicrobial peptides are essential for protecting the intestinal epithelium against bacteria, and their alteration is associated with ALD. The production of mucin by goblet cells specifically decreases in mice with alcohol-induced liver lesions depending on the IM (97).

Surprisingly, mice deficient for mucin production were protected against alcohol-induced liver lesions. This deficiency was associated with a large increase in defensin production, as well as lectins Reg3β and Reg3γ, increasing the killing of commensal bacteria and preventing bacterial overgrowth (107). Moreover, defensin, Reg3β, and Reg3γ levels decreased in mice fed alcohol in a mouse model of ALD (95), and mice deficient for Reg3β and Reg3γ showed increased adherent bacteria and a high level of bacterial translocation, promoting alcohol-induced liver lesions (108). Conversely, mice that overexpressed Reg3γ were protected from alcohol-induced hepatic toxicity, associated with decreased adherent bacteria and a low-level bacterial translocation. Moreover, mice harboring a specific IM, that were protected from the hepatic toxicity of alcohol, also expressed high levels of defensins (109). These data suggest that the control of bacterial overgrowth and adherent bacterial content is essential to the protective mechanisms against alcohol-induced liver toxicity.

Recent data have emphasized the role played by the IM in the sensing of nutrients and hormones via the gastrointestinal nervous system (110–112). The increase in intestinal permeability and dysbiosis in alcoholic patients was associated with higher scores of depression, anxiety, and alcohol craving (113). Alcoholic patients with gut permeability harbored a lower abundance of genera belonging to the *Ruminococcaceae* family (*Ruminococcus, Faecalibacterium, Subdoligranulum, Oscillibacter,* and *Anaerofilum*), as well as clostridia, than patients with less gut permeability. Conversely, the abundance of *Dorea* (*Lachnospiraceae*), *Blautia,* and *Megasphaera* was increased in these patients. VOC produced by these members of the IM were different in alcoholic patients harboring dysbiosis and gut leakiness, especially several indole and phenol species. This suggests that metabolites produced by the IM are involved not only in cell dysfunction and liver disease but also in the psychological symptoms of alcohol dependence (113).

Prebiotics, Probiotics, or Fecal Microbiota Transfer To Treat ALD

Several probiotics have been tested in rodent models and several human trials to improve ALD progression. The first use of probiotics in ALD was performed in a rodent model of alcohol intake by using *Lactobacillus* sp. strain GG (*Lactobacillus* GG), which improved gut leakiness and liver inflammation (114–116). The addition of oat fiber or a supernatant of *Lactobacillus* GG induced similar results, suggesting that bacterial products were partially involved in the protective mechanisms (94, 117, 118). VSL#3, a mixture of eight probiotic strains, also improved liver lesions in ALD in humans and rodents (119, 120). Several other probiotic strains have been tested and improved liver lesions in rodents. They are well summarized in a recent review (121). Prebiotic use was also tested and showed that FOS improved rodent alcohol-induced liver damage in a mouse model of alcoholic liver disease (95).

Altogether, these studies highlight the promise of controlling the IM by pre- or probiotic treatments, but further studies are needed to decipher the mechanisms involved in bacterium-related gut and liver damage.

ADVANCED LIVER DISEASE

Fibrosis

The composition and functions of the gut microbiota are altered in patients with fibrosis (122). Patients with a fibrosis score of 2 or more harbor more *Bacteroides* and *Ruminococcus* and fewer *Prevotella* bacteria than patients with a fibrosis score of 0 or 1. Moreover, genes related to carbohydrate, lipid, and amino acid metabolism are overrepresented in the microbiome of patients with stage 2 fibrosis or greater, indicating a shift in the metabolic functions of the gut microbiota (122).

The bile duct ligation mouse model in combination with an HFD was used to evaluate the consequences of fibrosis on the IM.

These mice developed higher hepatic stellate cell (major producers of the fibrotic matrix) activity, resulting in increased liver fibrosis. This was associated with dysbiosis, characterized by a marked increase in the abundance of *Enterobacteriaceae* (Gram negative) and the complete disappearance of *Bifidobacterium* (Gram positive) (123). The authors further selected the Gram-negative and Gram-positive fractions of the gut microbiota from the fibrogenic HFD/bile duct ligation mice and transplanted them into control mice. Mice receiving the Gram-negative fraction displayed increased liver injury, showing that dysbiosis may contribute not only to steatosis and inflammation but also to fibrogenesis in the liver (123).

Fibrosis has also been induced by injections of carbon tetrachloride (CCl_4), showing that the IM was modified during the process of fibrosis development. There was a specific decrease in the abundance of *Clostridium* spp. and, more generally, an increase in the ratio of aerobic to anaerobic bacteria, which correlated with a higher fibrosis score (124). Bacterial DNA found in the mesenteric lymph nodes, reflecting disruption of the gut barrier, was modified in rats with chemically induced fibrosis (125). Moreover, the absence of an IM worsened fibrosis development in germ-free mice, but the immaturity of their immune system may have also played a role in the evolution of the liver damage (126). Probiotic treatments, such as use of *Saccharomyces cerevisiae* subsp. *boulardii*, were associated with a slower progression of liver fibrosis (127), and VSL#3 prevented bacterial translocation (128). However, it is not possible to conclude whether these treatments played a role early in the inflammation stage to limit the progression to fibrosis.

Cirrhosis

Patients with cirrhosis have distinct fecal microbial communities relative to healthy individuals. Members of the phylum *Bacteroidetes* were less abundant in cirrhotic

patients (24 hepatitis B virus [HBV] and 12 alcohol-related cirrhosis patients), whereas *Proteobacteria* and *Fusobacteria* were more abundant (129) (Table 3). Among cirrhotic patients, the abundance of *Prevotellaceae* was greater in alcoholic patients than those infected with HBV. Moreover, the prevalence of potentially pathogenic bacteria, such as *Enterobacteriaceae* and *Streptococcaceae*, and the reduction of beneficial populations, such as *Lachnospiraceae*, in patients with cirrhosis may affect prognosis (129). In a more recent study, the functional diversity of the IM was shown to be significantly lower in patients with hepatitis B-related cirrhosis than in controls (130). Moreover, 54% of the cirrhotic patient enriched taxonomically assigned species are of buccal origin, suggesting an invasion of the gut from the mouth in liver cirrhosis (130).

The gut microbiome has been assessed in cirrhotic patients and compared to that of healthy individuals by metagenomic studies. The modified metabolic pathways showed an enrichment of genes involved in gluconeogenesis and lipid metabolism in the IM of cirrhotic patients and a decrease of genes involved in BA metabolism (131). Another study revealed specific clusters representing cognate bacterial species; 28 were enriched in cirrhotic patients and 38 in control individuals. Among bacterial genes, those involved in denitrification, assimilation or dissimilation of nitrate, gamma-aminobutyric acid biosynthesis, heme biosynthesis, and phosphotransferase systems were found to be associated with liver cirrhosis (130). Genetic and functional biomarkers specific for liver cirrhosis were revealed by a comparison with those for type 2 diabetes and inflammatory bowel disease. Fifteen biomarkers were specifically associated with cirrhosis. However, generalization of these results is difficult, as the number of patients was low and the cause of cirrhosis was restricted mainly to HBV infection (130).

Most cirrhotic patients are asymptomatic until they develop decompensated cirrhosis.

TABLE 3 Comparison of healthy microbiotas and microbiotas associated with cirrhosis[a]

Phylum	Family	Genus	Reference
Bacteroidetes ⇩			Healthy (*n* = 24)
[*Firmicutes*]	*Veillonellaceae* ⇧		Cirrhosis (*n* = 36: HBV = 24, Alc = 12)
	Streptococcaceae ⇧		Chen et al., 2011 (129)
	Lachnospiraceae ⇩		
Proteobacteria ⇧	**Enterobacteriaceae** ⇧		
Fusobacteria ⇧			
[*Bacteroidetes*]	*Rikenellaceae* ⇩		Healthy (*n* = 14)
[*Firmicutes*]	*Veillonellaceae* ⇧	*Blautia* ⇩	Cirrhosis (*n* = 47)
	Ruminococcaceae ⇩		Kakiyama et al., 2013 (101)
	Lachnospiraceae ⇩		
[*Proteobacteria*]	**Enterobacteriaceae** ⇧		
[*Bacteroidetes*]	*Porphyromonadaceae* ⇩		Healthy (*n* = 25)
[*Firmicutes*]	*Veillonellaceae* ⇩		Cirrhosis (*n* = 175: HCV = 75, Alc = 31, others = 71)
	Ruminococcaceae ⇩		Bajaj et al., 2014 (132, 137)
	Lachnospiraceae ⇩		
	Clostridiales XIV ⇩		
	Enterococcaceae ⇧		
	Staphylococcaceae ⇧		
[*Proteobacteria*]	**Enterobacteriaceae** ⇧		
Bacteroidetes ⇩	[*Bacteroidaceae*]	*Bacteroides* ⇩	Healthy (*n* = 83)
	[*Prevotellaceae*]	*Prevotella* ⇧	Cirrhosis (*n* = 98: HBV = 79, Alc = 10, others = 9)
	[*Rikenellaceae*]	*Alistipes* ⇩	Qin et al., 2014 (130)
[*Firmicutes*]	[*Veillonellaceae*]	*Veillonella* ⇧	
	[*Streptococcaceae*]	*Streptococcus* ⇧	
	[*Clostridiaceae*]	*Clostridium* ⇧	
	[*Lachnospiraceae*]	*Eubacterium* ⇩	
Proteobacteria ⇧			
Fusobacteria ⇧			

[a]Microbiota were analyzed using 16S deep sequencing, except in the study of Qin et al., which used metagenomics. Additional taxonomic information for discriminating taxa is in brackets. Taxa in boldface are those identified in more than one study.

The survival rate of cirrhotic patients is dependent on the associated complications, including episodes of hepatic encephalopathy (HE), ascites, or infections, which have been associated with specific bacterial communities (132).

In cirrhotic patients, HE was associated with a specific dysbiosis: a high level of *Enterobacteriaceae*, already associated with infection in decompensated cirrhosis, was also associated with HE (133). *Alcaligenaceae*, bacteria that are specifically involved in urea metabolism, were also more abundant in HE patients. In a prospective clinical trial, VSL#3 was found to be efficient in preventing hepatic encephalopathy in cirrhotic patients, suggesting that the dysbiosis in HE may have a causative role (134). Conversely,

this treatment did not affect the portal pressure (135).

A cirrhosis dysbiosis ratio (CDR) has been developed to evaluate the severity of cirrhosis (132). The CDR is a ratio between the abundance of *Clostridiales* (*Clostridium* cluster XIV), *Ruminococcaceae*, and *Lachnospiraceae* and that of *Bacteroidaceae* and *Enterobacteriaceae*. Healthy patients have a CDR of approximately 2, decreasing to 0.9 in patients with compensated cirrhosis and to 0.3 in cirrhotic patients with an infection. *Enterobacteriaceae* is the most prevalent family modified in the CDR and is specifically associated with the complications of cirrhosis due to the production of potent endotoxins. The level of fecal *Bacteroidaceae* and *Clostridium* cluster XIV may predict the risk of hospitalization in patients with cirrhosis, independently of other classical clinical predictors, such as the MELD (model for end-stage liver disease) score, HE, or the intake of proton pump inhibitors (136). These data prove the relationship between dysbiosis and the severity of cirrhosis. Moreover, a randomized clinical trial using *Lactobacillus* GG in cirrhotic patients demonstrated that altering the composition of the IM through the use of probiotics improved dysbiosis and endotoxemia (137).

Viable bacteria have been found in the ascites of patients with decompensated cirrhosis, including several species of *Propionibacterium*, *Pseudomonas*, and *Staphylococcus* recognized as commonly colonizing the skin (138). Thus, access to the peritoneal cavity is not limited to the translocation of bacteria from the gut. The quantity of bacteria in the ascites is not sufficient to induce spontaneous bacterial peritonitis, but there is a relationship between the bacterial species and the severity of the disease (138).

Bacterial metabolites are related to the abundance of the bacterial species and may have beneficial or deleterious effects. Secondary BAs are exclusively produced by the IM. Cirrhosis has been recently shown to be associated with the abundance of specific bacterial families and to be linked with a decrease in the amount of secondary BAs in the feces (101, 132). Moreover, BA levels can discriminate between patients with severe alcoholic hepatitis associated with cirrhosis and alcoholic patients without liver lesions (97). Further studies are needed to decipher the spectra of metabolites that mediate the deleterious effects of bacterial dysbiosis.

Hepatocellular Carcinoma

HCC occurs in the presence of chronic liver inflammation, typically in patients with cirrhosis (139). To understand the contribution of NAFLD or ALD to the development of HCC, other causes of liver disease need to be excluded, especially HBV or HCV infection.

TLR4 deficiency resulted in decreased promotion of HCC but did not affect HCC initiation in chemically induced HCC in adult mice, either by diethylnitrosamine (DEN) alone or by DEN and chronic CCL4 injections (140, 141). Sterilization of the gut by antibiotherapy decreased both HCC initiation and progression. Accordingly, germ-free mice showed an approximately 80% reduction of HCC (140). Altogether, these data show that the inhibition of the LPS/TLR4 pathway prevents HCC progression. However, opposite results were obtained in another model of HCC, using TLR4-deficient mice in which HCC was induced by the unique injection of DEN, 15 days after birth (142). These discrepancies can be explained by the high frequency of DNA mutations in this DEN model relative to DEN injections in adult rodents associated with the development of a chronic liver inflammation. In humans, only indirect evidence has been published and showed that TLR2, -4, and -9 overexpression was associated with a poor prognosis for HCC progression (143).

The role of the IM was recently assessed in obesity-associated HCC. HCC was chemically induced in mice using DMBA [7,12-dimethylbenz(a)anthracene] at the neonatal stage. The association of DMBA and HFD induced tumor development in the mice (65). The analysis of serum metabolites showed an increase in DCA levels in mice that developed tumors. The production of the secondary BA DCA by the IM was associated with the presence of *Clostridium* species that harbored a 7α-dehydroxylase function to metabolize primary BAs (144). DCA levels were lowered using UDCA or by chemical inhibition of 7α-dehydroxylase. Moreover, vancomycin, which targets Gram-positive bacteria, especially *Clostridium*, also decreased serum DCA levels. Under these conditions, lowering serum DCA levels reduced HCC development.

These findings provide new evidence that the IM could be involved in the initiation and progression of HCC.

CONCLUSION

The complex community of the intestinal bacteria influences both the normal and pathological states of the liver, and we are only beginning to understand the mechanisms involved in this relationship. In dysbiosis of the gut microbiota associated with metabolic or alcoholic liver diseases, the changes in bacterial gene expression or metabolite production may be more important than the changes in bacterial composition. Understanding the clinical significance of gut microbiota dysbiosis in the context of liver disease remains a challenge and must consider the possible association between host genetic or/and epigenetic changes that favor liver injury. Further studies are needed, combining metagenomics, metatranscriptomics, and metabolomics with longitudinal studies, along with standardization of these techniques, to better comprehend the role of microbiota changes in the development of liver disease.

Many studies already strongly suggest that targeting the IM through the use of pro-, pre-, and symbiotics, and possibly fecal transfer, may be an effective treatment for NAFLD and ALD. However, larger studies incorporating liver biopsies, standardized dose administration and duration, and an analysis of the impact on the gut microbiota are clearly needed. This should help to open new treatment strategies based on the modulation of the gut microbiota.

CITATION

Cassard A-M, Gérard P, Perlemuter G. 2017. Microbiota, liver diseases, and alcohol. Microbiol Spectrum 5(4):BAD-0007-2016.

REFERENCES

1. **Perlemuter G, Bigorgne A, Cassard-Doulcier AM, Naveau S.** 2007. Nonalcoholic fatty liver disease: from pathogenesis to patient care. *Nat Clin Pract Endocrinol Metab* **3**:458–469.

2. **Voican CS, Perlemuter G, Naveau S.** 2011. Mechanisms of the inflammatory reaction implicated in alcoholic hepatitis: 2011 update. *Clin Res Hepatol Gastroenterol* **35**:465–474.

3. **Voican CS, Njiké-Nakseu M, Boujedidi H, Barri-Ova N, Bouchet-Delbos L, Agostini H, Maitre S, Prévot S, Cassard-Doulcier AM, Naveau S, Perlemuter G.** 2015. Alcohol withdrawal alleviates adipose tissue inflammation in patients with alcoholic liver disease. *Liver Int* **35**:967–978.

4. **Hardy T, Oakley F, Anstee QM, Day CP.** 2016. Nonalcoholic fatty liver disease: pathogenesis and disease spectrum. *Annu Rev Pathol* **11**:151–496.

5. **Bedossa P.** 2013. Current histological classification of NAFLD: strength and limitations. *Hepatol Int* **7**(Suppl 2):765–770.

6. **European Association for the Study of the Liver–European Organisation for Research and Treatment of Cancer.** 2012. EASL-EORTC clinical practice guidelines: management of hepatocellular carcinoma. *J Hepatol* **56**:908–943.

7. **Paradis V, Zalinski S, Chelbi E, Guedj N, Degos F, Vilgrain V, Bedossa P, Belghiti J.** 2009. Hepatocellular carcinomas in patients with metabolic syndrome often develop without significant liver fibrosis: a pathological analysis. *Hepatology* **49**:851–859.

8. **Dugum M, McCullough A.** 2015. Diagnosis and management of alcoholic liver disease. *J Clin Transl Hepatol* **3**:109–116.

9. **Naveau S, Cassard-Doulcier AM, Njiké-Nakseu M, Bouchet-Delbos L, Barri-Ova N, Boujedidi H, Dauvois B, Balian A, Maitre S, Prévot S, Dagher I, Agostini H, Grangeot-Keros L, Emilie D, Perlemuter G.** 2010. Harmful effect of adipose tissue on liver lesions in patients with alcoholic liver disease. *J Hepatol* **52**:895–902.

10. **Saadeh S, Younossi ZM, Remer EM, Gramlich T, Ong JP, Hurley M, Mullen KD, Cooper JN, Sheridan MJ.** 2002. The utility of radiological imaging in nonalcoholic fatty liver disease. *Gastroenterology* **123**:745–750.

11. **Musso G.** 2011. The Finnish Diabetes Risk Score (FINDRISC) and other non-invasive scores for screening of hepatic steatosis and associated cardiometabolic risk. *Ann Med* **43**:413–417.

12. **Ekstedt M, Franzén LE, Mathiesen UL, Thorelius L, Holmqvist M, Bodemar G, Kechagias S.** 2006. Long-term follow-up of patients with NAFLD and elevated liver enzymes. *Hepatology* **44**:865–873.

13. **Adams LA, Lymp JF, St Sauver J, Sanderson SO, Lindor KD, Feldstein A, Angulo P.** 2005. The natural history of nonalcoholic fatty liver

disease: a population-based cohort study. *Gastroenterology* **129:**113–121.

14. **Angulo P, Kleiner DE, Dam-Larsen S, Adams LA, Bjornsson ES, Charatcharoenwitthaya P, Mills PR, Keach JC, Lafferty HD, Stahler A, Haflidadottir S, Bendtsen F.** 2015. Liver fibrosis, but no other histologic features, is associated with long-term outcomes of patients with nonalcoholic fatty liver disease. *Gastroenterology* **149:**389–397.e10.

15. **McPherson S, Hardy T, Henderson E, Burt AD, Day CP, Anstee QM.** 2015. Evidence of NAFLD progression from steatosis to fibrosing-steatohepatitis using paired biopsies: implications for prognosis and clinical management. *J Hepatol* **62:**1148–1155.

16. **Ratziu V, Giral P, Charlotte F, Bruckert E, Thibault V, Theodorou I, Khalil L, Turpin G, Opolon P, Poynard T.** 2000. Liver fibrosis in overweight patients. *Gastroenterology* **118:**1117–1123.

17. **Ertle J, Dechêne A, Sowa JP, Penndorf V, Herzer K, Kaiser G, Schlaak JF, Gerken G, Syn WK, Canbay A.** 2011. Non-alcoholic fatty liver disease progresses to hepatocellular carcinoma in the absence of apparent cirrhosis. *Int J Cancer* **128:**2436–2443.

18. **Promrat K, Kleiner DE, Niemeier HM, Jackvony E, Kearns M, Wands JR, Fava JL, Wing RR.** 2010. Randomized controlled trial testing the effects of weight loss on nonalcoholic steatohepatitis. *Hepatology* **51:**121–129.

19. **Kistler KD, Brunt EM, Clark JM, Diehl AM, Sallis JF, Schwimmer JB, NASH CRN Research Group.** 2011. Physical activity recommendations, exercise intensity, and histological severity of nonalcoholic fatty liver disease. *Am J Gastroenterol* **106:**460–468, quiz 469.

20. **Wu T, Gao X, Chen M, van Dam RM.** 2009. Long-term effectiveness of diet-plus-exercise interventions vs. diet-only interventions for weight loss: a meta-analysis. *Obes Rev* **10:**313–323.

21. **Hardy T, Anstee QM, Day CP.** 2015. Nonalcoholic fatty liver disease: new treatments. *Curr Opin Gastroenterol* **31:**175–183.

22. **Mackenzie TA, Zaha R, Smith J, Karagas MR, Morden NE.** 2016. Diabetes pharmacotherapies and bladder cancer: a medicare epidemiologic study. *Diabetes Ther* **7:**61–73.

23. **Shin NR, Lee JC, Lee HY, Kim MS, Whon TW, Lee MS, Bae JW.** 2014. An increase in the *Akkermansia* spp. population induced by metformin treatment improves glucose homeostasis in diet-induced obese mice. *Gut* **63:**727–735.

24. **Sanyal AJ, Chalasani N, Kowdley KV, McCullough A, Diehl AM, Bass NM, Neuschwander-Tetri BA, Lavine JE, Tonascia J, Unalp A, Van Natta M, Clark J, Brunt EM, Kleiner DE, Hoofnagle JH, Robuck PR, NASH Clinical Research Network.** 2010. Pioglitazone, vitamin E, or placebo for nonalcoholic steatohepatitis. *N Engl J Med* **362:**1675–1685.

25. **Neuschwander-Tetri BA, Loomba R, Sanyal AJ, Lavine JE, Van Natta ML, Abdelmalek MF, Chalasani N, Dasarathy S, Diehl AM, Hameed B, Kowdley KV, McCullough A, Terrault N, Clark JM, Tonascia J, Brunt EM, Kleiner DE, Doo E, NASH Clinical Research Network.** 2015. Farnesoid X nuclear receptor ligand obeticholic acid for non-cirrhotic, non-alcoholic steatohepatitis (FLINT): a multicentre, randomised, placebo-controlled trial. *Lancet* **385:**956–965.

26. **Lassailly G, Caiazzo R, Buob D, Pigeyre M, Verkindt H, Labreuche J, Raverdy V, Leteurtre E, Dharancy S, Louvet A, Romon M, Duhamel A, Pattou F, Mathurin P.** 2015. Bariatric surgery reduces features of nonalcoholic steatohepatitis in morbidly obese patients. *Gastroenterology* **149:** 379–388; quiz e315–376.

27. **Thursz MR, Forrest EH, Ryder S, STOPAH Investigators.** 2015. Prednisolone or pentoxifylline for alcoholic hepatitis. *N Engl J Med* **373:** 282–283.

28. **Mathurin P, Louvet A, Duhamel A, Nahon P, Carbonell N, Boursier J, Anty R, Diaz E, Thabut D, Moirand R, Lebrec D, Moreno C, Talbodec N, Paupard T, Naveau S, Silvain C, Pageaux GP, Sobesky R, Canva-Delcambre V, Dharancy S, Salleron J, Dao T.** 2013. Prednisolone with vs without pentoxifylline and survival of patients with severe alcoholic hepatitis: a randomized clinical trial. *JAMA* **310:**1033–1041.

29. **Thursz MR, Richardson P, Allison M, Austin A, Bowers M, Day CP, Downs N, Gleeson D, MacGilchrist A, Grant A, Hood S, Masson S, McCune A, Mellor J, O'Grady J, Patch D, Ratcliffe I, Roderick P, Stanton L, Vergis N, Wright M, Ryder S, Forrest EH, STOPAH Trial.** 2015. Prednisolone or pentoxifylline for alcoholic hepatitis. *N Engl J Med* **372:**1619–1628.

30. **Nguyen-Khac E, Thevenot T, Piquet MA, Benferhat S, Goria O, Chatelain D, Tramier B, Dewaele F, Ghrib S, Rudler M, Carbonell N, Tossou H, Bental A, Bernard-Chabert B, Dupas JL, AAH-NAC Study Group.** 2011. Glucocorticoids plus N-acetylcysteine in severe alcoholic hepatitis. *N Engl J Med* **365:**1781–1789.

31. **Thursz M, Morgan TR.** 2016. Treatment of severe alcoholic hepatitis. *Gastroenterology* **150:**1823–1834.

32. **Mathurin P, Moreno C, Samuel D, Dumortier J, Salleron J, Durand F, Castel H, Duhamel A, Pageaux GP, Leroy V, Dharancy S, Louvet A, Boleslawski E, Lucidi V, Gustot T, Francoz C, Letoublon C, Castaing D, Belghiti J, Donckier V, Pruvot FR, Duclos-Vallée JC.** 2011. Early liver transplantation for severe alcoholic hepatitis. *N Engl J Med* **365**:1790–1800.

33. **Zeng H, Liu J, Jackson MI, Zhao FQ, Yan L, Combs GF Jr.** 2013. Fatty liver accompanies an increase in lactobacillus species in the hind gut of C57BL/6 mice fed a high-fat diet. *J Nutr* **143**:627–631.

34. **Zhu L, Baker SS, Gill C, Liu W, Alkhouri R, Baker RD, Gill SR.** 2013. Characterization of gut microbiomes in nonalcoholic steatohepatitis (NASH) patients: a connection between endogenous alcohol and NASH. *Hepatology* **57**:601–609.

35. **Raman M, Ahmed I, Gillevet PM, Probert CS, Ratcliffe NM, Smith S, Greenwood R, Sikaroodi M, Lam V, Crotty P, Bailey J, Myers RP, Rioux KP.** 2013. Fecal microbiome and volatile organic compound metabolome in obese humans with nonalcoholic fatty liver disease. *Clin Gastroenterol Hepatol* **11**:868–875.e1–3.

36. **Jiang W, Wu N, Wang X, Chi Y, Zhang Y, Qiu X, Hu Y, Li J, Liu Y.** 2015. Dysbiosis gut microbiota associated with inflammation and impaired mucosal immune function in intestine of humans with non-alcoholic fatty liver disease. *Sci Rep* **5**:8096.

37. **Mouzaki M, Comelli EM, Arendt BM, Bonengel J, Fung SK, Fischer SE, McGilvray ID, Allard JP.** 2013. Intestinal microbiota in patients with nonalcoholic fatty liver disease. *Hepatology* **58**:120–127.

38. **Wong VW, Tse CH, Lam TT, Wong GL, Chim AM, Chu WC, Yeung DK, Law PT, Kwan HS, Yu J, Sung JJ, Chan HL.** 2013. Molecular characterization of the fecal microbiota in patients with nonalcoholic steatohepatitis—a longitudinal study. *PLoS One* **8**:e62885.

39. **Wang B, Jiang X, Cao M, Ge J, Bao Q, Tang L, Chen Y, Li L.** 2016. Altered fecal microbiota correlates with liver biochemistry in nonobese patients with non-alcoholic fatty liver disease. *Sci Rep* **6**:32002.

40. **Spencer MD, Hamp TJ, Reid RW, Fischer LM, Zeisel SH, Fodor AA.** 2011. Association between composition of the human gastrointestinal microbiome and development of fatty liver with choline deficiency. *Gastroenterology* **140**:976–986.

41. **Gérard P.** 2016. Gut microbiota and obesity. *Cell Mol Life Sci* **73**:147–162.

42. **Wang ZK, Yang YS, Chen Y, Yuan J, Sun G, Peng LH.** 2014. Intestinal microbiota pathogenesis and fecal microbiota transplantation for inflammatory bowel disease. *World J Gastroenterol* **20**:14805–14820.

43. **Claus SP, Ellero SL, Berger B, Krause L, Bruttin A, Molina J, Paris A, Want EJ, de Waziers I, Cloarec O, Richards SE, Wang Y, Dumas ME, Ross A, Rezzi S, Kochhar S, Van Bladeren P, Lindon JC, Holmes E, Nicholson JK.** 2011. Colonization-induced host-gut microbial metabolic interaction. *mBio* **2**:e00271-10.

44. **Henao-Mejia J, Elinav E, Jin C, Hao L, Mehal WZ, Strowig T, Thaiss CA, Kau AL, Eisenbarth SC, Jurczak MJ, Camporez JP, Shulman GI, Gordon JI, Hoffman HM, Flavell RA.** 2012. Inflammasome-mediated dysbiosis regulates progression of NAFLD and obesity. *Nature* **482**:179–185.

45. **Le Roy T, Llopis M, Lepage P, Bruneau A, Rabot S, Bevilacqua C, Martin P, Philippe C, Walker F, Bado A, Perlemuter G, Cassard-Doulcier AM, Gérard P.** 2013. Intestinal microbiota determines development of non-alcoholic fatty liver disease in mice. *Gut* **62**:1787–1794.

46. **Ferolla SM, Armiliato GN, Couto CA, Ferrari TC.** 2014. The role of intestinal bacteria overgrowth in obesity-related nonalcoholic fatty liver disease. *Nutrients* **6**:5583–5599.

47. **Miele L, Valenza V, La Torre G, Montalto M, Cammarota G, Ricci R, Masciana R, Forgione A, Gabrieli ML, Perotti G, Vecchio FM, Rapaccini G, Gasbarrini G, Day CP, Grieco A.** 2009. Increased intestinal permeability and tight junction alterations in nonalcoholic fatty liver disease. *Hepatology* **49**:1877–1887.

48. **Giorgio V, Miele L, Principessa L, Ferretti F, Villa MP, Negro V, Grieco A, Alisi A, Nobili V.** 2014. Intestinal permeability is increased in children with non-alcoholic fatty liver disease, and correlates with liver disease severity. *Dig Liver Dis* **46**:556–560.

49. **Cani PD, Amar J, Iglesias MA, Poggi M, Knauf C, Bastelica D, Neyrinck AM, Fava F, Tuohy KM, Chabo C, Waget A, Delmée E, Cousin B, Sulpice T, Chamontin B, Ferrières J, Tanti JF, Gibson GR, Casteilla L, Delzenne NM, Alessi MC, Burcelin R.** 2007. Metabolic endotoxemia initiates obesity and insulin resistance. *Diabetes* **56**:1761–1772.

50. **Poggi M, Bastelica D, Gual P, Iglesias MA, Gremeaux T, Knauf C, Peiretti F, Verdier M, Juhan-Vague I, Tanti JF, Burcelin R, Alessi MC.** 2007. C3H/HeJ mice carrying a toll-like receptor 4 mutation are protected against the development of insulin resistance in white adipose tissue in response to a high-fat diet. *Diabetologia* **50**:1267–1276.

51. **Ye D, Li FY, Lam KS, Li H, Jia W, Wang Y, Man K, Lo CM, Li X, Xu A.** 2012. Toll-like receptor-4 mediates obesity-induced non-alcoholic steatohepatitis through activation of X-box binding protein-1 in mice. *Gut* **61:** 1058–1067.

52. **Laugerette F, Vors C, Géloën A, Chauvin MA, Soulage C, Lambert-Porcheron S, Peretti N, Alligier M, Burcelin R, Laville M, Vidal H, Michalski MC.** 2011. Emulsified lipids increase endotoxemia: possible role in early postprandial low-grade inflammation. *J Nutr Biochem* **22:**53–59.

53. **Harte AL, da Silva NF, Creely SJ, McGee KC, Billyard T, Youssef-Elabd EM, Tripathi G, Ashour E, Abdalla MS, Sharada HM, Amin AI, Burt AD, Kumar S, Day CP, McTernan PG.** 2010. Elevated endotoxin levels in non-alcoholic fatty liver disease. *J Inflamm (Lond)* **7:**15.

54. **Verdam FJ, Rensen SS, Driessen A, Greve JW, Buurman WA.** 2011. Novel evidence for chronic exposure to endotoxin in human nonalcoholic steatohepatitis. *J Clin Gastroenterol* **45:**149–152.

55. **Yuan J, Baker SS, Liu W, Alkhouri R, Baker RD, Xie J, Ji G, Zhu L.** 2014. Endotoxemia unrequired in the pathogenesis of pediatric nonalcoholic steatohepatitis. *J Gastroenterol Hepatol* **29:**1292–1298.

56. **de Medeiros IC, de Lima JG.** 2015. Is nonalcoholic fatty liver disease an endogenous alcoholic fatty liver disease? - A mechanistic hypothesis. *Med Hypotheses* **85:**148–152.

57. **Volynets V, Küper MA, Strahl S, Maier IB, Spruss A, Wagnerberger S, Königsrainer A, Bischoff SC, Bergheim I.** 2012. Nutrition, intestinal permeability, and blood ethanol levels are altered in patients with nonalcoholic fatty liver disease (NAFLD). *Dig Dis Sci* **57:**1932–1941.

58. **Buchman AL, Dubin MD, Moukarzel AA, Jenden DJ, Roch M, Rice KM, Gornbein J, Ament ME.** 1995. Choline deficiency: a cause of hepatic steatosis during parenteral nutrition that can be reversed with intravenous choline supplementation. *Hepatology* **22:**1399–1403.

59. **Dumas ME, Barton RH, Toye A, Cloarec O, Blancher C, Rothwell A, Fearnside J, Tatoud R, Blanc V, Lindon JC, Mitchell SC, Holmes E, McCarthy MI, Scott J, Gauguier D, Nicholson JK.** 2006. Metabolic profiling reveals a contribution of gut microbiota to fatty liver phenotype in insulin-resistant mice. *Proc Natl Acad Sci USA* **103:**12511–12516.

60. **Hofmann AF, Hagey LR, Krasowski MD.** 2010. Bile salts of vertebrates: structural variation and possible evolutionary significance. *J Lipid Res* **51:**226–246.

61. **Ridlon JM, Kang DJ, Hylemon PB.** 2006. Bile salt biotransformations by human intestinal bacteria. *J Lipid Res* **47:**241–259.

62. **Hylemon PB, Zhou H, Pandak WM, Ren S, Gil G, Dent P.** 2009. Bile acids as regulatory molecules. *J Lipid Res* **50:**1509–1520.

63. **Gérard P.** 2013. Metabolism of cholesterol and bile acids by the gut microbiota. *Pathogens* **3:**14–24.

64. **Hofmann AF.** 2004. Detoxification of lithocholic acid, a toxic bile acid: relevance to drug hepatotoxicity. *Drug Metab Rev* **36:**703–722.

65. **Yoshimoto S, Loo TM, Atarashi K, Kanda H, Sato S, Oyadomari S, Iwakura Y, Oshima K, Morita H, Hattori M, Honda K, Ishikawa Y, Hara E, Ohtani N.** 2013. Obesity-induced gut microbial metabolite promotes liver cancer through senescence secretome. *Nature* **499:** 97–101.

66. **Stenman LK, Holma R, Forsgård R, Gylling H, Korpela R.** 2013. Higher fecal bile acid hydrophobicity is associated with exacerbation of dextran sodium sulfate colitis in mice. *J Nutr* **143:**1691–1697.

67. **Lepercq P, Gérard P, Béguet F, Raibaud P, Grill JP, Relano P, Cayuela C, Juste C.** 2004. Epimerization of chenodeoxycholic acid to ursodeoxycholic acid by *Clostridium baratii* isolated from human feces. *FEMS Microbiol Lett* **235:**65–72.

68. **Ritze Y, Bárdos G, Claus A, Ehrmann V, Bergheim I, Schwiertz A, Bischoff SC.** 2014. *Lactobacillus rhamnosus* GG protects against non-alcoholic fatty liver disease in mice. *PLoS One* **9:**e80169.

69. **Cano PG, Santacruz A, Trejo FM, Sanz Y.** 2013. *Bifidobacterium* CECT 7765 improves metabolic and immunological alterations associated with obesity in high-fat diet-fed mice. *Obesity (Silver Spring)* **21:**2310–2321.

70. **Gauffin Cano P, Santacruz A, Moya Á, Sanz Y.** 2012. *Bacteroides uniformis* CECT 7771 ameliorates metabolic and immunological dysfunction in mice with high-fat-diet induced obesity. *PLoS One* **7:**e41079.

71. **Okubo H, Sakoda H, Kushiyama A, Fujishiro M, Nakatsu Y, Fukushima T, Matsunaga Y, Kamata H, Asahara T, Yoshida Y, Chonan O, Iwashita M, Nishimura F, Asano T.** 2013. *Lactobacillus casei* strain Shirota protects against nonalcoholic steatohepatitis development in a rodent model. *Am J Physiol Gastrointest Liver Physiol* **305:**G911–G918.

72. **Nardone G, Compare D, Liguori E, Di Mauro V, Rocco A, Barone M, Napoli A, Lapi D,**

Iovene MR, Colantuoni A. 2010. Protective effects of *Lactobacillus paracasei* F19 in a rat model of oxidative and metabolic hepatic injury. *Am J Physiol Gastrointest Liver Physiol* 299:G669–G676.

73. Ma X, Hua J, Li Z. 2008. Probiotics improve high fat diet-induced hepatic steatosis and insulin resistance by increasing hepatic NKT cells. *J Hepatol* 49:821–830.

74. Li Z, Yang S, Lin H, Huang J, Watkins PA, Moser AB, Desimone C, Song XY, Diehl AM. 2003. Probiotics and antibodies to TNF inhibit inflammatory activity and improve nonalcoholic fatty liver disease. *Hepatology* 37:343–350.

75. Ma YY, Li L, Yu CH, Shen Z, Chen LH, Li YM. 2013. Effects of probiotics on nonalcoholic fatty liver disease: a meta-analysis. *World J Gastroenterol* 19:6911–6918.

76. Everard A, Belzer C, Geurts L, Ouwerkerk JP, Druart C, Bindels LB, Guiot Y, Derrien M, Muccioli GG, Delzenne NM, de Vos WM, Cani PD. 2013. Cross-talk between *Akkermansia muciniphila* and intestinal epithelium controls diet-induced obesity. *Proc Natl Acad Sci USA* 110:9066–9071.

77. Pachikian BD, Essaghir A, Demoulin JB, Catry E, Neyrinck AM, Dewulf EM, Sohet FM, Portois L, Clerbaux LA, Carpentier YA, Possemiers S, Bommer GT, Cani PD, Delzenne NM. 2013. Prebiotic approach alleviates hepatic steatosis: implication of fatty acid oxidative and cholesterol synthesis pathways. *Mol Nutr Food Res* 57:347–359.

78. Foschini MP, Macchia S, Losi L, Dei Tos AP, Pasquinelli G, Di Tommaso L, Del Duca S, Roncaroli F, Dal Monte PR. 1998. Identification of mitochondria in liver biopsies. A study by immunohistochemistry, immunogold and Western blot analysis. *Virchows Arch* 433:267–273.

79. Malaguarnera M, Vacante M, Antic T, Giordano M, Chisari G, Acquaviva R, Mastrojeni S, Malaguarnera G, Mistretta A, Li Volti G, Galvano F. 2012. *Bifidobacterium longum* with fructo-oligosaccharides in patients with non alcoholic steatohepatitis. *Dig Dis Sci* 57:545–553.

80. Eslamparast T, Poustchi H, Zamani F, Sharafkhah M, Malekzadeh R, Hekmatdoost A. 2014. Synbiotic supplementation in nonalcoholic fatty liver disease: a randomized, double-blind, placebo-controlled pilot study. *Am J Clin Nutr* 99:535–542.

81. Adachi Y, Moore LE, Bradford BU, Gao W, Thurman RG. 1995. Antibiotics prevent liver injury in rats following long-term exposure to ethanol. *Gastroenterology* 108:218–224.

82. Bode C, Kugler V, Bode JC. 1987. Endotoxemia in patients with alcoholic and non-alcoholic cirrhosis and in subjects with no evidence of chronic liver disease following acute alcohol excess. *J Hepatol* 4:8–14.

83. Mathurin P, Deng QG, Keshavarzian A, Choudhary S, Holmes EW, Tsukamoto H. 2000. Exacerbation of alcoholic liver injury by enteral endotoxin in rats. *Hepatology* 32:1008–1017.

84. Nanji AA, Khettry U, Sadrzadeh SM, Yamanaka T. 1993. Severity of liver injury in experimental alcoholic liver disease. Correlation with plasma endotoxin, prostaglandin E2, leukotriene B4, and thromboxane B2. *Am J Pathol* 142:367–373.

85. Keshavarzian A, Fields JZ, Vaeth J, Holmes EW. 1994. The differing effects of acute and chronic alcohol on gastric and intestinal permeability. *Am J Gastroenterol* 89:2205–2211.

86. Parlesak A, Schäfer C, Schütz T, Bode JC, Bode C. 2000. Increased intestinal permeability to macromolecules and endotoxemia in patients with chronic alcohol abuse in different stages of alcohol-induced liver disease. *J Hepatol* 32:742–747.

87. Rao R. 2009. Endotoxemia and gut barrier dysfunction in alcoholic liver disease. *Hepatology* 50:638–644.

88. Elamin EE, Masclee AA, Dekker J, Jonkers DM. 2013. Ethanol metabolism and its effects on the intestinal epithelial barrier. *Nutr Rev* 71:483–499.

89. Zhong W, Li Q, Xie G, Sun X, Tan X, Sun X, Jia W, Zhou Z. 2013. Dietary fat sources differentially modulate intestinal barrier and hepatic inflammation in alcohol-induced liver injury in rats. *Am J Physiol Gastrointest Liver Physiol* 305:G919–G932.

90. Grewal RK, Mahmood A. 2009. Ethanol induced changes in glycosylation of mucins in rat intestine. *Ann Gastroenterol* 22:178–183.

91. Ferrier L, Bérard F, Debrauwer L, Chabo C, Langella P, Buéno L, Fioramonti J. 2006. Impairment of the intestinal barrier by ethanol involves enteric microflora and mast cell activation in rodents. *Am J Pathol* 168:1148–1154.

92. Ulluwishewa D, Anderson RC, McNabb WC, Moughan PJ, Wells JM, Roy NC. 2011. Regulation of tight junction permeability by intestinal bacteria and dietary components. *J Nutr* 141:769–776.

93. Bull-Otterson L, Feng W, Kirpich I, Wang Y, Qin X, Liu Y, Gobejishvili L, Joshi-Barve S, Ayvaz T, Petrosino J, Kong M, Barker D, McClain C, Barve S. 2013. Metagenomic analyses of alcohol induced pathogenic alterations in the intestinal microbiome and the effect of *Lactobacillus rhamnosus* GG treatment. *PLoS One* 8:e53028.

94. Mutlu E, Keshavarzian A, Engen P, Forsyth CB, Sikaroodi M, Gillevet P. 2009. Intestinal dysbiosis: a possible mechanism of alcohol-induced endotoxemia and alcoholic steatohepatitis in rats. *Alcohol Clin Exp Res* **33:** 1836–1846.

95. Yan AW, Fouts DE, Brandl J, Stärkel P, Torralba M, Schott E, Tsukamoto H, Nelson KE, Brenner DA, Schnabl B. 2011. Enteric dysbiosis associated with a mouse model of alcoholic liver disease. *Hepatology* **53:**96–105.

96. Mutlu EA, Gillevet PM, Rangwala H, Sikaroodi M, Naqvi A, Engen PA, Kwasny M, Lau CK, Keshavarzian A. 2012. Colonic microbiome is altered in alcoholism. *Am J Physiol Gastrointest Liver Physiol* **302:**G966–G978.

97. Llopis M, Cassard AM, Wrzosek L, Boschat L, Bruneau A, Ferrere G, Puchois V, Martin JC, Lepage P, Le Roy T, Lefèvre L, Langelier B, Cailleux F, González-Castro AM, Rabot S, Gaudin F, Agostini H, Prévot S, Berrebi D, Ciocan D, Jousse C, Naveau S, Gérard P, Perlemuter G. 2016. Intestinal microbiota contributes to individual susceptibility to alcoholic liver disease. *Gut* **65:**830–839.

98. Dorrestein PC, Mazmanian SK, Knight R. 2014. Finding the missing links among metabolites, microbes, and the host. *Immunity* **40:**824–832.

99. Couch RD, Dailey A, Zaidi F, Navarro K, Forsyth CB, Mutlu E, Engen PA, Keshavarzian A. 2015. Alcohol induced alterations to the human fecal VOC metabolome. *PLoS One* **10:**e0119362.

100. Xie G, Zhong W, Li H, Li Q, Qiu Y, Zheng X, Chen H, Zhao X, Zhang S, Zhou Z, Zeisel SH, Jia W. 2013. Alteration of bile acid metabolism in the rat induced by chronic ethanol consumption. *FASEB J* **27:**3583–3593.

101. Kakiyama G, Pandak WM, Gillevet PM, Hylemon PB, Heuman DM, Daita K, Takei H, Muto A, Nittono H, Ridlon JM, White MB, Noble NA, Monteith P, Fuchs M, Thacker LR, Sikaroodi M, Bajaj JS. 2013. Modulation of the fecal bile acid profile by gut microbiota in cirrhosis. *J Hepatol* **58:**949–955.

102. Jones ML, Martoni CJ, Ganopolsky JG, Labbé A, Prakash S. 2014. The human microbiome and bile acid metabolism: dysbiosis, dysmetabolism, disease and intervention. *Expert Opin Biol Ther* **14:**467–482.

103. Lefebvre P, Cariou B, Lien F, Kuipers F, Staels B. 2009. Role of bile acids and bile acid receptors in metabolic regulation. *Physiol Rev* **89:**147–191.

104. Manley S, Ding W. 2015. Role of farnesoid X receptor and bile acids in alcoholic liver disease. *Acta Pharm Sin B* **5:**158–167.

105. Wu WB, Chen YY, Zhu B, Peng XM, Zhang SW, Zhou ML. 2015. Excessive bile acid activated NF-kappa B and promoted the development of alcoholic steatohepatitis in farnesoid X receptor deficient mice. *Biochimie* **115:**86–92.

106. Fouts DE, Torralba M, Nelson KE, Brenner DA, Schnabl B. 2012. Bacterial translocation and changes in the intestinal microbiome in mouse models of liver disease. *J Hepatol* **56:** 1283–1292.

107. Hartmann P, Chen P, Wang HJ, Wang L, McCole DF, Brandl K, Stärkel P, Belzer C, Hellerbrand C, Tsukamoto H, Ho SB, Schnabl B. 2013. Deficiency of intestinal mucin-2 ameliorates experimental alcoholic liver disease in mice. *Hepatology* **58:**108–119.

108. Wang L, Fouts DE, Stärkel P, Hartmann P, Chen P, Llorente C, DePew J, Moncera K, Ho SB, Brenner DA, Hooper LV, Schnabl B. 2016. Intestinal REG3 lectins protect against alcoholic steatohepatitis by reducing mucosa-associated microbiota and preventing bacterial translocation. *Cell Host Microbe* **19:**227–239.

109. Ferrere G, Wrzosek L, Cailleux F, Turpin W, Puchois V, Spatz M, Ciocan D, Rainteau D, Humbert L, Hugot C, Gaudin F, Noordine ML, Robert V, Berrebi D, Thomas M, Naveau S, Perlemuter G, Cassard AM. 2017. Fecal microbiota manipulation prevents dysbiosis and alcohol-induced liver injury in mice. *J Hepatol* **66:**806–815.

110. Little TJ, Feinle-Bisset C. 2011. Effects of dietary fat on appetite and energy intake in health and obesity–oral and gastrointestinal sensory contributions. *Physiol Behav* **104:**613–620.

111. Mithieux G. 2014. Crosstalk between gastrointestinal neurons and the brain in the control of food intake. *Best Pract Res Clin Endocrinol Metab* **28:**739–744.

112. Bauer KC, Huus KE, Finlay BB. 2016. Microbes and the mind: emerging hallmarks of the gut microbiota-brain axis. *Cell Microbiol* **18:**632–644.

113. Leclercq S, Matamoros S, Cani PD, Neyrinck AM, Jamar F, Stärkel P, Windey K, Tremaroli V, Bäckhed F, Verbeke K, de Timary P, Delzenne NM. 2014. Intestinal permeability, gut-bacterial dysbiosis, and behavioral markers of alcohol-dependence severity. *Proc Natl Acad Sci USA* **111:**E4485–E4493.

114. Forsyth CB, Farhadi A, Jakate SM, Tang Y, Shaikh M, Keshavarzian A. 2009. *Lactobacillus* GG treatment ameliorates alcohol-induced intestinal oxidative stress, gut leakiness, and liver injury in a rat model of alcoholic steatohepatitis. *Alcohol* **43:**163–172.

115. **Nanji AA, Khettry U, Sadrzadeh SM.** 1994. *Lactobacillus* feeding reduces endotoxemia and severity of experimental alcoholic liver (disease). *Proc Soc Exp Biol Med* **205**:243–247.

116. **Keshavarzian A, Choudhary S, Holmes EW, Yong S, Banan A, Jakate S, Fields JZ.** 2001. Preventing gut leakiness by oats supplementation ameliorates alcohol-induced liver damage in rats. *J Pharmacol Exp Ther* **299**:442–448.

117. **Wang Y, Kirpich I, Liu Y, Ma Z, Barve S, McClain CJ, Feng W.** 2011. *Lactobacillus rhamnosus* GG treatment potentiates intestinal hypoxia-inducible factor, promotes intestinal integrity and ameliorates alcohol-induced liver injury. *Am J Pathol* **179**:2866–2875.

118. **Wang Y, Liu Y, Kirpich I, Ma Z, Wang C, Zhang M, Suttles J, McClain C, Feng W.** 2013. *Lactobacillus rhamnosus* GG reduces hepatic TNFα production and inflammation in chronic alcohol-induced liver injury. *J Nutr Biochem* **24**:1609–1615.

119. **Chang B, Sang L, Wang Y, Tong J, Zhang D, Wang B.** 2013. The protective effect of VSL#3 on intestinal permeability in a rat model of alcoholic intestinal injury. *BMC Gastroenterol* **13**:151.

120. **Loguercio C, Federico A, Tuccillo C, Terracciano F, D'Auria MV, De Simone C, Del Vecchio Blanco C.** 2005. Beneficial effects of a probiotic VSL#3 on parameters of liver dysfunction in chronic liver diseases. *J Clin Gastroenterol* **39**: 540–543.

121. **Zhong W, Zhou Z.** 2014. Alterations of the gut microbiome and metabolome in alcoholic liver disease. *World J Gastrointest Pathophysiol* **5**: 514–522.

122. **Boursier J, Mueller O, Barret M, Machado M, Fizanne L, Araujo-Perez F, Guy CD, Seed PC, Rawls JF, David LA, Hunault G, Oberti F, Calès P, Diehl AM.** 2016. The severity of nonalcoholic fatty liver disease is associated with gut dysbiosis and shift in the metabolic function of the gut microbiota. *Hepatology* **63**:764–775.

123. **De Minicis S, Rychlicki C, Agostinelli L, Saccomanno S, Candelaresi C, Trozzi L, Mingarelli E, Facinelli B, Magi G, Palmieri C, Marzioni M, Benedetti A, Svegliati-Baroni G.** 2014. Dysbiosis contributes to fibrogenesis in the course of chronic liver injury in mice. *Hepatology* **59**:1738–1749.

124. **Gómez-Hurtado I, Santacruz A, Peiró G, Zapater P, Gutiérrez A, Pérez-Mateo M, Sanz Y, Francés R.** 2011. Gut microbiota dysbiosis is associated with inflammation and bacterial translocation in mice with CCl4-induced fibrosis. *PLoS One* **6**:e23037.

125. **Cuenca S, Sanchez E, Santiago A, El Khader I, Panda S, Vidal S, Camilo Nieto J, Juárez C, Sancho F, Guarner F, Soriano G, Guarner C, Manichanh C.** 2014. Microbiome composition by pyrosequencing in mesenteric lymph nodes of rats with CCl4-induced cirrhosis. *J Innate Immun* **6**:263–271.

126. **Mazagova M, Wang L, Anfora AT, Wissmueller M, Lesley SA, Miyamoto Y, Eckmann L, Dhungana S, Pathmasiri W, Sumner S, Westwater C, Brenner DA, Schnabl B.** 2015. Commensal microbiota is hepatoprotective and prevents liver fibrosis in mice. *FASEB J* **29**:1043–1055.

127. **Li M, Zhu L, Xie A, Yuan J.** 2015. Oral administration of *Saccharomyces boulardii* ameliorates carbon tetrachloride-induced liver fibrosis in rats via reducing intestinal permeability and modulating gut microbial composition. *Inflammation* **38**:170–179.

128. **Sánchez E, Nieto JC, Boullosa A, Vidal S, Sancho FJ, Rossi G, Sancho-Bru P, Oms R, Mirelis B, Juárez C, Guarner C, Soriano G.** 2015. VSL#3 probiotic treatment decreases bacterial translocation in rats with carbon tetrachloride-induced cirrhosis. *Liver Int* **35**:735–745.

129. **Chen Y, Yang F, Lu H, Wang B, Chen Y, Lei D, Wang Y, Zhu B, Li L.** 2011. Characterization of fecal microbial communities in patients with liver cirrhosis. *Hepatology* **54**:562–572.

130. **Qin N, Yang F, Li A, Prifti E, Chen Y, Shao L, Guo J, Le Chatelier E, Yao J, Wu L, Zhou J, Ni S, Liu L, Pons N, Batto JM, Kennedy SP, Leonard P, Yuan C, Ding W, Chen Y, Hu X, Zheng B, Qian G, Xu W, Ehrlich SD, Zheng S, Li L.** 2014. Alterations of the human gut microbiome in liver cirrhosis. *Nature* **513**:59–64.

131. **Wei X, Yan X, Zou D, Yang Z, Wang X, Liu W, Wang S, Li X, Han J, Huang L, Yuan J.** 2013. Abnormal fecal microbiota community and functions in patients with hepatitis B liver cirrhosis as revealed by a metagenomic approach. *BMC Gastroenterol* **13**:175.

132. **Bajaj JS, Heuman DM, Hylemon PB, Sanyal AJ, White MB, Monteith P, Noble NA, Unser AB, Daita K, Fisher AR, Sikaroodi M, Gillevet PM.** 2014. Altered profile of human gut microbiome is associated with cirrhosis and its complications. *J Hepatol* **60**:940–947.

133. **Bajaj JS, Ridlon JM, Hylemon PB, Thacker LR, Heuman DM, Smith S, Sikaroodi M, Gillevet PM.** 2012. Linkage of gut microbiome with cognition in hepatic encephalopathy. *Am J Physiol Gastrointest Liver Physiol* **302**:G168–G175.

134. **Lunia MK, Sharma BC, Sharma P, Sachdeva S, Srivastava S.** 2014. Probiotics prevent

hepatic encephalopathy in patients with cirrhosis: a randomized controlled trial. *Clin Gastroenterol Hepatol* **12**:1003–1008.e1.

135. **Jayakumar S, Carbonneau M, Hotte N, Befus AD, St Laurent C, Owen R, McCarthy M, Madsen K, Bailey RJ, Ma M, Bain V, Rioux K, Tandon P.** 2013. VSL#3 ® probiotic therapy does not reduce portal pressures in patients with decompensated cirrhosis. *Liver Int* **33**:1470–1477.

136. **Bajaj JS, Betrapally NS, Hylemon PB, Thacker LR, Daita K, Kang DJ, White MB, Unser AB, Fagan A, Gavis EA, Sikaroodi M, Dalmet S, Heuman DM, Gillevet PM.** 2015. Gut microbiota alterations can predict hospitalizations in cirrhosis independent of diabetes mellitus. *Sci Rep* **5**:18559.

137. **Bajaj JS, Heuman DM, Hylemon PB, Sanyal AJ, Puri P, Sterling RK, Luketic V, Stravitz RT, Siddiqui MS, Fuchs M, Thacker LR, Wade JB, Daita K, Sistrun S, White MB, Noble NA, Thorpe C, Kakiyama G, Pandak WM, Sikaroodi M, Gillevet PM.** 2014. Randomised clinical trial: *Lactobacillus* GG modulates gut microbiome, metabolome and endotoxemia in patients with cirrhosis. *Aliment Pharmacol Ther* **39**:1113–1125.

138. **Rogers GB, van der Gast CJ, Bruce KD, Marsh P, Collins JE, Sutton J, Wright M.** 2013. Ascitic microbiota composition is correlated with clinical severity in cirrhosis with portal hypertension. *PLoS One* **8**:e74884.

139. **Sherman M.** 2010. Epidemiology of hepatocellular carcinoma. *Oncology* **78**(Suppl 1):7–10.

140. **Dapito DH, Mencin A, Gwak GY, Pradere JP, Jang MK, Mederacke I, Caviglia JM, Khiabanian H, Adeyemi A, Bataller R, Lefkowitch JH, Bower M, Friedman R, Sartor RB, Rabadan R, Schwabe RF.** 2012. Promotion of hepatocellular carcinoma by the intestinal microbiota and TLR4. *Cancer Cell* **21**:504–516.

141. **Yu LX, Yan HX, Liu Q, Yang W, Wu HP, Dong W, Tang L, Lin Y, He YQ, Zou SS, Wang C, Zhang HL, Cao GW, Wu MC, Wang HY.** 2010. Endotoxin accumulation prevents carcinogen-induced apoptosis and promotes liver tumorigenesis in rodents. *Hepatology* **52**: 1322–1333.

142. **Wang Z, Yan J, Lin H, Hua F, Wang X, Liu H, Lv X, Yu J, Mi S, Wang J, Hu ZW.** 2013. Toll-like receptor 4 activity protects against hepatocellular tumorigenesis and progression by regulating expression of DNA repair protein Ku70 in mice. *Hepatology* **57**:1869–1881.

143. **Eiro N, Altadill A, Juarez LM, Rodriguez M, Gonzalez LO, Atienza S, Bermudez S, Fernandez-Garcia B, Fresno-Forcelledo MF, Rodrigo L, Vizoso FJ.** 2014. Toll-like receptors 3, 4 and 9 in hepatocellular carcinoma: relationship with clinicopathological characteristics and prognosis. *Hepatology Res* **44**:769–778.

144. **Wells JE, Hylemon PB.** 2000. Identification and characterization of a bile acid 7alpha-dehydroxylation operon in *Clostridium* sp. strain TO-931, a highly active 7alpha-dehydroxylating strain isolated from human feces. *Appl Environ Microbiol* **66**:1107–1113.

The Potential of Probiotics as a Therapy for Osteoporosis

9

FRASER L. COLLINS,[1] NAIOMY D. RIOS-ARCE,[1] JONATHAN D. SCHEPPER,[1] NARAYANAN PARAMESWARAN,[1] and LAURA R. MCCABE[1,2,3]

THE SKELETON

The adult human skeleton comprises 206 bones, excluding the sesamoid bones (1). The bones are subdivided into four general types: long bones, short bones, flat bones, and irregular bones. Long bones such as the femur are composed of a hollow diaphysis which flares at the end to form the metaphysis, the region below the growth plate, and the epiphysis, the region above the growth plate. The diaphysis, also known as the shaft, is mainly composed of dense, solid bone known as cortical bone, whereas the metaphysis and epiphysis contain a honeycomb-like network of interconnected trabecular plates surrounding bone marrow known as cancellous or trabecular bone (1).

Bone is critical for structural support and movement, protection of vital organs, and maintenance of mineral homeostasis and hematopoiesis. Bone is a dynamic organ and is continuously undergoing remodeling. Control of bone remodeling is a highly complex process that involves integrative signals from not only the different bone cells but also from other systems including immune, neuronal, and hormonal systems (2, 3). While it has been known for a long time that the gastrointestinal system plays a critical role in bone

[1]Department of Physiology; [2]Department of Radiology; [3]Biomedical Imaging Research Center, Michigan State University, East Lansing, MI 48824
Bugs as Drugs: Therapeutic Microbes for the Prevention and Treatment of Disease
Edited by Robert A. Britton and Patrice D. Cani
© 2018 American Society for Microbiology, Washington, DC
doi:10.1128/microbiolspec.BAD-0015-2016

homeostasis via regulation of calcium absorption, recent studies underscore the emerging role of the gut microbiota in regulating bone remodeling. Thus, modification of the gut microbiota by ingesting probiotics could be a viable therapeutic strategy to regulate bone remodeling under a variety of conditions that lead to bone loss and osteoporosis. In this review we provide a comprehensive analysis of recent studies that have examined the effectiveness of probiotics for the treatment of bone loss and osteoporosis.

Bone Remodeling

Throughout a lifetime the skeleton is subjected to a variety of stresses and strains leading to the formation of cracks and microdamage. To maintain its integrity, the skeleton is continuously remodeled; in the adult human skeleton, 5 to 10% of the existing bone is replaced every year (4). Remodeling is accomplished by the coupled activities of a group of cells collectively termed the bone remodeling unit (5). The cells that constitute the bone remodeling unit are the osteoblasts, cells that produce the organic bone matrix and facilitate bone mineralization (6); the osteoclasts, cells responsible for the degradation of bone and extracellular matrix (7); the osteocytes, osteoblast-derived cells that lie within the bone matrix and act as mechanosensors and endocrine cells (8); and the bone-lining cells that form the canopy of the trabecular bone remodeling compartment and help to couple bone formation to resorption (9). There are four distinct phases in the bone remodeling cycle: initiation, resorption, reversal, and formation (see Fig. 1 for more details).

Osteoclasts and Osteoblasts

Osteoclasts are the principal cells responsible for bone resorption, while osteoblasts mediate bone formation. The osteoclast is a terminally differentiated, highly motile, multinucleated cell formed by the fusion of monocyte/macrophage precursors derived from hematopoietic origin (10) (Fig. 2). In contrast, osteoblasts arise from mesenchymal stem cells, which are pluripotent cells that have the potential to differentiate into numerous cell types including adipocytes, chondrocytes, and osteoblasts (11) (Fig. 3). Control of osteoclast and osteoblast differentiation is regulated by numerous cytokines, hormones, growth factors, and transcription factors (12, 13).

Osteoimmunology

While cells of the osteoblast and osteoclast lineage modulate each other's differentiation and function through cell-cell contact and diffusible paracrine factors, it is now well recognized that immune cells, including lymphocytes (T and B) and dendritic cells, also play a key role in modulating bone remodeling in both health and disease. This modulation occurs via direct and indirect measures through expression of a large number of cytokines which can have both a pro-osteoclastogenic effect, resulting in bone loss, or a pro-osteogenic effect, resulting in bone formation (Fig. 4) (12, 14).

BONE DISEASE

Diseases of the bone are typically characterized by direct or indirect effect on the balance of remodeling, with increased or decreased bone resorption/formation. Osteoporosis is a typical example of an imbalance in resorption/formation that is skewed more toward bone loss. By definition, osteoporosis is characterized by low bone mass and microarchitectural deterioration of bone tissue with a consequent increase in bone fragility and susceptibility to fracture (15). It affects approximately 54 million Americans, with studies suggesting that one in three women and one in five men age 50 and older will break a bone due to osteoporosis (16). In 2005 more than 2 million incident fractures

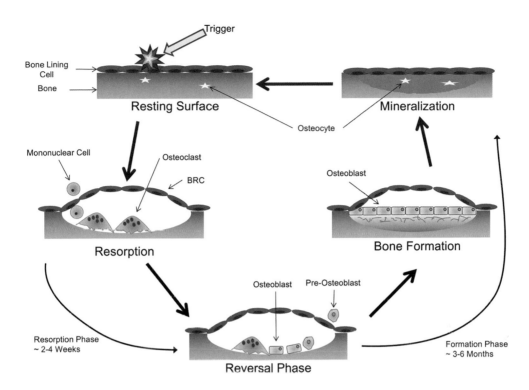

FIGURE 1 A simplified representation of the bone remodeling cycle. The initiation phase of bone remodeling is induced by mechanical strain, damage, or signals from cytokines or systemic factors. This generates local signals that lead to the bone-lining cells separating from the bone surface and forming a canopy over the site to be resorbed (90). Osteoclasts and their precursors are then recruited to the site of bone remodeling from the circulatory system via capillaries that are closely associated with the bone remodeling compartment (91). The signals for the initiation of osteoclast differentiation and resorption, macrophage colony stimulating factor and receptor activator of NF-κB ligand, are provided by cells of the osteoblast lineage, including osteocytes as well as T and B cells (91–94). Once the remodeling process is initiated, resorption of the bone occurs. Osteoclasts attach to the exposed surface of the mineralized matrix, where they polarize and form a sealed microenvironment. This sealed microenvironment is then acidified to break down the inorganic component of bone followed by release of the enzymes cathepsin K, matrix metalloproteinase-9 (MMP-9), and tartrate-resistant acid phosphatase, which break down the organic component (7, 95). Following resorption of the old damaged bone, the process undergoes reversal. Toward the end of the resorption phase of the bone remodeling cycle, mononuclear cells of the osteoblast lineage move into the resorption pit. These mononuclear cells remove the old demineralized collagen while laying down a new thin layer (96). During this phase the process of "coupling" bone resorption to bone formation occurs to ensure that the volume of bone removed is replaced. Coupling of bone resorption to bone formation is a multifaceted process with numerous regulator molecules derived from the matrix, secreted by cells, or membrane-bound contributing to the process (90, 97, 98). Bone formation is a two-step process and proceeds slowly, taking approximately 3 months (compared to resorption, which typically takes 3 weeks). The osteoblast first secretes the unmineralized osteoid, which is then mineralized through the incorporation of hydroxyapatite (99). When the osteoblasts have completed the matrix formation, they undergo a number of possible fates. The majority of osteoblasts become apoptotic; however, some get trapped in the mineralized matrix and undergo further differentiation into the osteocyte, while others may become inactive bone-lining cells (100). Through the production of sclerostin, an inhibitor of Wnt signaling, the osteocyte can regulate the amount of new bone formation that takes place (8).

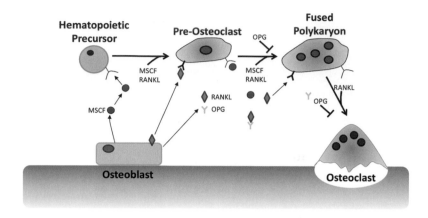

FIGURE 2 **Osteoclast differentiation is the process by which mononuclear cells undergo fusion into the multinucleated osteoclast. Three cytokines are critical for osteoclast differentiation: MCSF, RANKL, and OPG, a soluble decoy receptor for RANKL (101–104). In the initial stages of differentiation, precursor cells proliferate in response to MCSF signaling through its receptor c-FMS (105). RANKL, expressed as a membrane-bound or soluble form, then binds to its receptor, RANK, which is present on the precursor cells (106, 107). This results in the transcription and activation of numerous osteoclast-specific genes: cathepsin K, tartrate-resistant acid phosphatase (an osteoclast marker), calcitonin receptor, and B3 integrin (108). The precursor cells then migrate along chemokine gradients and fuse together to form the multinucleated osteoclast. Control of osteoclast differentiation is via the soluble receptor OPG, which competes with RANK for RANKL binding, thus inhibiting osteoclast differentiation (109, 110). Abbreviations: MCSF, macrophage colony stimulating factor; RANK(L), receptor activator of NF-κB (ligand); OPG, osteoprotegerin.**

were reported in the United States alone, at a cost of approximately $17 billion. This number is predicted to rise in excess of $25 billion by 2025 (17). Osteoporosis can be defined as two forms: primary osteoporosis, which occurs as part of the normal human aging process, and secondary osteoporosis, when bone loss is caused by a medical condition/disease or treatment.

Primary Osteoporosis

In females, the onset of menopause is a major factor that contributes to development of postmenopausal osteoporosis. Loss of estrogen gives rise to two stages of bone loss: an early rapid loss of trabecular and cortical bone due to increased osteoclast activity and decreased osteoclast apoptosis, and a second slower prolonged loss due to decreased osteoblast activity (18). The mechanisms behind this uncoupling of bone resorption and

bone formation are complex and multifactorial. Loss of estrogen has been observed to increase expression of proinflammatory and osteogenic cytokines, namely, interleukin-1 (IL-1), IL-6, IL-7, tumor necrosis factor alpha (TNFα), macrophage colony-stimulating factor (MCSF), and receptor activator of NF-κB ligand (RANKL) from osteoblasts, as well as T cells and B cells (19–23). Of these cells, T lymphocytes are believed to play a particularly critical role in the bone loss associated with estrogen deficiency. This was demonstrated using T-cell-deficient mice that were protected from ovariectomy (OVX)-induced bone loss (24). Furthermore, dysregulation of T cell CD40L signaling following estrogen deficiency leads to increased stromal cell expression of osteoclastogenic cytokines while decreasing expression of osteoprotegerin (OPG) (25). Aside from its pro-osteoclastogenic effects, the increased expression of TNFα following estrogen deficiency has also been

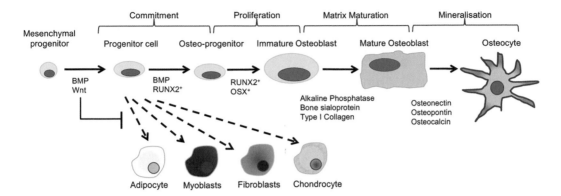

FIGURE 3 Osteoblast differentiation. Signaling by members of the canonical Wnt/β-catenin pathway such as Wnt10b, BMP2, and BMP4 directs the mesenchymal stem cell fate toward the osteoblast lineage. This is achieved by suppressing the adipogenic transcription factors C/EBPα and PPARγ while inducing the osteogenic transcription factors Runx2 and osterix (28, 111, 112). This immature osteoblast still has the potential to divide and express low levels of alkaline phosphatase activity, as well as to synthesize type I collagen, which makes up to 90% of the organic component of bone (113). Differentiation to the nonproliferating mature cuboidal osteoblast that actively mineralizes bone matrix is dependent on the transcription factor osterix (114). Before the newly laid matrix can be mineralized, however, it must first undergo maturation. Matrix maturation is associated with increased expression of alkaline phosphatase and several noncollagen proteins, including osteocalcin, osteopontin, and bone sialoprotein (115). Mineralization of bone is completed by the incorporation of hydroxyapatite [$Ca_{10}(PO_4)_6(OH)_2$] into the newly deposited osteoid. Membrane-bound extracellular bodies (extracellular matrix vesicles) released from the osteoblast facilitate initial mineral deposition by accumulating calcium and phosphate ions in a protected environment. Clusters of these ions come together to form the first stable crystals. Addition of ions to these crystals follows, resulting in their growth (99, 116). At the completion of bone formation, a subset of osteoblasts can undergo further differentiation, upon being entombed in the bone matrix, and become osteocytes. The remaining osteoblasts are thought to either undergo apoptosis or become inactive bone-lining cells (100).

shown to increase expression of sclerostin, a secreted wingless-related integration site (Wnt) antagonist (26). The subsequent decrease in Wnt signaling results in a shift of mesenchymal stem cell differentiation away from osteoblasts and toward adipocytes, resulting in reduced bone formation (27, 28). Changes in death receptor signaling on osteoclasts and osteoblasts following estrogen deficiency are thought to contribute further to the overall bone loss. OVX has been shown to increase osteoblast expression of Fas (CD95), a well-characterized death receptor, resulting in suppressed osteoblast differentiation and increased apoptosis (29). Interestingly, Fas-deficient mice are protected from OVX-induced bone loss due to enhanced osteoblast differentiation and activity (30).

Secondary Osteoporosis

Secondary osteoporosis is bone loss caused by a variety of medical and pathological factors including but not limited to smoking, type 1 diabetes (T1D), hyperparathyroidism, inflammatory bowel disease (IBD), arthritis, and glucocorticoid treatment. The incidence of secondary osteoporosis is difficult to discern, but it has been suggested to occur in almost two-thirds of men and one-fifth of postmenopausal women with osteoporosis (31, 32). Various gastrointestinal diseases are known to cause secondary osteoporosis, particularly IBD; up to three-quarters of IBD patients may have reduced bone mineral density (32). Several mechanisms contribute to the bone loss in IBD patients,

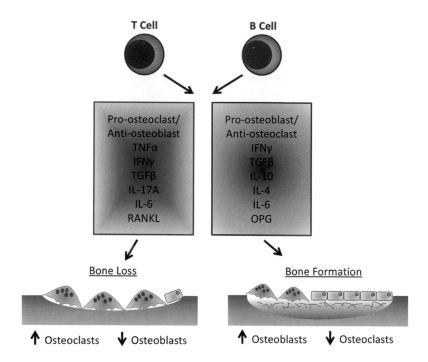

FIGURE 4 Cross-talk between osteoclasts, osteoblasts, and the immune system. Activated T lymphocytes, specifically T helper 17 cells, have been identified as osteoclastogenic through the expression of RANKL and the cytokine interleukin (IL)-17, which induces RANKL expression on osteoblasts (117). Furthermore, expression of IL-17 enhances local inflammation, driving expression of other proinflammatory cytokines and promoting additional RANKL expression (12). In addition to IL-17, T cell TNFα production has been demonstrated to affect the balance of bone remodeling. Increased T cell TNFα enhances osteoclastogenesis while inhibiting osteoblast differentiation and collagen synthesis (24, 118, 119). In addition to pro-osteoclastogenic cytokines, T-lymphocytes also secrete IL-10, IL-4, and interferon (IFN)-γ that are potentially antiosteoclastogenic (12, 120). A role for B-lymphocytes in bone homeostasis has been suggested because B cell-deficient mice exhibit an osteoporotic phenotype (110). B-lymphocytes are responsible for 64% of total bone marrow OPG production, with 45% of this derived from mature B cells (110).

including malnutrition; malabsorption of vitamin D, calcium, and vitamin K; immobilization; and increased expression of inflammatory cytokines such as TNFα, IL-1β, and IL-6 (33).

The autoimmune disease T1D is also associated with secondary osteoporosis (34, 35). Through the use of T1D animal models, several mechanisms that may contribute to T1D osteoporosis have been identified. In the streptozotocin-induced murine model of T1D, gene expression of TNFα, IL-1β, and IL-6 in the bone marrow is upregulated, leading to increased osteoblast death directly (36) and suppressed Wnt10b expression (37,

38). Suppression of Wnt10b is known to further decrease osteoblast viability, maturation, and lineage selection. Consistent with this finding, expression of the critical osteoblast transcription factor Runx2 is reduced, while the adipogenic markers, aP2 (FABP4) and PPARγ, are increased in T1D mouse bone (37). These data suggest that an anabolic defect is a major contributor to the secondary osteoporosis observed in T1D.

Osteoporosis Treatments

Numerous therapies have been developed for the treatment of osteoporosis, with the aim of reducing bone loss and correcting the imbalance in bone remodeling. In addition to lifestyle modifications (increased physical activity, reduced alcohol intake, and cessation of smoking), current baseline therapies for the prevention and treatment of osteoporosis comprise vitamin D and calcium supplementation (39). In patients that have a higher risk of fracture, pharmacological interventions are employed. The drugs fall into two classes: (i) drugs that inhibit bone resorption (antiresorptive) and (ii) drugs that stimulate bone formation (anabolic) (see Table 1).

Of the antiresorptive drugs, bisphosphonates constitute the largest class. Bisphosphonates can be administered orally or intravenously and have a high affinity for bone. In addition, they are inexpensive and have a long safety record. Bisphosphonates inhibit osteoclast activity either by a direct toxic effect or by altering their cytoskeleton (40). Antiresorptive drugs, however, have unintended effects in some patients, including upper gastrointestinal irritation from oral bisphosphonates, as well as osteonecrosis of the jaw and atypical subtrochanteric femoral fractures (41).

While numerous antiresorptive drugs exist, in the United States there is only one approved anabolic drug that builds up new bone: parathyroid hormone (PTH). PTH is used as either a full-length (PTH 1-84) or N-terminal fragment (teriparatide, PTH 1-34). PTH treatment is administered daily via a subcutaneous injection and stimulates increased bone density through an increase in the bone remodeling rate which favors bone formation. Therapeutic courses of PTH are limited to 24 months due to safety concerns related to an increase in the risk of osteosarcoma as well as the high cost of the drug (41, 42).

These limitations in treatments for osteoporosis underscore the need for novel therapies that have fewer side effects. Interestingly, recent studies have identified the intestinal microbiota as an important link in modulating bone health (43–45). The focus of this article is on probiotics and bone health. In the next subsections, we will examine how the microbiota and its modulation by probiotics are beneficial in osteoporosis, at least in animal models of disease.

THE MICROBIOTA

It is now clear from both human and animal studies that the intestinal microbiota is needed for the health of its host and plays a crucial role in many aspects of host physiology, including metabolism, nutrition, pathogen resistance, and immune function. While different parts of the intestinal tract exhibit different densities of microbiota, the colon usually has the highest content, 10^{11} CFU/ml (46). The human body is thought be a host for ~100 trillion microbes from ~1,000 species and 28 phyla (47). In addition to the sheer number of microbes, outnumbering the host cell number (estimated at ~60 trillion), gut microbiota also express 100-fold more genes compared to the human genome (47). Thus, as the microbiome coevolves with us, changes in that population can have both beneficial and harmful consequences on human health (48). Therefore, gaining knowledge of the microbiome-host relationship with respect to physiology is critical not only to understand disease pathogenesis but also to target the microbiome for therapeutic purposes.

TABLE 1 Established treatments for osteoporosis[a]

Effect	Treatment
Antiresorptive	Bisphosphonates
	Raloxifene
	HRT
	Denosumab
Bone forming	Teriparatide (parathyroid hormone)
Other	Calcium
	Vitamin D
	Strontium ranelate
	Calcitonin
	Calcitriol
	Exercise

[a]Table modified from references 121 and 122.

Role of the Intestinal Microbiota in Influencing Bone

Previous studies have clearly demonstrated that the intestinal tract can profoundly influence the health of the bone. One way this occurs is through the regulation of mineral absorption, which is required for healthy bone and includes calcium, phosphorus, and magnesium. In addition, endocrine factors that influence the absorption of these minerals as well as gut-derived factors such as incretins and serotonin can also influence bone turnover (49, 50). More recent studies using germfree mice and probiotics have demonstrated the influence of the intestinal microbiome in modulating bone physiology (51, 52).

Early evidence that the intestinal microbiota could affect bone was provided by Sjögren et al. (51). In their study, germfree mice, conventional mice, and germfree mice colonized with a normal microbiota were used to investigate the role of the microbiota in bone health. Bone mass was observed to be higher in germfree mice compared to that of the conventional mice; germfree mice additionally had reduced numbers of osteoclasts per bone surface and decreased frequency of $CD4^+$ T cells and osteoclast precursors in their bone marrow. These findings were normalized following colonization of the germfree intestine with a conventional microbiota. However, the exact role that the microbiota plays in the development of bone is not without controversy, because subsequent studies have either shown no difference in bone density between conventional mice and germfree mice (52) or showed that while initial colonization acutely reduces bone density, long-term colonization results in an increase in bone formation (53). This suggests that the effects of the microbiota on bone health are complex and time-dependent. The evidence for a role of probiotic supplementation in modulating bone health, however, is much stronger. Numerous studies have revealed that modulating the intestinal microbiota with probiotic bacteria can have a beneficial effect. These studies will be discussed in detail later in the article.

PROBIOTICS

Probiotics are defined as dietary supplements that contain live nonpathogenic microorganisms that when administered in adequate amounts can be beneficial in the treatment as well as in the prevention of pathological conditions (54). Many genera of bacteria such as *Lactobacillus, Enterococcus, Bacillus, Escherichia,* and *Bifidobacterium* have been used for their beneficial effects as probiotics. Although most probiotics are bacteria, yeasts such as *Saccharomyces* have also been found to have probiotic characteristics (55). Probiotic bacteria are naturally found in the mucous membranes such as the mouth, skin, and urinary and genital organs, and in the intestines. They are also commonly found in dietary supplements, fermented products (e.g., meat, milk products, beer), and nonconventional products such as toothpaste and ice cream. The Food and Agriculture Organization of the United Nations/World Health Organization has developed guidelines for the assessment and use of probiotic bacteria for consumption (56). For a microbe to be classified as probiotic it needs to present specific characteristics such as survival in the gastrointestinal system (acid and bile tolerance), phenotype and genotype stability, adhesion to the mucosal surface, antibiotic resistance, production of antimicrobial substances, and the ability to inhibit known pathogens. In addition, probiotic bacteria or their fermented products cannot be harmful to the host and cannot induce an immune system response unless it is induced against pathogenic microorganisms, and bacteria that contain transmissible drug resistance genes should not be used.

In recent years, multiple studies have been published indicating the potential benefits of probiotic supplementation on bone health in both healthy and pathological states. These beneficial effects have been observed with multiple strains of bacteria and in numerous experimental animal models of disease (Table 2). The mechanism through which probiotics exert their effects, however, hasn't been fully elucidated. It is known that probiotics can influence the gut through regulation of luminal pH, secretion of antimicrobial peptides, enhancement of barrier function by increasing mucus production, and modulation of the host immune system, and by modifying the gut microflora (57–60). Which of these mechanisms are important for the beneficial effects on bone is not yet well known.

Probiotics and Bone in Nonpathological Animal Models

Healthy nonpathogenic animal models have been used to evaluate the safety, efficacy, and mechanism of probiotic supplementation. Interestingly, the effect of probiotics under healthy nonpathological conditions has been shown to be dependent on many variables including the strain and sex of the animal.

In a study using *Lactobacillus reuteri* ATCC 6475, oral administration of the probiotic for a period of 4 weeks to specific-pathogen-free healthy male mice, but not female mice, resulted in a significant increase in femoral and vertebral trabecular bone density, trabecular number, trabecular thickness, bone mineral content, and bone mineral density when compared to untreated controls (61). This increase in bone density was attributed to an increase in osteoblast bone formation as evidenced by elevated levels of the osteoblast marker osteocalcin and increased bone formation rate; no difference was observed in serum tartrate resistant acid phosphatase (TRAP) levels. While the mechanism of action was not fully identified in this study, supplementation with *L. reuteri* 6475 was observed to decrease expression of the inflammatory cytokine TNFα in the jejunum

and ileum (61). Interestingly, while intact healthy female mice did not respond to oral *L. reuteri* in terms of bone health, further studies revealed that they subsequently responded to the probiotic if their health status was skewed toward a mild inflammatory state (62). This mild inflammatory state was induced via a dorsal surgical incision (DSI) and following probiotic supplementation resulted in the female mice exhibiting increased bone density. However, this took longer than the males (8-week treatment in females versus 4 weeks in males). In addition to an increase in femoral trabecular bone density, DSI female mice (treated with probiotic) exhibited higher trabecular number as well as mineral apposition rate compared with nontreated DSI female mice and treated intact female mice (62). These results suggest that under naive healthy conditions, females are likely at their maximal anti-inflammatory state, and therefore *L. reuteri* is unable to influence inflammation and bone formation. However, slight inflammation induced by DSI skews the females (in spite of intact estrogen) toward a proinflammatory state, so *L. reuteri* is able to have a beneficial effect on bone density. However, the precise mechanisms of *L. reuteri* 6475 effects on bone density are still under investigation.

In studies parallel to the mouse model, treatment of rats with yogurt containing *Lactobacillus casei*, *L. reuteri*, and *Lactobacillus gasseri* increased calcium absorption, resulting in elevated bone mineral content (BMC) compared to the control (63). Likewise, supplementation of growing rats with *Lactobacillus rhamnosus* (HN001) improved magnesium and calcium retention (64). In addition to different strains of *Lactobacillus*, beneficial effects on bone have also been observed with *Bifidobacterium longum*. Supplementation of male rats with *B. longum* (ATCC 15707) for 28 days showed an increase in calcium, phosphorus, and magnesium content in the tibia and higher percentage fracture strength than untreated rats (65). In a separate study rats fed a high-cholesterol

TABLE 2 Effect of probiotics on bone (animal studies)

Probiotic strain	Animal model	Duration	Analysis method	Bone effects	Reference
Bacillus licheniformis and *Bacillus subtilis*	Broiler	6 weeks	Measuring calipers	↑ Tibia lateral and medial wall thickness	79
Brewer's yeast	Broiler	9 weeks	Visual	↓ Tibial dyschondroplasia	80
Lactobacillus	Broiler	28 days	Atomic absorption spectrophotometry Phosphomolybdic acid method	↑ Ca and P retention	75
Lactobacillus reuteri (ATCC 6475)	Male mice	4 weeks	μCT	↑ Bone volume fraction ↑ Trabecular number ↑ Trabecular thickness ↑ Bone mineral content ↑ Bone mineral density ↑ Osteocalcin ↑ Bone formation rate	61
	Female mice (OVX)	4 weeks	μCT	↑ Bone volume fraction ↑ Bone mineral content ↑ Bone mineral density ↓ RANKL gene expression ↓ TRAP5 expression	67
	Female mice (dorsal surgery)	8 weeks	μCT	↑ Bone volume fraction ↑ Mineral apposition rate ↓ RANKL gene expression ↑ OPG gene expression ↑ IL-10 gene expression	62
	Male mice (streptozotocin-induced T1D)	4 weeks	μCT	↑ Bone volume fraction ↑ Bone mineral content ↑ Bone mineral density ↑ Mineral apposition rate ↑ Serum osteocalcin ↑ Wnt10b expression	38

Probiotic	Animal model	Duration	Method	Effects	Reference
Lactobacillus casei, *L. reuteri*, and *Lactobacillus gasseri*	Rats			↑ Bone mineral content	63
Bifidobacterium longum-fermented broccoli	Male Wistar rats	12 weeks	Histology	↑ Ca absorption ↓ TRAP$^+$ osteoclasts	66
B. longum (ATCC 15707)	Male Wistar rats	28 days	Texture analyzer Plasma emission spectrophotometry	↑ Tibial Ca, P, and Mg content ↑ Fracture strength	65
Lactobacillus rhamnosus (HN001)	Male Sprague-Dawley rats	3 weeks	DEXA^a	↑ Ca and Mg retention	64
	Female Sprague-Dawley rats (OVX)	3 months	DEXA	↓ Bone loss	64
	Female mice (OVX)	4 weeks	µCT	↑ Bone volume fraction ↑ Serum osteocalcin ↓ RANKL gene expression ↓ TNFα gene expression ↓ IL-17 gene expression	52
Lactobacillus paracasei (NTU 101) or *Lactobacillus plantarum* (NTU 102)-fermented soy milk	Female mice (OVX)	8 weeks	µCT Scanning electron microscopy	↑ Bone volume fraction ↑ Trabecular number	69
L. paracasei or *L. paracasei* and *L. plantarum*	Female mice (OVX)	6 weeks	µCT	↑ Cortical bone mineral content ↑ Cortical area ↑ OPG expression	68
L. casei 393-fermented milk	Female Sprague-Dawley rats (OVX)	6 weeks	DEXA Texture analyzer plasma emission spectrophotometry	↑ Bone mineral density ↑ Fracture strength ↑ Ca content ↓ TRAP activity	82
Lactobacillus helveticus-fermented milk	Spontaneously hypertensive male rats	14 weeks	DEXA Plasma emission spectrophotometry	↑ Bone mineral density ↑ Bone mineral content	87
L. casei and *Lactobacillus acidophilus*	Female Wistar rat (adjuvant-induced arthritis)	12 days	X ray	↓ Bone loss	123
Enterococcus faecium (with methotrexate)	Male Lewis rat (adjuvant-induced arthritis)	50 days	DEXA X ray	↑ Anti-inflammatory effects ↑ Anti-arthritic effects	124

^{a}DEXA, dual-energy X-ray absorptiometry.

diet supplemented with *B. longum*-fermented broccoli for 12 weeks presented a reduction in the number of TRAP-positive osteoclasts compared with untreated rats (66).

Probiotics and Bone Health in Animal Models of Osteoporosis

A number of studies have utilized animal models to investigate whether probiotics can be used to prevent both primary and secondary osteoporotic bone loss (38, 52, 67, 68). These studies have mainly used different species of the genera *Lactobacillus* and *Bifidobacterium*.

Primary osteoporosis

In a recent study from our lab (67) the bacterium *L. reuteri* ATCC 6475 was used in the primary osteoporosis mouse menopause (OVX) model. Twelve-week-old BALB/c mice were provided with *L. reuteri* ATCC 6475 three times a week by gavage (1×10^9 CFU/ml) and constantly in their drinking water (1.5×10^8 CFU/ml) for 4 weeks following OVX surgery, and the femoral and vertebral bones were analyzed by micro-computed tomography (μCT). OVX mice supplemented with *L. reuteri* were found to be completely protected from bone loss, resulting in a bone volume/total volume (BV/TV) that was comparable to the control mice. Furthermore, significant increases in trabecular bone mineral density and BMC were observed in the OVX treated mice compared to the OVX controls. The protective effect of *L. reuteri* was attributed to a decrease in bone mRNA levels of RANKL and TRAP5. Serum TRAP5 levels were also modestly changed by *L. reuteri* treatment. However, osteoblast markers such as osteocalcin were not affected. These results suggested that the protective effect of *L. reuteri* observed in this model is via an anti-osteoclastogenic effect. This was supported by *ex vivo* bone marrow cultures, in which the osteoclastogenic potential of the OVX *L. reuteri*-treated bone marrow was signifi-

cantly reduced compared to the OVX bone marrow cultures. These data support an earlier study by Chiang and Pan (69), who revealed that OVX mice treated with either *Lactobacillus paracasei* (101 nephelometric turbidity units)-fermented or *Lactobacillus plantarum* (102 nephelometric turbidity units)-fermented soy milk had significantly increased BV/TV and trabecular number compared to OVX controls.

Further support for the beneficial effects of *Lactobacillus* treatment preventing estrogen-deficiency-induced trabecular bone loss has been provided by Li et al. (52). In their study they utilized both the OVX model in specific-pathogen-free mice as well as an ovarian sex steroid inhibitor (leuprolide) in germfree mice. These animals were treated with either *L. rhamnosus* GG (LGG) or the commercially available probiotic supplement VSL#3 (containing four species of *Lactobacillus*, three species of *Bifidobacterium*, and *Streptococcus salivarius* subsp. *thermophilus* [70]). In both models LGG and VSL#3 markedly prevented the decrease in femoral bone density and trabecular thickness and number compared with the untreated controls. Importantly, nonprobiotic bacteria such as *Escherichia coli* DH5alpha and the LGG pili mutant (LGG [ΔSpaC]) did not provide any protection from bone loss. While the mechanism of action was not fully elucidated in this study, CTX levels in the serum, a marker of osteoclast bone resorption, were decreased in the OVX + LGG and VSL#3 cohorts but not in the nonprobiotic groups (52). This suggests that, as with the other studies in the OVX model of bone loss, probiotics mediate their effects on OVX-induced bone loss by inhibiting osteoclast activity.

In an analogous study by Ohlsson et al. (68), mice were treated with either a single *L. paracasei* strain (DSM 13434) or a mixture of three strains (*L. paracasei* DSM 13434 and *L. plantarum* DSM 15312 and DSM 1531) in their drinking water for 2 weeks prior and for 4 weeks after OVX surgery. *L. paracasei* DSM 13434 and the multiple strains increased cortical bone mineral content compared to the vehicle-treated OVX mice. Serum levels of the resorption marker C-terminal telopeptides and the urinary fractional excretion of calcium were decreased, as was the cortical bone RANKL/OPG ratio in the probiotic-treated groups compared with the vehicle-treated group. However, mRNA levels of three osteoblast-associated genes (osterix, Col1α1, and osteocalcin) were not affected by the different probiotics. Together, these results further support the notion that probiotics prevent bone loss in estrogen-deficient mice by regulating osteoclast resorption but not osteoblast bone formation.

The effectiveness of probiotics to inhibit OVX-induced bone loss has also been investigated in other animal models. In the OVX rat model the effect of *B. longum* on bone density, bone mineral content, bone remodeling, bone structure, and osteoclast/osteoblast gene expression markers was investigated. Rats were treated with *B. longum* for 16 weeks after OVX surgery. The *B. longum*-supplemented group presented an increase in bone density, trabecular number, and thickness. Femoral strength was also enhanced by *B. longum* supplementation. When compared to the sham group, OVX decreased osteoblast but increased osteoclast surface over bone surface in the femur. These effects were prevented by the *B. longum* treatment, in addition to decreasing levels of serum C-terminal telopeptide, suggesting that similar to the mouse OVX model, probiotics modulate osteoclast formation and activity in the rat OVX model (71).

Secondary osteoporosis

While the majority of studies have so far investigated the beneficial effects of probiotic supplementation on primary osteoporosis, few studies have investigated the potential effect on conditions of secondary osteoporosis. Specifically, in the context of T1D-induced bone loss our lab has revealed some potentially exciting results with the use of probiotic treatment (38).

T1D is a metabolic disease caused by insulin secretion deficiency. Hyperglycemia as well as other metabolic impairments have devastating consequences to several organs including the skeleton. In contrast to primary osteoporosis, T1D-induced osteoporosis is characterized by a dysregulation of osteoblast number and activity as well as increased bone marrow adiposity; however, osteoclast activity seems to be mostly unaffected (72). Similar to the effects of *L. reuteri* in the mouse OVX model, administration of *L. reuteri* was effective in preventing streptozotocin-induced T1D-mediated bone loss in male C57BL/6 (14 weeks old) mice. After 4 weeks (post-streptozotocin injection), diabetic mice displayed a 35% reduction in bone volume fraction, an effect that was inhibited by *L. reuteri* treatment. This was further supported by the trabecular bone parameter data, which revealed that *L. reuteri* treatment prevented the reduction in trabecular number and the increase in trabecular spacing induced by T1D. Evidence that T1D bone loss was due to reduced osteoblast activity was revealed by decreased serum markers of bone formation such as osteocalcin and by a reduced mineral apposition rate. *L. reuteri* 6475 treatment enhanced mouse serum osteocalcin levels and mineral apposition rate, suggesting that in this model, unlike the OVX model, *L. reuteri* has an anabolic bone-forming effect (38).

Probiotics and Bone Health in Livestock

The treatment of low bone density in humans is not the only potential use of probiotics. Skeletal abnormalities affecting the quality and output of livestock cost the agricultural sector millions of dollars per annum (73). This is especially true in the poultry industry, where the burden of having to produce large, fast-growing, and affordable broilers in large-scale rearing facilities has resulted in the development of bone pathologies (74). While traditionally, these impediments were treated with growth factors, antibiotics, and veterinary medicines, public opinion and government regulations have changed, meaning alternatives such as probiotics are required.

The treatment of chickens with probiotic supplementation in feed has been shown to provide numerous benefits including improved weight gain, reduced mortality, increased egg size, decreased incidence of *Salmonella* infection, and improved bone health (75–80). In one study supplementation of the diet with *Bacillus licheniformis* and *Bacillus subtilis* significantly increased the thicknesses of the tibia lateral and medial walls. The probiotic-supplemented diet also slightly improved tibia yield stress and modulus of elasticity. However, the percentage of calcium on the bone was not affected by probiotic consumption, suggesting that the increase in bone density was independent of bone calcium content (79). These data supported an earlier study that observed an increase in bone strength and lower incidence of tibial dyschondroplasia in chickens receiving brewer's yeast (80). These studies indicate that in addition to the potential treatment of human bone pathologies, probiotics can be utilized for the improvement of livestock.

Probiotics Mechanism of Action

The mechanisms through which probiotic bacteria exert a beneficial effect on bone density are still being investigated. However, both *in vitro* and *in vivo* studies have highlighted a complex and multifaceted process by which probiotic bacteria can exert an influence on the host (Fig. 5a,b).

In vitro studies

In vitro studies using probiotics or probiotic-fermented products have been performed to determine whether probiotic secretory products can directly affect the bone cells. These studies have revealed that osteoclast differentiation from monocytic-macrophages was significantly inhibited when cultured with *L. reuteri*-conditioned media. This suggests

that the probiotic releases an antiosteoclastogenic factor that modulates osteoclastogenesis (67). Similar to its effects on osteoclast differentiation, a secreted component of *L. reuteri* was sufficient to reverse TNFα-induced suppression of Wnt10b expression in the MC3T3 preosteoblast cell line (38). The ability of *L. reuteri* to secrete a modulatory factor is supported by an earlier study which demonstrated that *L. reuteri* secretes histamine, which is capable of suppressing TNFα production from human monocytoid cells (81). Further evidence for probiotics having a direct effect on bone cells has been observed with *Lactobacillus helveticus* and *L. casei*. In MC3T3-E1 cultures *L. casei*-fermented milk increased proliferation in a dose-dependent manner (82). Also, addition of *L. helveticus*-fermented milk products to primary bone marrow cultures increased calcium accumulation in osteoblast cultures, suggesting that it has the potential to increase osteoblast differentiation. Remarkably, *L. helveticus*-fermented milk products had no effect on osteoclast differentiation (83), suggesting that different species/strains of bacteria may have cell-specific effects.

In vivo studies

The mechanism by which probiotic bacteria exert their effect on bone *in vivo* is not very well known and is most likely complex, with multiple bacterial components affecting different pathways within the host. Bacteria have been shown to synthesize numerous vitamins and enzymes that are required for matrix formation and bone growth, including vitamins D, K, and C and folate (84, 85). Furthermore, bacteria of the genus *Bifidobacterium* produce short-chain fatty acids that can reduce the intestinal tract pH, subsequently increasing the absorption of minerals (86).

Studies performed with *L. reuteri* 6475 have highlighted that this probiotic is capable of systemically suppressing the gene expression of proinflammatory and pro-osteoclastogenic cytokines, in both the intestine and the bone

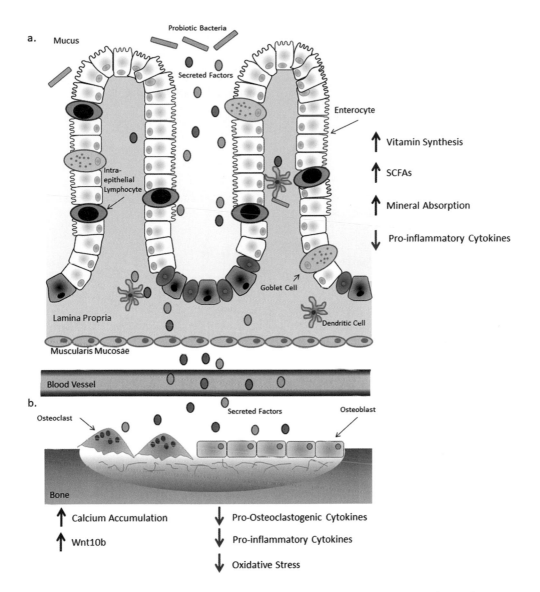

FIGURE 5 Potential mechanism by which probiotic bacteria benefit bone. (a) Probiotic bacteria or their secreted factors interact with the intestinal epithelial barrier and cells in the lamina propria. Within the lamina propria the probiotic bacteria/secreted factors interact with antigen-presenting cells such dendritic cells, modulating their immune response. This results in a reduction of inflammatory cytokines, leading to an uptake in minerals from the intestinal lumen. (b) The bacterial secreted factors then pass into the bloodstream and are transported to the bone. Here they can interact with osteoclasts and osteoblasts as well as immune cells. This could then reduce expression of proinflammatory and pro-osteoclastogenic cytokines and oxidative stress while enhancing mineral apposition and Wnt10b expression. This modulation results in reduced osteoclast formation, subsequently leading to increased levels of bone.

marrow (61, 62, 67). This anti-inflammatory effect has also been observed with other species of *Lactobacilli*. Both LGG and VSL#3 were shown to reduce expression of TNFα, IL-17, and RANKL in cells isolated from the small intestine and bone marrow of OVX mice (52). By reducing intestinal inflammation, the probiotic bacteria may directly enhance the transport of calcium across the intestinal barrier.

It is likely that different probiotic bacterial strains act via distinct and/or overlapping mechanisms. For example, while *L. helveticus* has been suggested to enhance bone density by increasing calcium uptake, studies have shown that it is also able to produce the bioactive peptides isoleucyl-prolyl-proline and valyl-prolyl-proline. These peptides are capable of inhibiting the angiotensin-converting enzyme, preventing the formation of angiotensin II, a stimulator of osteoclast resorption, from angiotensin I (83, 87).

In contrast, *B. longum* has been shown to reduce periodontal oxidative stress by decreasing NF-κB gene expression (66). Estrogen deficiency is associated with an increase in oxidative stress which can potentially inhibit osteoblast differentiation while enhancing osteoclast differentiation (18, 88, 89). This suggests that *B. longum* can potentially stimulate osteoblastogenesis while inhibiting osteoclastogenesis.

CONCLUSIONS

Osteoporosis is a devastating complication of the skeleton that has a profound influence on quality of life. It is critical that we continue to develop new, safe, and effective strategies to prevent or treat osteoporosis associated with different conditions and variables (age, biological sex, disease, genetic background). The effect of probiotics in animal models suggests that oral probiotic supplementation could be a safe and effective alternative for preventing bone loss in various conditions in humans, including menopause and T1D, as well as for

enhancing bone density under healthy or modestly inflamed conditions.

ACKNOWLEDGMENTS

We acknowledge support from grants R01 DK101050 from the National Institute of Diabetes and Digestive and Kidney Diseases (NIDDK) and R01 AT007695 from the National Center for Complementary and Alternative Medicine (NCCAM), National Institutes of Health.

CITATION

Collins FL, Rios-Arce ND, Schepper JD, Parameswaran N, McCabe LR. 2017. The potential of probiotics as a therapy for osteoporosis. Microbiol Spectrum 5(4):BAD-0015-2016.

REFERENCES

1. **Rizzo DC.** 2015. *Fundamentals of Anatomy and Physiology*. Cengage Learning, Boston, MA.
2. **Turner RT, Kalra SP, Wong CP, Philbrick KA, Lindenmaier LB, Boghossian S, Iwaniec UT.** 2013. Peripheral leptin regulates bone formation. *J Bone Miner Res* **28:**22–34.
3. **Wong IPL, Driessler F, Khor EC, Shi YC, Hörmer B, Nguyen AD, Enriquez RF, Eisman JA, Sainsbury A, Herzog H, Baldock PA.** 2012. Peptide YY regulates bone remodeling in mice: a link between gut and skeletal biology. *PLoS One* **7:**e40038.
4. **Takayanagi H.** 2009. Osteoimmunology and the effects of the immune system on bone. *Nat Rev Rheumatol* **5:**667–676.
5. **Hauge EM, Qvesel D, Eriksen EF, Mosekilde L, Melsen F.** 2001. Cancellous bone remodeling occurs in specialized compartments lined by cells expressing osteoblastic markers. *J Bone Miner Res* **16:**1575–1582.
6. **Karsenty G, Kronenberg HM, Settembre C.** 2009. Genetic control of bone formation. *Annu Rev Cell Dev Biol* **25:**629–648.
7. **Teitelbaum SL.** 2007. Osteoclasts: what do they do and how do they do it? *Am J Pathol* **170:**427–435.
8. **Bonewald LF, Johnson ML.** 2008. Osteocytes, mechanosensing and Wnt signaling. *Bone* **42:**606–615.

9. **Andersen TL, Sondergaard TE, Skorzynska KE, Dagnaes-Hansen F, Plesner TL, Hauge EM, Plesner T, Delaisse JM.** 2009. A physical mechanism for coupling bone resorption and formation in adult human bone. *Am J Pathol* **174:**239–247.

10. **Xing L, Schwarz EM, Boyce BF.** 2005. Osteoclast precursors, RANKL/RANK, and immunology. *Immunol Rev* **208:**19–29.

11. **Pittenger MF, Mackay AM, Beck SC, Jaiswal RK, Douglas R, Mosca JD, et al.** 2013. Multilineage potential of adult human mesenchymal stem cells. *Science* **284:**143–147.

12. **Takayanagi H.** 2010. New immune connections in osteoclast formation. *Ann N Y Acad Sci* **1192:**117–123.

13. **Long F.** 2011. Building strong bones: molecular regulation of the osteoblast lineage. *Nat Rev Mol Cell Biol* **13:**27–38.

14. **Matsuo K, Irie N.** 2008. Osteoclast-osteoblast communication. *Arch Biochem Biophys* **473:**201–209.

15. **Am J Med.** 1993. Consensus development conference: diagnosis, prophylaxis, and treatment of osteoporosis. *Am J Med* **94:**646–650.

16. **International Osteoporosis Foundation.** 2015. *Facts and Statistics.* https://www.iofbonehealth.org/facts-statistics.

17. **Burge R, Dawson-Hughes B, Solomon DH, Wong JB, King A, Tosteson A.** 2007. Incidence and economic burden of osteoporosis-related fractures in the United States, 2005–2025. *J Bone Miner Res* **22:**465–475.

18. **Manolagas SC.** 2010. From estrogen-centric to aging and oxidative stress: a revised perspective of the pathogenesis of osteoporosis. *Endocr Rev* **31:**266–300.

19. **Pfeilschifter J, Köditz R, Pfohl M, Schatz H.** 2002. Changes in proinflammatory cytokine activity after menopause. *Endocr Rev* **23:**90–119.

20. **Bismar H, Diel I, Ziegler R, Pfeilschifter J.** 1995. Increased cytokine secretion by human bone marrow cells after menopause or discontinuation of estrogen replacement. *J Clin Endocrinol Metab* **80:**3351–3355.

21. **D'Amelio P, Grimaldi A, Di Bella S, Brianza SZ, Cristofaro MA, Tamone C, Giribaldi G, Ulliers D, Pescarmona GP, Isaia G.** 2008. Estrogen deficiency increases osteoclastogenesis up-regulating T cells activity: a key mechanism in osteoporosis. *Bone* **43:**92–100.

22. **Weitzmann MN, Roggia C, Toraldo G, Weitzmann L, Pacifici R.** 2002. Increased production of IL-7 uncouples bone formation from bone resorption during estrogen deficiency. *J Clin Invest* **110:**1643–1650.

23. **Eghbali-Fatourechi G, Khosla S, Sanyal A, Boyle WJ, Lacey DL, Riggs BL.** 2003. Role of RANK ligand in mediating increased bone resorption in early postmenopausal women. *J Clin Invest* **111:**1221–1230.

24. **Cenci S, Weitzmann MN, Roggia C, Namba N, Novack D, Woodring J, Pacifici R.** 2000. Estrogen deficiency induces bone loss by enhancing T-cell production of TNF-alpha. *J Clin Invest* **106:**1229–1237.

25. **Li JY, Tawfeek H, Bedi B, Yang X, Adams J, Gao KY, Zayzafoon M, Weitzmann MN, Pacifici R.** 2011. Ovariectomy disregulates osteoblast and osteoclast formation through the T-cell receptor CD40 ligand. *Proc Natl Acad Sci USA* **108:**768–773.

26. **Kim BJ, Bae SJ, Lee SY, Lee YS, Baek JE, Park SY, Lee SH, Koh JM, Kim GS.** 2012. TNF-α mediates the stimulation of sclerostin expression in an estrogen-deficient condition. *Biochem Biophys Res Commun* **424:**170–175.

27. **Foo C, Frey S, Yang HH, Zellweger R, Filgueira L.** 2007. Downregulation of beta-catenin and transdifferentiation of human osteoblasts to adipocytes under estrogen deficiency. *Gynecol Endocrinol* **23:**535–540.

28. **Bennett CN, Longo KA, Wright WS, Suva LJ, Lane TF, Hankenson KD, MacDougald OA.** 2005. Regulation of osteoblastogenesis and bone mass by Wnt10b. *Proc Natl Acad Sci USA* **102:**3324–3329.

29. **García-Moreno C, Catalán MP, Ortiz A, Alvarez L, De la Piedra C.** 2004. Modulation of survival in osteoblasts from postmenopausal women. *Bone* **35:**170–177.

30. **Kovacic N, Grcevic D, Katavic V, Lukic IK, Grubisic V, Mihovilovic K, Cvija H, Croucher PI, Marusic A.** 2010. Fas receptor is required for estrogen deficiency-induced bone loss in mice. *Lab Invest* **90:**402–413.

31. **Fitzpatrick LA.** 2002. Secondary causes of osteoporosis. *Mayo Clin Proc* **77:**453–468.

32. **Painter SE, Kleerekoper M, Camacho PM.** 2006. Secondary osteoporosis: a review of the recent evidence. *Endocr Pract* **12:**436–445.

33. **Ghishan FK, Kiela PR.** 2011. Advances in the understanding of mineral and bone metabolism in inflammatory bowel diseases. *Am J Physiol Gastrointest Liver Physiol* **300:**G191–G201.

34. **Levin ME, Boisseau VC, Avioli LV.** 1976. Effects of diabetes mellitus on bone mass in juvenile and adult-onset diabetes. *N Engl J Med* **294:**241–245.

35. **Coe LM, Zhang J, McCabe LR.** 2013. Both spontaneous Ins2(+/−) and streptozotocin-induced type I diabetes cause bone loss in young mice. *J Cell Physiol* **228:**689–695.

36. **Coe LM, Irwin R, Lippner D, McCabe LR.** 2011. The bone marrow microenvironment contributes to type I diabetes induced osteoblast death. *J Cell Physiol* **226:**477–483.

37. **Motyl KJ, Botolin S, Irwin R, Appledorn DM, Kadakia T, Amalfitano A, Schwartz RC, McCabe LR.** 2009. Bone inflammation and altered gene expression with type I diabetes early onset. *J Cell Physiol* **218:**575–583.

38. **Zhang J, Motyl KJ, Irwin R, MacDougald OA, Britton RA, McCabe LR.** 2015. Loss of bone and Wnt10b expression in male type 1 diabetic mice is blocked by the probiotic *L. reuteri. Endocrinology* **156:**3169–3182.

39. **Kanis JA, McCloskey EV, Johansson H, Cooper C, Rizzoli R, Reginster JY, Scientific Advisory Board of the European Society for Clinical and Economic Aspects of Osteoporosis and Osteoarthritis (ESCEO), Committee of Scientific Advisors of the International Osteoporosis Foundation (IOF).** 2013. European guidance for the diagnosis and management of osteoporosis in postmenopausal women. *Osteoporos Int* **24:**23–57.

40. **Papapoulos SE.** 2008. Bisphosphonates: how do they work? *Best Pract Res Clin Endocrinol Metab* **22:**831–847.

41. **Reid IR.** 2015. Efficacy, effectiveness and side effects of medications used to prevent fractures. *J Intern Med* **277:**690–706.

42. **Sambrook P, Cooper C.** 2006. Osteoporosis. *Lancet* **367:**2010–2018.

43. **Jones RM, Mulle JG, Pacifici R.** 2017. Osteomicrobiology: the influence of gut microbiota on bone in health and disease. *Bone.* [Epub ahead of print.]

44. **Ohlsson C, Sjögren K.** 2015. Effects of the gut microbiota on bone mass. *Trends Endocrinol Metab* **26:**69–74.

45. **McCabe L, Britton RA, Parameswaran N.** 2015. Prebiotic and probiotic regulation of bone health: role of the intestine and its microbiome. *Curr Osteoporos Rep* **13:**363–371.

46. **Loh G, Blaut M.** 2012. Role of commensal gut bacteria in inflammatory bowel diseases. *Gut Microbes* **3:**544–555.

47. **Fukuda S, Ohno H.** 2014. Gut microbiome and metabolic diseases. *Semin Immunopathol* **36:**103–114.

48. **Ley RE, Turnbaugh PJ, Klein S, Gordon JI.** 2006. Microbial ecology: human gut microbes associated with obesity. *Nature* **444:**1022–1023.

49. **Baggio LL, Drucker DJ.** 2007. Biology of incretins: GLP-1 and GIP. *Gastroenterology* **132:**2131–2157.

50. **Yadav VK, Ryu JH, Suda N, Tanaka KF, Gingrich JA, Schütz G, Glorieux FH, Chiang CY, Zajac JD, Insogna KL, Mann JJ, Hen R, Ducy P, Karsenty G.** 2008. Lrp5 controls bone formation by inhibiting serotonin synthesis in the duodenum. *Cell* **135:**825–837.

51. **Sjögren K, Engdahl C, Henning P, Lerner UH, Tremaroli V, Lagerquist MK, Bäckhed F, Ohlsson C.** 2012. The gut microbiota regulates bone mass in mice. *J Bone Miner Res* **27:**1357–1367.

52. **Li J-Y, Chassaing B, Tyagi AM, Vaccaro C, Luo T, Adams J, Darby TM, Weitzmann MN, Mulle JG, Gewirtz AT, Jones RM, Pacifici R.** 2016. Sex steroid deficiency-associated bone loss is microbiota dependent and prevented by probiotics. *J Clin Invest* **126:**2049–2063.

53. **Yan J, Herzog JW, Tsang K, Brennan CA, Bower MA, Garrett WS, Sartor BR, Aliprantis AO, Charles JF.** 2016. Gut microbiota induce IGF-1 and promote bone formation and growth. *Proc Natl Acad Sci USA* **113:**E7554–E7563.

54. **Araya M, Morelli L, Reid G, Sanders ME, Stanton C.** 2002. *Guidelines for the Evaluation of Probiotics in Food.* FAO/WHO, London, Ontario, Canada.

55. **Czerucka D, Piche T, Rampal P.** 2007. Review article: yeast as probiotics: *Saccharomyces boulardii. Aliment Pharmacol Ther* **26:**767–778.

56. **FAO and WHO.** 2006. *Probiotics in Food.* Food and Nutrition Paper 85. FAO/WHO, Rome, Italy.

57. **Broekaert IJ, Nanthakumar NN, Walker WA.** 2007. Secreted probiotic factors ameliorate enteropathogenic infection in zinc-deficient human Caco-2 and T84 cell lines. *Pediatr Res* **62:**139–144.

58. **Matsuguchi T, Takagi A, Matsuzaki T, Nagaoka M, Ishikawa K, Yokokura T, Yoshikai Y.** 2003. Lipoteichoic acids from *Lactobacillus* strains elicit strong tumor necrosis factor alpha-inducing activities in macrophages through Toll-like receptor 2. *Clin Diagn Lab Immunol* **10:**259–266.

59. **Nishimura J.** 2014. Exopolysaccharides produced from *Lactobacillus delbrueckii* subsp. *bulgaricus. Adv Microbiol* **4:**1017–1023.

60. **Sougioultzis S, Simeonidis S, Bhaskar KR, Chen X, Anton PM, Keates S, Pothoulakis C, Kelly CP.** 2006. *Saccharomyces boulardii* produces a soluble anti-inflammatory factor that inhibits NF-kappaB-mediated IL-8 gene expression. *Biochem Biophys Res Commun* **343:**69–76.

61. **McCabe LR, Irwin R, Schaefer L, Britton RA.** 2013. Probiotic use decreases intestinal inflammation and increases bone density in healthy male but not female mice. *J Cell Physiol* **228:**1793–1798.

62. **Collins FL, Irwin R, Bierhalter H, Schepper J, Britton RA, Parameswaran N, McCabe**

LR. 2016. *Lactobacillus reuteri* 6475 increases bone density in intact females only under an inflammatory setting. *PLoS One* **11**:e0153180.

63. **Ghanem KZ, Badawy IH, Abdel-Salam AM.** 2004. Influence of yoghurt and probiotic yoghurt on the absorption of calcium, magnesium, iron and bone mineralization in rats. *Milchwissenschaft* **59**:472–475.

64. **Kruger MC, Fear A, Chua W-H, Plimmer GG, Schollum LM.** 2009. The effect of *Lactobacillus rhamnosus* HN001 on mineral absorption and bone health in growing male and ovariectomised female rats. *Dairy Sci Technol* **89**:219–231.

65. **Rodrigues FC, Castro AS, Rodrigues VC, Fernandes SA, Fontes EA, de Oliveira TT, Martino HS, de Luces Fortes Ferreira CL.** 2012. Yacon flour and *Bifidobacterium longum* modulate bone health in rats. *J Med Food* **15**:664–670.

66. **Tomofuji T, Ekuni D, Azuma T, Irie K, Endo Y, Yamamoto T, Ishikado A, Sato T, Harada K, Suido H, Morita M.** 2012. Supplementation of broccoli or *Bifidobacterium longum*-fermented broccoli suppresses serum lipid peroxidation and osteoclast differentiation on alveolar bone surface in rats fed a high-cholesterol diet. *Nutr Res* **32**:301–307.

67. **Britton RA, Irwin R, Quach D, Schaefer L, Zhang J, Lee T, Parameswaran N, McCabe LR.** 2014. Probiotic *L. reuteri* treatment prevents bone loss in a menopausal ovariectomized mouse model. *J Cell Physiol* **229**:1822–1830.

68. **Ohlsson C, Engdahl C, Fåk F, Andersson A, Windahl SH, Farman HH, Movérare-Skrtic S, Islander U, Sjögren K.** 2014. Probiotics protect mice from ovariectomy-induced cortical bone loss. *PLoS One* **9**:e92368.

69. **Chiang SS, Pan TM.** 2011. Antiosteoporotic effects of *Lactobacillus*-fermented soy skim milk on bone mineral density and the microstructure of femoral bone in ovariectomized mice. *J Agric Food Chem* **59**:7734–7742.

70. **Caballero-Franco C, Keller K, De Simone C, Chadee K.** 2007. The VSL#3 probiotic formula induces mucin gene expression and secretion in colonic epithelial cells. *Am J Physiol Gastrointest Liver Physiol* **292**:G315–G322.

71. **Parvaneh K, Ebrahimi M, Sabran MR, Karimi G, Hwei ANM, Abdul-Majeed S, et al.** 2015. Probiotics (*Bifidobacterium longum*) increase bone mass density and upregulate *Sparc* and *Bmp-2* genes in rats with bone loss resulting from ovariectomy. *Biomed Res Int* **2015**:1–10.

72. **McCabe L, Zhang J, Raehtz S.** 2011. Understanding the skeletal pathology of type 1 and 2 diabetes mellitus. *Crit Rev Eukaryot Gene Expr* **21**:187–206.

73. **Payne JM.** 1977. *Metabolic Diseases in Farm Animals.* Butterworth-Heinemann, London, United Kingdom.

74. **Sullivan TW.** 1994. Skeletal problems in poultry: estimated annual cost and descriptions. *Poult Sci* **73**:879–882.

75. **Nahashon SN, Nakaue HS, Mirosh LW.** 1994. Production variables and nutrient retention in single comb white Leghorn laying pullets fed diets supplemented with direct-fed microbials. *Poult Sci* **73**:1699–1711.

76. **Jin LZ, Ho YW, Abdullah N, Jalaludin S.** 1997. Probiotics in poultry: modes of action. *Worlds Poult Sci J* **53**:351–368.

77. **Nava GM, Bielke LR, Callaway TR, Castañeda MP.** 2005. Probiotic alternatives to reduce gastrointestinal infections: the poultry experience. *Anim Health Res Rev* **6**:105–118.

78. **Khan RU, Naz S.** 2013. The applications of probiotics in poultry production. *Worlds Poult Sci J* **69**:621–632.

79. **Mutuş R, Kocabagli N, Alp M, Acar N, Eren M, Gezen SS.** 2006. The effect of dietary probiotic supplementation on tibial bone characteristics and strength in broilers. *Poult Sci* **85**:1621–1625.

80. **Plavnik I, Scott ML.** 1980. Effects of additional vitamins, minerals, or brewer's yeast upon leg weaknesses in broiler chickens. *Poult Sci* **59**:459–464.

81. **Thomas CM, Hong T, van Pijkeren JP, Hemarajata P, Trinh DV, Hu W, Britton RA, Kalkum M, Versalovic J.** 2012. Histamine derived from probiotic *Lactobacillus reuteri* suppresses TNF via modulation of PKA and ERK signaling. *PLoS One* **7**:e31951.

82. **Kim JG, Lee E, Kim SH, Whang KY, Oh S, Imm JY.** 2009. Effects of a *Lactobacillus casei* 393 fermented milk product on bone metabolism in ovariectomised rats. *Int Dairy J* **19**:690–695.

83. **Narva M, Halleen J, Väänänen K, Korpela R.** 2004. Effects of *Lactobacillus helveticus* fermented milk on bone cells *in vitro*. *Life Sci* **75**:1727–1734.

84. **Crittenden RG, Martinez NR, Playne MJ.** 2003. Synthesis and utilisation of folate by yoghurt starter cultures and probiotic bacteria. *Int J Food Microbiol* **80**:217–222.

85. **Arunachalam KD.** 1999. Role of bifidobacteria in nutrition, medicine and technology. *Nutr Res* **19**:1559–1597.

86. **Campbell JM, Fahey GC Jr, Wolf BW.** 1997. Selected indigestible oligosaccharides affect large bowel mass, cecal and fecal short-chain fatty acids, pH and microflora in rats. *J Nutr* **127**:130–136.

87. **Narva M, Collin M, Lamberg-Allardt C, Kärkkäinen M, Poussa T, Vapaatalo H, Korpela R.** 2004. Effects of long-term intervention with *Lactobacillus helveticus*-fermented

milk on bone mineral density and bone mineral content in growing rats. *Ann Nutr Metab* **48:** 228–234.

88. **Bai XC, Lu D, Bai J, Zheng H, Ke ZY, Li XM, Luo SQ.** 2004. Oxidative stress inhibits osteoblastic differentiation of bone cells by ERK and NF-kappaB. *Biochem Biophys Res Commun* **314:**197–207.

89. **Suda N, Morita I, Kuroda T, Murota S.** 1993. Participation of oxidative stress in the process of osteoclast differentiation. *Biochim Biophys Acta* **1157:**318–323.

90. **Sims NA, Martin TJ.** 2014. Coupling the activities of bone formation and resorption: a multitude of signals within the basic multicellular unit. *Bonekey Rep* **3:**481.

91. **Kristensen HB, Andersen TL, Marcussen N, Rolighed L, Delaisse JM.** 2013. Increased presence of capillaries next to remodeling sites in adult human cancellous bone. *J Bone Miner Res* **28:**574–585.

92. **Nakashima T, Hayashi M, Fukunaga T, Kurata K, Oh-Hora M, Feng JQ, Bonewald LF, Kodama T, Wutz A, Wagner EF, Penninger JM, Takayanagi H.** 2011. Evidence for osteocyte regulation of bone homeostasis through RANKL expression. *Nat Med* **17:**1231–1234.

93. **Fuller K, Wong B, Fox S, Choi Y, Chambers TJ.** 1998. TRANCE is necessary and sufficient for osteoblast-mediated activation of bone resorption in osteoclasts. *J Exp Med* **188:**997–1001.

94. **Yoshida H, Hayashi S, Kunisada T, Ogawa M, Nishikawa S, Okamura H, Sudo T, Shultz LD, Nishikawa S.** 1990. The murine mutation osteopetrosis is in the coding region of the macrophage colony stimulating factor gene. *Nature* **345:**442–444.

95. **Teitelbaum SL.** 2000. Bone resorption by osteoclasts. *Science* **289:**1504–1508.

96. **Everts V, Delaissé JM, Korper W, Jansen DC, Tigchelaar-Gutter W, Saftig P, Beertsen W.** 2002. The bone lining cell: its role in cleaning Howship's lacunae and initiating bone formation. *J Bone Miner Res* **17:**77–90.

97. **Edwards CM, Mundy GR.** 2008. Eph receptors and ephrin signaling pathways: a role in bone homeostasis. *Int J Med Sci* **5:**263–272.

98. **Tang Y, Wu X, Lei W, Pang L, Wan C, Shi Z, Zhao L, Nagy TR, Peng X, Hu J, Feng X, Van Hul W, Wan M, Cao X.** 2009. TGF-beta1-induced migration of bone mesenchymal stem cells couples bone resorption with formation. *Nat Med* **15:**757–765.

99. **Anderson HC.** 2003. Matrix vesicles and calcification. *Curr Rheumatol Rep* **5:**222–226.

100. **Bonewald LF.** 2011. The amazing osteocyte. *J Bone Miner Res* **26:**229–238.

101. **Tanaka S, Takahashi N, Udagawa N, Tamura T, Akatsu T, Stanley ER, Kurokawa T, Suda T.** 1993. Macrophage colony-stimulating factor is indispensable for both proliferation and differentiation of osteoclast progenitors. *J Clin Invest* **91:**257–263.

102. **Lacey DL, Timms E, Tan HL, Kelley MJ, Dunstan CR, Burgess T, Elliott R, Colombero A, Elliott G, Scully S, Hsu H, Sullivan J, Hawkins N, Davy E, Capparelli C, Eli A, Qian YX, Kaufman S, Sarosi I, Shalhoub V, Senaldi G, Guo J, Delaney J, Boyle WJ.** 1998. Osteoprotegerin ligand is a cytokine that regulates osteoclast differentiation and activation. *Cell* **93:**165–176.

103. **Kong YY, Yoshida H, Sarosi I, Tan HL, Timms E, Capparelli C, Morony S, Oliveira-dos-Santos AJ, Van G, Itie A, Khoo W, Wakeham A, Dunstan CR, Lacey DL, Mak TW, Boyle WJ, Penninger JM.** 1999. OPGL is a key regulator of osteoclastogenesis, lymphocyte development and lymph-node organogenesis. *Nature* **397:**315–323.

104. **Simonet WS, Lacey DL, Dunstan CR, Kelley M, Chang MS, Lüthy R, Nguyen HQ, Wooden S, Bennett L, Boone T, Shimamoto G, DeRose M, Elliott R, Colombero A, Tan HL, Trail G, Sullivan J, Davy E, Bucay N, Renshaw-Gegg L, Hughes TM, Hill D, Pattison W, Campbell P, Sander S, Van G, Tarpley J, Derby P, Lee R, Boyle WJ.** 1997. Osteoprotegerin: a novel secreted protein involved in the regulation of bone density. *Cell* **89:**309–319.

105. **Dai X-M, Ryan GR, Hapel AJ, Dominguez MG, Russell RG, Kapp S, Sylvestre V, Stanley ER.** 2002. Targeted disruption of the mouse colony-stimulating factor 1 receptor gene results in osteopetrosis, mononuclear phagocyte deficiency, increased primitive progenitor cell frequencies, and reproductive defects. *Blood* **99:**111–120.

106. **Hsu H, Lacey DL, Dunstan CR, Solovyev I, Colombero A, Timms E, Tan HL, Elliott G, Kelley MJ, Sarosi I, Wang L, Xia XZ, Elliott R, Chiu L, Black T, Scully S, Capparelli C, Morony S, Shimamoto G, Bass MB, Boyle WJ.** 1999. Tumor necrosis factor receptor family member RANK mediates osteoclast differentiation and activation induced by osteoprotegerin ligand. *Proc Natl Acad Sci USA* **96:**3540–3545.

107. **Dougall WC, Glaccum M, Charrier K, Rohrbach K, Brasel K, De Smedt T, Daro E, Smith J, Tometsko ME, Maliszewski CR, Armstrong A, Shen V, Bain S, Cosman D, Anderson D, Morrissey PJ, Peschon JJ, Schuh J.** 1999. RANK is essential for osteoclast and lymph node development. *Genes Dev* **13:** 2412–2424.

108. **Asagiri M, Takayanagi H.** 2007. The molecular understanding of osteoclast differentiation. *Bone* **40:**251–264.

109. **Udagawa N, Takahashi N, Yasuda H, Mizuno A, Itoh K, Ueno Y, Shinki T, Gillespie MT, Martin TJ, Higashio K, Suda T.** 2000. Osteoprotegerin produced by osteoblasts is an important regulator in osteoclast development and function. *Endocrinology* **141:**3478–3484.

110. **Li Y, Toraldo G, Li A, Yang X, Zhang H, Qian WP, Weitzmann MN.** 2007. B cells and T cells are critical for the preservation of bone homeostasis and attainment of peak bone mass *in vivo. Blood* **109:**3839–3848.

111. **Ducy P, Zhang R, Geoffroy V, Ridall AL, Karsenty G.** 1997. Osf2/Cbfa1: a transcriptional activator of osteoblast differentiation. *Cell* **89:**747–754.

112. **Nakashima K, Zhou X, Kunkel G, Zhang Z, Deng JM, Behringer RR, de Crombrugghe B.** 2002. The novel zinc finger-containing transcription factor osterix is required for osteoblast differentiation and bone formation. *Cell* **108:**17–29.

113. **Boskey AL.** 2013. Bone composition: relationship to bone fragility and antiosteoporotic drug effects. *Bonekey Rep* **2:**447.

114. **Yang X, Matsuda K, Bialek P, Jacquot S, Masuoka HC, Schinke T, Li L, Brancorsini S, Sassone-Corsi P, Townes TM, Hanauer A, Karsenty G.** 2004. ATF4 is a substrate of RSK2 and an essential regulator of osteoblast biology: implication for Coffin-Lowry syndrome. *Cell* **117:**387–398.

115. **Clarke B.** 2008. Normal bone anatomy and physiology. *Clin J Am Soc Nephrol* **3**(Suppl 3): S131–S139.

116. **Robey P, Boskey A.** 2006. Extracellular matrix and biomineralization of bone, p 12–19. *In* Favus MJ (ed), *Primer on the Metabolic Bone Diseases and Disorders of Mineral Metabolism,* 6th ed. American Society for Bone and Mineral Research, Washington, DC.

117. **Sato K, Suematsu A, Okamoto K, Yamaguchi A, Morishita Y, Kadono Y, Tanaka S, Kodama T, Akira S, Iwakura Y, Cua DJ, Takayanagi H.** 2006. Th17 functions as an osteoclastogenic helper T cell subset that links T cell activation and bone destruction. *J Exp Med* **203:**2673–2682.

118. **Gilbert L, He X, Farmer P, Boden S, Kozlowski M, Rubin J, Nanes MS.** 2000. Inhibition of osteoblast differentiation by tumor necrosis factor-alpha. *Endocrinology* **141:**3956–3964.

119. **Centrella M, McCarthy TL, Canalis E.** 1988. Tumor necrosis factor-alpha inhibits collagen synthesis and alkaline phosphatase activity independently of its effect on deoxyribonucleic acid synthesis in osteoblast-enriched bone cell cultures. *Endocrinology* **123:**1442–1448.

120. **Takayanagi H, Ogasawara K, Hida S, Chiba T, Murata S, Sato K, Takaoka A, Yokochi T, Oda H, Tanaka K, Nakamura K, Taniguchi T.** 2000. T-cell-mediated regulation of osteoclastogenesis by signalling cross-talk between RANKL and IFN-gamma. *Nature* **408:**600–605.

121. **Eastell R.** 2005. Osteoporosis. *Medicine (Baltimore)* **33:**61–65.

122. **Khosla S, Amin S, Orwoll E.** 2008. Osteoporosis in men. *Endocr Rev* **29:**441–464.

123. **Amdekar S, Kumar A, Sharma P, Singh R, Singh V.** 2012. *Lactobacillus* protected bone damage and maintained the antioxidant status of liver and kidney homogenates in female wistar rats. *Mol Cell Biochem* **368:**155–165.

124. **Rovenský J, Svík K, Matha V, Istok R, Ebringer L, Ferencík M, Stancíková M.** 2004. The effects of *Enterococcus faecium* and selenium on methotrexate treatment in rat adjuvant-induced arthritis. *Clin Dev Immunol* **11:**267–273.

Ecological Therapeutic Opportunities for Oral Diseases

10

ANILEI HOARE,[1] PHILIP D. MARSH,[2] and PATRICIA I. DIAZ[1]

INTRODUCTION

The oral microbiome is formed by hundreds of microbial species, including bacteria, fungi, archaea, and viruses, which coexist in specific and organized arrangements in the different habitats of the oral cavity (1–8). Oral subhabitats include the mucosa, covered by keratinized and nonkeratinized stratified squamous epithelium, the papillary surface of the tongue dorsum, and the hard structures of teeth, which comprise those above (supragingival) and those below (subgingival) the gingival margin. The distinct environmental characteristics found in each of these habitats promote the development of unique microbial communities that, although living in close proximity, can be clearly discriminated from each other (9–12). Moreover, the microbial composition of these communities is critical to oral health, with the main oral diseases characterized by deleterious alterations in microbiome community structure at specific subhabitats (13, 14).

As in other human mucosal compartments, an understanding of the composition of health- and disease-associated communities, together with the development of treatments to attempt the restoration of healthy communities in diseased individuals, has been the subject of increasing research. In this

[1]Division of Periodontology, Department of Oral Health and Diagnostic Sciences, UConn Health, Farmington, CT 06030; [2]Division of Oral Biology, School of Dentistry, University of Leeds, Leeds, United Kingdom

Bugs as Drugs: Therapeutic Microbes for the Prevention and Treatment of Disease
Edited by Robert A. Britton and Patrice D. Cani
© 2018 American Society for Microbiology, Washington, DC
doi:10.1128/microbiolspec.BAD-0006-2016

review, we present an overview of the main oral diseases and a critical evaluation of potential microbial-based therapies. We conclude with a perspective on what we believe are key points regarding the etiology of oral diseases that need to be taken into account when developing microbial-based therapeutics for oral conditions.

ECOLOGICAL FACTORS MEDIATING THE ASSEMBLY OF ORAL COMMUNITIES

The oral cavity subhabitats are colonized by uniquely adapted microbial communities. As other accessible surfaces of the human body, like skin, upper respiratory tract, gastrointestinal tract, and vagina, the oral cavity is colonized soon after birth (15). The oral microbiome is one of the most complex and diverse microbial communities, harboring hundreds of species (2, 16). The distribution of such species within oral subhabitats is determined by a number of factors, such as (i) the characteristics of the surfaces available for attachment, (ii) oxygen availability, (iii) exposure to nutrients from the diet of the host, and (iv) exposure to host products delivered by saliva and gingival crevicular fluid. Microbial successions and interspecies interactions also shape the development of oral communities.

Two different types of surfaces, hard and soft, are available for colonization in the oral cavity. The presence of hard, nonshedding surfaces is a unique feature of the mouth, as tooth surfaces (and dentures) allow the development of permanent communities and substantial biomass unless disrupted by regular oral hygiene; in contrast, soft mucosal surfaces promote constant community turnover due to epithelial cell shedding. Both types of surfaces are constantly bathed by saliva, with salivary glycoproteins and proteins adsorbing in a selective way to create a conditioning film. The glycoproteins and proteins in the conditioning film serve as ligands attracting specific species from the genera *Streptococcus, Actinomyces, Capnocytophaga, Eikenella, Haemophilus, Prevotella, Propionibacterium,* and *Veillonella,* among others, which are considered early colonizers (17, 18). These microorganisms possess specific arrangements of surface ligands (usually proteins) that allow their adherence (19). Species such as *Streptococcus mitis* and *Streptococcus sanguinis* recognize sialic acid residues present in adsorbed salivary mucins (20–23). Other species, such as *Actinomyces* spp., produce enzymes that actively modify adsorbed glycoproteins, exposing specific saccharide residues (cryptic receptors), which mediate their own attachment (24, 25). Additionally, most of the indigenous streptococci express polypeptides of the AgI/II family that mediate the recognition of salivary glycoproteins such as gp-340 and their adhesion to epithelial cells (26–28). This group of peptides is also involved in streptococcal attachment to extracellular matrix components such as fibronectin, collagen, and laminin (29, 30), which are exposed when epithelial integrity is disrupted. Thus, selective recognition by early colonizers of molecules exposed at the different surfaces determines and confers specificity to early microbial colonization events.

The attachment of early colonizers to tooth surfaces provides new ligands for the colonization of other species that successively adhere, giving place to the formation of a biofilm (31). Interspecies communication and microbial succession also constitute important aspects of community assembly at different oral surfaces. Classic studies on the physical interactions (coaggregation and coadhesion) among oral species have demonstrated that bacterial-bacterial and fungal-bacterial cell recognition and attachment are highly specific (32–36). Indeed, analysis of dental plaque shows that oral microbial assemblages are specifically organized structures in which individual taxa are arranged in a way suggestive of their functional niche in the consortium (6, 8, 37, 38). For example, in a nine-taxon consortium recently identified in supragingival plaque, filamentous corynebacteria occupied the central position, with other taxa radially arranged around them. Anaerobic taxa tended to be in the interior, whereas facultative or obligate aerobes were located at the periphery of the consortium. Consumers and producers of certain metabolites, such as lactate, tended to be near each other (6). Such highly organized spatial arrangements are likely to result from and facilitate a great variety of interspecies interactions, including the formation of metabolic networks (17).

Interactions among neighboring microbial species in oral communities could be synergistic or antagonistic in nature. One example of synergism in the oral cavity is the collective degradation of salivary glycoproteins by microbial consortia, in which complementary enzymatic activities allow the utilization of mucins in saliva as an energy source, as no microorganism possesses the diverse array of enzymes needed for their complete breakdown (39). Also, several examples of food chains in which a metabolic product of one species is utilized as a primary energy source by a partner species have been documented (40–42). Antagonistic interactions mediated by the production of bacteriocins and hydrogen peroxide may also affect community assembly (43–48).

The interaction of communities with the host also plays a key role in community development. Multiple factors found in the mucosa, saliva, and gingival crevicular fluid (GCF), a serum-like exudate constantly flowing between the gingiva and teeth, modulate the growth of the resident microbiota at the different surfaces (49–52). Antimicrobial peptides of the β-defensin family are found in various locations of the oral cavity such as oral mucosa, gingiva, tongue epithelium, and salivary glands (53). These peptides are believed to selectively control the growth of resident microorganisms (49). In saliva, multiple antimicrobial activities have been described, such as the inhibitory effect of histatins against *Candida* and *Streptococcus*; the antimicrobial activity of cystatins on *Porphyromonas gingivalis*, and cathelicidin LL-37

activity against *Candida* spp. (54–57). Other molecules such as lactoferrin, lysozyme, and a variety of antimicrobial peptides present in saliva may also influence the composition of the microbial community (for a review, see Marsh et al. [52]). Finally, elements of the complement system found in GCF may modulate colonization of the subgingival sulcus (50, 58).

Depending on the location in the oral cavity, the sources of nutrients for microorganisms also differ. In exposed surfaces such as tongue, mucosa, and supragingival surfaces of teeth, dietary products as well as saliva components are the main available nutritional sources, while in the subgingival crevice the resident microorganisms obtain nutrients mainly from GCF. Saliva contains glycoproteins such as mucins, amylase, and immunoglobulin A (IgA) (52, 59), while GCF contains many serum-derived proteins, such as hemoglobin-derived peptides, IgM, IgG, and albumin, which serve as nutrients for subgingival species (50, 60–62). Bacteria from supragingival plaque use host glycoproteins as a major energy source and function as a microbial community to sequentially degrade these structurally complex molecules (39, 63). Enrichment cultivation studies in serum and evaluation of the growth of bacteria in the presence of serum proteins suggest that the protein- and iron-rich GCF promotes the growth of Gram-negative anaerobic proteolytic taxa, which characterize subgingival plaque (61, 64–66). In contrast, dietary carbohydrates affect mostly the community structure of supragingival plaque, with their frequent intake promoting an enrichment of species with an efficient carbohydrate metabolism and an ability to grow well at acidic pH values (67, 68).

Oxygen availability is another important factor driving the selective colonization of microbes in the oral cavity, since it varies widely among the different surfaces found in the mouth. The gingival crevice constitutes a highly reduced area with E_h levels as low as −300 mV as a consequence of low tension of oxygen (69–71). Therefore, this environment selects mostly obligately anaerobic species, while supragingival plaque is enriched with aerobic and facultative microorganisms. Anaerobic bacteria also are found in greater proportions in the tongue crypts, which serve as an anaerobic "pocket-like" reservoir for microbes (72).

ECOLOGICAL ASPECTS OF ORAL DISEASE ETIOLOGY

The three main oral diseases, that is, caries, periodontal diseases, and oral candidiasis, are associated with dysbiosis of the resident oral microbiome. In the three conditions, there is an overgrowth of certain indigenous microorganisms, which become the dominant species at the affected site at the expense of health-associated taxa. Figure 1 summarizes the factors mediating microbiome shifts in these three conditions.

Caries

Caries is the localized demineralization of dental hard tissues by acidic by-products derived from bacterial fermentation of dietary carbohydrates (73). If not controlled, the disease progresses, resulting in the cavitation of the affected tooth, potentially allowing microbial colonization of the tooth pulpal tissue (74). Dental caries is a multifactorial disease in which the frequent intake of dietary carbohydrates and the subsequent generation of a low environmental pH drive alterations in the composition and metabolic properties of the bacterial communities in dental plaque, leading to the enrichment of acid-producing (acidogenic) and acid-tolerant (aciduric) microorganisms (39, 75). The ecological plaque hypothesis, proposed to explain caries etiology, summarizes these dynamics (39). Prior to the onset of the disease, acidogenic bacteria present in the dental biofilm metabolize dietary fermentable sugars. The acid produced changes the local

environment, driving an ecological shift in the resident microbiota that favors the selection of aciduric species, which are able to tolerate, grow in, and continue to produce acid in low-pH environments. With the frequent intake of dietary sugars and a more acidogenic and aciduric microbiome, the plaque pH is therefore maintained at low levels, promoting enamel demineralization (76).

Despite intersubject variability, cariogenic plaques are enriched by a common but limited number of acidogenic/aciduric species compared to healthy subjects. Among these species, *Streptococcus mutans* shows the greater correlation with both onset and progression of caries (14, 77–79). However, besides *S. mutans*, an increased abundance of other streptococci as well as species of *Actinomyces, Atopobium, Lactobacillus, Bifidobacterium, Propionibacterium*, and *Scardovia* has also been associated with caries lesions (14, 77, 80–87). A recent microbiome evaluation by Gross et al. (14) reported that *S. mutans* was the dominant species in many, but not all, subjects with caries. A different species from the mutans group of streptococci (MS) (*Streptococcus sobrinus*), a phylotype from the salivarius group of streptococci (*Streptococcus vestibularis/salivarius*), and a species from the mitis group of streptococci (*Streptococcus parasanguinis*) were also found in high levels in subjects with caries, especially in individuals with no or low levels of *S. mutans* (14). These findings indicate that the acidogenic activity of plaque is probably more important for lesion development than the presence of specific bacterial species. Thus, given the right ecological pressure, other species different from *S. mutans*, but with aciduric and acidogenic characteristics, could become significant contributors to the disease.

Periodontal Diseases

Periodontal diseases are inflammatory conditions that affect the supporting structures of teeth. The interplay between biofilms that accumulate at the gingival margin and the

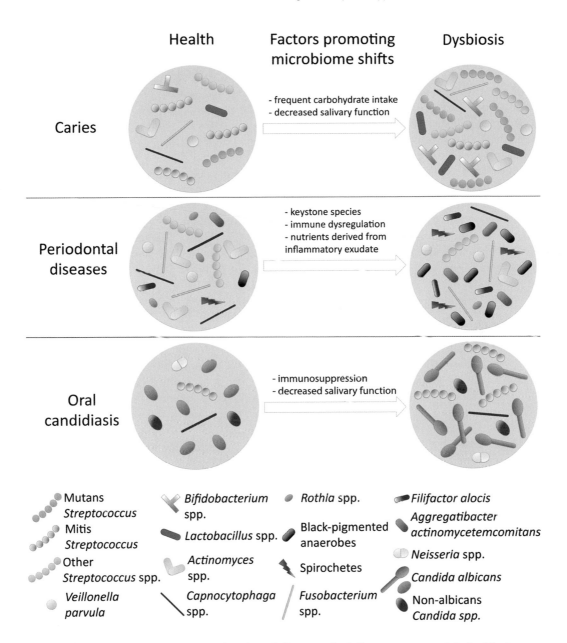

FIGURE 1 Dsybiotic changes associated with oral diseases. Oral diseases are associated with changes in microbiome community structure. Examples of microbiome community shifts and the main factors promoting the establishment of the dysbiotic microbiota are depicted for caries, periodontal diseases, and oral candidiasis.

resulting local immune responses results in gingival inflammation, that is, gingivitis. Further inflammation, as observed in periodontitis, results in the destruction of the connective tissue attachment, alveolar bone resorption, and eventual tooth loss (88). Periodontitis can be broadly classified as aggressive or chronic, based on clinical presentation and progression rate. Compared to more aggressive forms, chronic periodontitis is generally detected in older subjects, has slower rates of progression and destruction, and is associated with thicker and more-complex biofilms (89). Aggressive periodontitis is further divided into localized and generalized forms, the former typically affecting specific teeth (90).

The transition from health to periodontitis is characterized by shifts in the community structure of the subgingival microbiome, probably as a result of the interaction between resident communities and the inflammatory response of the host (13, 88, 91). Health-associated subgingival communities are enriched in Gram-positive taxa, such as *Rothia* spp. and *Actinomyces* spp., while gingivitis communities are enriched with mostly Gram-negative species from the genera *Prevotella*, *Selenomonas*, and *Fusobacterium*, among others (92–94). Further microbiome shifts occur as periodontitis develops with the establishment of a highly diverse community enriched in species such as *P. gingivalis*, *Tannerella forsythia*, *Treponema* spp., *Filifactor alocis*, and *Fretibacterium* spp., among many others (13, 95, 96, 97). Moreover, the aggressive form of periodontitis is characterized by elevated proportions of *Aggregatibacter actinomycetemcomitans* in addition to some of the mentioned bacterial species typically enriched in chronic periodontitis (98–102).

The exact mechanisms behind microbiome shifts associated with periodontal diseases have not been completely elucidated, but it is likely that both microbial and host forces drive the community structure changes. Currently, the most accepted hypothesis of periodontal disease etiology is the polymicrobial synergy and dysbiosis model (88, 103). According to this model, low levels of keystone species such as *P. gingivalis* enhance microbial community virulence by disabling immune surveillance mechanisms in the gingival sulcus, allowing overall community overgrowth, which promotes inflammation. Inflammation further modifies the community selecting for "inflammophilic" organisms, which are those capable of metabolism of proteinaceous substrates derived from tissue

breakdown and from GCF, the flow of which is increased in disease. Inflammation and dysbiosis reinforce each other, eventually causing destruction of periodontal tissues (88). Several mechanisms have been described to mediate the keystone pathogen-driven dysregulation of the host response. *P. gingivalis* has been shown to dysregulate proinflammatory signals in epithelial cells, such as the neutrophil chemokine interleukin-8 (IL-8) and the T-cell chemokine CXCL10/IP-10 (104, 105). Also, *P. gingivalis*, together with *Prevotella intermedia* and *T. forsythia*, dysregulates via several mechanisms the complement pathway (88, 106–109), with animal models showing that complement plays an essential role in the pathogenesis of periodontitis (110). Therefore, synergic interactions between species in the community, the decreased effectiveness of host surveillance mechanisms, and the resulting enhancement of overall community growth with subsequent inflammatory responses conducive to connective tissue attachment and bone loss are likely to contribute to the onset of periodontitis.

Oral Candidiasis

Oral candidiasis is the superficial inflammation of the oral mucosa due to the overgrowth of *Candida* spp. (111). Clinical presentations of the primary forms of oral candidiasis include (i) acute pseudomembranous candidiasis; (ii) chronic erythematous candidiasis; (iii) acute erythematous candidiasis; and (iv) chronic hyperplastic candidiasis (112). *Candida albicans* is the most predominant species associated with oral candidiasis, followed by *Candida glabrata*, *Candida tropicalis*, *Candida parapsilosis*, *Candida kefyr*, *Candida dubliniensis*, *Candida lusitaniae* (currently *Clavispora lusitaniae*), *Candida krusei* (currently *Pichia kudriazevii* and *Issatchenkia orientalis*), and *Candida guilliermondii* (currently *Meyerozyma guilliermondii*) (113). However, the sole presence of these species in the oral cavity is not enough for disease onset. Oral candidiasis development is driven mostly by conditions that compromise the systemic immune response such as organ transplantation, HIV infection, chemotherapy, radiotherapy, and advanced age. Other local contributory factors that may promote *Candida* overgrowth include wearing a removable prosthesis, poor oral hygiene, tobacco use, and hyposalivation (111). Saliva seems to be a key element in the control of *Candida* overgrowth, since it has components such as soluble IgA and mucins that bind and clear the fungi from the oral cavity, as well as histatin 5 and calprotectin, which have potent antifungal activities (114).

Contrary to other mucosal compartments, no clear relationship between the disruption of the bacterial component of the oral microbiome by the use of antibiotics and the overgrowth of *Candida* spp. in the oral cavity has been established. Our current understanding of fungal-bacterial ecology in relation to oral health and disease is limited. Current *in vitro* studies and animal models suggest that the interactions between *C. albicans* and bacterial partners such as oral streptococci may be synergistic rather than antagonistic (115–117). However, no longitudinal studies involving humans and evaluating fungal and bacterial microbiome interactions during oral candidiasis progression exist.

OVERVIEW OF MECHANISMS BEHIND COMMON MICROBIAL THERAPEUTIC APPROACHES

Microbial therapeutics include several approaches aimed at restoring the ecological balance through the use of viable cells. Such strategies have been applied with successful results mainly in gastrointestinal diseases and range from targeting specific species to the replacement of the entire microbiota. Among the strategies that use live cells as therapeutic agents and have been considered in the context of oral diseases are (i) use of probiotics, (ii) bacterial replacement, and (iii) use of predatory bacteria and bacteriophages.

Probiotics

The World Health Organization and the Food and Agriculture Organization of the United Nations define probiotics as "Live microorganisms which, when administered in adequate amounts, confer a health benefit on the host." Some of the desirable characteristics of a probiotic strain include non-pathogenicity and safety for the patient, genetic stability, and ability to survive processing and administration conditions. Other characteristics such as being able to adhere to mucus and/or human epithelial cells, having antimicrobial activity against potentially pathogenic bacteria, and/or the ability to reduce pathogen adhesion to surfaces may also be desirable (118).

Although the exact molecular mechanisms of action of probiotics are largely unknown, the proposed mechanisms can be summarized in three general areas: (i) enhancement of mucosal barrier function, (ii) modulation of the immune response, and (iii) antagonism of pathogens either by the production of antimicrobial compounds or through competition for mucosal binding sites (119, 120). The enhancement of the mucosal barrier is thought to be mediated by the interaction of microorganism-associated molecular patterns with specific epithelial cell receptors (119). Also, several specific bacterial molecules have been shown to direct the expression of tight-junction proteins protecting epithelial cells from apoptosis and promoting cellular proliferation (121), suppress intestinal inflammation through the activation of the histamine H2 receptor (122), and reduce the recruitment of T helper 17 (Th17) cells downregulating interleukin 17 (IL-17) cytokine production (123). Fungal probiotics such as *Saccharomyces boulardii* (*Saccharomyces cerevisiae* var. *boulardii*) have been shown to improve gut barrier function and decrease the inflammation tone, reducing body weight, fat mass, and hepatic steatosis in obese and type 2 diabetic mice (124–127). Another example of an immunomodulatory probiotic effect is the production of a cell surface-associated exopolysaccharide by *Bifidobacterium breve* that protects against infection with enteric pathogens in mice by inducing alterations in antibody production (128).

The direct antagonist effects of probiotics on potentially pathogenic species are possibly mediated by competition for nutrients or adherence and via direct antimicrobial activity (129–132). Although some direct probiotic-pathogen interactions have been documented, whether probiotics need to change the composition of the microbiota to exert their effect remains controversial. Probiotic-induced changes in microbial composition towards beneficial bacteria have been shown in both obesity and hepatocellular carcinoma models (123, 124), while McNulty et al. (133) showed that the metabolic function of the community changed without alterations in community membership after treatment of mice with a mixture of probiotics.

A list of instances in which probiotic use is most accepted as some beneficial effect has been found includes treatment of infectious childhood diarrhea, prevention of antibiotic-associated diarrhea, prevention and maintenance of remission in pouchitis, treatment and maintenance of remission in ulcerative colitis, treatment and prevention of atopic eczema associated with cow's milk allergy, and hepatic liver disease. The recommendations for use of probiotics are strain specific, and these strains include mostly *Lactobacillus* and *Bifidobacterium* spp. (134–136).

Bacterial Replacement Therapies

Bacterial replacement therapies are based on the utilization of indigenous bacteria, usually genetically modified, to colonize human tissues and thereby prevent the outgrowth of disease-associated microorganisms (137, 138). The "effector" bacterial strain is normally an isolate from a human reservoir modified using genetic tools with the purpose of incorporating some beneficial properties. Desirable characteristics for an effector mi-

crobial strain have been summarized as the following: (i) specifically active against target pathogens without significantly disturbing the balance of the existing microbial ecosystem, (ii) indigenous to, and able to survive in, the selected habitat and/or ecosystem and not elsewhere, (iii) nonpathogenic (or weakly opportunistic) for the host species, (iv) susceptible to low-risk antibiotics such as penicillin so that the strain can be later eliminated if desired, (v) easily propagated and readily prepared in a stable form for commercial distribution, (vi) easily identifiable among the resident microbiota, (vii) not causing systemic toxicity or immunological sensitization in the host or leading to selection of resistant microorganisms, (viii) capable of persisting in the host tissues to effect long-term protection (138).

In comparison to probiotics, less research has been conducted to create and evaluate genetically modified effector strains to prevent or treat human disease. Examples of studies using this approach include the evaluation of the role of genetically modified strains of *S. mutans* in the prevention and/or treatment of caries (139, 140). Additionally, studies have been published evaluating the effect of nongenetically modified strains that may outcompete pathogens when administered; for example, a nasal spray containing a mixture of *S. sanguinis*, *S. mitis*, and *Streptococcus oralis* showed promise as a therapeutic alternative for acute otitis media in children (141).

A relatively new strategy that utilizes the bacterial replacement principles for the treatment of dysbiotic disorders is whole-microbiome transplantation, also called eco-therapeutics. This strategy has been directed mainly towards the restoration of the intestinal microbiota after antibiotic treatment, which alters the indigenous community structure and allows colonization by pathogens such as *Clostridium difficile* (142). Ecotherapeutics include mostly fecal transplantation, which consists of administration of stool from a healthy donor to the symptomatic patient (143). Fecal transplantation has been tested as a therapy for *C. difficile*-associated diarrhea with excellent clinical results, showing restoration of bacterial diversity in stool samples and a decrease in symptomatology with a performance far superior to that of vancomycin treatment, which has been the standard of care (144, 145). Also, some promising results have been obtained for other conditions such as metabolic syndrome, obesity, ulcerative colitis, and irritable bowel syndrome (146–150).

Transplantation of selected members of the community also appears as a future viable alternative for the treatment of some dysbiotic diseases. The identification of specific strains with a probiotic-like capacity within the indigenous microbiome and subsequent administration seems a promising strategy. Experiments in mice have shown that oral administration of a cocktail of human intestinal clostridia was able to induce regulatory T cells and anti-inflammatory molecules and attenuated disease in models of colitis and allergic diarrhea (151). Another approach involves the identification of indigenous microorganisms that confer resistance to infection by exogenous pathogens after antibiotic treatment and that could thus be administered prophylactically with the aim of enriching them in the microbiome. For instance, the bile acid 7α-dehydroxylating intestinal bacterium *Clostridium scindens* has been shown to be associated with resistance to *C. difficile* infection when it forms part of the native gut microbiome, and it enhances resistance to postantibiotic infection when administered exogenously (152). These studies highlight the possibility of using indigenous effector bacteria that specifically modulate the inflammatory response and/or antagonize pathogenic strains and are habitat specific.

Predatory Bacteria and Bacteriophages

Predatory bacteria consist of a diverse group of obligatory predators widely distributed in aquatic and terrestrial environments (153).

The most studied strain is *Bdellovibrio bacteriovorus* HD100, which is a predator for Gram-negative species. After attaching to its prey, the predator invades its periplasmic space and multiplies while destroying its cytoplasm. Once the multiplication cycle is completed, the predator destroys the rest of the prey's cell and releases its progeny (154).

Beside *B. bacteriovorus*, a number of strains of predatory bacteria called bdellovibrio-and-like-organisms (BALOs) have received attention as antibacterial agents for the control of pathogenic bacteria. Among the characteristics that make these species good candidates for the control of diseases are (i) being non-pathogenic and nontoxic in several mammalians models, (ii) being potentially well tolerated by humans, (iii) being able to attack a wide range of Gram-negative bacteria, (iv) being able to attack both planktonic and biofilm cells, and (v) being able to attack their prey even in the presence of Gram-positive bacteria (155).

The characteristics listed above make BALOs candidate antibacterial agents for the treatment of a number of Gram-negative-bacterium-associated diseases. Several studies have reported the killing activity of BALOs against a wide range of bacteria such as *Helicobacter pylori* and *Campylobacter jejuni* (156), as well as against bacteria associated with ocular infections (157) and periodontitis (158, 159). However, no human studies have been performed with BALOs, and only one study has demonstrated efficacy *in vivo*, showing that both cecal inflammation and colonization by *Salmonella enterica* serovar Enteritidis were reduced in chicken treated with *Bdellovibrio* (160).

Bacteriophages are viral particles that infect bacteria, leading either to lytic or lysogenic cycles. Lytic (virulent) phages, once replicated and assembled, rapidly destroy the bacterial cell, releasing their progeny (161). Because of their ability to kill bacteria, lytic phages have been historically used for treating infectious diseases such as dysentery and skin and urinary tract infections, among others (reviewed by Abedon et al. [162]). Several studies have been conducted with phages to prevent the formation of *in vitro* biofilms of *Pseudomonas aeruginosa*. Although initially promising results were obtained in one of these studies, regrowth of the biofilm after 24 h of phage administration was observed (151). As an alternative, cocktails of phages or combinations of the viral particles with other antimicrobial agents were investigated with better efficiency at destroying biofilms (163–165). The efficacy of phage cocktails has also been tested in human trials for otitis and wound infections, which showed some clinical improvements and no adverse effects (166, 167).

APPLICATION OF MICROBIAL-BASED THERAPIES TO ORAL DISEASES

Current strategies for treatment of caries and periodontal diseases are focused on the mechanical removal of dental plaque and associated deposits, complemented with the use of antimicrobial compounds and, in the case of caries, with diet modification, topical fluoride application, and if needed, restoration of damaged tooth structures (73, 168–170). The main limitation of such strategies is that only a temporary modification of the pathogenic communities is achieved after therapy, with the disease-associated microbiota, in some individuals, recovering shortly after the initial therapeutic intervention (86, 171, 172). It is also not clear whether the oral microbiome is completely restored, even in the short term, by these treatment strategies to a composition similar to that of a healthy subject that never experienced the disease. Oral candidiasis is treated mostly with antifungal agents, some of which select for strains of *Candida* spp. resistant to such antimicrobial agents (173, 174). Therefore, there is a current need for preventive and therapeutic strategies for oral diseases that aim at restoring a healthy microbiome and increase its resistance to dysbiotic perturbations.

Microbial Therapeutics for Caries

Attempts have been made to apply replacement therapies for the management of dental caries using potential effector strains with decreased acidogenicity, such as an *S. mutans* strain defective in intracellular polysaccharide (IPS) metabolism (140), a noncariogenic *S. salivarius* strain called TOVE-R (175), and an *S. mutans* strain deficient in lactate dehydrogenase activity (176). These strains were used in studies that evaluated their antagonistic activity against native acidogenic *S. mutans* and other caries-associated species, their ability to persistently colonize the oral cavity, their safety and noncariogenicity, and the possibility to be eradicated if needed (139, 175, 177, 178).

The group of Jason M. Tanzer conducted studies with both an *S. mutans* defective in IPS metabolism and the noncariogenic *S. salivarius* TOVE-R. The IPS-deficient *S. mutans* mutant was shown to prevent the colonization by two caries-associated strains of *S. mutans* and *S. sobrinus* in *S. mutans*-free conventional rats (140), but no further studies were conducted. *S. salivarius* TOVE-R was demonstrated to partially displace both *S. mutans* and *S. sobrinus* pathogenic strains in a rat model, accompanied by a decrease in caries experience (175, 179). Some *in vitro* studies were conducted to characterize its mechanism of action (180), but probably because of lack of genetic information on the strain, further studies in humans were not performed.

The group of Jeffrey D. Hillman isolated the *S. mutans* strain JH1001, which produced a bacteriocin, mutacin 1140, able to inhibit the *in vitro* growth of a wide range of bacteria including caries-associated species of *Streptococcus*, *Actinomyces*, and *Lactobacillus* (176, 181). The effector strain failed to consistently colonize the human oral cavity; thus, a mutant that produced higher levels of mutacin 1140 was constructed, thereby improving its colonization and competition with indigenous *S. mutans* (177, 182). Subsequent genetic modifications of the bacteriocin-producing strain were conducted, obtaining a less cariogenic strain due to deletion of lactate dehydrogenase activity (139). Further mutations were later introduced, consisting of the deletion of the *dal* gene, involved in D-alanine biosynthesis, and the *comE* gene, involved in the uptake of environmental DNA (178). The last strain (A2JM) was expected to be noncariogenic, able to displace oral cariogenic microorganisms, less prone to transformation, and dependent on the exogenous addition of D-alanine, a property that allows control of its growth in the host via the exogenous administration of the amino acid. Although subsequent studies showed that it was possible to eradicate the effector strain A2JM in a rat model, the genetically modified strain did not have greater genetic stability than the parental strain, and no studies in humans have been reported (178).

The evaluation of the effectiveness of probiotics as anticariogenic agents has been the subject of high attention for the last 20 years. Despite an increasing number of publications in the field, only a small proportion of these studies have evaluated the effects of probiotics in human clinical trials. Stensson et al. (183) showed that the administration of *Lactobacillus reuteri* during the first year of life was associated with a decrease in caries prevalence at 9 years of age. Moreover, studies have shown that the administration of *Lactobacillus* and/or *Bifidobacterium* strains has a positive short-term effect in decreasing MS counts in saliva (184–199). Other studies, however, have found that MS counts in plaque and/or saliva samples do not change or increase after probiotic intake (200–204). Also, changes in acidogenicity were not observed in plaque or saliva after probiotic use (201, 202). Long-term evaluation of probiotic administration has also shown contradictory results. While a reduction in caries incidence and/or MS counts was shown to occur after 10 or 12 months of ingestion of lactobacilli (205, 206), intervention early in life with *Lactobacillus* or *Bifidobacterium* spp. had no effect on the occurrence of caries and/or on MS counts up to 4 years after the administration (207, 208). Even though the study of potentially probiotic bacteria focuses mostly on lactobacilli, other human indigenous species from the genera *Pediococcus*, *Leuconostoc*, and *Streptococcus* have also been proposed to have probiotic effects against caries (209, 210). *S. salivarius* M18 and a mouthwash containing a mixture of *S. oralis* KJ3sm, *Streptococcus uberis* KJ2sm, and *Streptococcus rattus* JH145 (a spontaneous lactic acid-deficient mutant) have been shown to decrease levels of MS (211, 212). Gruner et al. (213) recently performed a meta-analysis with the data available from randomized controlled trials published between 1967 and June 2015 regarding the use of probiotics in caries, considering human studies that included a control group of either placebo or alternative treatments. Although the analysis showed that probiotics were associated with reductions in the counts of *S. mutans*, the authors found no significant reduction in caries experience, concluding that currently there is no sufficient evidence for recommending probiotics in either prevention or treatment of caries.

More recently, investigations on caries have focused on finding a rationally designed strategy to alter tooth plaque metabolism towards that of a microbial community compatible with health. Clinical studies in children with different caries experiences have shown that plaque alkali production may be related to caries susceptibility, with plaque from healthy children showing a greater ability to produce alkali via the arginine deaminase system (ADS) than plaque from children with caries lesions (214, 215). A limited number of oral species are capable of metabolizing arginine via the ADS with alkali generation. Most species identified belong to the genus *Streptococcus*, with *S. sanguinis* strains being very prevalent among ADS-positive isolates (216). Moreover, a highly arginolytic strain of *Streptococcus* belonging to a potentially novel species was isolated from supragingival plaque of a caries-free individual. The strain not only expressed the ADS pathway at high levels under a variety of conditions but also effectively inhibited the growth of, and two intercellular signaling pathways important in, *S. mutans* (217). These studies show that strains capable of alkali production via arginine may be important contributors to the stability of healthy communities and have prompted investigators to consider if the exogenous administration of arginine may have a beneficial effect in enriching for a health-compatible dental plaque community. Indeed, a clinical study showed that the use of an arginine-containing toothpaste significantly increased ADS activity in plaque of caries-active individuals and shifted the bacterial composition to a healthier community, more similar to that of caries-free individuals (218). These investigations show that arginine could potentially serve as an anticariogenic agent and that perhaps the combination of exogenous arginine administration and enrichment of the microbiome with ADS-positive strains could potentially have a health benefit.

In summary, the management of caries with bacterial replacement therapies based on genetically modified strains has not advanced into clinical trials. Meanwhile, several clinical studies have been conducted with various probiotic combinations, but results are mixed and so far are insufficient for recommending their use in caries management. The use of probiotics for caries prevention does not seem to be derived from a clear rationale, as probiotics may not antagonize the local acidogenic microbiota and the strains themselves have a potential for acidogenicity. Recent efforts focused on defining the metabolic properties of microbial communities associated with health seem to offer more promise, with therapies aimed at the enrichment of alkali production via arginine metabolism representing a more rational alternative.

Microbial Therapeutics for Periodontal Diseases

In the case of periodontal diseases, oral or exogenous probiotic strains have been evaluated under the assumption that they could help in the suppression of periodontitis-associated species by the production of antimicrobial substances or via competitive-exclusion mechanisms and also contribute to modulation of immune responses (219, 220). Different bacterial strains have shown beneficial immunomodulatory effects with respect to the periodontium. These include species like *S. salivarius* and *Streptococcus cristatus* in *in vitro* studies (221–223) and *Lactobacillus brevis* CD2 in animal models and in humans with periodontitis (224, 225). *S. cristatus* has been shown to attenuate the expression of cytokines such as IL-8, IL-1α, IL-6, and tumor necrosis factor alpha in epithelial cells in response to *Fusobacterium nucleatum* (222, 223), while *S. salivarius* K12 has been shown to inhibit the secretion of IL-8 in response to several microorganism-associated molecular patterns (221). In both mice and humans, *L. brevis* has been shown to decrease levels of inflammatory markers like prostaglandin E-2, gamma interferon, tumor necrosis factor alpha, IL-1β, IL-6, and IL-17A (224, 225).

The antimicrobial effects of probiotic-like strains against bacterial species associated with periodontal diseases have also been studied. Among these, a hydrogen peroxide-producing *S. sanguinis* strain has been shown to suppress *A. actinomycetemcomitans* *in vitro* and antagonize its colonization in gnobiotic rats (226). *In vitro* studies have also shown that species such as *S. sanguinis*, *S. cristatus*, *S. salivarius*, and *S. mitis* inhibit colonization of epithelial cells by *A. actinomycetemcomitans* (227, 228), while in another study *S. sanguinis*, *S. salivarius*, *S. mitis*, *Actinomyces naeslundii*, and *Haemophilus parainfluenzae* reduced the adhesion of *P. gingivalis* to the bottom plate of a parallel-plate flow chamber but failed to significantly inhibit *A. actinomycetemcomitans* (229). *Bifidobacterium* species isolated from saliva samples of periodontally healthy individuals have also been shown to inhibit *P. gingivalis* growth, possibly by competing for vitamin K (230).

Human clinical studies on the effect of *Lactobacillus* spp. probiotics in the treatment of chronic periodontitis have reported statistically significant improvements in periodontal clinical parameters such as plaque index, bleeding on probing, and pocket depth and/or reduction of periodontitis-associated species when utilized alone (231, 232) or as an adjunct to periodontal treatment, in comparison to a control group (232–234). However, another study reported that the adjunctive use of a probiotic tablet containing *Streptococcus oralis* KJ3, *Streptococcus uberis* KJ2, and *Streptococcus rattus* JH145 did not significantly improve the therapeutic outcomes of scaling and root planing when compared to the placebo group (235). In subjects with gingivitis, the use of probiotics has shown a positive clinical effect in some studies (236–238), while Iniesta et al. (239) reported decreased levels of *P. intermedia* in saliva and *P. gingivalis* in subgingival plaque but no improvements in plaque and gingival indexes after probiotic administration. Moreover, in healthy children subjected to complete oral prophylaxes followed by probiotic administration in the form of curd, no differences in gingival health were observed in comparison to the control (240). Other studies report that probiotic administration has a positive effect in reducing inflammatory markers in GCF or decreasing levels of periodontitis-associated microorganisms (241–243).

The previously mentioned meta-analysis by Gruner et al. (213) of data available on probiotics trials between 1967 and June 2015 also included periodontal diseases as an outcome. This evaluation revealed that while the use of probiotics for periodontal disease management did not significantly affect the counts of *A. actinomycetemcomitans*, *P. gingivalis*, and *P. intermedia*, it improved two clinical markers indicative of inflammation, i.e., bleeding on probing and gingival index, and helped in reduction of pocket probing depth (213). In summary, most studies report a small but potentially beneficial effect of the use of probiotics in reducing risk factors associated with periodontal diseases or when used as adjuncts to periodontal therapy, with most positive outcomes associated with the use of lactobacilli.

Attempts to recolonize the subgingival environment with health-associated bacteria as part of periodontal therapy were conducted by Teughels et al. (244), who evaluated the effect of administering a mixture of *S. sanguinis*, *S. salivarius*, and *S. mitis* strains as adjuvants in subgingival artificially created pockets in beagle dogs. Four months after the pockets were induced, different treatments consisting of either subgingival scaling and root planing (Rp), root planing and a single topical application of the streptococcus mixture (Rp$_{single}$), or root planing followed by three successive topical applications of the bacterial mixture (Rp$_{multi}$) were evaluated. The effect of each treatment was evaluated after 12 weeks, and the results were compared with those for an untreated control group. Although significant reductions in pocket depth, bleeding on probing, and clinical attachment level were observed in the three treatment groups, the improvements were greatest in the Rp$_{multi}$ group. The Rp$_{multi}$ dogs also showed the most dramatic reduction in anaerobic and black-pigmented species including *Porphyromonas gulae* (a canine form of *P. gingivalis*), *P. intermedia*, and *Campylobacter rectus* and a lesser tendency for reemergence of these pathogens after 12 weeks (244), together with a significant increase in bone density (245). Although the authors did not evaluate whether the streptococci actually colonized the subgingival environment, it is worth noting that streptococci represent a minor genus in dogs (246, 247), and therefore the administration of human streptococci to dogs could be considered an exogenous microbial implantation rather than a restoration of the indigenous microbiota. These experiments constitute perhaps one of the few attempts to evaluate if enrichment of the microbiome with species associated with periodontal health could have a beneficial effect.

Despite the knowledge that periodontitis is associated with a profound dysbiosis of the subgingival microbiome, no attempts at whole subgingival microbiome transplantation as a treatment of periodontal disease are found in the literature. Only one report shows research towards a possible application of microbiota transplantation in the oral cavity (248). In this study, the authors tested an antimicrobial approach to decrease the oral bacterial load in preparation for future whole-microbiome transplantation. The report shows that the use of sodium hypochlorite was effective at reducing the numbers of oral bacteria and its antimicrobial effect could be inactivated by a nontoxic sodium ascorbate-ascorbic acid buffer.

A potentially interesting approach that has been evaluated in the context of periodontal diseases is the use of BALOs, since periodontitis-associated dysbiosis is due mostly to an overgrowth of Gram-negative species. *B. bacteriovorus* HD100 has been shown to significantly reduce the number of viable *A. actinomycetemcomitans* cells in both planktonic and biofilm *in vitro* cultures (249). The eradication of *A. actinomycetemcomitans* from biofilms by predators, however, is not complete, but the combination of BALOs with an exopolysaccharide-hydrolyzing enzyme has been shown to be more effective at decreasing the levels of *A. actinomycetemcomitans* (158). Other studies have shown that different strains of *B. bacteriovorus* may be required to effectively antagonize other Gram-negative species such as *P. intermedia*, *P. gingivalis*, and *Capnocytophaga sputigena* (158, 159). Moreover, the presence of saliva and other nontarget bacteria such as the Gram-positive health-associated *A. naeslundii* has been shown to be noninhibitory to the predatory activity (159). The effect of *Bdellovibrio* has also been tested in a more complex context such as a six-species community formed by *P. intermedia*, *A. actinomycetemcomitans*, *P. gingivalis*, *F. nucleatum*, *S. mitis*, and *A. naeslundii*, as well as against saliva or subgingival plaque samples. In both

cases, although it was observed that the efficiency of predation decreased as the complexity of the models increased, the predator was effective at decreasing the levels of *F. nucleatum* and *A. actinomycetemcomitans*, but other species such as *P. gingivalis* were not affected (250). Importantly, the predatory activity of BALOs was shown to be completely abolished under oxygen-limiting conditions since BALOs are strict aerobes (159, 251). This is a relevant aspect and questions their true potential to eliminate periodontitis-associated species in the reduced conditions that exist in periodontal pockets. In summary, although BALOs show promising *in vitro* results, especially in the control of *A. actinomycetemcomitans*, their effectiveness has not been tested *in vivo*.

Evaluations of the oral virome have revealed that the oral cavity harbors a great amount of bacteriophages (252–254). Although some efforts have been conducted to elucidate the contribution of viruses in the shifts associated with oral diseases, their role in dysbiosis remains unknown (255, 256). Differences in virome community structure were found between healthy and periodontal disease environments in both subgingival and supragingival plaque but not in saliva, with higher proportions of lysogenic *Syphoviridae* in health, while lytic viruses from the *Myoviridae* family were enriched in disease (256). These observations suggest that an altered virome is part of the dysbiosis associated with periodontitis. Despite the potential use of phages as antimicrobial agents against oral pathogens, only a few studies have focused on discovering phages for the control of periodontal dysbiosis (257, 258). Phages isolated from saliva and wastewater from dental chair drainages showed antimicrobial activity against planktonic *F. nucleatum* or *A. actinomycetemcomitans* in *in vitro* biofilms, suggesting a potential application in gingivitis or aggressive periodontitis, which are diseases associated with these respective species (257, 258).

Microbial Therapeutics for Oral Candidiasis

Several *in vitro* studies show that probiotics may affect the virulence potential of *C. albicans*. *Lactobacillus* spp. and *S. salivarius* have been shown to negatively impact *C. albicans* yeast-to-hypha differentiation and/or biofilm formation (259, 260). The mechanism of action would not depend on probiotic-yeast contact, because the use of sterile-filtered supernatant obtained from *S. salivarius* and *Lactobacillus* spp. significantly downregulates, in *C. albicans*, genes critical for the yeast-hypha transition, biofilm formation, host cell invasion, and virulence (261, 262). Also, the treatment of an engineered human oral mucosa tissue model with *Bacillus subtilis* has been shown to decrease *C. albicans* attachment (263).

Animal models have been used to demonstrate potential antagonistic effects of probiotic-like strains on *C. albicans*. *L. acidophilus* protected *Galleria mellonella* larvae against experimental candidiasis (262), while in immunosuppressed mice, *L. rhamnosus* reduced oral *C. albicans* colonization to a higher extent than the antifungal nystatin (264). Moreover, oral administration of *L. acidophilus* to mice has been shown to significantly shorten the duration of *C. albicans* colonization in the mouth, possibly due to an immunomodulatory effect (265). It has also been shown that the application of heat-killed *Enterococcus faecalis* to the tongue of immunosuppressed mice reduces both symptoms and *Candida* counts (266).

Human studies support the mentioned *in vitro* and animal studies, with positive reported effects for probiotic intake with regards to the risk of developing oral candidiasis. Salivary levels of yeast in elderly subjects have been shown to decrease compared to basal levels after probiotic intake (267–269), together with a significant increase in anti-*Candida* IgA levels (269). In patients diagnosed with oral candidiasis, the local administration of a mixture of *Bifidobacterium longum*, *Lactobacillus bulgaricus*, and *Streptococcus thermophilus* was shown to improve oral pain and reduce the prevalence of *Candida* spp. compared with conventional antifungal therapies (270). Moreover, in asymptomatic denture wearers harboring oral *Candida* spp., yeast detection was reduced in the probiotic group compared to the placebo group (271).

LIMITATIONS OF CURRENT MICROBIAL THERAPEUTIC APPROACHES FOR ORAL DISEASES AND PERSPECTIVES FOR DEVELOPMENT OF NEW STRATEGIES

Positive but discrete results have been reported for the management of oral diseases using microbial-based therapies. Most microbial-based therapies evaluated in clinical studies are in the probiotic category, with studies showing some small clinical benefits but lack of defined mechanisms of action. The use of probiotic-like strains seems more beneficial for periodontal diseases and oral candidiasis than for caries (213, 270, 271). Both periodontal diseases and candidiasis are associated with an increased inflammatory response (88, 111), and it is likely that probiotic-mediated immune modulation mediates such favorable effects. It is not clear, however, if the probiotic strains are indeed incorporated into the local microbiota, whether their effect is related to their direct interaction with oral tissues, or if their effects are related to interactions with distant mucosal cells in the gastrointestinal tract and systemic immune modulation. It is also worth noting that although most clinical studies reviewed showed trends towards a positive effect of probiotics as adjuncts to periodontal therapy and in reducing oral yeast carriage, adequately powered and high-quality clinical studies are scarce. Furthermore, the effect size in all studies testing probiotics seems rather small, questioning the clinical relevance of their administration.

The development of more rationally designed microbial-based therapies for oral diseases is still in its infancy but offers more promise than the indiscriminate use of non-specific probiotic strains. Oral diseases are associated with dysbiosis, and therefore, preservation or restoration of the homeo-static state promoted by a health-associated community is the ultimate preventive and therapeutic goal. As reviewed in Fig. 1, unique mechanisms mediate the microbiome shifts associated with caries, periodontal dis-eases, and oral candidiasis. It is conceivable that microbial therapeutics could contribute to the prevention and treatment of these conditions via promotion of the growth of a health-associated community. The implanta-tion of selected oral strains representing health-associated taxa and the reimplanta-tion of a sample from the same patient but enriched with health-promoting strains are alternatives, as is whole-microbiome trans-plantation. One of the challenges, however, of using microbial-based therapies in the mouth compared to the gut is the potential for the rapid loss of the microbial species from the oral cavity by swallowing before they have had a chance to become established and/or exert an effect. The potential advantage of using indigenous oral species as microbial therapeutics is their great potential to colo-nize the specific habitat from which were they were extracted, compared to exogenous strains. It is, however, clear that even if a health-associated community is obtained via such transplantation approaches or through selected killing of disease-associated species, a long-term effect would not be attained un-less the environmental and host-related risk factors shown in Fig. 1 are modified. Micro-bial therapeutics are therefore conceivable only within the context of a more holistic pre-ventive approach involving several strategies.

In the case of caries, research involving microbial-based therapies has focused on competition and/or suppression of *S. mutans*. However, it is important to recognize that in the absence of *S. mutans*, other acidogenic/aciduric species could become enriched given the right environmental pressure (frequent carbohydrate intake). Thus, more attention should be paid to the control of the acidifi-cation of dental biofilms rather than to the elimination of specific species. A conceivable microbial-based therapy for caries could be the enrichment of the microbiome with in-digenous strains that counteract acid produc-tion and therefore promote health-associated species, such as the recently isolated argino-lytic strain of *Streptococcus* (217). Exogenous administration of such strains together with arginine oral supplementation may prove beneficial for caries prevention. The ques-tion, however, is whether such a strain, al-though native to the oral cavity of humans, can effectively colonize another host with an already-assembled, organized, and inter-acting microbiome community in which the specific niche is already occupied. Also, since the highly arginolytic strain is also a strepto-coccus, it is possible that under carbohydrate pressure it may become acidogenic. It is thus clear that even if such a microbial-based ther-apy becomes a reality for caries management, it should be part of a holistic preventive ap-proach with a focus on carbohydrate intake modification (Fig. 2).

In the case of periodontal diseases, cur-rent traditional therapies are directed to-wards controlling the subgingival microbial load. The use of mechanical and chemical means to control biofilm accretion is effec-tive at preventing gingivitis and maintain-ing periodontal stability after therapy in most patients suffering from the disease but constitutes by no means a highly effective strategy as it depends on patient compli-ance. Desirable microbial-based therapeutics for periodontal diseases would be those that prevent the microbiome shifts associated with dysbiosis. In this respect, strategies to antagonize the establishment of keystone pathogens such as *P. gingivalis* are desirable; however, more knowledge is required regard-ing interbacterial interactions in subgingival plaque and the identification of antagonistic species. For instance, *P. gingivalis* has the abil-ity to sense extracellular arginine deiminase

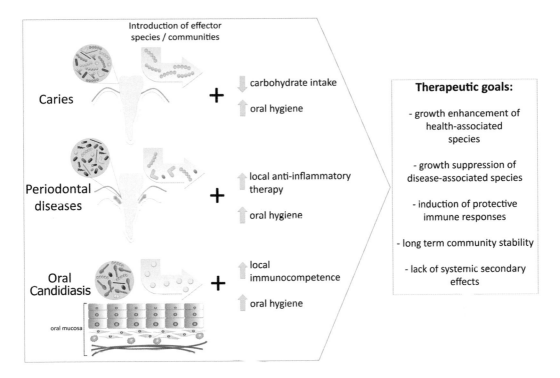

FIGURE 2 Potential beneficial effects of microbial therapies in the management of oral diseases. The desirable effects of the introduction of effector species/communities together with complementary therapies are shown for caries, periodontal diseases, and oral candidiasis.

produced by *S. cristatus* and *S. intermedius*, responding by downregulating the expression of key surface structures required for colonization (272, 273). Indeed, a negative correlation between the distribution of *S. cristatus* and *P. gingivalis* has been observed in subgingival plaque, suggesting that this antagonistic interaction may be important during *in vivo* community maturation (274). Moreover, understanding subgingival microbiome metabolic dynamics could uncover species that are important for overall community stability and increase the resilience of a health-associated community. This implies the application of a systems biology approach to study the microbiome, focusing on the construction and analysis of *in silico* system-level metabolic models (275). Our field currently has information derived from omics studies that can be used to reconstitute the metabolic frameworks of oral bacteria

in relation to oral diseases. Such metabolic models may allow prediction of the role that each species may have in the health- and/or disease-associated consortia (5, 276–278). As with caries, however, microbial therapeutics for periodontal diseases may be just a part of a broader approach that should also include immune modulation, as it seems that microbiome shifts associated with periodontitis are initially the result of immune dysregulation and are perpetuated by uncontrolled inflammation (Fig. 2). Examples of targeted anti-inflammatory strategies against periodontitis include resolvins, anti-complement, and anti-IL-17, which directly address the disease immune-mediated pathophysiology (110, 279).

Although highly experimental, whole oral microbiome transplantation is a strategy that should be tested in the context of oral diseases. Such treatment may have an application in the restoration of homeostasis in patients suffering from periodontitis in which a profound microbiome shift has led to the establishment of a resilient pathogenic community. It should be considered, however, that the transplantation of an entire community may generate unexpected outcomes, such as nonspecific immune responses, either local as a result of the community implantation in the oral cavity or systemic if certain species migrate to extraoral sites. Another nondesired effect may be unexpected interactions between the implanted microbiota components and the indigenous species that could favor the growth of potentially pathogenic species. The question about what constitutes a healthy community is also an aspect that needs to be considered. Both community composition and function in the donor need to be evaluated before transplantation, but there are no specific thresholds to define a health-promoting microbiome. On the other hand, an advantage of whole-microbiome transplantation is that an entire community may have more chances to establish itself and compete with a pathogenic community than the administration of selected species. Disruption of the native pathogenic community would probably be necessary for the establishment of the transplanted one, and therefore, whole-microbiome transplantation should be part of a treatment approach aimed at decreasing the microbial load by mechanical means or antimicrobial strategies. Also important for the long-term stability of the transplanted health-associated community would be that environmental factors such as the inflammatory exudate are controlled, as eventually the newly established community could also become dysbiotic.

In the case of oral candidiasis, little knowledge is available regarding the role of other microbiome members on *Candida* overgrowth. While it is clear that immune dysregulation at the oral mucosal barrier promotes the outgrowth of *C. albicans*, the main species associated with candidiasis, it is less clear whether bacteria or other oral fungi contribute to or antagonize *Candida* growth.

Such information can be obtained from longitudinal studies evaluating microbiome dynamics during oral candidiasis and would be essential for the possible development of microbial-based therapeutic adjuvants to prevent or treat candidiasis. Once again, such microbial adjuvants would require enhancement of mucosal immunocompetence in a combined strategy to prevent candidiasis (Fig. 2).

CONCLUDING REMARKS

In this review, we discuss current approaches based on the use of live microbial strains for the manipulation of oral microbial populations to maintain host-microbe homeostasis. Novel strategies that consider not only the composition of communities associated with disease but also the pathogenic functions may be more promising for the management of oral dysbiosis. However, the design of such strategies necessitates a deeper understanding of the intermicrobial interactions involved in the transitions from health to disease and the functions important to maintain the stability and that confer resilience to health-associated communities. Any microbial-based therapeutic strategy aimed at oral conditions, however, should be part of a holistic approach to control the environmental factors that are primarily responsible for microbiome shifts.

ACKNOWLEDGMENTS

We acknowledge support from grants R01 DE021578 and R21 DE023967 from the National Institute of Dental and Craniofacial Research (NIDCR), National Institutes of Health.

CITATION

Hoare A, Marsh PD, Diaz PI. 2017. Ecological therapeutic opportunities for oral diseases. Microbiol Spectrum 5(4):BAD-0006-2016.

REFERENCES

1. **Chen T, Yu WH, Izard J, Baranova OV, Lakshmanan A, Dewhirst FE.** 2010. The Human Oral Microbiome Database: a web accessible resource for investigating oral microbe taxonomic and genomic information. *Database (Oxford)* **2010:** baq013.

2. **Dewhirst FE, Chen T, Izard J, Paster BJ, Tanner AC, Yu WH, Lakshmanan A, Wade WG.** 2010. The human oral microbiome. *J Bacteriol* **192:**5002–5017.

3. **Dupuy AK, David MS, Li L, Heider TN, Peterson JD, Montano EA, Dongari-Bagtzoglou A, Diaz PI, Strausbaugh LD.** 2014. Redefining the human oral mycobiome with improved practices in amplicon-based taxonomy: discovery of *Malassezia* as a prominent commensal. *PLoS One* **9:**e90899.

4. **Lepp PW, Brinig MM, Ouverney CC, Palm K, Armitage GC, Relman DA.** 2004. Methanogenic *Archaea* and human periodontal disease. *Proc Natl Acad Sci USA* **101:**6176–6181.

5. **Yost S, Duran-Pinedo AE, Teles R, Krishnan K, Frias-Lopez J.** 2015. Functional signatures of oral dysbiosis during periodontitis progression revealed by microbial metatranscriptome analysis. *Genome Med* **7:**27.

6. **Mark Welch JL, Rossetti BJ, Rieken CW, Dewhirst FE, Borisy GG.** 2016. Biogeography of a human oral microbiome at the micron scale. *Proc Natl Acad Sci USA* **113:**E791–E800.

7. **Zijnge V, van Leeuwen MB, Degener JE, Abbas F, Thurnheer T, Gmür R, Harmsen HJ.** 2010. Oral biofilm architecture on natural teeth. *PLoS One* **5:**e9321.

8. **Marsh PD, Moter A, Devine DA.** 2011. Dental plaque biofilms: communities, conflict and control. *Periodontol 2000* **55:**16–35.

9. **Aas JA, Paster BJ, Stokes LN, Olsen I, Dewhirst FE.** 2005. Defining the normal bacterial flora of the oral cavity. *J Clin Microbiol* **43:**5721–5732.

10. **Diaz PI, Dupuy AK, Abusleme L, Reese B, Obergfell C, Choquette L, Dongari-Bagtzoglou A, Peterson DE, Terzi E, Strausbaugh LD.** 2012. Using high throughput sequencing to explore the biodiversity in oral bacterial communities. *Mol Oral Microbiol* **27:**182–201.

11. **Frandsen EV, Pedrazzoli V, Kilian M.** 1991. Ecology of viridans streptococci in the oral cavity and pharynx. *Oral Microbiol Immunol* **6:**129–133.

12. **Xu X, He J, Xue J, Wang Y, Li K, Zhang K, Guo Q, Liu X, Zhou Y, Cheng L, Li M, Li Y, Li Y, Shi W, Zhou X.** 2015. Oral cavity contains distinct niches with dynamic microbial communities. *Environ Microbiol* **17:**699–710.

13. **Abusleme L, Dupuy AK, Dutzan N, Silva N, Burleson JA, Strausbaugh LD, Gamonal J, Diaz PI.** 2013. The subgingival microbiome in health and periodontitis and its relationship with community biomass and inflammation. *ISME J* **7:**1016–1025.

14. **Gross EL, Beall CJ, Kutsch SR, Firestone ND, Leys EJ, Griffen AL.** 2012. Beyond *Streptococcus mutans*: dental caries onset linked to multiple species by 16S rRNA community analysis. *PLoS One* **7:**e47722.

15. **Cephas KD, Kim J, Mathai RA, Barry KA, Dowd SE, Meline BS, Swanson KS.** 2011. Comparative analysis of salivary bacterial microbiome diversity in edentulous infants and their mothers or primary care givers using pyrosequencing. *PLoS One* **6:**e23503.

16. **Huttenhower C, et al, Human Microbiome Project Consortium.** 2012. Structure, function and diversity of the healthy human microbiome. *Nature* **486:**207–214.

17. **Kolenbrander PE, Andersen RN, Blehert DS, Egland PG, Foster JS, Palmer RJ Jr.** 2002. Communication among oral bacteria. *Microbiol Mol Biol Rev* **66:**486–505.

18. **Palmer RJ Jr, Gordon SM, Cisar JO, Kolenbrander PE.** 2003. Coaggregation-mediated interactions of streptococci and actinomyces detected in initial human dental plaque. *J Bacteriol* **185:**3400–3409.

19. **Nobbs AH, Lamont RJ, Jenkinson HF.** 2009. *Streptococcus* adherence and colonization. *Microbiol Mol Biol Rev* **73:**407–450.

20. **Levine MJ, Herzberg MC, Levine MS, Ellison SA, Stinson MW, Li HC, van Dyke T.** 1978. Specificity of salivary-bacterial interactions: role of terminal sialic acid residues in the interaction of salivary glycoproteins with *Streptococcus sanguis* and *Streptococcus mutans*. *Infect Immun* **19:**107–115.

21. **McBride BC, Gisslow MT.** 1977. Role of sialic acid in saliva-induced aggregation of *Streptococcus sanguis*. *Infect Immun* **18:** 35–40.

22. **Murray PA, Levine MJ, Reddy MS, Tabak LA, Bergey EJ.** 1986. Preparation of a sialic acid-binding protein from *Streptococcus mitis* KS32AR. *Infect Immun* **53:**359–365.

23. **Murray PA, Levine MJ, Tabak LA, Reddy MS.** 1982. Specificity of salivary-bacterial interactions. II. Evidence for a lectin on *Streptococcus sanguis* with specificity for a NeuAc alpha 2, 3Gal beta 1, 3GalNAc sequence. *Biochem Biophys Res Commun* **106:**390–396.

24. **Ellen RP, Fillery ED, Chan KH, Grove DA.** 1980. Sialidase-enhanced lectin-like mechanism for *Actinomyces viscosus* and *Actinomy-*

ces naeslundii hemagglutination. *Infect Immun* **27**:335–343.

25. **Gibbons RJ, Hay DI, Childs WC III, Davis G.** 1990. Role of cryptic receptors (cryptitopes) in bacterial adhesion to oral surfaces. *Arch Oral Biol* **35**(Suppl):107S–114S.

26. **Loimaranta V, Jakubovics NS, Hytönen J, Finne J, Jenkinson HF, Strömberg N.** 2005. Fluid- or surface-phase human salivary scavenger protein gp340 exposes different bacterial recognition properties. *Infect Immun* **73**: 2245–2252.

27. **Jakubovics NS, Kerrigan SW, Nobbs AH, Strömberg N, van Dolleweerd CJ, Cox DM, Kelly CG, Jenkinson HF.** 2005. Functions of cell surface-anchored antigen I/II family and Hsa polypeptides in interactions of *Streptococcus gordonii* with host receptors. *Infect Immun* **73**:6629–6638.

28. **Jenkinson HF, Lamont RJ.** 1997. Streptococcal adhesion and colonization. *Crit Rev Oral Biol Med* **8**:175–200.

29. **Busscher HJ, van de Belt-Gritter B, Dijkstra RJ, Norde W, Petersen FC, Scheie AA, van der Mei HC.** 2007. Intermolecular forces and enthalpies in the adhesion of *Streptococcus mutans* and an antigen I/II-deficient mutant to laminin films. *J Bacteriol* **189**:2988–2995.

30. **Love RM, McMillan MD, Jenkinson HF.** 1997. Invasion of dentinal tubules by oral streptococci is associated with collagen recognition mediated by the antigen I/II family of polypeptides. *Infect Immun* **65**:5157–5164.

31. **Kolenbrander PE, Palmer RJ Jr, Periasamy S, Jakubovics NS.** 2010. Oral multispecies biofilm development and the key role of cell-cell distance. *Nat Rev Microbiol* **8**:471–480.

32. **Gibbons RJ, Nygaard M.** 1970. Interbacterial aggregation of plaque bacteria. *Arch Oral Biol* **15**:1397–1400.

33. **Cisar JO, Kolenbrander PE, McIntire FC.** 1979. Specificity of coaggregation reactions between human oral streptococci and strains of *Actinomyces viscosus* or *Actinomyces naeslundii*. *Infect Immun* **24**:742–752.

34. **Kolenbrander PE, Andersen RN, Holdeman LV.** 1985. Coaggregation of oral *Bacteroides* species with other bacteria: central role in coaggregation bridges and competitions. *Infect Immun* **48**:741–746.

35. **Kolenbrander PE, Andersen RN, Moore LV.** 1989. Coaggregation of *Fusobacterium nucleatum, Selenomonas flueggei, Selenomonas infelix, Selenomonas noxia,* and *Selenomonas sputigena* with strains from 11 genera of oral bacteria. *Infect Immun* **57**:3194–3203.

36. **Jenkinson HF, Lala HC, Shepherd MG.** 1990. Coaggregation of *Streptococcus sanguis* and other streptococci with *Candida albicans*. *Infect Immun* **58**:1429–1436.

37. **Listgarten MA.** 1976. Structure of the microbial flora associated with periodontal health and disease in man. A light and electron microscopic study. *J Periodontol* **47**:1–18.

38. **Ozok AR, Persoon IF, Huse SM, Keijser BJ, Wesselink PR, Crielaard W, Zaura E.** 2012. Ecology of the microbiome of the infected root canal system: a comparison between apical and coronal root segments. *Int Endod J* **45**: 530–541.

39. **Bradshaw DJ, Homer KA, Marsh PD, Beighton D.** 1994. Metabolic cooperation in oral microbial communities during growth on mucin. *Microbiology* **140**:3407–3412.

40. **Kuramitsu HK, He X, Lux R, Anderson MH, Shi W.** 2007. Interspecies interactions within oral microbial communities. *Microbiol Mol Biol Rev* **71**:653–670.

41. **Grenier D, Mayrand D.** 1986. Nutritional relationships between oral bacteria. *Infect Immun* **53**:616–620.

42. **Grenier D.** 1992. Nutritional interactions between two suspected periodontopathogens, *Treponema denticola* and *Porphyromonas gingivalis*. *Infect Immun* **60**:5298–5301.

43. **Chikindas ML, Novák J, Driessen AJ, Konings WN, Schilling KM, Caufield PW.** 1995. Mutacin II, a bactericidal antibiotic from *Streptococcus mutans*. *Antimicrob Agents Chemother* **39**:2656–2660.

44. **Donoghue HD, Tyler JE.** 1975. Antagonisms amongst streptococci isolated from the human oral cavity. *Arch Oral Biol* **20**:381–387.

45. **Grenier D.** 1996. Antagonistic effect of oral bacteria towards *Treponema denticola*. *J Clin Microbiol* **34**:1249–1252.

46. **Kaewsrichan J, Douglas CW, Nissen-Meyer J, Fimland G, Teanpaisan R.** 2004. Characterization of a bacteriocin produced by *Prevotella nigrescens* ATCC 25261. *Lett Appl Microbiol* **39**:451–458.

47. **Kreth J, Merritt J, Shi W, Qi F.** 2005. Competition and coexistence between *Streptococcus mutans* and *Streptococcus sanguinis* in the dental biofilm. *J Bacteriol* **187**:7193–7203.

48. **Liu X, Ramsey MM, Chen X, Koley D, Whiteley M, Bard AJ.** 2011. Real-time mapping of a hydrogen peroxide concentration profile across a polymicrobial bacterial biofilm using scanning electrochemical microscopy. *Proc Natl Acad Sci USA* **108**:2668–2673.

49. **Greer A, Zenobia C, Darveau RP.** 2013. Defensins and LL-37: a review of function

in the gingival epithelium. *Periodontol 2000* **63**:67–79.

50. **Huynh AH, Veith PD, McGregor NR, Adams GG, Chen D, Reynolds EC, Ngo LH, Darby IB.** 2015. Gingival crevicular fluid proteomes in health, gingivitis and chronic periodontitis. *J Periodontal Res* **50**:637–649.

51. **van 't Hof W, Veerman EC, Nieuw Amerongen AV, Ligtenberg AJ.** 2014. Antimicrobial defense systems in saliva. *Monogr Oral Sci* **24**:40–51.

52. **Marsh PD, Do T, Beighton D, Devine DA.** 2016. Influence of saliva on the oral microbiota. *Periodontol 2000* **70**:80–92.

53. **Mathews M, Jia HP, Guthmiller JM, Losh G, Graham S, Johnson GK, Tack BF, McCray PB Jr.** 1999. Production of beta-defensin antimicrobial peptides by the oral mucosa and salivary glands. *Infect Immun* **67**:2740–2745.

54. **Blankenvoorde MF, van't Hof W, Walgreen-Weterings E, van Steenbergen TJ, Brand HS, Veerman EC, Nieuw Amerongen AV.** 1998. Cystatin and cystatin-derived peptides have antibacterial activity against the pathogen *Porphyromonas gingivalis*. *Biol Chem* **379**:1371–1375.

55. **den Hertog AL, van Marle J, van Veen HA, Van't Hof W, Bolscher JG, Veerman EC, Nieuw Amerongen AV.** 2005. Candidacidal effects of two antimicrobial peptides: histatin 5 causes small membrane defects, but LL-37 causes massive disruption of the cell membrane. *Biochem J* **388**:689–695.

56. **MacKay BJ, Denepitiya L, Iacono VJ, Krost SB, Pollock JJ.** 1984. Growth-inhibitory and bactericidal effects of human parotid salivary histidine-rich polypeptides on *Streptococcus mutans*. *Infect Immun* **44**:695–701.

57. **Pollock JJ, Denepitiya L, MacKay BJ, Iacono VJ.** 1984. Fungistatic and fungicidal activity of human parotid salivary histidine-rich polypeptides on *Candida albicans*. *Infect Immun* **44**:702–707.

58. **Hajishengallis G, Abe T, Maekawa T, Hajishengallis E, Lambris JD.** 2013. Role of complement in host-microbe homeostasis of the periodontium. *Semin Immunol* **25**:65–72.

59. **Carpenter GH.** 2013. The secretion, components, and properties of saliva. *Annu Rev Food Sci Technol* **4**:267–276.

60. **Ngo LH, Veith PD, Chen YY, Chen D, Darby IB, Reynolds EC.** 2010. Mass spectrometric analyses of peptides and proteins in human gingival crevicular fluid. *J Proteome Res* **9**:1683–1693.

61. **ter Steeg PF, van der Hoeven JS, de Jong MH, van Munster PJJ, Jansen MJH.** 1988. Modelling the gingival pocket by enrichment of subgingival microflora in human serum in chemostats. *Microb Ecol Health Dis* **1**:73–84.

62. **ter Steeg PF, van der Hoeven JS, Bakkeren JAJM.** 1989. Immunoglobulin G cleaving species in serum-degrading consortia of periodontal bacteria. *Microb Ecol Health Dis* **2**:163–169.

63. **Glenister DA, Salmon KE, Smith K, Beighton D, Keevil CW.** 1988. Enhanced growth of complex communities of dental plaque bacteria in mucin-limited continuous culture. *Microb Ecol Health Dis* **1**:31–38.

64. **ter Steeg PF, Van der Hoeven JS, de Jong MH, van Munster PJ, Jansen MJ.** 1987. Enrichment of subgingival microflora on human serum leading to accumulation of *Bacteroides* species, peptostreptococci and *Fusobacteria*. *Antonie van Leeuwenhoek* **53**:261–272.

65. **Grenier D, Imbeault S, Plamondon P, Grenier G, Nakayama K, Mayrand D.** 2001. Role of gingipains in growth of *Porphyromonas gingivalis* in the presence of human serum albumin. *Infect Immun* **69**:5166–5172.

66. **Grenier D, Mayrand D, McBride BC.** 1989. Further studies on the degradation of immunoglobulins by black-pigmented *Bacteroides*. *Oral Microbiol Immunol* **4**:12–18.

67. **Bradshaw DJ, Marsh PD.** 1998. Analysis of pH-driven disruption of oral microbial communities in vitro. *Caries Res* **32**:456–462.

68. **Bradshaw DJ, McKee AS, Marsh PD.** 1989. Effects of carbohydrate pulses and pH on population shifts within oral microbial communities in vitro. *J Dent Res* **68**:1298–1302.

69. **Gibbons RJ, Houte JV.** 1975. Bacterial adherence in oral microbial ecology. *Annu Rev Microbiol* **29**:19–44.

70. **Mettraux GR, Gusberti FA, Graf H.** 1984. Oxygen tension (pO2) in untreated human periodontal pockets. *J Periodontol* **55**:516–521.

71. **Kenney EB, Ash MM Jr.** 1969. Oxidation reduction potential of developing plaque, periodontal pockets and gingival sulci. *J Periodontol* **40**:630–633.

72. **Mager DL, Ximenez-Fyvie LA, Haffajee AD, Socransky SS.** 2003. Distribution of selected bacterial species on intraoral surfaces. *J Clin Periodontol* **30**:644–654.

73. **Selwitz RH, Ismail AI, Pitts NB.** 2007. Dental caries. *Lancet* **369**:51–59.

74. **Fontana M, Young DA, Wolff MS, Pitts NB, Longbottom C.** 2010. Defining dental caries for 2010 and beyond. *Dent Clin North Am* **54**:423–440.

75. **van Houte J.** 1994. Role of micro-organisms in caries etiology. *J Dent Res* **73**:672–681.

76. **Marsh PD.** 2003. Are dental diseases examples of ecological catastrophes? *Microbiology* **149:** 279–294.

77. **Becker MR, Paster BJ, Leys EJ, Moeschberger ML, Kenyon SG, Galvin JL, Boches SK, Dewhirst FE, Griffen AL.** 2002. Molecular analysis of bacterial species associated with childhood caries. *J Clin Microbiol* **40:**1001–1009.

78. **Loesche WJ, Rowan J, Straffon LH, Loos PJ.** 1975. Association of *Streptococcus mutants* with human dental decay. *Infect Immun* **11:**1252–1260.

79. **Marchant S, Brailsford SR, Twomey AC, Roberts GJ, Beighton D.** 2001. The predominant microflora of nursing caries lesions. *Caries Res* **35:**397–406.

80. **Aas JA, Griffen AL, Dardis SR, Lee AM, Olsen I, Dewhirst FE, Leys EJ, Paster BJ.** 2008. Bacteria of dental caries in primary and permanent teeth in children and young adults. *J Clin Microbiol* **46:**1407–1417.

81. **Belda-Ferre P, Alcaraz LD, Cabrera-Rubio R, Romero H, Simón-Soro A, Pignatelli M, Mira A.** 2012. The oral metagenome in health and disease. *ISME J* **6:**46–56.

82. **Kanasi E, Dewhirst FE, Chalmers NI, Kent R Jr, Moore A, Hughes CV, Pradhan N, Loo CY, Tanner AC.** 2010. Clonal analysis of the microbiota of severe early childhood caries. *Caries Res* **44:**485–497.

83. **Loesche WJ, Eklund S, Earnest R, Burt B.** 1984. Longitudinal investigation of bacteriology of human fissure decay: epidemiological studies in molars shortly after eruption. *Infect Immun* **46:**765–772.

84. **Munson MA, Banerjee A, Watson TF, Wade WG.** 2004. Molecular analysis of the microflora associated with dental caries. *J Clin Microbiol* **42:**3023–3029.

85. **Preza D, Olsen I, Aas JA, Willumsen T, Grinde B, Paster BJ.** 2008. Bacterial profiles of root caries in elderly patients. *J Clin Microbiol* **46:** 2015–2021.

86. **Tanner AC, Kent RL Jr, Holgerson PL, Hughes CV, Loo CY, Kanasi E, Chalmers NI, Johansson I.** 2011. Microbiota of severe early childhood caries before and after therapy. *J Dent Res* **90:**1298–1305.

87. **van Ruyven FO, Lingström P, van Houte J, Kent R.** 2000. Relationship among mutans streptococci, "low-pH" bacteria, and lodophilic polysaccharide-producing bacteria in dental plaque and early enamel caries in humans. *J Dent Res* **79:**778–784.

88. **Lamont RJ, Hajishengallis G.** 2015. Polymicrobial synergy and dysbiosis in inflammatory disease. *Trends Mol Med* **21:**172–183.

89. **Armitage GC, Cullinan MP.** 2010. Comparison of the clinical features of chronic and aggressive periodontitis. *Periodontol 2000* **53:** 12–27.

90. **Lang N, Bartold PM, Cullinan M, Jeffcoat M, Mombelli A, Murakami S, Page R, Papapanou P, Tonetti M, Van Dyke T.** 1999. Consensus report: aggressive periodontitis. *Ann Periodontol* **4:**53.

91. **Diaz PI, Hoare A, Hong BY.** 2016. Subgingival microbiome shifts and community dynamics in periodontal diseases. *J Calif Dent Assoc* **44:**421–435.

92. **Kistler JO, Booth V, Bradshaw DJ, Wade WG.** 2013. Bacterial community development in experimental gingivitis. *PLoS One* **8:**e71227.

93. **Huang S, Li R, Zeng X, He T, Zhao H, Chang A, Bo C, Chen J, Yang F, Knight R, Liu J, Davis C, Xu J.** 2014. Predictive modeling of gingivitis severity and susceptibility via oral microbiota. *ISME J* **8:**1768–1780.

94. **Loe H, Theilade E, Jensen SB.** 1965. Experimental gingivitis in man. *J Periodontol* **36:**177–187.

95. **Griffen AL, Beall CJ, Campbell JH, Firestone ND, Kumar PS, Yang ZK, Podar M, Leys EJ.** 2012. Distinct and complex bacterial profiles in human periodontitis and health revealed by 16S pyrosequencing. *ISME J* **6:** 1176–1185.

96. **Hong BY, Furtado Araujo MV, Strausbaugh LD, Terzi E, Ioannidou E, Diaz PI.** 2015. Microbiome profiles in periodontitis in relation to host and disease characteristics. *PLoS One* **10:**e0127077.

97. **Kirst ME, Li EC, Alfant B, Chi YY, Walker C, Magnusson I, Wang GP.** 2015. Dysbiosis and alterations in predicted functions of the subgingival microbiome in chronic periodontitis. *Appl Environ Microbiol* **81:**783–793.

98. **Fine DH, Kaplan JB, Kachlany SC, Schreiner HC.** 2006. How we got attached to *Actinobacillus actinomycetemcomitans*: a model for infectious diseases. *Periodontol 2000* **42:**114–157.

99. **Kamma JJ, Nakou M, Gmür R, Baehni PC.** 2004. Microbiological profile of early onset/aggressive periodontitis patients. *Oral Microbiol Immunol* **19:**314–321.

100. **Lourenço TG, Heller D, Silva-Boghossian CM, Cotton SL, Paster BJ, Colombo AP.** 2014. Microbial signature profiles of periodontally healthy and diseased patients. *J Clin Periodontol* **41:**1027–1036.

101. **Oliveira RR, Fermiano D, Feres M, Figueiredo LC, Teles FR, Soares GM, Faveri M.** 2016. Levels of candidate periodontal pathogens in subgingival biofilm. *J Dent Res* **95:**711–718.

102. **Haubek D, Ennibi OK, Poulsen K, Vaeth M, Poulsen S, Kilian M.** 2008. Risk of aggressive periodontitis in adolescent carriers of the JP2 clone of *Aggregatibacter* (*Actinobacillus*) *actinomycetemcomitans* in Morocco: a prospective longitudinal cohort study. *Lancet* **371:**237–242.

103. **Hajishengallis G, Lamont RJ.** 2012. Beyond the red complex and into more complexity: the polymicrobial synergy and dysbiosis (PSD) model of periodontal disease etiology. *Mol Oral Microbiol* **27:**409–419.

104. **Jauregui CE, Wang Q, Wright CJ, Takeuchi H, Uriarte SM, Lamont RJ.** 2013. Suppression of T-cell chemokines by *Porphyromonas gingivalis*. *Infect Immun* **81:**2288–2295.

105. **Takeuchi H, Hirano T, Whitmore SE, Morisaki I, Amano A, Lamont RJ.** 2013. The serine phosphatase SerB of *Porphyromonas gingivalis* suppresses IL-8 production by dephosphorylation of NF-κB RelA/p65. *PLoS Pathog* **9:** e1003326.

106. **Popadiak K, Potempa J, Riesbeck K, Blom AM.** 2007. Biphasic effect of gingipains from *Porphyromonas gingivalis* on the human complement system. *J Immunol* **178:**7242–7250.

107. **Jusko M, Potempa J, Karim AY, Ksiazek M, Riesbeck K, Garred P, Eick S, Blom AM.** 2012. A metalloproteinase karilysin present in the majority of *Tannerella forsythia* isolates inhibits all pathways of the complement system. *J Immunol* **188:**2338–2349.

108. **Potempa M, Potempa J, Kantyka T, Nguyen KA, Wawrzonek K, Manandhar SP, Popadiak K, Riesbeck K, Eick S, Blom AM.** 2009. Interpain A, a cysteine proteinase from *Prevotella intermedia*, inhibits complement by degrading complement factor C3. *PLoS Pathog* **5:** e1000316.

109. **Maekawa T, Krauss JL, Abe T, Jotwani R, Triantafilou M, Triantafilou K, Hashim A, Hoch S, Curtis MA, Nussbaum G, Lambris JD, Hajishengallis G.** 2014. *Porphyromonas gingivalis* manipulates complement and TLR signaling to uncouple bacterial clearance from inflammation and promote dysbiosis. *Cell Host Microbe* **15:**768–778.

110. **Maekawa T, Abe T, Hajishengallis E, Hosur KB, DeAngelis RA, Ricklin D, Lambris JD, Hajishengallis G.** 2014. Genetic and intervention studies implicating complement C3 as a major target for the treatment of periodontitis. *J Immunol* **192:**6020–6027.

111. **Lalla RV, Patton LL, Dongari-Bagtzoglou A.** 2013. Oral candidiasis: pathogenesis, clinical presentation, diagnosis and treatment strategies. *J Calif Dent Assoc* **41:**263–268.

112. **Williams D, Lewis M.** 2011. Pathogenesis and treatment of oral candidosis. *J Oral Microbiol* **3.**

113. **Muadcheingka T, Tantivitayakul P.** 2015. Distribution of *Candida albicans* and non-*albicans Candida* species in oral candidiasis patients: correlation between cell surface hydrophobicity and biofilm forming activities. *Arch Oral Biol* **60:**894–901.

114. **Salvatori O, Puri S, Tati S, Edgerton M.** 2016. Innate immunity and saliva in *Candida albicans*-mediated oral diseases. *J Dent Res* **95:**365–371.

115. **Diaz PI, Xie Z, Sobue T, Thompson A, Biyikoglu B, Ricker A, Ikonomou L, Dongari-Bagtzoglou A.** 2012. Synergistic interaction between *Candida albicans* and commensal oral streptococci in a novel in vitro mucosal model. *Infect Immun* **80:**620–632.

116. **Xu H, Sobue T, Thompson A, Xie Z, Poon K, Ricker A, Cervantes J, Diaz PI, Dongari-Bagtzoglou A.** 2014. Streptococcal co-infection augments *Candida* pathogenicity by amplifying the mucosal inflammatory response. *Cell Microbiol* **16:**214–231.

117. **Bamford CV, d'Mello A, Nobbs AH, Dutton LC, Vickerman MM, Jenkinson HF.** 2009. *Streptococcus gordonii* modulates *Candida albicans* biofilm formation through intergeneric communication. *Infect Immun* **77:**3696–3704.

118. **FAO/WHO J.** 2002. *Report of a Joint FAO/ WHO Expert Consultation on Guidelines for the Evaluation of Probiotics in Food.* World Health Organization and Food and Agriculture Organization of the United Nations, Ontario, Canada.

119. **Bron PA, van Baarlen P, Kleerebezem M.** 2011. Emerging molecular insights into the interaction between probiotics and the host intestinal mucosa. *Nat Rev Microbiol* **10:**66–78.

120. **Lebeer S, Vanderleyden J, De Keersmaecker SC.** 2008. Genes and molecules of lactobacilli supporting probiotic action. *Microbiol Mol Biol Rev* **72:**728–764.

121. **Yan F, Cao H, Cover TL, Whitehead R, Washington MK, Polk DB.** 2007. Soluble proteins produced by probiotic bacteria regulate intestinal epithelial cell survival and growth. *Gastroenterology* **132:**562–575.

122. **Gao C, Major A, Rendon D, Lugo M, Jackson V, Shi Z, Mori-Akiyama Y, Versalovic J.** 2015. Histamine H2 receptor-mediated suppression of intestinal inflammation by probiotic *Lactobacillus reuteri*. *MBio* **6:**e01358-15.

123. **Li J, Sung CY, Lee N, Ni Y, Pihlajamäki J, Panagiotou G, El-Nezami H.** 2016. Probiotics modulated gut microbiota suppresses hepato-

cellular carcinoma growth in mice. *Proc Natl Acad Sci USA* **113**:E1306–E1315.

124. **Everard A, Matamoros S, Geurts L, Delzenne NM, Cani PD.** 2014. *Saccharomyces boulardii* administration changes gut microbiota and reduces hepatic steatosis, low-grade inflammation, and fat mass in obese and type 2 diabetic db/db mice. *MBio* **5**:e01011-4.

125. **Jahn HU, Ullrich R, Schneider T, Liehr RM, Schieferdecker HL, Holst H, Zeitz M.** 1996. Immunological and trophical effects of *Saccharomyces boulardii* on the small intestine in healthy human volunteers. *Digestion* **57**:95–104.

126. **Martins FS, Vieira AT, Elian SD, Arantes RM, Tiago FC, Sousa LP, Araújo HR, Pimenta PF, Bonjardim CA, Nicoli JR, Teixeira MM.** 2013. Inhibition of tissue inflammation and bacterial translocation as one of the protective mechanisms of *Saccharomyces boulardii* against *Salmonella* infection in mice. *Microbes Infect* **15**:270–279.

127. **Justino PF, Melo LF, Nogueira AF, Costa JV, Silva LM, Santos CM, Mendes WO, Costa MR, Franco AX, Lima AA, Ribeiro RA, Souza MH, Soares PM.** 2014. Treatment with *Saccharomyces boulardii* reduces the inflammation and dysfunction of the gastrointestinal tract in 5-fluorouracil-induced intestinal mucositis in mice. *Br J Nutr* **111**:1611–1621.

128. **Fanning S, Hall LJ, Cronin M, Zomer A, MacSharry J, Goulding D, Motherway MO, Shanahan F, Nally K, Dougan G, van Sinderen D.** 2012. Bifidobacterial surface-exopolysaccharide facilitates commensal-host interaction through immune modulation and pathogen protection. *Proc Natl Acad Sci USA* **109**:2108–2113.

129. **Asahara T, Shimizu K, Nomoto K, Hamabata T, Ozawa A, Takeda Y.** 2004. Probiotic bifidobacteria protect mice from lethal infection with Shiga toxin-producing *Escherichia coli* O157:H7. *Infect Immun* **72**:2240–2247.

130. **Klaenhammer TR.** 1988. Bacteriocins of lactic acid bacteria. *Biochimie* **70**:337–349.

131. **Lee YK, Lim CY, Teng WL, Ouwehand AC, Tuomola EM, Salminen S.** 2000. Quantitative approach in the study of adhesion of lactic acid bacteria to intestinal cells and their competition with enterobacteria. *Appl Environ Microbiol* **66**:3692–3697.

132. **Mack DR, Ahrne S, Hyde L, Wei S, Hollingsworth MA.** 2003. Extracellular MUC3 mucin secretion follows adherence of *Lactobacillus* strains to intestinal epithelial cells in vitro. *Gut* **52**:827–833.

133. **McNulty NP, Yatsunenko T, Hsiao A, Faith JJ, Muegge BD, Goodman AL, Henrissat B, Oozeer R, Cools-Portier S, Gobert G, Chervaux C, Knights D, Lozupone CA, Knight R, Duncan AE, Bain JR, Muehlbauer MJ, Newgard CB, Heath AC, Gordon JI.** 2011. The impact of a consortium of fermented milk strains on the gut microbiome of gnotobiotic mice and monozygotic twins. *Sci Transl Med* **3**:106ra106.

134. **Floch MH, Walker WA, Madsen K, Sanders ME, Macfarlane GT, Flint HJ, Dieleman LA, Ringel Y, Guandalini S, Kelly CP, Brandt LJ.** 2011. Recommendations for probiotic use-2011 update. *J Clin Gastroenterol* **45**(Suppl):S168–S171.

135. **Floch MH.** 2014. Recommendations for probiotic use in humans-a 2014 update. *Pharmaceuticals (Basel)* **7**:999–1007.

136. **Floch MH, Walker WA, Sanders ME, Nieuwdorp M, Kim AS, Brenner DA, Qamar AA, Miloh TA, Guarino A, Guslandi M, Dieleman LA, Ringel Y, Quigley EM, Brandt LJ.** 2015. Recommendations for probiotic use—2015 update: proceedings and consensus opinion. *J Clin Gastroenterol* **49**(Suppl 1):S69–S73.

137. **Allaker RP, Douglas CW.** 2009. Novel antimicrobial therapies for dental plaque-related diseases. *Int J Antimicrob Agents* **33**:8–13.

138. **Tagg JR, Dierksen KP.** 2003. Bacterial replacement therapy: adapting 'germ warfare' to infection prevention. *Trends Biotechnol* **21**:217–223.

139. **Hillman JD, Brooks TA, Michalek SM, Harmon CC, Snoep JL, van Der Weijden CC.** 2000. Construction and characterization of an effector strain of *Streptococcus mutans* for replacement therapy of dental caries. *Infect Immun* **68**:543–549.

140. **Tanzer JM, Fisher J, Freedman ML.** 1982. Preemption of *Streptococcus mutans* 10449S colonization by its mutant 805. *Infect Immun* **35**:138–142.

141. **Roos K, Håkansson EG, Holm S.** 2001. Effect of recolonisation with "interfering" alpha streptococci on recurrences of acute and secretory otitis media in children: randomised placebo controlled trial. *BMJ* **322**:210–212.

142. **Pamer EG.** 2016. Resurrecting the intestinal microbiota to combat antibiotic-resistant pathogens. *Science* **352**:535–538.

143. **Petrof EO, Claud EC, Gloor GB, Allen-Vercoe E.** 2013. Microbial ecosystems therapeutics: a new paradigm in medicine? *Benef Microbes* **4**:53–65.

144. **van Nood E, Vrieze A, Nieuwdorp M, Fuentes S, Zoetendal EG, de Vos WM, Visser CE, Kuijper EJ, Bartelsman JF, Tijssen JG, Speelman P, Dijkgraaf MG, Keller JJ.** 2013. Duodenal infusion of donor feces for recurrent *Clostridium difficile*. *N Engl J Med* **368**:407–415.

145. **Shahinas D, Silverman M, Sittler T, Chiu C, Kim P, Allen-Vercoe E, Weese S, Wong A, Low DE, Pillai DR.** 2012. Toward an understanding of changes in diversity associated with fecal microbiome transplantation based on 16S rRNA gene deep sequencing. *MBio* **3:** e00338-12.

146. **Al-Dasooqi N, Sonis ST, Bowen JM, Bateman E, Blijlevens N, Gibson RJ, Logan RM, Nair RG, Stringer AM, Yazbeck R, Elad S, Lalla RV, Mucositis Study Group of Multinational Association of Supportive Care in Cancer/International Society of Oral Oncology (MASCC/ISOO).** 2013. Emerging evidence on the pathobiology of mucositis. *Support Care Cancer* **21:** 2075–2083.

147. **Borody TJ, Warren EF, Leis S, Surace R, Ashman O.** 2003. Treatment of ulcerative colitis using fecal bacteriotherapy. *J Clin Gastroenterol* **37:**42–47.

148. **Moayyedi P, Surette MG, Kim PT, Libertucci J, Wolfe M, Onischi C, Armstrong D, Marshall JK, Kassam Z, Reinisch W, Lee CH.** 2015. Fecal microbiota transplantation induces remission in patients with active ulcerative colitis in a randomized controlled trial. *Gastroenterology* **149:**102–109.e6.

149. **Pinn DM, Aroniadis OC, Brandt LJ.** 2014. Is fecal microbiota transplantation the answer for irritable bowel syndrome? A single-center experience. *Am J Gastroenterol* **109:**1831–1832.

150. **Vrieze A, Van Nood E, Holleman F, Salojarvi J, Kootte RS, Bartelsman JF, Dallinga-Thie GM, Ackermans MT, Serlie MJ, Oozeer R, Derrien M, Druesne A, Van Hylckama Vlieg JE, Bloks VW, Groen AK, Heilig HG, Zoetendal EG, Stroes ES, de Vos WM, Hoekstra JB, Nieuwdorp M.** 2012. Transfer of intestinal microbiota from lean donors increases insulin sensitivity in individuals with metabolic syndrome. *Gastroenterology* **143:**913–916.e7.

151. **Atarashi K, Tanoue T, Oshima K, Suda W, Nagano Y, Nishikawa H, Fukuda S, Saito T, Narushima S, Hase K, Kim S, Fritz JV, Wilmes P, Ueha S, Matsushima K, Ohno H, Olle B, Sakaguchi S, Taniguchi T, Morita H, Hattori M, Honda K.** 2013. Treg induction by a rationally selected mixture of clostridia strains from the human microbiota. *Nature* **500:**232–236.

152. **Buffie CG, Bucci V, Stein RR, McKenney PT, Ling L, Gobourne A, No D, Liu H, Kinnebrew M, Viale A, Littmann E, van den Brink MR, Jenq RR, Taur Y, Sander C, Cross JR, Toussaint NC, Xavier JB, Pamer EG.** 2015. Precision microbiome reconstitution restores bile acid mediated resistance to *Clostridium difficile*. *Nature* **517:**205–208.

153. **Martin MO.** 2002. Predatory prokaryotes: an emerging research opportunity. *J Mol Microbiol Biotechnol* **4:**467–477.

154. **Sockett RE, Lambert C.** 2004. *Bdellovibrio* as therapeutic agents: a predatory renaissance? *Nat Rev Microbiol* **2:**669–675.

155. **Dwidar M, Monnappa AK, Mitchell RJ.** 2012. The dual probiotic and antibiotic nature of *Bdellovibrio bacteriovorus*. *BMB Rep* **45:**71–78.

156. **Markelova NI.** 2010. Interaction of *Bdellovibrio bacteriovorus* with *Campylobacter jejuni* and *Helicobacter pylori*. *Mikrobiologiia* **79:**779–781. (In Russian.)

157. **Shanks RM, Davra VR, Romanowski EG, Brothers KM, Stella NA, Godboley D, Kadouri DE.** 2013. An eye to a kill: using predatory bacteria to control Gram-negative pathogens associated with ocular infections. *PLoS One* **8:**e66723.

158. **Dashiff A, Kadouri DE.** 2011. Predation of oral pathogens by *Bdellovibrio bacteriovorus* 109J. *Mol Oral Microbiol* **26:**19–34.

159. **Van Essche M, Quirynen M, Sliepen I, Loozen G, Boon N, Van Eldere J, Teughels W.** 2011. Killing of anaerobic pathogens by predatory bacteria. *Mol Oral Microbiol* **26:**52–61.

160. **Atterbury RJ, Hobley L, Till R, Lambert C, Capeness MJ, Lerner TR, Fenton AK, Barrow P, Sockett RE.** 2011. Effects of orally administered *Bdellovibrio bacteriovorus* on the wellbeing and *Salmonella* colonization of young chicks. *Appl Environ Microbiol* **77:**5794–5803.

161. **Guttman B, Raya R, Kutter E.** 2005. Basic phage biology, p 29–66. *In* Kutter E, Sulakvelidze A (ed), *Bacteriophages: Biology and Applications*. CRC Press LLC, Boca Raton, FL.

162. **Abedon ST, Kuhl SJ, Blasdel BG, Kutter EM.** 2011. Phage treatment of human infections. *Bacteriophage* **1:**66–85.

163. **Fu W, Forster T, Mayer O, Curtin JJ, Lehman SM, Donlan RM.** 2010. Bacteriophage cocktail for the prevention of biofilm formation by *Pseudomonas aeruginosa* on catheters in an in vitro model system. *Antimicrob Agents Chemother* **54:**397–404.

164. **Hall AR, De Vos D, Friman VP, Pirnay JP, Buckling A.** 2012. Effects of sequential and simultaneous applications of bacteriophages on populations of *Pseudomonas aeruginosa* in vitro and in wax moth larvae. *Appl Environ Microbiol* **78:**5646–5652.

165. **Torres-Barceló C, Arias-Sánchez FI, Vasse M, Ramsayer J, Kaltz O, Hochberg ME.** 2014. A window of opportunity to control the bacterial pathogen *Pseudomonas aeruginosa* combining antibiotics and phages. *PLoS One* **9:**e106628.

166. **Wright A, Hawkins CH, Anggård EE, Harper DR.** 2009. A controlled clinical trial of a

therapeutic bacteriophage preparation in chronic otitis due to antibiotic-resistant *Pseudomonas aeruginosa*; a preliminary report of efficacy. *Clin Otolaryngol* **34**:349–357.

167. **Rose T, Verbeken G, Vos DD, Merabishvili M, Vaneechoutte M, Lavigne R, Jennes S, Zizi M, Pirnay JP.** 2014. Experimental phage therapy of burn wound infection: difficult first steps. *Int J Burns Trauma* **4**:66–73.

168. **Armitage GC, Robertson PB.** 2009. The biology, prevention, diagnosis and treatment of periodontal diseases: scientific advances in the United States. *J Am Dent Assoc* **140** (Suppl 1):36S–43S.

169. **Weyant RJ, Tracy SL, Anselmo TT, Beltrán-Aguilar ED, Donly KJ, Frese WA, Hujoel PP, Iafolla T, Kohn W, Kumar J, Levy SM, Tinanoff N, Wright JT, Zero D, Aravamudhan K, Frantsve-Hawley J, Meyer DM, American Dental Association Council on Scientific Affairs Expert Panel on Topical Fluoride Caries Preventive Agents.** 2013. Topical fluoride for caries prevention: executive summary of the updated clinical recommendations and supporting systematic review. *J Am Dent Assoc* **144**:1279–1291.

170. **Sharma G, Puranik MP, K R S.** 2015. Approaches to arresting dental caries: an update. *J Clin Diagn Res* **9**:ZE08–ZE11.

171. **Haffajee AD, Uzel NG, Arguello EI, Torresyap G, Guerrero DM, Socransky SS.** 2004. Clinical and microbiological changes associated with the use of combined antimicrobial therapies to treat "refractory" periodontitis. *J Clin Periodontol* **31**:869–877.

172. **Bizzarro S, Laine ML, Buijs MJ, Brandt BW, Crielaard W, Loos BG, Zaura E.** 2016. Microbial profiles at baseline and not the use of antibiotics determine the clinical outcome of the treatment of chronic periodontitis. *Sci Rep* **6**:20205.

173. **Ford CB, Funt JM, Abbey D, Issi L, Guiducci C, Martinez DA, Delorey T, Li BY, White TC, Cuomo C, Rao RP, Berman J, Thompson DA, Regev A.** 2015. The evolution of drug resistance in clinical isolates of *Candida albicans*. *eLife* **4**:e00662.

174. **Kalantar E, Marashi SM, Pormazaheri H, Mahmoudi E, Hatami S, Barari MA, Naseh MH, Asadi M.** 2015. First experience of *Candida* non-*albicans* isolates with high antibiotic resistance pattern caused oropharyngeal candidiasis among cancer patients. *J Cancer Res Ther* **11**:388–390.

175. **Tanzer JM, Kurasz AB, Clive J.** 1985. Competitive displacement of mutans streptococci and inhibition of tooth decay by *Streptococcus salivarius* TOVE-R. *Infect Immun* **48**:44–50.

176. **Hillman JD.** 1978. Lactate dehydrogenase mutants of *Streptococcus mutans*: isolation and preliminary characterization. *Infect Immun* **21**:206–212.

177. **Hillman JD, Dzuback AL, Andrews SW.** 1987. Colonization of the human oral cavity by a *Streptococcus mutans* mutant producing increased bacteriocin. *J Dent Res* **66**:1092–1094.

178. **Hillman JD, Mo J, McDonell E, Cvitkovitch D, Hillman CH.** 2007. Modification of an effector strain for replacement therapy of dental caries to enable clinical safety trials. *J Appl Microbiol* **102**:1209–1219.

179. **Tanzer JM, Kurasz AB, Clive J.** 1985. Inhibition of ecological emergence of mutans streptococci naturally transmitted between rats and consequent caries inhibition by *Streptococcus salivarius* TOVE-R infection. *Infect Immun* **49**:76–83.

180. **Kurasz AB, Tanzer JM, Bazer L, Savoldi E.** 1986. In vitro studies of growth and competition between *S. salivarius* TOVE-R and mutans streptococci. *J Dent Res* **65**:1149–1153.

181. **Hillman JD, Johnson KP, Yaphe BI.** 1984. Isolation of a *Streptococcus mutans* strain producing a novel bacteriocin. *Infect Immun* **44**: 141–144.

182. **Hillman JD, Yaphe BI, Johnson KP.** 1985. Colonization of the human oral cavity by a strain of *Streptococcus mutans*. *J Dent Res* **64**:1272–1274.

183. **Stensson M, Koch G, Coric S, Abrahamsson TR, Jenmalm MC, Birkhed D, Wendt LK.** 2014. Oral administration of *Lactobacillus reuteri* during the first year of life reduces caries prevalence in the primary dentition at 9 years of age. *Caries Res* **48**:111–117.

184. **Ahola AJ, Yli-Knuuttila H, Suomalainen T, Poussa T, Ahlström A, Meurman JH, Korpela R.** 2002. Short-term consumption of probiotic-containing cheese and its effect on dental caries risk factors. *Arch Oral Biol* **47**:799–804.

185. **Bhalla M, Ingle NA, Kaur N, Yadav P.** 2015. Mutans streptococci estimation in saliva before and after consumption of probiotic curd among school children. *J Int Soc Prev Community Dent* **5**:31–34.

186. **Caglar E, Sandalli N, Twetman S, Kavaloglu S, Ergeneli S, Selvi S.** 2005. Effect of yogurt with *Bifidobacterium* DN-173 010 on salivary mutans streptococci and lactobacilli in young adults. *Acta Odontol Scand* **63**:317–320.

187. **Caglar E, Cildir SK, Ergeneli S, Sandalli N, Twetman S.** 2006. Salivary mutans streptococci and lactobacilli levels after ingestion of the probiotic bacterium *Lactobacillus reuteri*

ATCC 55730 by straws or tablets. *Acta Odontol Scand* **64:**314–318.

188. Caglar E, Kavaloglu SC, Kuscu OO, Sandalli N, Holgerson PL, Twetman S. 2007. Effect of chewing gums containing xylitol or probiotic bacteria on salivary mutans streptococci and lactobacilli. *Clin Oral Investig* **11:**425–429.

189. Caglar E, Kuscu OO, Selvi Kuvvetli S, Kavaloglu Cildir S, Sandalli N, Twetman S. 2008. Short-term effect of ice-cream containing *Bifidobacterium lactis* Bb-12 on the number of salivary mutans streptococci and lactobacilli. *Acta Odontol Scand* **66:**154–158.

190. Campus G, Cocco F, Carta G, Cagetti MG, Simark-Mattson C, Strohmenger L, Lingström P. 2014. Effect of a daily dose of *Lactobacillus brevis* CD2 lozenges in high caries risk schoolchildren. *Clin Oral Investig* **18:**555–561.

191. Chuang LC, Huang CS, Ou-Yang LW, Lin SY. 2011. Probiotic *Lactobacillus paracasei* effect on cariogenic bacterial flora. *Clin Oral Investig* **15:**471–476.

192. Cildir SK, Germec D, Sandalli N, Ozdemir FI, Arun T, Twetman S, Caglar E. 2009. Reduction of salivary mutans streptococci in orthodontic patients during daily consumption of yoghurt containing probiotic bacteria. *Eur J Orthod* **31:**407–411.

193. Jindal G, Pandey RK, Agarwal J, Singh M. 2011. A comparative evaluation of probiotics on salivary mutans streptococci counts in Indian children. *Eur Arch Paediatr Dent* **12:**211–215.

194. Juneja A, Kakade A. 2012. Evaluating the effect of probiotic containing milk on salivary mutans streptococci levels. *J Clin Pediatr Dent* **37:**9–14.

195. Nikawa H, Makihira S, Fukushima H, Nishimura H, Ozaki Y, Ishida K, Darmawan S, Hamada T, Hara K, Matsumoto A, Takemoto T, Aimi R. 2004. *Lactobacillus reuteri* in bovine milk fermented decreases the oral carriage of mutans streptococci. *Int J Food Microbiol* **95:**219–223.

196. Singh RP, Damle SG, Chawla A. 2011. Salivary mutans streptococci and lactobacilli modulations in young children on consumption of probiotic ice-cream containing *Bifidobacterium lactis* Bb12 and *Lactobacillus acidophilus* La5. *Acta Odontol Scand* **69:**389–394.

197. Srivastava S, Saha S, Kumari M, Mohd S. 2016. Effect of probiotic curd on salivary pH and *Streptococcus mutans*: a double blind parallel randomized controlled trial. *J Clin Diagn Res* **10:**ZC13–ZC16.

198. Teanpaisan R, Piwat S. 2014. *Lactobacillus paracasei* SD1, a novel probiotic, reduces mutans streptococci in human volunteers: a randomized placebo-controlled trial. *Clin Oral Investig* **18:**857–862.

199. Nishihara T, Suzuki N, Yoneda M, Hirofuji T. 2014. Effects of *Lactobacillus salivarius*-containing tablets on caries risk factors: a randomized open-label clinical trial. *BMC Oral Health* **14:**110.

200. Aminabadi NA, Erfanparast L, Ebrahimi A, Oskouei SG. 2011. Effect of chlorhexidine pretreatment on the stability of salivary lactobacilli probiotic in six- to twelve-year-old children: a randomized controlled trial. *Caries Res* **45:**148–154.

201. Keller MK, Twetman S. 2012. Acid production in dental plaque after exposure to probiotic bacteria. *BMC Oral Health* **12:**44.

202. Marttinen A, Haukioja A, Karjalainen S, Nylund L, Satokari R, Öhman C, Holgerson P, Twetman S, Söderling E. 2012. Short-term consumption of probiotic lactobacilli has no effect on acid production of supragingival plaque. *Clin Oral Investig* **16:**797–803.

203. Nozari A, Motamedifar M, Seifi N, Hatamizargaran Z, Ranjbar MA. 2015. The effect of Iranian customary used probiotic yogurt on the children's salivary cariogenic microflora. *J Dent (Shiraz)* **16:**81–86.

204. Pinto GS, Cenci MS, Azevedo MS, Epifanio M, Jones MH. 2014. Effect of yogurt containing *Bifidobacterium animalis* subsp. *lactis* DN-173010 probiotic on dental plaque and saliva in orthodontic patients. *Caries Res* **48:** 63–68.

205. Rodríguez G, Ruiz B, Faleiros S, Vistoso A, Marró ML, Sánchez J, Urzúa I, Cabello R. 2016. Probiotic compared with standard milk for high-caries children: a cluster randomized trial. *J Dent Res* **95:**402–407.

206. Näse L, Hatakka K, Savilahti E, Saxelin M, Pönkä A, Poussa T, Korpela R, Meurman JH. 2001. Effect of long-term consumption of a probiotic bacterium, *Lactobacillus rhamnosus* GG, in milk on dental caries and caries risk in children. *Caries Res* **35:**412–420.

207. Hasslöf P, West CE, Videhult FK, Brandelius C, Stecksén-Blicks C. 2013. Early intervention with probiotic *Lactobacillus paracasei* F19 has no long-term effect on caries experience. *Caries Res* **47:**559–565.

208. Taipale T, Pienihäkkinen K, Alanen P, Jokela J, Söderling E. 2013. Administration of *Bifidobacterium animalis* subsp. *lactis* BB-12 in early childhood: a post-trial effect on caries occurrence at four years of age. *Caries Res* **47:**364–372.

209. Bosch M, Nart J, Audivert S, Bonachera MA, Alemany AS, Fuentes MC, Cuñé J. 2012. Isolation and characterization of probiotic

strains for improving oral health. *Arch Oral Biol* **57**:539–549.

210. Terai T, Okumura T, Imai S, Nakao M, Yamaji K, Ito M, Nagata T, Kaneko K, Miyazaki K, Okada A, Nomura Y, Hanada N. 2015. Screening of probiotic candidates in human oral bacteria for the prevention of dental disease. *PLoS One* **10**:e0128657.

211. Burton JP, Drummond BK, Chilcott CN, Tagg JR, Thomson WM, Hale JD, Wescombe PA. 2013. Influence of the probiotic *Streptococcus salivarius* strain M18 on indices of dental health in children: a randomized double-blind, placebo-controlled trial. *J Med Microbiol* **62**:875–884.

212. Zahradnik RT, Magnusson I, Walker C, McDonell E, Hillman CH, Hillman JD. 2009. Preliminary assessment of safety and effectiveness in humans of ProBiora3, a probiotic mouthwash. *J Appl Microbiol* **107**:682–690.

213. Gruner D, Paris S, Schwendicke F. 2016. Probiotics for managing caries and periodontitis: systematic review and meta-analysis. *J Dent* **48**:16–25.

214. Nascimento MM, Liu Y, Kalra R, Perry S, Adewumi A, Xu X, Primosch RE, Burne RA. 2013. Oral arginine metabolism may decrease the risk for dental caries in children. *J Dent Res* **92**:604–608.

215. do Nascimento C, Ferreira de Albuquerque Junior R, Issa JP, Ito IY, Lovato da Silva CH, de Freitas Oliveira Paranhos H, de Souza RF. 2009. Use of the DNA Checkerboard hybridization method for detection and quantitation of *Candida* species in oral microbiota. *Can J Microbiol* **55**:622–626.

216. Huang X, Schulte RM, Burne RA, Nascimento MM. 2015. Characterization of the arginolytic microflora provides insights into pH homeostasis in human oral biofilms. *Caries Res* **49**:165–176.

217. Huang X, Palmer SR, Ahn SJ, Richards VP, Williams ML, Nascimento MM, Burne RA. 2016. A highly arginolytic *Streptococcus* species that potently antagonizes *Streptococcus mutans*. *Appl Environ Microbiol* **82**:2187–2201.

218. Nascimento MM, Browngardt C, Xiaohui X, Klepac-Ceraj V, Paster BJ, Burne RA. 2014. The effect of arginine on oral biofilm communities. *Mol Oral Microbiol* **29**:45–54.

219. Roberts FA, Darveau RP. 2002. Beneficial bacteria of the periodontium. *Periodontol 2000* **30**:40–50.

220. Teughels W, Loozen G, Quirynen M. 2011. Do probiotics offer opportunities to manipulate the periodontal oral microbiota? *J Clin Periodontol* **38**(Suppl 11):159–177.

221. Cosseau C, Devine DA, Dullaghan E, Gardy JL, Chikatamarla A, Gellatly S, Yu LL, Pistolic J, Falsafi R, Tagg J, Hancock RE. 2008. The commensal *Streptococcus salivarius* K12 downregulates the innate immune responses of human epithelial cells and promotes host-microbe homeostasis. *Infect Immun* **76**:4163–4175.

222. Zhang G, Chen R, Rudney JD. 2008. *Streptococcus cristatus* attenuates *Fusobacterium nucleatum*-induced interleukin-8 expression in oral epithelial cells. *J Periodontal Res* **43**:408–416.

223. Zhang G, Rudney JD. 2011. *Streptococcus cristatus* attenuates *Fusobacterium nucleatum*-induced cytokine expression by influencing pathways converging on nuclear factor-κB. *Mol Oral Microbiol* **26**:150–163.

224. Riccia DN, Bizzini F, Perilli MG, Polimeni A, Trinchieri V, Amicosante G, Cifone MG. 2007. Anti-inflammatory effects of *Lactobacillus brevis* (CD2) on periodontal disease. *Oral Dis* **13**:376–385.

225. Maekawa T, Hajishengallis G. 2014. Topical treatment with probiotic *Lactobacillus brevis* CD2 inhibits experimental periodontal inflammation and bone loss. *J Periodontal Res* **49**:785–791.

226. Hillman JD, Shivers M. 1988. Interaction between wild-type, mutant and revertant forms of the bacterium *Streptococcus sanguis* and the bacterium *Actinobacillus actinomycetemcomitans* in vitro and in the gnotobiotic rat. *Arch Oral Biol* **33**:395–401.

227. Sliepen I, Van Essche M, Loozen G, Van Eldere J, Quirynen M, Teughels W. 2009. Interference with *Aggregatibacter actinomycetemcomitans*: colonization of epithelial cells under hydrodynamic conditions. *Oral Microbiol Immunol* **24**:390–395.

228. Teughels W, Kinder Haake S, Sliepen I, Pauwels M, Van Eldere J, Cassiman JJ, Quirynen M. 2007. Bacteria interfere with *A. actinomycetemcomitans* colonization. *J Dent Res* **86**:611–617.

229. Van Hoogmoed CG, Geertsema-Doornbusch GI, Teughels W, Quirynen M, Busscher HJ, Van der Mei HC. 2008. Reduction of periodontal pathogens adhesion by antagonistic strains. *Oral Microbiol Immunol* **23**:43–48.

230. Hojo K, Nagaoka S, Murata S, Taketomo N, Ohshima T, Maeda N. 2007. Reduction of vitamin K concentration by salivary *Bifidobacterium* strains and their possible nutritional competition with *Porphyromonas gingivalis*. *J Appl Microbiol* **103**:1969–1974.

231. Vicario M, Santos A, Violant D, Nart J, Giner L. 2013. Clinical changes in periodontal sub-

jects with the probiotic *Lactobacillus reuteri* Prodentis: a preliminary randomized clinical trial. *Acta Odontol Scand* 71:813–819.

232. **Vivekananda MR, Vandana KL, Bhat KG.** 2010. Effect of the probiotic *Lactobacilli reuteri* (Prodentis) in the management of periodontal disease: a preliminary randomized clinical trial. *J Oral Microbiol* 2:5344.

233. **Morales A, Carvajal P, Silva N, Hernandez M, Godoy C, Rodriguez G, Cabello R, Garcia-Sesnich J, Hoare A, Diaz PI, Gamonal J.** 2016. Clinical effects of *Lactobacillus rhamnosus* in non-surgical treatment of chronic periodontitis: a randomized placebo-controlled trial with 1-year follow-up. *J Periodontol* 87:944–952.

234. **Teughels W, Durukan A, Ozcelik O, Pauwels M, Quirynen M, Haytac MC.** 2013. Clinical and microbiological effects of *Lactobacillus reuteri* probiotics in the treatment of chronic periodontitis: a randomized placebo-controlled study. *J Clin Periodontol* 40:1025–1035.

235. **Lalcman I, Yilmaz E, Ozcelik O, Haytac C, Pauwels M, Herrero ER, Slomka V, Quirynen M, Alkaya B, Teughels W.** 2015. The effect of a streptococci containing probiotic in periodontal therapy: a randomized controlled trial. *J Clin Periodontol* 42:1032–1041.

236. **Krasse P, Carlsson B, Dahl C, Paulsson A, Nilsson A, Sinkiewicz G.** 2006. Decreased gum bleeding and reduced gingivitis by the probiotic *Lactobacillus reuteri*. *Swed Dent J* 30:55–60.

237. **Twetman S, Derawi B, Keller M, Ekstrand K, Yucel-Lindberg T, Stecksen-Blicks C.** 2009. Short-term effect of chewing gums containing probiotic *Lactobacillus reuteri* on the levels of inflammatory mediators in gingival crevicular fluid. *Acta Odontol Scand* 67:19–24.

238. **Slawik S, Staufenbiel I, Schilke R, Nicksch S, Weinspach K, Stiesch M, Eberhard J.** 2011. Probiotics affect the clinical inflammatory parameters of experimental gingivitis in humans. *Eur J Clin Nutr* 65:857–863.

239. **Iniesta M, Herrera D, Montero E, Zurbriggen M, Matos AR, Marín MJ, Sánchez-Beltrán MC, Llama-Palacio A, Sanz M.** 2012. Probiotic effects of orally administered *Lactobacillus reuteri*-containing tablets on the subgingival and salivary microbiota in patients with gingivitis. A randomized clinical trial. *J Clin Periodontol* 39:736–744.

240. **Karuppaiah RM, Shankar S, Raj SK, Ramesh K, Prakash R, Kruthika M.** 2013. Evaluation of the efficacy of probiotics in plaque reduction and gingival health maintenance among school children—a randomized control trial. *J Int Oral Health* 5:33–37.

241. **Mayanagi G, Kimura M, Nakaya S, Hirata H, Sakamoto M, Benno Y, Shimauchi H.** 2009. Probiotic effects of orally administered *Lactobacillus salivarius* WB21-containing tablets on periodontopathic bacteria: a double-blinded, placebo-controlled, randomized clinical trial. *J Clin Periodontol* 36:506–513.

242. **Staab B, Eick S, Knöfler G, Jentsch H.** 2009. The influence of a probiotic milk drink on the development of gingivitis: a pilot study. *J Clin Periodontol* 36:850–856.

243. **Shimauchi H, Mayanagi G, Nakaya S, Minamibuchi M, Ito Y, Yamaki K, Hirata H.** 2008. Improvement of periodontal condition by probiotics with *Lactobacillus salivarius* WB21: a randomized, double-blind, placebo-controlled study. *J Clin Periodontol* 35:897–905.

244. **Teughels W, Newman MG, Coucke W, Haffajee AD, Van Der Mei HC, Haake SK, Schepers E, Cassiman JJ, Van Eldere J, van Steenberghe D, Quirynen M.** 2007. Guiding periodontal pocket recolonization: a proof of concept. *J Dent Res* 86:1078–1082.

245. **Nackaerts O, Jacobs R, Quirynen M, Rober M, Sun Y, Teughels W.** 2008. Replacement therapy for periodontitis: pilot radiographic evaluation in a dog model. *J Clin Periodontol* 35:1048–1052.

246. **Dewhirst FE, Klein EA, Thompson EC, Blanton JM, Chen T, Milella L, Buckley CM, Davis IJ, Bennett ML, Marshall-Jones ZV.** 2012. The canine oral microbiome. *PLoS One* 7:e36067.

247. **Sturgeon A, Stull JW, Costa MC, Weese JS.** 2013. Metagenomic analysis of the canine oral cavity as revealed by high-throughput pyrosequencing of the 16S rRNA gene. *Vet Microbiol* 162:891–898.

248. **Pozhitkov AE, Leroux BG, Randolph TW, Beikler T, Flemmig TF, Noble PA.** 2015. Towards microbiome transplant as a therapy for periodontitis: an exploratory study of periodontitis microbial signature contrasted by oral health, caries and edentulism. *BMC Oral Health* 15:125.

249. **Van Essche M, Quirynen M, Sliepen I, Van Eldere J, Teughels W.** 2009. *Bdellovibrio bacteriovorus* attacks *Aggregatibacter actinomycetemcomitans*. *J Dent Res* 88:182–186.

250. **Loozen G, Boon N, Pauwels M, Slomka V, Rodrigues Herrero E, Quirynen M, Teughels W.** 2015. Effect of *Bdellovibrio bacteriovorus* HD100 on multispecies oral communities. *Anaerobe* 35(Pt A):45–53.

251. **Schoeffield AJ, Williams HN, Turng B, Fackler WA Jr.** 1996. A comparison of the survival of intraperiplasmic and attack phase *Bdellovibrios* with reduced oxygen. *Microb Ecol* 32:35–46.

252. **Abeles SR, Pride DT.** 2014. Molecular bases and role of viruses in the human microbiome. *J Mol Biol* **426:**3892–3906.

253. **Edlund A, Santiago-Rodriguez TM, Boehm TK, Pride DT.** 2015. Bacteriophage and their potential roles in the human oral cavity. *J Oral Microbiol* **7:**27423.

254. **Pride DT, Salzman J, Haynes M, Rohwer F, Davis-Long C, White RA III, Loomer P, Armitage GC, Relman DA.** 2012. Evidence of a robust resident bacteriophage population revealed through analysis of the human salivary virome. *ISME J* **6:**915–926.

255. **Hitch G, Pratten J, Taylor PW.** 2004. Isolation of bacteriophages from the oral cavity. *Lett Appl Microbiol* **39:**215–219.

256. **Ly M, Abeles SR, Boehm TK, Robles-Sikisaka R, Naidu M, Santiago-Rodriguez T, Pride DT.** 2014. Altered oral viral ecology in association with periodontal disease. *MBio* **5:**e01133-14.

257. **Machuca P, Daille L, Vinés E, Berrocal L, Bittner M.** 2010. Isolation of a novel bacteriophage specific for the periodontal pathogen *Fusobacterium nucleatum*. *Appl Environ Microbiol* **76:**7243–7250.

258. **Castillo-Ruiz M, Vinés ED, Montt C, Fernández J, Delgado JM, Hormazábal JC, Bittner M.** 2011. Isolation of a novel *Aggregatibacter actinomycetemcomitans* serotype b bacteriophage capable of lysing bacteria within a biofilm. *Appl Environ Microbiol* **77:**3157–3159.

259. **Ishijima SA, Hayama K, Burton JP, Reid G, Okada M, Matsushita Y, Abe S.** 2012. Effect of *Streptococcus salivarius* K12 on the in vitro growth of *Candida albicans* and its protective effect in an oral candidiasis model. *Appl Environ Microbiol* **78:**2190–2199.

260. **Matsubara VH, Wang Y, Bandara HM, Mayer MP, Samaranayake LP.** 2016. Probiotic lactobacilli inhibit early stages of *Candida albicans* biofilm development by reducing their growth, cell adhesion, and filamentation. *Appl Microbiol Biotechnol* **100:**6415–6426.

261. **James KM, MacDonald KW, Chanyi RM, Cadieux PA, Burton JP.** 2016. Inhibition of *Candida albicans* biofilm formation and modulation of gene expression by probiotic cells and supernatant. *J Med Microbiol* **65:**328–336.

262. **Vilela SF, Barbosa JO, Rossoni RD, Santos JD, Prata MC, Anbinder AL, Jorge AO, Junqueira JC.** 2015. *Lactobacillus acidophilus* ATCC 4356 inhibits biofilm formation by *C. albicans* and attenuates the experimental candidiasis in *Galleria mellonella*. *Virulence* **6:**29–39.

263. **Zhao C, Lv X, Fu J, He C, Hua H, Yan Z.** 2016. In vitro inhibitory activity of probiotic products against oral *Candida* species. *J Appl Microbiol* **121:**254–262.

264. **Matsubara VH, Silva EG, Paula CR, Ishikawa KH, Nakamae AE.** 2012. Treatment with probiotics in experimental oral colonization by *Candida albicans* in murine model (DBA/2). *Oral Dis* **18:**260–264.

265. **Elahi S, Pang G, Ashman R, Clancy R.** 2005. Enhanced clearance of *Candida albicans* from the oral cavities of mice following oral administration of *Lactobacillus acidophilus*. *Clin Exp Immunol* **141:**29–36.

266. **Ishijima SA, Hayama K, Ninomiya K, Iwasa M, Yamazaki M, Abe S.** 2014. Protection of mice from oral candidiasis by heat-killed *Enterococcus faecalis*, possibly through its direct binding to *Candida albicans*. *Med Mycol J* **55:**E9–E19.

267. **Hatakka K, Ahola AJ, Yli-Knuuttila H, Richardson M, Poussa T, Meurman JH, Korpela R.** 2007. Probiotics reduce the prevalence of oral *Candida* in the elderly--a randomized controlled trial. *J Dent Res* **86:**125–130.

268. **Kraft-Bodi E, Jørgensen MR, Keller MK, Kragelund C, Twetman S.** 2015. Effect of probiotic bacteria on oral *Candida* in frail elderly. *J Dent Res* **94**(Suppl):181S–186S.

269. **Mendonça FH, Santos SS, Faria IS, Gonçalves e Silva CR, Jorge AO, Leão MV.** 2012. Effects of probiotic bacteria on *Candida* presence and IgA anti-*Candida* in the oral cavity of elderly. *Braz Dent J* **23:**534–538.

270. **Li D, Li Q, Liu C, Lin M, Li X, Xiao X, Zhu Z, Gong Q, Zhou H.** 2014. Efficacy and safety of probiotics in the treatment of *Candida*-associated stomatitis. *Mycoses* **57:**141–146.

271. **Ishikawa KH, Mayer MP, Miyazima TY, Matsubara VH, Silva EG, Paula CR, Campos TT, Nakamae AE.** 2015. A multispecies probiotic reduces oral *Candida* colonization in denture wearers. *J Prosthodont* **24:**194–199.

272. **Xie H, Lin X, Wang BY, Wu J, Lamont RJ.** 2007. Identification of a signalling molecule involved in bacterial intergeneric communication. *Microbiology* **153:**3228–3234.

273. **Christopher AB, Arndt A, Cugini C, Davey ME.** 2010. A streptococcal effector protein that inhibits *Porphyromonas gingivalis* biofilm development. *Microbiology* **156:**3469–3477.

274. **Wang BY, Wu J, Lamont RJ, Lin X, Xie H.** 2009. Negative correlation of distributions of *Streptococcus cristatus* and *Porphyromonas gingivalis* in subgingival plaque. *J Clin Microbiol* **47:**3902–3906.

275. **Borenstein E.** 2012. Computational systems biology and in silico modeling of the human microbiome. *Brief Bioinform* **13:**769–780.

276. **Takahashi N.** 2015. Oral microbiome metabolism: from "who are they?" to "what are they doing?". *J Dent Res* **94:**1628–1637.

277. **Duran-Pinedo AE, Chen T, Teles R, Starr JR, Wang X, Krishnan K, Frias-Lopez J.** 2014. Community-wide transcriptome of the oral microbiome in subjects with and without periodontitis. *ISME J* **8:**1659–1672.

278. **Jorth P, Turner KH, Gumus P, Nizam N, Buduneli N, Whiteley M.** 2014. Metatran-scriptomics of the human oral microbiome during health and disease. *MBio* **5:**e01012-14.

279. **Hasturk H, Kantarci A, Goguet-Surmenian E, Blackwood A, Andry C, Serhan CN, Van Dyke TE.** 2007. Resolvin E1 regulates inflammation at the cellular and tissue level and restores tissue homeostasis in vivo. *J Immunol* **179:**7021–7029.

C. CONTROL OF INFECTIOUS DISEASE BY MICROBES

Control of *Clostridium difficile* Infection by Defined Microbial Communities

11

JAMES COLLINS[1] and JENNIFER M. AUCHTUNG[1]

INTRODUCTION

Each year in the United States, billions of dollars are spent combating almost half a million *Clostridium difficile* infections (CDIs) and trying to reduce the ~29,000 patient deaths in which *C. difficile* has an attributed role (1). In Europe, disease prevalence varies by country and level of surveillance, though yearly costs are estimated at €3 billion (2). One factor contributing to the significant health care burden of *C. difficile* is the relatively high frequency of recurrent CDIs (3). Recurrent CDI, i.e., a second episode of symptomatic CDI occurring within 8 weeks of successful initial CDI treatment, occurs in ~25% of patients, with 35 to 65% of these patients experiencing multiple episodes of recurrent disease (4, 5). Using microbial communities to treat recurrent CDI, either as whole fecal transplants or as defined consortia of bacterial isolates, has shown great success (in the case of fecal transplants) or potential promise (in the case of defined consortia of isolates). This review will briefly summarize the epidemiology and physiology of *C. difficile* infection, describe our current understanding of how fecal microbiota transplants treat recurrent CDI, and outline potential ways that knowledge can be used to rationally design and test alternative microbe-based therapeutics.

[1]Alkek Center for Metagenomics and Microbiome Research and Department of Molecular Virology and Microbiology, Baylor College of Medicine, Houston, TX 77030
Bugs as Drugs: Therapeutic Microbes for the Prevention and Treatment of Disease
Edited by Robert A. Britton and Patrice D. Cani
© 2018 American Society for Microbiology, Washington, DC
doi:10.1128/microbiolspec.BAD-0009-2016

HISTORY OF *C. DIFFICILE* INFECTION

A strictly anaerobic, spore-forming, Gram-positive bacillus, *C. difficile* (originally named *Bacillus difficilis*) was first identified in healthy neonates in 1935 (6). It was not until the late 1970s, however, that the role of *C. difficile* as an etiological agent of antibiotic-associated diarrhea and pseudomembranous colitis was described (7–10). Throughout the 1980s and 1990s the clinical importance of *C. difficile* remained limited. When encountered, disease was often mild and easily controlled with antibiotics (Table 1). In the early 2000s, a new lineage of *C. difficile* strains (equivalently known as ribotype 027, restriction endonuclease analysis group BI, or North American pulsed-field electrophoresis 1) emerged that was linked to increased disease severity, morbidity, and mortality (11, 12) (Fig. 1). In the following years, the ribotype 027 lineage spread throughout North America and Europe (13, 14), paralleling increases in the overall incidence and severity of *C. difficile* infection (CDI). Strains of the ribotype 027 lineage have often been described as "hypervirulent" (11, 15). Studies have pointed to increased toxin production (16), production of a binary toxin (17), fluoroquinolone resistance (14), increased frequency of sporulation (18), enhanced ecological fitness (19), and a higher correlation with recurrent infection (20, 21) as potential mechanisms that led to increased incidence and/or severity of infections associated with ribotype 027 strains. However, some "hypervirulent" attributes of ribotype 027 vary across strains (e.g., degree of toxin production and sporulation [22]) or are found in ribotypes not typically associated with increased disease severity (e.g., fluoroquinolone resistance [23]), making it difficult to pinpoint specific mechanisms responsible for increased incidence and/or severity of infection with ribotype 027 strains. Correspondingly, some clinical studies (24–26) failed to reproduce statistically significant increases in severe CDI in patients infected with ribotype 027 observed in other studies (13, 27, 28). Finally, even as the frequency of ribotype 027-associated CDI has stabilized or decreased in some regions (29, 30), the overall frequency of CDI has remained high, with other *C. difficile* ribotypes increasing in prevalence (29–32). The picture emerging from these diverse and sometimes

TABLE 1 Stratification of disease severity associated with *C. difficile* colonization (44, 45)

Classification	Diagnostic criteria
Asymptomatic carriage/colonization	Positive identification of *C. difficile* (toxigenic or nontoxigenic) without clinical symptoms
Mild to moderate CDI	≥3 unformed stools in 24 hours
	Positive identification of toxigenic *C. difficile*
	White blood cell (WBC) count <15,000 and serum creatinine levels <1.5× premorbid level
Severe CDI	Positive identification of toxigenic *C. difficile* and/or evidence of pseudomembranous colitis
	WBC count ≥15,000 cells/μl, serum albumin <3 g/dl, and/or serum creatinine level ≥1.5× premorbid level
Severe, complicated CDI (sometimes referred to as "fulminant") (45)	Hypotension, shock, ileus, or megacolon
	Other systemic signs of severe infection (144) including:
	Admission to intensive care unit
	Altered mental status
	Fever ≥38.5°C
	WBC <2,000 or >30,000/μl
	Lactate >2.2 mmol/liter
	Evidence of end-organ damage
	Positive identification of toxigenic *C. difficile*
rCDI	Recurrence of symptoms within 8 weeks of successful *C. difficile* treatment

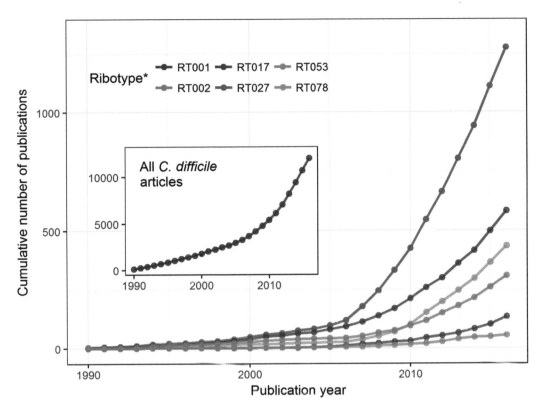

FIGURE 1 Cumulative number of *C. difficile* articles in PubMed. Total article number includes all articles with "difficile" in either the title or abstract. *Ribotype articles are those that have "difficile" and the ribotype (or alternative nomenclature) in the title or abstract; e.g., RT027 articles were classified as such if they had "difficile" AND "Ribotype 027" OR "RT027" OR "Sequence Type 1" OR "NAP1" etc. Although not a definitive measure of global ribotype abundance, these data can serve as a proxy for the relative frequency of outbreaks associated with specific ribotypes.

conflicting studies is that although the spread of the ribotype 027 lineage significantly contributed to the initial increase in CDI, factors in addition to the ribotype of the infecting strain contribute to the continued prevalence of CDI, which remains a significant threat to public health.

C. DIFFICILE CARRIAGE AND DISEASE

Traditionally, CDI has not been considered a risk to healthy individuals. Infection is usually preceded by disruption of the "healthy" gut microbiome through antibiotic use (33). Meta-analyses examining the risk of CDI

following antibiotic use found clindamycin to be the greatest hazard followed by carbapenems, fluoroquinolones, and cephalosporins; more moderate risks were associated with macrolides, sulfonamides, and penicillins; and no risk was associated with tetracyclines (34–36). Use of proton pump inhibitors (37), inflammatory bowel disease (38), and advancing age (39) are also risk factors, likely due to changes to the gut microbiota (40, 41), and in the latter case, reduced efficacy of the immune system (39). However, increases in the rates of community-acquired CDI have also demonstrated that CDI can occur in relatively healthy populations previously thought to be at low risk for infection, including people who had not been exposed to antibiotics within the previous 3 months (reviewed in 31, 42), revealing that there remain additional, previously unrecognized risk factors for CDI.

Once a susceptible individual is exposed to *C. difficile*, multiple outcomes are possible (Table 1). Asymptomatic carriage occurs in a subset of susceptible individuals. Symptomatic CDI can manifest with increasing degrees of severity, which influences approaches used to treat disease. Following the resolution of symptomatic disease, asymptomatic shedding of spores in stool can persist for up to 6 weeks (43). A brief description of treatment modalities is given later in the review to provide context for the use of microbial-based therapies for treatment of CDI. However, because neither author is a clinician, we point to several recent reviews (44–46) written by clinicians experienced in diagnosis and treatment of *C. difficile* that provide excellent detailed descriptions of the diagnosis and treatment of CDI in adults.

Asymptomatic Carriage in Infants

Infants (<1 year of age) are frequently asymptomatic carriers of *C. difficile*, with a wide range of carriage rates reported (2 to 100% [47–51]). The mechanisms that mediate high levels of asymptomatic carriage in infants are unclear, though the immature microbiome likely plays a role. During the first year of life, the infant gastrointestinal microbiome undergoes successional maturation, transitioning from a low-complexity community, dominated by facultative anaerobes and aerobic bacteria, to a complex community dominated by obligate anaerobes and more similar to the adult gastrointestinal microbiome (52, 53). Hypotheses for how infant carriage rates remain on the whole asymptomatic include the failure of the immature infant immune system to activate an inflammatory response, protective maternal antibodies transferred in breast milk, and/or the inability of toxins to interact appropri-

ately with receptors and cause disease (reviewed in references 50 and 54). Additional studies, including those that utilize physiologically relevant models of the infant gastrointestinal tract, are needed to delineate mechanisms through which infants are asymptomatically colonized with *C. difficile*.

Asymptomatic Carriage in Adults

Carriage rates decrease with increasing age (49, 50), with asymptomatic carriage rates in healthy adults reported between 0 and 15% (50, 55–57). Patients in long-term care facilities have a higher average asymptomatic carriage rate at 14.8% (95% CI 7.6 to 24.0%), though it is hard to discern if this is due to a change in the cohort physiology (microbiota, immune response), the environment, or both (58). Asymptomatic carriage is often limited in duration (reviewed in reference 56) and has been associated with a lower likelihood of developing symptomatic CDI (59, 60).

Potential Mechanisms Underlying Asymptomatic Carriage

Two small studies have suggested that differences in the host microbiota could be a potential mechanism that distinguishes between asymptomatic carriage and disease (61, 62). By comparing microbial community composition between four patients with CDI, four asymptomatically colonized patients, and noncolonized controls, Vincent et al. (62) found that organisms classified as members of the *Clostridiales incertae sedis* XI family, *Eubacterium* species, or *Clostridium* species other than *C. difficile* were enriched in asymptomatically colonized patients compared to patients with symptomatic CDI. By comparing eight symptomatically infected patients, eight asymptomatically colonized *C. difficile* patients, and healthy controls, Zhang et al. (61) observed trends toward increased levels of *Bacteroides*, *Lachnospiraceae incertae sedis*, and *Clostridium* XIVa species and statistically significant decreases in the levels of *Escherichia/Shigella* species in asymptomatically colonized patients compared to healthy controls. Both asymptomatically colonized patients and patients with CDI also had significantly decreased microbial diversity compared to healthy controls. Although the authors reached different conclusions as to the potential driving forces responsible for microbiome composition differences, both studies observed increased levels of specific *Clostridiales* family members in asymptomatically colonized patients relative to symptomatic CDI patients and healthy controls. Although preliminary, these data suggest that expansion of these *Clostridiales* members may limit *C. difficile* pathogenesis, either by regulating levels of *C. difficile* and/or its toxin or by blocking pathogenic interactions between *C. difficile* and the host epithelium and/or immune system.

Variation in immune response is another potential mechanism that distinguishes symptomatic from asymptomatic carriage of *C. difficile*. A study by Kyne et al. (63) compared adults who became colonized with *C. difficile* upon admission to the hospital and either developed *C. difficile*-associated diarrhea or remained asymptomatic. Asymptomatic patients mounted a higher serum IgG response to toxin A than patients who developed *C. difficile*-associated diarrhea. This difference was only observed in patients newly exposed to *C. difficile*; patients in long-stay hospitalization that were either asymptomatically colonized or suffering from *C. difficile*-associated diarrhea had similar levels of serum IgG to toxin A (64), suggesting that the timing of immune response following initial CDI may be more important than the ability to mount a serum IgG response. Furthermore, patients that mount a more robust antitoxin immune response in the early stages of CDI are less likely to experience recurrent disease (65). This property has been exploited with the recent FDA approval of a monoclonal antibody to toxin B,

Zinplava (bezlotoxumab), developed by Merck. In a 12-week trial, patients administered Zinplava in combination with standard of care antibacterial drugs (metronidazole, vancomycin, or fidaxomicin) saw a 10% absolute reduction in CDI recurrence (40% relative risk reduction) compared to placebo. However, an increase (3-fold) in heart failure was also observed in patients with a prior history of heart failure (http://www.fda.gov/Drugs/InformationOnDrugs/ucm528793.htm). Merck has also developed an antibody to toxin A (actoxumab), but it provided no additional benefit over Zinplava.

MECHANISMS GOVERNING *C. DIFFICILE* INFECTION AND DISEASE

C. difficile Life Cycle

Two physiologically distinct cell types are important in mediating CDI and disease—vegetative cells and spores. Actively growing, vegetative cells are the primary mediators of disease. In this state, *C. difficile* cells are capable of producing two large exotoxins: toxin A (TcdA, 308 kDa) and toxin B (TcdB, 270 kDa) (66). Toxins A and B are both glucosyltransferases that inactivate Rho- and Ras-family GTPases within target epithelial cells; the ensuing disruption of signaling pathways causes a loss of structural integrity and cell death via apoptosis (reviewed in 67, 68). Both toxins are also capable of inducing host proinflammatory signaling pathways (reviewed in 69, 70). At higher concentrations, toxin B can induce production of reactive oxygen species through induction of NADPH-oxidase complexes, which leads to necrosis (71). Toxin A has also been shown to induce production of reactive oxygen species (72, 73), though the mechanism of induction is unknown. A subset of *C. difficile* strains also produce a third toxin, binary toxin (CDT; composed of a 53-kDa enzymatic component, CDTa, and a 98.8-kDa binding component, CDTb), which ADP-ribosylates actin, leading to its depolymerization, and may contribute to more severe disease (reviewed in 74).

During CDI, a subset of vegetative cells differentiate into endospores (75, 76). Metabolically dormant, spores are intrinsically resistant to prolonged oxygen exposure, desiccation, low pH, bleach-free cleaning agents (such as the ethanol hand-wash commonly seen in hospitals), antibiotics, and heat that would kill vegetative cells (77, 78). These characteristics make the spore the primary infectious and transmissible morphotype (79). Upon ingestion, spores pass undamaged through the low-pH environment of the stomach and along the gastrointestinal tract to the lower intestine, the putative germination site (76, 80, 81). To resume active growth, spores germinate in response to multiple environmental signals.

The principal germinants of *C. difficile* are the primary bile salt, cholate, and its derivatives (taurocholate, deoxycholate, glycocholate), which act in combination with glycine, and potentially other amino acids (L-alanine, L-arginine, L-phenylalanine, L-cysteine, β-alanine, L-norvaline, and γ-aminobutyric acid [82]) to promote efficient germination (80, 83). Germination is competitively inhibited by a second primary bile salt, chenodeoxycholate, its derivative (lithocholate), and other analogs (84, 85).

Cholate and chenodeoxycholate are produced in the liver and conjugated to either glycine or taurine (reviewed in 86). Following transport to the gallbladder for storage, bile salts are secreted into the duodenum to aid in digestion. The majority of bile salts are reabsorbed in the small intestine, though a portion (<10%) continue into the colon (87), where they are subject to microbiota-driven transformations (86). Bile salt hydrolases, encoded by several different members of the gastrointestinal community, cleave the taurine- and glycine-conjugated primary bile salts into unconjugated bile salts (cholate and chenodeoxycholate) and free taurine or glycine (86). Enzymes for a second modifica-

tion step, 7α-dehydroxylation of cholate and chenodeoxycholate to deoxycholate and lithocholate, are encoded by a limited number of bacterial species present in the colonic microbiome (86).

Potential Mechanisms of Colonization Resistance

Patients receiving broad-spectrum antibiotic treatment show marked alterations and loss of diversity in their gut microbiota (e.g., 88, 89). Concomitant to the loss of microbial diversity is a notable shift in bile salt composition from secondary bile salts, deoxycholate and lithocholate, to primary bile salts (90–92). Changes in the ratios of bile salts have important consequences for both germination and outgrowth of vegetative *C. difficile* cells. As described above, increases in the levels of cholate and taurocholate favor germination. Although increases in chenodeoxycholate could competitively inhibit germination, absorption of chenodeoxycholate by the colonic epithelium, which occurs 10 times faster than cholate (93), likely reduces levels of chenodeoxycholate below that needed for inhibition (85). Both lithocholate and deoxycholate inhibit growth of vegetative *C. difficile* (80, 94, 95). Antibiotic treatment is known to reduce the levels of organisms that are capable of 7α-dehydroxylation (90, 95–97). Addition of *Clostridium scindens*, a member of the human microbiome that is capable of 7α-dehydroxylation of primary bile salts (85 and references therein), partially restored the ability of an antibiotic-disrupted mouse microbiome to resist CDI (95).

In addition to disrupting bile salt metabolism, the large changes in microbial diversity that accompany antibiotic treatment significantly alter other features of the gastrointestinal environment that could help mediate colonization resistance. Studies of mice have demonstrated that antibiotic treatment leads to profound shifts in the levels and types of metabolites present in the cecal contents and feces (90, 98). Loss of organisms important for consumption of simple sugars and sugar alcohols liberates carbohydrates that can be metabolized by *C. difficile* (90, 99, 100). In mouse, hamster, and chemostat models of CDI, competition for nutrients appears to play a role in the inhibition of *C. difficile* growth by the microbiome (90, 99, 101, 102). Decreased microbial fermentation following antibiotic treatment also lowers the levels of short chain fatty acids (90, 103), which may provide a more favorable environment for *C. difficile* growth. Physiologically relevant butyrate levels have been shown to inhibit *C. difficile* growth *in vitro* (104), and higher short chain fatty acid levels correlate with growth inhibition in porcine (105) and murine (90) models. Bacteriocins targeting Gram-positive organisms, including *C. difficile* (e.g., nisin, lacticin 3147 [106, 107]), or narrowly targeting *C. difficile* (thuricin CD [108]) are another potential mechanism for preventing *C. difficile* colonization that could be encoded by antibiotic-susceptible members of the microbiome. Finally, the commensal microbiome plays a significant role in maintaining intestinal homeostasis, promoting barrier integrity, and educating the immune system (109, 110). Immune responses to CDI can play a role in limiting *C. difficile* disease (e.g., interleukin-25-mediated recruitment of eosinophils) or causing more severe disease outcomes (e.g., interleukin-23-mediated neutrophil recruitment and histopathology [111, 112]) and may also differentiate patients who develop *C. difficile* disease from asymptomatic carriers (reviewed in 70, 113).

In summary, disruption of the gut microbiota by use of broad-spectrum antibiotics causes dramatic changes that inhibit the ability of the host to resist colonization by *C. difficile*. Antibiotic treatment alters the bile salt composition in the intestinal lumen, leading to conditions that promote spore germination. Decreases in secondary bile salts, as well as the presence of fermentable carbohydrates and the absence of potentially inhibitory molecules produced by the microbiome, provide a niche in which *C. difficile* can replicate and cause disease. Disrupted interactions between the microbiome, the host epithelium, and the host immune system due to dysbiosis inhibit other host-encoded mechanisms to limit CDI and disease. In cases of recurrent CDI, it appears that colonization resistance cannot be restored without further intervention (Fig. 2). One approach that has shown significant success in restoring colonization resistance and ameliorating CDI is fecal microbiota transplantation (FMT). Better understanding how FMT ameliorates disease should provide insights into the rational design of defined communities for treatment of recurrent CDI.

FMT

The historical treatment for primary, nonsevere CDI involves oral administration (over 10 to 14 days) of either metronidazole or vancomycin (45). In most cases, this is sufficient for full resolution of disease. For ~25% of patients, however, at least one recurrence of disease is observed, and of those patients up to 35 to 65% will suffer multiple episodes, developing chronic, recurrent disease (rCDI) (4, 5). Relapses can be caused by the initial infective strain or by reinfection from another *C. difficile* strain acquired from the environment (114–118). Administering a tapering or pulsed course of vancomycin can reduce rCDI occurrences (119), presumably by killing off vegetative cells as they germinate from the spore form. Recently, the narrow-spectrum antibiotic fidaxomicin has been approved for CDI treatment. Fidaxomicin is noninferior to vancomycin for CDI treatment and results in fewer relapses of disease (120). Whereas a course of metronidazole or vancomycin can be relatively inexpensive ($35 to $700, respectively), fidaxomicin can cost $3,360 for a 10-day course (121). This has led to some reluctance to prescribe fidaxomicin, but it has been argued that compared to the expense (financial and to the

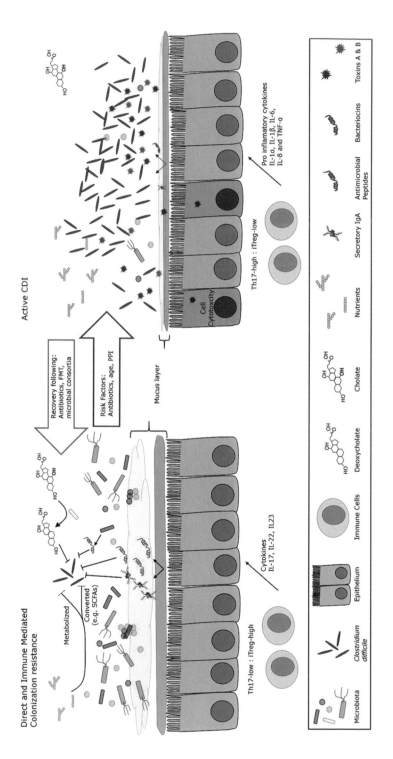

FIGURE 2 Under normal circumstances the gastrointestinal tract is able to resist infection by *C. difficile*. This is thought to be accomplished by a combination of factors mediated by the host and colonization resistance due to the indigenous microbiota. These mechanisms, expanded on in the main text, include (i) competition for nutrients and their conversion into metabolites inhibitory to *C. difficile*, (ii) microbial conversion of primary to secondary bile salts such as deoxycholate which can induce germination of *C. difficile* spores but prevent the growth of vegetative *C. difficile*, (iii) production of antimicrobial peptides and bacteriocins by the host microbiota, and (iv) a balanced host immune response that includes production of immunoglobulins, accumulation of protective iTreg cells in the lamina propria, and release of anti-inflammatory cytokines. Upon disruption of these resistance mechanisms, primarily through antibiotic use, there is an accumulation of proinflammatory Th17 cells and a reduction in bacterial diversity. In this state *C. difficile* is able to invade and proliferate, causing toxin-mediated damage to the epithelium. In many cases, following suitable antibiotic treatment for CDI the indigenous microbiota is able to recover and reestablish colonization resistance. However, in a significant number of cases this does not occur and patients are liable to suffer relapse. FMT has been shown to be remarkably successful for treating these patients, likely because multiple facets of colonization resistance are restored.

health of the patient) associated with rCDI, fidaxomicin is the superior first-line treatment option (122). Despite the increased efficacy of fidaxomicin, >10% of patients will develop recalcitrant rCDI (123).

Because of the limited options available for pharmaceutical treatment of rCDI, interest in alternative treatments has increased. FMT is one therapy that has risen in prominence since the early 2010s, due primarily to its startlingly high efficacy (over 90% success rate reported in some studies [124, 125]). FMT, however, is not a new idea. The earliest known roots can be traced back to the consumption of "yellow soup" in 4th century China by patients suffering from food poisoning or severe diarrhea (126), and FMT has been utilized by veterinarians since the 1600s when it was described by Italian anatomist Fabricius Aquapendente for treating ruminants (4). The first reported use of FMT in humans as a treatment for pseudomembranous colitis (potentially caused by *C. difficile*) occurred in 1958 (127), and its first definitive use against CDI was reported in the early 1980s (128).

Over the past 5 years, several controlled trials have been reported that evaluate the efficacy of FMT and explore how different variables impact outcome. We summarize some of the key outcomes of these studies below and discuss key variables (FMT donors, FMT recipients, and mode of administration) with their potential to influence efficacy. These data are presented to provide context for the discussion of therapeutic microbes and are not intended as guidelines for treatment. More comprehensive evaluations of FMT, including guides for clinicians on how to implement FMT, have been recently published (129, 130).

Key Variables with Potential to Influence the Success of FMT

FMT donors
The goal of FMT is to cure patients with recalcitrant rCDI by reintroducing a diverse microbiome within the colon, restoring a state of colonization resistance. There is, however, inherent risk in the transfer of biological material between donor and patient. Because of the potential to transmit infectious agents, donor stool samples are often screened for *C. difficile* toxin, enteric bacterial pathogens, parasites, and rotavirus; while blood samples from potential donors are screened for hepatitis A, B, and C, as well as HIV and syphilis, the regulatory requirements governing these tests vary (reviewed in references 131 and 132).

The role of the gastrointestinal microbiome has been increasingly studied in recent years, highlighting potential complications with wholesale transfer of microbial communities between individuals. Studies have linked the gut microbiome in numerous conditions including (but not limited to) depression (133), inflammatory bowel disease (134), and metabolic syndrome (135). An obesity phenotype has been shown to be transmissible in animal studies (136), and at least one case study infers that this can also take place in humans (137).

Donors can be split into two main groups: universal and patient-selected. Universal donors enable expedited treatment by providing a bank of processed fecal material that has already undergone a rigorous screening process (e.g., references 138, 139). This option requires preplanning and protocols to be in place within the medical establishment (discussed in 140) and has recently been standardized by Rebiotix in their formulation RBX2660 (141), which is currently advancing to phase 3 clinical development following successful treatment in phase 2B trials (78.8% treatment). Patient-selected donors are usually family members or close friends (e.g., 138). There is also the potential for patients to acquire untested stool from friends or family and to self-administer using one of the methods easily obtainable online (e.g., http://thepowerofpoop.com/epatients/fecal-transplant-instructions/). This practice is unadvisable and considered especially risky.

TABLE 2 Results of FMT in severely ill patients

Complication/extenuating factors	Success rate	Reference
Severe CDI: hypoalbuminemia (<3 g/dl) with peripheral white blood cell (WBC) count >15,000/µl and/or abdominal tenderness	91% (primary cure rate)	144
Complicated CDI: occurrence of 1 or more of the following as a consequence of CDI: admission to the intensive care unit, altered mental status, hypotension, fever >38.5°C, ileus, WBC <2,000 or >30,000/µl, lactate >2.2 mmol/liter, or evidence of end-organ damage	66% (primary cure rate)	144
Fulminant, life-threatening CDI	Case report	173
Fulminant CDI in an allogeneic stem cell transplant patient	Case report	174
Fulminant, life-threatening CDI with toxic megacolon	Case report	175

Even with well-screened samples, there is the possibility of low amounts of highly contagious infectious agents slipping through undetected (142).

FMT recipients

Patient criteria for FMT typically require symptomatic, toxin-positive *C. difficile* disease that has recurred at least once following cessation of antibiotic treatment (124, 138, 139, 143, 144). Reports suggest that FMT can be both safe and effective in severely ill patients (Table 2), though further clinical enquiry is required. Contraindications for the use of FMT differ by hospital but often include age <18 years, medical frailty (life expectancy from non-CDI disease <1 year), prolonged compromised immunity because of recent chemotherapy, the presence of HIV infection with CD4 count of less than 240, neutropenia (<0.5 × 10^9/liter), peripheral white blood cells (>30 × 10^9/liter), toxic megacolon, pregnancy, and corticosteroid use (124, 138, 143). A more complete understanding of patient populations most likely to benefit from FMT is continuing to develop as new studies are completed. The fact that some groups have reported successful FMT to children (145) and patients with severe disease (Table 2), criteria used by other groups as contraindications to treatment, indicates that these treatment considerations are continuing to evolve and outlines the need for increased controlled trials.

Route of administration

The majority of reported FMT procedures have been performed with fresh stool suspensions, though there appears to be no significant difference in infection clearance for fresh versus frozen samples (143). FMT for rCDI has been reported to be successful whether administered via a top-down nasogastric (146) or capsule (139) route or bottom-up colonoscopy (147) or enema (148), though a slight increase in efficacy has been observed with lower gastrointestinal delivery (see Table 3) (149, 150). Self-administered enemas can also be highly efficacious (151) and may be preferred by some patients because they can be performed at home (ideally in consultation with a medical professional and with a

TABLE 3 Comparison of rates of success and adverse events as a function of route of delivery for FMT

Delivery	Success rate[a]	Adverse events[b]	Serious adverse events[c]
Upper gastrointestinal	83.5%	43.6%	2.0%
Lower gastrointestinal	85.1%	17.7%	6.1%

[a]Success rate indicates 90-day cure rate of rCDI based on multistudy data in Furuya-Kanamori et al. (150).
[b]Adverse events include any unfavorable and unintended sign (including an abnormal laboratory finding), symptom, or disease temporally associated with FMT.
[c]Serious adverse events include death, life-threatening experience, inpatient hospitalization or prolongation of existing hospitalization, persistent or significant disability or incapacity, congenital anomaly or birth defect, or an important medical event (152). Adverse event data include multiple, rCDI and non-rCDI-related, FMT studies.

sample that has been screened for infectious agents). Adverse effects associated with FMT route of delivery (reviewed in 152; summarized in Table 3) should be taken into account along with success rates. One problem, regardless of administration route, is the potential for injury caused by endoscopic tools. Encapsulated FMT (shown to be successful in limited studies) may therefore be an attractive option, although use is limited in patients susceptible to esophageal reflux (139).

Recolonization of the Gastrointestinal Tract After FMT

Human stool is a complex mixture of bacteria, archaea, human colonocytes, fungi, protists, viruses (human, bacterial, and archaeal), metabolites, antibodies, and other proteins (reviewed in 153). The *Firmicutes* and *Bacteroidetes* are the dominant phyla in healthy individuals (though this is not the case for some traditional hunter gathers [154]), yet their ratios differ among people (155). Despite microbial community variation, metabolic pathways present within the microbial gene pool remain evenly distributed across healthy individuals (155). Patients with rCDI, in contrast, have a markedly reduced microbial diversity that differs significantly from healthy samples (156). At the phylum level, the microbiota of rCDI patients is dominated by *Proteobacteria*, with an abundance of *Enterobacteriaceae* often observed (157–159). Following FMT, there is an immediate shift in the patient gut microbiota to look more like the donor. Posttransplant samples are enriched for *Bacteroidetes*, while the overall abundance of *Proteobacteria* is significantly reduced. This suppression of *Proteobacteria* populations may play an important role in resetting intestinal immune homeostasis, because several species of *Proteobacteria* are capable of thriving in the inflamed intestine and perpetuating continued inflammation (reviewed in 160). The stability and similarity of recipients' micro-

biota following transplant when compared to the donor can vary, suggesting that some microbiota compositions may be more stable (160). In a recent study utilizing shotgun metagenomic sequencing to examine microbial colonization following FMT, Lee et al. (161) observed a significant increase in *Bacteroidetes* posttransplant and, interestingly, a negative correlation between genes involved in sporulation and successful colonization of the FMT recipient. This suggests that alternative treatments that rely heavily or solely on spore-forming bacteria (such as Seres Therapeutics SER-109, described in detail below) may suffer from limited colonization efficiency.

Alternatives to FMT

Despite its efficacy, the mechanisms that underlie successful FMT are not well understood. FMT mediates restoration of a diverse microbial population within recipients, but it is not clear whether the curative effect of FMT is due solely to the bacteria present. Although very few serious adverse events have been reported following FMT (noted above and in Table 3), it is unclear what long-term impacts fecal microbiota transplantation may have on the recipient. For these reasons, several alternative microbiota-driven approaches are being investigated.

Tvede and Rask-Madsen described the use of a defined consortium of 10 bacterial isolates to treat rCDI in five patients (162). They observed 100% efficacy with loss of *C. difficile* and its toxin and no recurrence during the 1-year follow-up period. The authors' proposed mechanism, based on *in vitro* antagonism studies and stool cultures before and after treatment, was that *Blautia producta*, *Escherichia coli*, and *Clostridium bifermentans* present in the consortium could directly antagonize *C. difficile*, which itself was actively inhibiting the survival of *Bacteroides* strains. In the absence of *C. difficile*, the levels of *Bacteroides* increased, which may be important for maintenance of colonization resistance. Follow-up studies from this group have not been reported, although a consortium based upon their work is being evaluated in an ongoing clinical trial (NCT01868373).

In 2013, Elaine Petrof and her colleagues reported the successful use of a consortium of 33 human fecal isolates to treat two patients with rCDI (163). They analyzed the change in microbiome composition before and after treatment by ion torrent sequencing of the V6 region of the 16S rRNA gene and observed that 50 to 70% of sequence reads were identical to the 16S genes present in the organisms in their consortium in the first 2 weeks following treatment. Although the persistence of sequences identical to the treatment consortium declined over time (both patients were treated with antibiotics for other conditions), neither patient experienced a disease recurrence. Follow-up studies using a mouse model of *C. difficile* colitis indicated that their synthetic consortium, now named MET-1, limits CDI by inhibiting toxigenicity of TcdA (164). Somewhat surprisingly, MET-1 had no impact on levels of *C. difficile* in the mouse model. A larger human clinical trial (NCT01372943) is ongoing and will provide additional insights into the efficacy of MET-1 when tested against a larger patient population.

Seres Therapeutics has developed preparations of *Firmicutes* spores isolated from human fecal donors (SER-109) to treat rCDI. These preparations, which vary from donor to donor, are composed of 50 ± 8 distinct operational taxonomic units ($\geq$97% identity) based upon Illumina sequencing of the V4 region of the 16S rRNA genes (165). Results from phase II clinical trials demonstrated a 96.7% success rate at 8 weeks post treatment (no CDI in 29 of 30 patients), although three successfully treated patients had recurrence of CDI (one following antibiotic treatment) in the 8- to 24-week follow-up period (165). Microbial community analyses of patient samples before and after treatment demonstrated significant changes. In addition to an overall increase in microbial diversity and

the expected increases in the proportion of *Firmicutes* (present in the SER-109 consortium), the authors observed increases in the proportion of *Bacteroidetes* sequences and decreases in the number of *Klebsiella* sequences in treated patients.

Interesting parallels can be drawn with the work of Tvede and Rask-Madsen, who proposed that suppression of *C. difficile* by two species in the *Firmicutes* phylum (*B. producta* and *C. bifermentans*) allowed re-emergence of *Bacteroides* species which were being suppressed by *C. difficile*. The 89-subject phase II trial of SER-109, however, did not show a reduced relative risk of recurrence of CDI. Subsequent reanalysis of the data by Seres Health suggests there may have been false-positive CDI diagnosis of patients at the time of enrollment and potentially during putative relapse due to nucleic acid amplification test-based testing without ensuing cytotoxin assays. In these cases, a positive result indicates that *C. difficile* cytotoxin genes are present but not necessarily that *C. difficile* is the source of clinical symptoms. (Although there is some support for diagnosis based solely on a positive nucleic acid amplification test in the presence of symptoms, other experts recommend a multistep approach to distinguish asymptomatic from symptomatic colonization (reviewed in 45). The analysis also suggested that the 1×10^8 spores received by patients in the phase II trial (phase I recipients received doses from 3×10^7 to 2×10^9 spores) may have been suboptimal—possibly due to the limited colonization efficiency of spore-forming bacteria (161). Despite the setback, Seres Health recently announced (12 June 2017) the initiation of a phase III SER-109 clinical study (ECOSPOR III) in patients with multiply recurrent CDI. This study will aim to enroll 320 patients and utilize a cytotoxin assay to diagnose *C. difficile* rather than PCR as well as an increased treatment dose.

In 2014, as a follow-up to a smaller 2009 study, Johan Bakken reported on the combined use of probiotic kefir with tapered reduction of vancomycin or metronidazole as an alternative treatment for rCDI (166, 167). In Bakken's study, a commercially available preparation of kefir produced by Lifeway (11 bacterial and 1 yeast species) was self-administered by patients three times per day for 6 weeks during staggered vancomycin/metronidazole withdrawal. Kefir self-administration continued for 2 months following the end of antibiotics. All 25 patients were free of symptoms at the end of the staggered antibiotic withdrawal, and 21 of 25 patients remained asymptomatic for 9 months following the end of the study. Despite no reported adverse effects in CDI patients in either study, the same probiotic kefir when used in a mouse model of CDI was found to exacerbate disease, highlighting the difficulty in studying translational therapies in animal models (168).

Gerding and colleagues have also evaluated the ability of nontoxigenic *C. difficile* administration to prevent and/or resolve rCDI (169). In their study, patients who had a primary episode of CDI or a single recurrence of CDI were recruited and treated with preparations of nontoxigenic spores for 7 to 14 days (based on treatment group). The recurrence rate in patients receiving nontoxigenic *C. difficile* spores was 11%, compared to 30% for placebo-treated patients. Treatment with nontoxigenic *C. difficile* holds promise, and success may be improved by changes in administration or by coupling it with other microbe-based therapeutics to more fully restore colonization resistance. One concern with this approach, however, is the ability of nontoxigenic strains to acquire the pathogenicity locus encoding toxins A and B from pathogenic strains via horizontal gene transfer (170).

Many microbial-based treatments for *C. difficile* target rCDI, but there is also an opportunity for these treatments to be used for *C. difficile* prophylaxis. A number of commercially available probiotic preparations have been used for *C. difficile* prophylaxis in several institutions, with reported decreases in the overall rate of CDI (reviewed in reference 171), although there is still not sufficient consensus to recommend widespread use of probiotics in CDI prophylaxis (reviewed in reference 172).

CONCLUSIONS

An intact gut microbiome exerts wide-ranging influence on both the host and its constituent members. Complex carbohydrates are fermented to produce short-chain fatty acids that can both inhibit certain bacterial species and provide energy to the cells that line the intestine; epithelial barrier integrity is promoted, bile salts are modified, and myriad communication signals and bacteriocins are produced. These factors, and others, result in a state of colonization resistance that prevents CDI. Upon significant disruption, some or all of these factors are lost, leaving the host susceptible to CDI. For most patients, antibiotic treatment is sufficient to cure CDI, and the gut microbiome eventually returns to a state of restored functionality and colonization resistance. However, for a significant minority, the microbiota fails to recover, and recurrent disease occurs. For these patients, the transfer of an exogenous source of microbes via FMT has proved to be extremely efficacious. The discovery and application of specific consortia of microbes that can be administered in a drug-like fashion has proven to be more elusive, but by targeting those microbes that can recapitulate the microbiome functionality there is great promise for the near future.

ACKNOWLEDGMENTS

The authors acknowledge Vince Young (University of Michigan) for helpful comments on the manuscript. This work was supported by seed funding from Baylor College of Medicine and by National Institute of Allergy and Infectious Diseases Grants AI121522 and AI234290 to Robert Britton.

CITATION

Collins J, Auchtung JM. 2017. Control of *Clostridium difficile* infection by defined microbial communities. Microbiol Spectrum 5(5):BAD-0009-2016.

REFERENCES

1. **Lessa FC, Mu Y, Bamberg WM, Beldavs ZG, Dumyati GK, Dunn JR, Farley MM, Holzbauer SM, Meek JI, Phipps EC, Wilson LE, Winston LG, Cohen JA, Limbago BM, Fridkin SK, Gerding DN, McDonald LC.** 2015. Burden of *Clostridium difficile* infection in the United States. *N Engl J Med* **372:**2369–2370.

2. **Jones AM, Kuijper EJ, Wilcox MH.** 2013. *Clostridium difficile*: a European perspective. *J Infect* **66:**115–128.

3. **Shah DN, Aitken SL, Barragan LF, Bozorgui S, Goddu S, Navarro ME, Xie Y, DuPont HL, Garey KW.** 2016. Economic burden of primary compared with recurrent *Clostridium difficile* infection in hospitalized patients: a prospective cohort study. *J Hosp Infect* **93:**286–289.

4. **Borody TJ, Warren EF, Leis SM, Surace R, Ashman O, Siarakas S.** 2004. Bacteriotherapy using fecal flora: toying with human motions. *J Clin Gastroenterol* **38:**475–483.

5. **Johnson S.** 2009. Recurrent *Clostridium difficile* infection: a review of risk factors, treatments, and outcomes. *J Infect* **58:**403–410.

6. **Hall IC, O'Toole E.** 1935. Intestinal flora in newborn infants: with a description of a new pathogenic anaerobe, *Bacillus difficilis*. *Am J Dis Child* **49:**390–402.

7. **Bartlett JG, Onderdonk AB, Cisneros RL, Kasper DL.** 1977. Clindamycin-associated colitis due to a toxin-producing species of *Clostridium* in hamsters. *J Infect Dis* **136:**701–705.

8. **George RH, Symonds JM, Dimock F, Brown JD, Arabi Y, Shinagawa N, Keighley MR, Alexander-Williams J, Burdon DW.** 1978. Identification of *Clostridium difficile* as a cause of pseudomembranous colitis. *BMJ* **1:**695.

9. **George WL, Sutter VL, Goldstein EJ, Ludwig SL, Finegold SM.** 1978. Aetiology of antimicrobial-agent-associated colitis. *Lancet* **1:**802–803.

10. **Larson HE, Price AB, Honour P, Borriello SP.** 1978. *Clostridium difficile* and the aetiology of pseudomembranous colitis. *Lancet* **1:**1063–1066.

11. **Pépin J, Valiquette L, Cossette B.** 2005. Mortality attributable to nosocomial *Clostridium difficile*-associated disease during an epidemic caused by a hypervirulent strain in Quebec. *CMAJ* **173:**1037–1042.

12. **Loo VG, Poirier L, Miller MA, Oughton M, Libman MD, Michaud S, Bourgault AM, Nguyen T, Frenette C, Kelly M, Vibien A, Brassard P, Fenn S, Dewar K, Hudson TJ, Horn R, René P, Monczak Y, Dascal A.** 2005. A predominantly clonal multi-institutional outbreak of *Clostridium difficile*-associated diarrhea with high morbidity and mortality. *N Engl J Med* **353:**2442–2449.

13. **McDonald LC, Killgore GE, Thompson A, Owens RC Jr, Kazakova SV, Sambol SP, Johnson S, Gerding DN.** 2005. An epidemic, toxin gene-variant strain of *Clostridium difficile*. *N Engl J Med* **353:**2433–2441.

14. **He M, Miyajima F, Roberts P, Ellison L, Pickard DJ, Martin MJ, Connor TR, Harris SR, Fairley D, Bamford KB, D'Arc S, Brazier J, Brown D, Coia JE, Douce G, Gerding D, Kim HJ, Koh TH, Kato H, Senoh M, Louie T, Michell S, Butt E, Peacock SJ, Brown NM, Riley T, Songer G, Wilcox M, Pirmohamed M, Kuijper E, Hawkey P, Wren BW, Dougan G, Parkhill J, Lawley TD.** 2013. Emergence and global spread of epidemic healthcare-associated *Clostridium difficile*. *Nat Genet* **45:**109–113.

15. **Ghose C.** 2013. *Clostridium difficile* infection in the twenty-first century. *Emerg Microbes Infect* **2:**e62.

16. **Warny M, Pepin J, Fang A, Killgore G, Thompson A, Brazier J, Frost E, McDonald LC.** 2005. Toxin production by an emerging strain of *Clostridium difficile* associated with outbreaks of severe disease in North America and Europe. *Lancet* **366:**1079–1084.

17. **Cowardin CA, Buonomo EL, Saleh MM, Wilson MG, Burgess SL, Kuehne SA, Schwan C, Eichhoff AM, Koch-Nolte F, Lyras D, Aktories K, Minton NP, Petri WA Jr.** 2016. The binary toxin CDT enhances *Clostridium difficile* virulence by suppressing protective colonic eosinophilia. *Nat Microbiol* **1:**16108.

18. **Merrigan M, Venugopal A, Mallozzi M, Roxas B, Viswanathan VK, Johnson S, Gerding DN, Vedantam G.** 2010. Human hypervirulent *Clostridium difficile* strains exhibit increased sporulation as well as robust toxin production. *J Bacteriol* **192:**4904–4911.

19. **Robinson CD, Auchtung JM, Collins J, Britton RA.** 2014. Epidemic *Clostridium difficile* strains demonstrate increased competitive fitness compared to nonepidemic isolates. *Infect Immun* **82:**2815–2825.

20. **Marsh JW, Arora R, Schlackman JL, Shutt KA, Curry SR, Harrison LH.** 2012. Association of relapse of *Clostridium difficile* disease with BI/NAP1/027. *J Clin Microbiol* **50:**4078–4082.

21. **Richardson C, Kim P, Lee C, Bersenas A, Weese JS.** 2015. Comparison of *Clostridium*

difficile isolates from individuals with recurrent and single episode of infection. *Anaerobe* **33**:105–108.

22. **Carlson PE Jr, Walk ST, Bourgis AE, Liu MW, Kopliku F, Lo E, Young VB, Aronoff DM, Hanna PC.** 2013. The relationship between phenotype, ribotype, and clinical disease in human *Clostridium difficile* isolates. *Anaerobe* **24**:109–116.

23. **Spigaglia P, Barbanti F, Mastrantonio P, Brazier JS, Barbut F, Delmée M, Kuijper E, Poxton IR, European Study Group on Clostridium difficile (ESGCD).** 2008. Fluoroquinolone resistance in *Clostridium difficile* isolates from a prospective study of *C. difficile* infections in Europe. *J Med Microbiol* **57**:784–789.

24. **Sirard S, Valiquette L, Fortier LC.** 2011. Lack of association between clinical outcome of *Clostridium difficile* infections, strain type, and virulence-associated phenotypes. *J Clin Microbiol* **49**:4040–4046.

25. **Walk ST, Micic D, Jain R, Lo ES, Trivedi I, Liu EW, Almassalha LM, Ewing SA, Ring C, Galecki AT, Rogers MA, Washer L, Newton DW, Malani PN, Young VB, Aronoff DM.** 2012. *Clostridium difficile* ribotype does not predict severe infection. *Clin Infect Dis* **55**:1661–1668.

26. **Aitken SL, Alam MJ, Khaleduzzaman M, Walk ST, Musick WL, Pham VP, Christensen JL, Atmar RL, Xie Y, Garey KW.** 2015. In the endemic setting, *Clostridium difficile* ribotype 027 is virulent but not hypervirulent. *Infect Control Hosp Epidemiol* **36**:1318–1323.

27. **Walker AS, Eyre DW, Wyllie DH, Dingle KE, Griffiths D, Shine B, Oakley S, O'Connor L, Finney J, Vaughan A, Crook DW, Wilcox MH, Peto TE, Infections in Oxfordshire Research Database.** 2013. Relationship between bacterial strain type, host biomarkers, and mortality in *Clostridium difficile* infection. *Clin Infect Dis* **56**:1589–1600.

28. **Rao K, Micic D, Natarajan M, Winters S, Kiel MJ, Walk ST, Santhosh K, Mogle JA, Galecki AT, LeBar W, Higgins PD, Young VB, Aronoff DM.** 2015. *Clostridium difficile* ribotype 027: relationship to age, detectability of toxins A or B in stool with rapid testing, severe infection, and mortality. *Clin Infect Dis* **61**:233–241.

29. **Wilcox MH, Shetty N, Fawley WN, Shemko M, Coen P, Birtles A, Cairns M, Curran MD, Dodgson KJ, Green SM, Hardy KJ, Hawkey PM, Magee JG, Sails AD, Wren MW.** 2012. Changing epidemiology of *Clostridium difficile* infection following the introduction of a national ribotyping-based surveillance scheme in England. *Clin Infect Dis* **55**:1056–1063.

30. **Jassem AN, Prystajecky N, Marra F, Kibsey P, Tan K, Umlandt P, Janz L, Champagne S,**

Gamage B, Golding GR, Mulvey MR, Henry B, Hoang LM. 2016. Characterization of *Clostridium difficile* strains in British Columbia, Canada: a shift from NAP1 majority (2008) to novel strain types (2013) in one region. *Can J Infect Dis Med Microbiol* **2016**:8207418.

31. **DePestel DD, Aronoff DM.** 2013. Epidemiology of *Clostridium difficile* infection. *J Pharm Pract* **26**:464–475.

32. **Waslawski S, Lo ES, Ewing SA, Young VB, Aronoff DM, Sharp SE, Novak-Weekley SM, Crist AE Jr, Dunne WM, Hoppe-Bauer J, Johnson M, Brecher SM, Newton DW, Walk ST.** 2013. *Clostridium difficile* ribotype diversity at six health care institutions in the United States. *J Clin Microbiol* **51**:1938–1941.

33. **Slimings C, Riley TV.** 2014. Antibiotics and hospital-acquired *Clostridium difficile* infection: update of systematic review and meta-analysis. *J Antimicrob Chemother* **69**:881–891.

34. **Brown KA, Khanafer N, Daneman N, Fisman DN.** 2013. Meta-analysis of antibiotics and the risk of community-associated *Clostridium difficile* infection. *Antimicrob Agents Chemother* **57**:2326–2332.

35. **Deshpande A, Pasupuleti V, Thota P, Pant C, Rolston DD, Sferra TJ, Hernandez AV, Donskey CJ.** 2013. Community-associated *Clostridium difficile* infection and antibiotics: a meta-analysis. *J Antimicrob Chemother* **68**:1951–1961.

36. **Vardakas KZ, Trigkidis KK, Boukouvala E, Falagas ME.** 2016. *Clostridium difficile* infection following systemic antibiotic administration in randomised controlled trials: a systematic review and meta-analysis. *Int J Antimicrob Agents* **48**:1–10.

37. **Janarthanan S, Ditah I, Adler DG, Ehrinpreis MN.** 2012. *Clostridium difficile*-associated diarrhea and proton pump inhibitor therapy: a meta-analysis. *Am J Gastroenterol* **107**:1001–1010.

38. **Rao K, Higgins PDR.** 2016. Epidemiology, diagnosis, and management of *Clostridium difficile* infection in patients with inflammatory bowel disease. *Inflamm Bowel Dis* **22**:1744–1754.

39. **Shin JH, High KP, Warren CA.** 2016. Older is not wiser, immunologically speaking: effect of aging on host response to *Clostridium difficile* infections. *J Gerontol A Biol Sci Med Sci* **71**:916–922.

40. **Claesson MJ, Jeffery IB, Conde S, Power SE, O'Connor EM, Cusack S, Harris HM, Coakley M, Lakshminarayanan B, O'Sullivan O, Fitzgerald GF, Deane J, O'Connor M, Harnedy N, O'Connor K, O'Mahony D, van Sinderen D, Wallace M, Brennan L, Stanton C, Marchesi JR, Fitzgerald AP, Shanahan F, Hill C, Ross**

RP, O'Toole PW. 2012. Gut microbiota composition correlates with diet and health in the elderly. *Nature* **488:**178–184 10.1038/nature11319.

41. **Seto CT, Jeraldo P, Orenstein R, Chia N, DiBaise JK.** 2014. Prolonged use of a proton pump inhibitor reduces microbial diversity: implications for *Clostridium difficile* susceptibility. *Microbiome* **2:**42. (Erratum, **4:**10. doi:10.1186/s40168-016-0158-1.)

42. **Bloomfield LE, Riley TV.** 2016. Epidemiology and risk factors for community-associated *Clostridium difficile* infection: a narrative review. *Infect Dis Ther* **5:**231–251.

43. **Sethi AK, Al-Nassir WN, Nerandzic MM, Bobulsky GS, Donskey CJ.** 2010. Persistence of skin contamination and environmental shedding of *Clostridium difficile* during and after treatment of *C. difficile* infection. *Infect Control Hosp Epidemiol* **31:**21–27.

44. **Cohen SH, Gerding DN, Johnson S, Kelly CP, Loo VG, McDonald LC, Pepin J, Wilcox MH, Society for Healthcare Epidemiology of America, Infectious Diseases Society of America.** 2010. Clinical practice guidelines for *Clostridium difficile* infection in adults: 2010 update by the society for healthcare epidemiology of America (SHEA) and the infectious diseases society of America (IDSA). *Infect Control Hosp Epidemiol* **31:**431–455.

45. **Bagdasarian N, Rao K, Malani PN.** 2015. Diagnosis and treatment of *Clostridium difficile* in adults: a systematic review. *JAMA* **313:**398–408.

46. **Fehér C, Mensa J.** 2016. A comparison of current guidelines of five international societies on *Clostridium difficile* infection management. *Infect Dis Ther* **5:**207–230.

47. **Larson HE, Barclay FE, Honour P, Hill ID.** 1982. Epidemiology of *Clostridium difficile* in infants. *J Infect Dis* **146:**727–733.

48. **Collignon A, Ticchi L, Depitre C, Gaudelus J, Delmée M, Corthier G.** 1993. Heterogeneity of *Clostridium difficile* isolates from infants. *Eur J Pediatr* **152:**319–322.

49. **Matsuki S, Ozaki E, Shozu M, Inoue M, Shimizu S, Yamaguchi N, Karasawa T, Yamagishi T, Nakamura S.** 2005. Colonization by *Clostridium difficile* of neonates in a hospital, and infants and children in three day-care facilities of Kanazawa, Japan. *Int Microbiol* **8:**43–48.

50. **Jangi S, Lamont JT.** 2010. Asymptomatic colonization by *Clostridium difficile* in infants: implications for disease in later life. *J Pediatr Gastroenterol Nutr* **51:**2–7.

51. **Rousseau C, Poilane I, De Pontual L, Maherault AC, Le Monnier A, Collignon A.** 2012. *Clostridium difficile* carriage in healthy infants in the

community: a potential reservoir for pathogenic strains. *Clin Infect Dis* **55:**1209–1215.

52. **Koenig JE, Spor A, Scalfone N, Fricker AD, Stombaugh J, Knight R, Angenent LT, Ley RE.** 2011. Succession of microbial consortia in the developing infant gut microbiome. *Proc Natl Acad Sci USA* **108**(Suppl 1):4578–4585.

53. **Bäckhed F, Roswall J, Peng Y, Feng Q, Jia H, Kovatcheva-Datchary P, Li Y, Xia Y, Xie H, Zhong H, Khan MT, Zhang J, Li J, Xiao L, Al-Aama J, Zhang D, Lee YS, Kotowska D, Colding C, Tremaroli V, Yin Y, Bergman S, Xu X, Madsen L, Kristiansen K, Dahlgren J, Wang J.** 2015. Dynamics and stabilization of the human gut microbiome during the first year of life. *Cell Host Microbe* **17:**852.

54. **McFarland LV, Brandmarker SA, Guandalini S.** 2000. Pediatric *Clostridium difficile*: a phantom menace or clinical reality? *J Pediatr Gastroenterol Nutr* **31:**220–231.

55. **Kato H, Kita H, Karasawa T, Maegawa T, Koino Y, Takakuwa H, Saikai T, Kobayashi K, Yamagishi T, Nakamura S.** 2001. Colonisation and transmission of *Clostridium difficile* in healthy individuals examined by PCR ribotyping and pulsed-field gel electrophoresis. *J Med Microbiol* **50:**720–727.

56. **Furuya-Kanamori L, Marquess J, Yakob L, Riley TV, Paterson DL, Foster NF, Huber CA, Clements AC.** 2015. Asymptomatic *Clostridium difficile* colonization: epidemiology and clinical implications. *BMC Infect Dis* **15:**516.

57. **Tian T-T, Zhao JH, Yang J, Qiang CX, Li ZR, Chen J, Xu KY, Ciu QQ, Li RX.** 2016. Molecular characterization of *Clostridium difficile* isolates from human subjects and the environment. *PLoS One* **11:**e0151964.

58. **Ziakas PD, Zacharioudakis IM, Zervou FN, Grigoras C, Pliakos EE, Mylonakis E.** 2015. Asymptomatic carriers of toxigenic *C. difficile* in long-term care facilities: a meta-analysis of prevalence and risk factors. *PLoS One* **10:** e0117195-14.

59. **Samore MH, DeGirolami PC, Tlucko A, Lichtenberg DA, Melvin ZA, Karchmer AW.** 1994. *Clostridium difficile* colonization and diarrhea at a tertiary care hospital. *Clin Infect Dis* **18:**181–187.

60. **Shim JK, Johnson S, Samore MH, Bliss DZ, Gerding DN.** 1998. Primary symptomless colonisation by *Clostridium difficile* and decreased risk of subsequent diarrhoea. *Lancet* **351:**633–636.

61. **Zhang L, Dong D, Jiang C, Li Z, Wang X, Peng Y.** 2015. Insight into alteration of gut microbiota in *Clostridium difficile* infection

and asymptomatic *C. difficile* colonization. *Anaerobe* **34:**1–7.

62. **Vincent C, Miller MA, Edens TJ, Mehrotra S, Dewar K, Manges AR.** 2016. Bloom and bust: intestinal microbiota dynamics in response to hospital exposures and *Clostridium difficile* colonization or infection. *Microbiome* **4:**12.

63. **Kyne L, Warny M, Qamar A, Kelly CP.** 2000. Asymptomatic carriage of *Clostridium difficile* and serum levels of IgG antibody against toxin A. *N Engl J Med* **342:**390–397.

64. **Sánchez-Hurtado K, Corretge M, Mutlu E, McIlhagger R, Starr JM, Poxton IR.** 2008. Systemic antibody response to *Clostridium difficile* in colonized patients with and without symptoms and matched controls. *J Med Microbiol* **57:**717–724.

65. **Solomon K.** 2013. The host immune response to *Clostridium difficile* infection. *Ther Adv Infect Dis* **1:**19–35.

66. **Martin-Verstraete I, Peltier J, Dupuy B.** 2016. The regulatory networks that control *Clostridium difficile* toxin synthesis. *Toxins (Basel)* **8:**153.

67. **Pruitt RN, Lacy DB.** 2012. Toward a structural understanding of *Clostridium difficile* toxins A and B. *Front Cell Infect Microbiol* **2:**28.

68. **Jank T, Belyi Y, Aktories K.** 2015. Bacterial glycosyltransferase toxins. *Cell Microbiol* **17:**1752–1765.

69. **Janoir C.** 2016. Virulence factors of *Clostridium difficile* and their role during infection. *Anaerobe* **37:**13–24.

70. **Péchiné S, Collignon A.** 2016. Immune responses induced by *Clostridium difficile*. *Anaerobe* **41:**68–78.

71. **Farrow MA, Chumbler NM, Lapierre LA, Franklin JL, Rutherford SA, Goldenring JR, Lacy DB.** 2013. *Clostridium difficile* toxin B-induced necrosis is mediated by the host epithelial cell NADPH oxidase complex. *Proc Natl Acad Sci USA* **110:**18674–18679.

72. **Qiu B, Pothoulakis C, Castagliuolo I, Nikulasson S, LaMont JT.** 1999. Participation of reactive oxygen metabolites in *Clostridium difficile* toxin A-induced enteritis in rats. *Am J Physiol* **276:** G485–G490.

73. **Kim H, Rhee SH, Kokkotou E, Na X, Savidge T, Moyer MP, Pothoulakis C, LaMont JT.** 2005. *Clostridium difficile* toxin A regulates inducible cyclooxygenase-2 and prostaglandin E2 synthesis in colonocytes via reactive oxygen species and activation of p38 MAPK. *J Biol Chem* **280:**21237–21245.

74. **Gerding DN, Johnson S, Rupnik M, Aktories K.** 2014. *Clostridium difficile* binary toxin CDT: mechanism, epidemiology, and potential clinical importance. *Gut Microbes* **5:**15–27.

75. **Janoir C, Denève C, Bouttier S, Barbut F, Hoys S, Caleechum L, Chapetón-Montes D, Pereira FC, Henriques AO, Collignon A, Monot M, Dupuy B.** 2013. Adaptive strategies and pathogenesis of *Clostridium difficile* from *in vivo* transcriptomics. *Infect Immun* **81:**3757–3769.

76. **Koenigsknecht MJ, Theriot CM, Bergin IL, Schumacher CA, Schloss PD, Young VB.** 2015. Dynamics and establishment of *Clostridium difficile* infection in the murine gastrointestinal tract. *Infect Immun* **83:**934–941.

77. **Jump RLP, Pultz MJ, Donskey CJ.** 2007. Vegetative *Clostridium difficile* survives in room air on moist surfaces and in gastric contents with reduced acidity: a potential mechanism to explain the association between proton pump inhibitors and *C. difficile*-associated diarrhea? *Antimicrob Agents Chemother* **51:**2883–2887.

78. **Carroll KC, Bartlett JG.** 2011. Biology of *Clostridium difficile*: implications for epidemiology and diagnosis. *Annu Rev Microbiol* **65:**501–521.

79. **Deakin LJ, Clare S, Fagan RP, Dawson LF, Pickard DJ, West MR, Wren BW, Fairweather NF, Dougan G, Lawley TD.** 2012. The *Clostridium difficile* spo0A gene is a persistence and transmission factor. *Infect Immun* **80:**2704–2711.

80. **Sorg JA, Sonenshein AL.** 2008. Bile salts and glycine as cogerminants for *Clostridium difficile* spores. *J Bacteriol* **190:**2505–2512.

81. **Theriot CM, Bowman AA, Young VB.** 2016. Antibiotic-induced alterations of the gut microbiota alter secondary bile acid production and allow for *Clostridium difficile* spore germination and outgrowth in the large intestine. *MSphere* **1:**e00045-15.

82. **Howerton A, Ramirez N, Abel-Santos E.** 2011. Mapping interactions between germinants and *Clostridium difficile* spores. *J Bacteriol* **193:**274–282.

83. **Bhattacharjee D, Francis MB, Ding X, McAllister KN, Shrestha R, Sorg JA.** 2015. Reexamining the germination phenotypes of several *Clostridium difficile* strains suggests another role for the CspC germinant receptor. *J Bacteriol* **198:**777–786.

84. **Sorg JA, Sonenshein AL.** 2009. Chenodeoxycholate is an inhibitor of *Clostridium difficile* spore germination. *J Bacteriol* **191:**1115–1117.

85. **Sorg JA, Sonenshein AL.** 2010. Inhibiting the initiation of *Clostridium difficile* spore germination using analogs of chenodeoxycholic acid, a bile acid. *J Bacteriol* **192:**4983–4990.

86. **Ridlon JM, Kang DJ, Hylemon PB.** 2006. Bile salt biotransformations by human intestinal bacteria. *J Lipid Res* **47:**241–259.

87. **Dawson PA, Lan T, Rao A.** 2009. Bile acid transporters. *J Lipid Res* **50:**2340–2357.

88. **Young VB, Schmidt TM.** 2004. Antibiotic-associated diarrhea accompanied by large-scale alterations in the composition of the fecal microbiota. *J Clin Microbiol* **42:**1203–1206.

89. **Dethlefsen L, Huse S, Sogin ML, Relman DA.** 2008. The pervasive effects of an antibiotic on the human gut microbiota, as revealed by deep 16S rRNA sequencing. *PLoS Biol* **6:**e280.

90. **Theriot CM, Koenigsknecht MJ, Carlson PE Jr, Hatton GE, Nelson AM, Li B, Huffnagle GB, Z Li J, Young VB.** 2014. Antibiotic-induced shifts in the mouse gut microbiome and metabolome increase susceptibility to *Clostridium difficile* infection. *Nat Commun* **5:**3114.

91. **Zhang Y, Limaye PB, Renaud HJ, Klaassen CD.** 2014. Effect of various antibiotics on modulation of intestinal microbiota and bile acid profile in mice. *Toxicol Appl Pharmacol* **277:**138–145.

92. **Allegretti JR, Kearney S, Li N, Bogart E, Bullock K, Gerber GK, Bry L, Clish CB, Alm E, Korzenik JR.** 2016. Recurrent *Clostridium difficile* infection associates with distinct bile acid and microbiome profiles. *Aliment Pharmacol Ther* **43:**1142–1153.

93. **Mekhjian HS, Phillips SF, Hofmann AF.** 1979. Colonic absorption of unconjugated bile acids: perfusion studies in man. *Dig Dis Sci* **24:**545–550.

94. **Wilson KH.** 1983. Efficiency of various bile salt preparations for stimulation of *Clostridium difficile* spore germination. *J Clin Microbiol* **18:**1017–1019.

95. **Buffie CG, Bucci V, Stein RR, McKenney PT, Ling L, Gobourne A, No D, Liu H, Kinnebrew M, Viale A, Littmann E, van den Brink MR, Jenq RR, Taur Y, Sander C, Cross JR, Toussaint NC, Xavier JB, Pamer EG.** 2015. Precision microbiome reconstitution restores bile acid mediated resistance to *Clostridium difficile*. *Nature* **517:**205–208.

96. **Samuel P, Holtzman CM, Meilman E, Sekowski I.** 1973. Effect of neomycin and other antibiotics on serum cholesterol levels and on 7alpha-dehydroxylation of bile acids by the fecal bacterial flora in man. *Circ Res* **33:**393–402.

97. **Giel JL, Sorg JA, Sonenshein AL, Zhu J.** 2010. Metabolism of bile salts in mice influences spore germination in *Clostridium difficile*. *PLoS One* **5:**e8740.

98. **Antunes LCM, Han J, Ferreira RB, Lolić P, Borchers CH, Finlay BB.** 2011. Effect of antibiotic treatment on the intestinal metabolome. *Antimicrob Agents Chemother* **55:**1494–1503.

99. **Wilson KH, Perini F.** 1988. Role of competition for nutrients in suppression of *Clostridium difficile* by the colonic microflora. *Infect Immun* **56:**2610–2614.

100. **Scaria J, Chen JW, Useh N, He H, McDonough SP, Mao C, Sobral B, Chang YF.** 2014. Comparative nutritional and chemical phenome of *Clostridium difficile* isolates determined using phenotype microarrays. *Int J Infect Dis* **27:**20–25.

101. **Ng KM, Ferreyra JA, Higginbottom SK, Lynch JB, Kashyap PC, Gopinath S, Naidu N, Choudhury B, Weimer BC, Monack DM, Sonnenburg JL.** 2013. Microbiota-liberated host sugars facilitate post-antibiotic expansion of enteric pathogens. *Nature* **502:**96–99.

102. **Nagaro KJ, Phillips ST, Cheknis AK, Sambol SP, Zukowski WE, Johnson S, Gerding DN.** 2013. Nontoxigenic *Clostridium difficile* protects hamsters against challenge with historic and epidemic strains of toxigenic BI/NAP1/027 C. difficile. *Antimicrob Agents Chemother* **57:**5266–5270.

103. **Høverstad T, Carlstedt-Duke B, Lingaas E, Midtvedt T, Norin KE, Saxerholt H, Steinbakk M.** 1986. Influence of ampicillin, clindamycin, and metronidazole on faecal excretion of short-chain fatty acids in healthy subjects. *Scand J Gastroenterol* **21:**621–626.

104. **Rolfe RD.** 1984. Role of volatile fatty acids in colonization resistance to *Clostridium difficile*. *Infect Immun* **45:**185–191.

105. **May T, Mackie RI, Fahey GC Jr, Cremin JC, Garleb KA.** 1994. Effect of fiber source on short-chain fatty acid production and on the growth and toxin production by *Clostridium difficile*. *Scand J Gastroenterol* **29:**916–922.

106. **Rea MC, Dobson A, O'Sullivan O, Crispie F, Fouhy F, Cotter PD, Shanahan F, Kiely B, Hill C, Ross RP.** 2011. Effect of broad- and narrow-spectrum antimicrobials on *Clostridium difficile* and microbial diversity in a model of the distal colon. *Proc Natl Acad Sci USA* **108**(Suppl 1):4639–4644.

107. **Mathur H, Rea MC, Cotter PD, Ross RP, Hill C.** 2014. The potential for emerging therapeutic options for *Clostridium difficile* infection. *Gut Microbes* **5:**696–710.

108. **Rea MC, Sit CS, Clayton E, O'Connor PM, Whittal RM, Zheng J, Vederas JC, Ross RP, Hill C.** 2010. Thuricin CD, a posttranslationally modified bacteriocin with a narrow spectrum of activity against *Clostridium difficile*. *Proc Natl Acad Sci USA* **107:**9352–9357.

109. **Hasegawa M, Kamada N, Jiao Y, Liu MZ, Núñez G, Inohara N.** 2012. Protective role of commensals against *Clostridium difficile* infec-

tion via an IL-1β-mediated positive-feedback loop. *J Immunol* **189**:3085–3091.

110. **Hooper LV, Littman DR, Macpherson AJ.** 2012. Interactions between the microbiota and the immune system. *Science* **336**:1268–1273.

111. **Buonomo EL, Madan R, Pramoonjago P, Li L, Okusa MD, Petri WA Jr.** 2013. Role of interleukin 23 signaling in *Clostridium difficile* colitis. *J Infect Dis* **208**:917–920.

112. **McDermott AJ, Falkowski NR, McDonald RA, Pandit CR, Young VB, Huffnagle GB.** 2016. Interleukin-23 (IL-23), independent of IL-17 and IL-22, drives neutrophil recruitment and innate inflammation during *Clostridium difficile* colitis in mice. *Immunology* **147**:114–124.

113. **Bibbò S, Lopetuso LR, Ianiro G, Di Rienzo T, Gasbarrini A, Cammarota G.** 2014. Role of microbiota and innate immunity in recurrent *Clostridium difficile* infection. *J Immunol Res* **2014**:462740.

114. **Wilcox MH, Fawley WN, Settle CD, Davidson A.** 1998. Recurrence of symptoms in *Clostridium difficile* infection: relapse or reinfection? *J Hosp Infect* **38**:93–100.

115. **Barbut F, Richard A, Hamadi K, Chomette V, Burghoffer B, Petit JC.** 2000. Epidemiology of recurrences or reinfections of *Clostridium difficile*-associated diarrhea. *J Clin Microbiol* **38**:2386–2388.

116. **Tang-Feldman Y, Mayo S, Silva J Jr, Cohen SH.** 2003. Molecular analysis of *Clostridium difficile* strains isolated from 18 cases of recurrent *Clostridium difficile*-associated diarrhea. *J Clin Microbiol* **41**:3413–3414.

117. **Kamboj M, Khosa P, Kaltsas A, Babady NE, Son C, Sepkowitz KA.** 2011. Relapse versus reinfection: surveillance of *Clostridium difficile* infection. *Clin Infect Dis* **53**:1003–1006.

118. **Figueroa I, Johnson S, Sambol SP, Goldstein EJ, Citron DM, Gerding DN.** 2012. Relapse versus reinfection: recurrent *Clostridium difficile* infection following treatment with fidaxomicin or vancomycin. *Clin Infect Dis* **55** (Suppl 2):S104–S109.

119. **McFarland LV, Elmer GW, Surawicz CM.** 2002. Breaking the cycle: treatment strategies for 163 cases of recurrent *Clostridium difficile* disease. *Am J Gastroenterol* **97**:1769–1775.

120. **Louie TJ, Miller MA, Mullane KM, Weiss K, Lentnek A, Golan Y, Gorbach S, Sears P, Shue YK, OPT-80-003 Clinical Study Group.** 2011. Fidaxomicin versus vancomycin for *Clostridium difficile* infection. *N Engl J Med* **364**:422–431.

121. **Dhiren P, Goldman-Levine JD.** 2011. Fidaxomicin (Dificid) for *Clostridium difficile* infection. *Med Lett Drugs Ther* **53**:73–74.

122. **Watt M, McCrea C, Johal S, Posnett J, Nazir J.** 2016. A cost-effectiveness and budget impact analysis of first-line fidaxomicin for patients with *Clostridium difficile* infection (CDI) in Germany. *Infection* **44**:599–606.

123. **Louie TJ, Cannon K, Byrne B, Emery J, Ward L, Eyben M, Krulicki W.** 2012. Fidaxomicin preserves the intestinal microbiome during and after treatment of *Clostridium difficile* infection (CDI) and reduces both toxin reexpression and recurrence of CDI. *Clin Infect Dis* **55**(Suppl 2): S132–S142.

124. **van Nood E, Vrieze A, Nieuwdorp M, Fuentes S, Zoetendal EG, de Vos WM, Visser CE, Kuijper EJ, Bartelsman JF, Tijssen JG, Speelman P, Dijkgraaf MG, Keller JJ.** 2013. Duodenal infusion of donor feces for recurrent *Clostridium difficile*. *N Engl J Med* **368**:407–415.

125. **Sofi AA, Silverman AL, Khuder S, Garborg K, Westerink JM, Nawras A.** 2013. Relationship of symptom duration and fecal bacteriotherapy in *Clostridium difficile* infection-pooled data analysis and a systematic review. *Scand J Gastroenterol* **48**:266–273.

126. **Zhang F, Luo W, Shi Y, Fan Z, Ji G.** 2012. Should we standardize the 1,700-year-old fecal microbiota transplantation? *Am J Gastroenterol* **107**:1755–1756.

127. **Eiseman B, Silen W, Bascom GS, Kauvar AJ.** 1958. Fecal enema as an adjunct in the treatment of pseudomembranous enterocolitis. *Surgery* **44**:854–859.

128. **Schwan A, Sjölin S, Trottestam U, Aronsson B.** 1983. Relapsing *Clostridium difficile* enterocolitis cured by rectal infusion of homologous faeces. *Lancet* **322**:845.

129. **Kelly CR, Kahn S, Kashyap P, Laine L, Rubin DT, Atreja A, Moore T, Wu G.** 2015. Update on fecal microbiota transplantation 2015: indications, methodologies, mechanisms, and outlook. *Gastroenterology* **149**:223–237.

130. **Moore T, Rodriguez A, Bakken JS.** 2014. Fecal microbiota transplantation: a practical update for the infectious disease specialist. *Clin Infect Dis* **58**:541–545.

131. **Lagier J-C.** 2014. Faecal microbiota transplantation: from practice to legislation before considering industrialization. *Clin Microbiol Infect* **20**:1112–1118.

132. **National Institute for Health Care and Excellence Interventional Procedures Programme.** 2014. *Interventional procedure overview of faecal microbiota transplant for recurrent* Clostridium difficile *infection.* https://www.nice.org.uk/guidance/ipg485.

133. **Collins SM, Surette M, Bercik P.** 2012. The interplay between the intestinal microbiota and the brain. *Nat Rev Microbiol* **10:**735–742.

134. **Sartor RB.** 2008. Microbial influences in inflammatory bowel diseases. *Gastroenterology* **134:**577–594.

135. **Woting A, Blaut M.** 2016. The intestinal microbiota in metabolic disease. *Nutrients* **8:**202.

136. **Ridaura VK, et al.** 2013. Gut microbiota from twins discordant for obesity modulate metabolism in mice. *Science* **341:**1241214.

137. **Alang N, Kelly CR.** 2015. Weight gain after fecal microbiota transplantation. *Open Forum Infect Dis* **2**(1):ofv004.

138. **Hamilton MJ, Weingarden AR, Sadowsky MJ, Khoruts A.** 2012. Standardized frozen preparation for transplantation of fecal microbiota for recurrent *Clostridium difficile* infection. *Am J Gastroenterol* **107:**761–767.

139. **Youngster I, Russell GH, Pindar C, Ziv-Baran T, Sauk J, Hohmann EL.** 2014. Oral, capsulized, frozen fecal microbiota transplantation for relapsing *Clostridium difficile* infection. *JAMA* **312:**1772–1778.

140. **Kelly CR, Kunde SS, Khoruts A.** 2014. Guidance on preparing an investigational new drug application for fecal microbiota transplantation studies. *Clin Gastroenterol Hepatol* **12:**283–288.

141. **Orenstein R, Dubberke E, Hardi R, Ray A, Mullane K, Pardi DS, Ramesh MS, PUNCH CD Investigators.** 2016. Safety and durability of RBX2660 (microbiota suspension) for recurrent *Clostridium difficile* infection: results of the PUNCH CD study. *Clin Infect Dis* **62:**596–602.

142. **Schwartz M, Gluck M, Koon S.** 2013. Norovirus gastroenteritis after fecal microbiota transplantation for treatment of *Clostridium difficile* infection despite asymptomatic donors and lack of sick contacts. *Am J Gastroenterol* **108:**1367.

143. **Lee CH, Steiner T, Petrof EO, Smieja M, Roscoe D, Nematallah A, Weese JS, Collins S, Moayyedi P, Crowther M, Ropeleski MJ, Jayaratne P, Higgins D, Li Y, Rau NV, Kim PT.** 2016. Frozen vs fresh fecal microbiota transplantation and clinical resolution of diarrhea in patients with recurrent *Clostridium difficile* infection: a randomized clinical trial. *JAMA* **315:**142–148.

144. **Agrawal M, Aroniadis OC, Brandt LJ, Kelly C, Freeman S, Surawicz C, Broussard E, Stollman N, Giovanelli A, Smith B, Yen E, Trivedi A, Hubble L, Kao D, Borody T, Finlayson S, Ray A, Smith R.** 2016. The long-term efficacy and safety of fecal microbiota transplant for recurrent, severe, and complicated *Clostridium diffi-*

cile infection in 146 elderly individuals. *J Clin Gastroenterol* **50:**403–407.

145. **Pierog A, Mencin A, Reilly NR.** 2014. Fecal microbiota transplantation in children with recurrent *Clostridium difficile* infection. *Pediatr Infect Dis J* **33:**1198–1200.

146. **Aas J, Gessert CE, Bakken JS.** 2003. Recurrent *Clostridium difficile* colitis: case series involving 18 patients treated with donor stool administered via a nasogastric tube. *Clin Infect Dis* **36:**580–585.

147. **Kelly CR, de Leon L, Jasutkar N.** 2012. Fecal microbiota transplantation for relapsing *Clostridium difficile* infection in 26 patients: methodology and results. *J Clin Gastroenterol* **46:**145–149.

148. **Kassam Z, Hundal R, Marshall JK, Lee CH.** 2012. Fecal transplant via retention enema for refractory or recurrent *Clostridium difficile* infection. *Arch Intern Med* **172:**191–193.

149. **Kassam Z, Lee CH, Yuan Y, Hunt RH.** 2013. Fecal microbiota transplantation for *Clostridium difficile* infection: systematic review and meta-analysis. *Am J Gastroenterol* **108:**500–508.

150. **Furuya-Kanamori L, Doi SA, Paterson DL, Helms SK, Yakob L, McKenzie SJ, Garborg K, Emanuelsson F, Stollman N, Kronman MP, Clark J, Huber CA, Riley TV, Clements AC.** 2017. Upper versus lower gastrointestinal delivery for transplantation of fecal microbiota in recurrent or refractory *Clostridium difficile* infection: a collaborative analysis of individual patient data from 14 studies. *J Clin Gastroenterol* **51:**145–150.

151. **Silverman MS, Davis I, Pillai DR.** 2010. Success of self-administered home fecal transplantation for chronic *Clostridium difficile* infection. *Clin Gastroenterol Hepatol* **8:**471–473.

152. **Wang S, Xu M, Wang W, Cao X, Piao M, Khan S, Yan F, Cao H, Wang B.** 2016. Systematic review: adverse events of fecal microbiota transplantation. *PLoS One* **11:**e0161174.

153. **Bojanova DP, Bordenstein SR.** 2016. Fecal transplants: what is being transferred? *PLoS Biol* **14:**e1002503–e1002512.

154. **Schnorr SL, Candela M, Rampelli S, Centanni M, Consolandi C, Basaglia G, Turroni S, Biagi E, Peano C, Severgnini M, Fiori J, Gotti R, De Bellis G, Luiselli D, Brigidi P, Mabulla A, Marlowe F, Henry AG, Crittenden AN.** 2014. Gut microbiome of the Hadza hunter-gatherers. *Nat Commun* **5:**3654.

155. **Human Microbiome Project Consortium.** 2012. Structure, function and diversity of the healthy human microbiome. *Nature* **486:**207–214.

156. **Chang JY, Antonopoulos DA, Kalra A, Tonelli A, Khalife WT, Schmidt TM, Young VB.** 2008. Decreased diversity of the fecal microbiome in recurrent *Clostridium difficile*-associated diarrhea. *J Infect Dis* **197**:435–438.

157. **Hamilton MJ, Weingarden AR, Unno T, Khoruts A, Sadowsky MJ.** 2013. High-throughput DNA sequence analysis reveals stable engraftment of gut microbiota following transplantation of previously frozen fecal bacteria. *Gut Microbes* **4**:125–135.

158. **Fuentes S, et al.** 2014. Reset of a critically disturbed microbial ecosystem: faecal transplant in recurrent *Clostridium difficile* infection. *ISME J* **8**:1621–1633.

159. **Seekatz AM, Theriot CM, Molloy CT, Wozniak KL, Bergin IL, Young VB.** 2015. Fecal microbiota transplantation eliminates *Clostridium difficile* in a murine model of relapsing disease. *Infect Immun* **83**:3838–3846.

160. **Bäumler AJ, Sperandio V.** 2016. Interactions between the microbiota and pathogenic bacteria in the gut. *Nature* **535**:85–93.

161. **Lee STM, Kahn SA, Delmont TO, Shaiber A, Esen ÖC, Hubert NA, Morrison HG, Antonopoulos DA, Rubin DT, Eren AM.** 2017. Tracking microbial colonization in fecal microbiota transplantation experiments via genome-resolved metagenomics. *Microbiome* **5**:50.

162. **Tvede M, Rask-Madsen J.** 1989. Bacteriotherapy for chronic relapsing *Clostridium difficile* diarrhoea in six patients. *Lancet* **333**:1156–1160.

163. **Petrof EO, Gloor GB, Vanner SJ, Weese SJ, Carter D, Daigneault MC, Brown EM, Schroeter K, Allen-Vercoe E.** 2013. Stool substitute transplant therapy for the eradication of *Clostridium difficile* infection: 'RePOOPulating' the gut. *Microbiome* **1**:3.

164. **Martz SL, et al.** 2017. A human gut ecosystem protects against C. difficile disease by targeting TcdA. *J Gastroenterol* **52**:452–465.

165. **Khanna S, Pardi DS, Kelly CR, Kraft CS, Dhere T, Henn MR, Lombardo MJ, Vulic M, Ohsumi T, Winkler J, Pindar C, McGovern BH, Pomerantz RJ, Aunins JG, Cook DN, Hohmann EL.** 2016. A novel microbiome therapeutic increases gut microbial diversity and prevents recurrent *Clostridium difficile* infection. *J Infect Dis* **214**:173–181.

166. **Bakken JS.** 2009. Resolution of recurrent *Clostridium difficile*-associated diarrhea using staggered antibiotic withdrawal and kefir. *Minn Med* **92**:38–40.

167. **Bakken JS.** 2014. Staggered and tapered antibiotic withdrawal with administration of kefir for recurrent *Clostridium difficile* infection. *Clin Infect Dis* **59**:858–861.

168. **Spinler JK, Brown A, Ross CL, Boonma P, Conner ME, Savidge TC.** 2016. Administration of probiotic kefir to mice with *Clostridium difficile* infection exacerbates disease. *Anaerobe* **40**:54–57.

169. **Gerding DN, Meyer T, Lee C, Cohen SH, Murthy UK, Poirier A, Van Schooneveld TC, Pardi DS, Ramos A, Barron MA, Chen H, Villano S.** 2015. Administration of spores of nontoxigenic *Clostridium difficile* strain M3 for prevention of recurrent *C difficile* infection: a randomized clinical trial. *JAMA* **313**:1719.

170. **Brouwer MSM, Roberts AP, Hussain H, Williams RJ, Allan E, Mullany P.** 2013. Horizontal gene transfer converts non-toxigenic *Clostridium difficile* strains into toxin producers. *Nat Commun* **4**:2601.

171. **Spinler JK, Ross CL, Savidge TC.** 2016. Probiotics as adjunctive therapy for preventing *Clostridium difficile* infection: what are we waiting for? *Anaerobe* **41**:51–57.

172. **Rao K, Young VB.** 2017. Probiotics for prevention of *Clostridium difficile* infection in hospitalized patients: is the jury still out? *Gastroenterology* **152**:1817–1819.

173. **You DM, Franzos MA, Holman RP.** 2008. Successful treatment of fulminant *Clostridium difficile* infection with fecal bacteriotherapy. *Ann Intern Med* **148**:632–633.

174. **Neemann K, Eichele DD, Smith PW, Bociek R, Akhtari M, Freifeld A.** 2012. Fecal microbiota transplantation for fulminant *Clostridium difficile* infection in an allogeneic stem cell transplant patient. *Transpl Infect Dis* **14**:E161–E165.

175. **Gweon TG, Lee KJ, Kang DH, Park SS, Kim KH, Seong HJ, Ban TH, Moon SJ, Kim JS, Kim SW.** 2015. A case of toxic megacolon caused by *Clostridium difficile* infection and treated with fecal microbiota transplantation. *Gut Liver* **9**:247–250.

Fecal Microbiota Transplantation: Therapeutic Potential for a Multitude of Diseases beyond *Clostridium difficile*

12

GUIDO J. BAKKER[1] and MAX NIEUWDORP[1,2,3]

INTRODUCTION

The human intestinal tract contains trillions of bacteria, collectively called the gut microbiota. The majority of bacteria belong to the Gram-negative phyla *Bacteroidetes* and *Proteobacteria* and the Gram-positive phyla *Firmicutes* and *Actinobacteria* (1). In humans, the diversity of the gut microbiota and the abundance of species increase rapidly after birth and, after 2 to 4 years, remain relatively stable throughout adult life (2). Nevertheless, shifts in gut microbiota composition may occur, especially after use of antibiotics. Even a short course of antibiotics can result in perturbations that last for several years (3, 4).

The gut microbiota has several beneficial functions. For example, a stable gut community offers resistance against colonization by pathogenic bacteria. When the intestinal microbiota composition is disturbed, a decrease in bacterial diversity and subsequent decrease in colonization resistance are thought to allow pathogenic bacteria, which are normally found in low numbers, to expand and cause disease. The most illustrative example of this is *Clostridium difficile* infection (CDI) after use of antibiotics (5).

[1]Department of Internal and Vascular Medicine, Academic Medical Center, Meibergdreef 9, 1105 AZ, Amsterdam, Netherlands; [2]Wallenberg Laboratory, Department of Molecular and Clinical Medicine, Sahlgrenska Academy, University of Gothenburg, Gothenburg, Sweden; [3]Department of Internal Medicine, VU University Medical Center, Amsterdam, Netherlands

Bugs as Drugs: Therapeutic Microbes for the Prevention and Treatment of Disease
Edited by Robert A. Britton and Patrice D. Cani
© 2018 American Society for Microbiology, Washington, DC
doi:10.1128/microbiolspec.BAD-0008-2017

In order to restore a balanced gut micro-biota composition, fecal microbiota transplan-tation (FMT), the transfer of fecal material containing bacteria from a healthy donor into a diseased patient, has been developed. Having been used for centuries and previ-ously referred to as "fecal bacteriotherapy," "fecal transfusion," "stool transplantation," or "fecal enema," FMT has emerged as a ther-apeutic option for a wide range of diseases. Moreover, FMT may be used as a research tool to search for novel therapeutic targets. In this chapter, we focus on the therapeutic potential of FMT.

HISTORY OF FMT

The use of FMT for human disease goes back many centuries. During the Dong Jin Dynasty, in the 4th century AD, the tradi-tional Chinese medicine doctor Ge Hong first described the oral ingestion of human fecal suspension in his handbook "Zhou Hou Bei Ji Fang" ("Handy Therapy for Emergencies"). It was used to successfully treat patients who had food poisoning or severe diarrhea. In the 16th century, in the traditional Chinese medi-cine book "Ben Cao Gang Mu" ("Compendium of Materia Medica"), another well-known Chinese doctor, Li Shizhen, documented treat-ment of severe diarrhea, fever, pain, vomiting, and constipation using several different prep-arations, including dry feces, fermented and fresh fecal suspensions, and infant feces. For aesthetic considerations, these treatments were aptly given original names, such as "yellow soup" and "golden syrup" (6). During World War II, German soldiers in Africa were recom-mended by Bedouins to treat bacterial dysen-tery with "consumption of fresh, warm camel feces" (7).

The first description of FMT in modern medicine dates back to 1958. Dr. Ben Eiseman, an American surgeon, used fecal enemas to treat four patients who had developed fulmi-nant pseudomembranous enterocolitis after antibiotic use; the treatment resulted in a

rapid resolution of symptoms (8). Although not known as a cause at that time, it is likely that these patients were suffering from CDI. In 2013, the first randomized controlled trial (RCT) using FMT in CDI patients was pub-lished (9). Since then, FMT has been inves-tigated as a possible therapy in a variety of diseases.

PRACTICAL FMT GUIDELINES

In the past years, FMT has become a boom-ing practice, ranging from highly organized stool banking programs to individual treat-ments with patient-identified donors, and even to harmful do-it-yourself practices. Most pub-lished protocols and recommendations regard-ing FMT methodology are based on opinions, common sense, and anecdotal experiences. Thus, regarding donor selection, preparation of fecal samples, and administration of the solution, large differences in FMT methods still exist among centers worldwide. In 2011, the FMT Workgroup described a general protocol for FMT (10). Moreover, recently a European consensus report on clinical in-dications, applications, and methodological aspects of FMT was published (11). Here, we provide practical guidelines regarding FMT for CDI and research purposes based on these protocols. These steps are based on what has been described but not necessarily rigorously tested.

In all cases of planned FMT, local ethical approval and patient and donor informed consent should be obtained. Moreover, FMT should be performed only in specialized centers with extensive prior experience. In the case of CDI, a fecal transplantation expert and an infectious disease expert should be consulted to consider other treatment op-tions and determine patient eligibility.

Donor Selection

It is important to carefully screen potential fecal donors for pathogens to prevent dis-

TABLE 1 Recommended analyses for screening of fecal donors[a]

History
  Antibiotic use in past 3 months
  Atopy, allergies, or autoimmune diseases
  Blood transfusions
  Gastrointestinal illness (IBD, IBS, colorectal polyps, or cancer)
  Incarceration, tattoos, or body piercings in past 6 months
  Infectious diseases (HBV, HCV, HIV, HTLV, malaria, trypanosomiasis, tuberculosis, rotavirus, *Giardia lamblia*)
  Metabolic disorders (morbid obesity, diabetes)
  Neurologic disorders
  Previous reception of tissue/organ transplant
  Previous reception of blood products
  Risky sexual behavior
  Travel history
  Use of any medication or illegal drugs
Stool testing
  Adenovirus 40/41
  Adenovirus non-41/41
  Aeromonas spp.
  Astrovirus
  Blastocystis hominis
  Clostridium difficile
  Cryptosporidium spp.
  Dientamoeba fragilis
  ESBL-producing *Enterobacteriaceae*
  Entamoeba histolytica
  Enterovirus
  Giardia lamblia
  Helicobacter pylori
  Isospora spp.
  Microscopy for parasites, cysts, and ova
  Microsporidium spp.
  Norovirus type I and II
  Pathogenic *Campylobacter* spp.
  Plesiomonas shigelloides
  Rotavirus
  Salmonella spp.
  Sapovirus
  Shiga toxin-producing *Escherichia coli*
  Shigella spp.
  Vancomycin-resistant *Enterococcus* spp.
  Yersinia spp.
Serologic testing
  CMV
  EBV
  Entamoeba histolytica
  Hepatitis A, B, C, E virus
  HIV
  HTLV
  Strongyloides spp.
  Treponema pallidum

ease transmission to the recipient. Structured questionnaires can be used to estimate the risk of recently acquired pathogens that might not be detected in laboratory analysis. These questionnaires should at least contain questions regarding travel history, sexual behavior, medical history, use of medication, recreational drug use, and risk factors for communicable diseases such as recent tattoos or piercings. Donors that have had antibiotic exposure in the past 3 to 6 months, gastrointestinal (GI) illness, diarrhea, or medication use should be excluded. Apart from questionnaires, potential donors should undergo blood and stool testing for infectious diseases. In Table 1, we list the pathogens that should be tested.

It is unpractical and expensive to screen donors shortly before every donation. Therefore, we propose to screen donors once every 6 months in the absence of overseas travel and illness. After traveling or illness, donors should be rescreened before being allowed to donate.

Donors should preferably be aged less than 60 years. However, this recommendation should not be mandatory, in order not to foreclose the use of intimate healthy partners merely because of age. It is unclear whether the use of feces from related donors improves the therapeutic potential of FMT, although this choice may be driven by specific needs, such as when there is a potential advantage of choosing unrelated donors to treat conditions with a pathogenic genetic basis. Two recent meta-analyses investigating the effect of FMT on CDI showed differential effects on resolution compared to nonrelated donor FMT (12, 13). For practical reasons (e.g., when using stools from donor banks), it may be more convenient to use donor feces from non-

---

[a]A questionnaire and extensive screening of donor blood and feces are recommended. In the case of any positive result, a consultation with the clinical microbiologist is required to determine the eligibility of the donor. IBD, inflammatory bowel disease; IBS, irritable bowel syndrome; CMV, cytomegalovirus; EBV, Epstein-Barr virus; HTLV, human T-lymphotropic virus.

related donors. However, if a patient wishes to receive FMT from a related donor, there is evidence to abstain from this. In clinical studies, investigators should choose either related or nonrelated donors in all participants to improve homogeneity in the findings.

Preparation of the Fecal Sample

During preparation of the fecal sample, several precautions must be taken to ensure the safety of staff. For example, specimens must be contained in an airtight container and further processed under a hood, as stool is a level 2 biohazard. Preferably, processing should occur in an anaerobic chamber to protect obligate anaerobic bacteria. However, many studies showed beneficial effects of FMT despite processing the sample in an aerobic chamber, so this is not a necessity.

A stool sample weighing at least 30 g should be mixed with up to 500 ml of diluent, usually sterile saline. However, it is worth noting that bacterial counts are more relevant to measuring dosing than stool weight, as they can vary ~10-fold even for the same donors on different days, so that 30 g on one day may actually be equivalent to 3 g (or 300 g) on another day. Homogenization can be done manually or using a dedicated blender. The sample should be filtered or centrifuged to remove large particles such as undigested food. The final amount of bacterial solution that is administered should be 200 to 500 ml.

The use of ethanol in the preparation of the suspension is still controversial. Despite encouraging phase 1 findings (14), an ethanol-treated mix of sporulating bacteria failed to treat recurrent CDI in a phase 2 study (15). It is plausible that ethanol, apart from killing pathogens, can also severely alter the composition of the commensal microbiota, possibly eliminating critical elements such as bacteriophages, fungi, and nonsporulating bacterial components.

It is expected that storing the sample decreases the viability and diversity of the bacteria. After obtaining the sample, it can be stored at 4°C until further processing. Storing the sample at 4°C for 8 h was shown to reduce diversity by 10% (16). Thus, we recommend to minimize the time from production of the sample to administration of the solution and preferably to keep it under 6 h.

As an alternative to fresh feces, frozen stool samples can be used. In CDI, a randomized, open-label, controlled study showed that using frozen FMT was safe and effective (17). Later, a double-blind RCT showed that frozen FMT was not inferior to fresh FMT in patients with CDI (18).

The FMT approach based on frozen feces is essential for the development of a stool bank and is the optimal way to standardize the FMT process and to allow the availability of stool on demand. Moreover, a frozen stool bank allows fecal donors to be recruited and thoroughly screened ahead of time, in a methodical manner, without time pressure, and with the potential advantage to reduce the costs associated with donor screening, as one donor can serve for multiple FMT donations. Finally, stool banks may improve the accessibility of FMT to centers that otherwise would be unable to provide the service due to inadequate resources to conduct donor recruitment/screening and FMT processing.

Indeed, several countries have created a stool bank in which frozen stool samples are stored for later use in FMT. Practical guidelines that can be used in establishing a frozen stool bank have been published elsewhere (19).

Administration of the Fecal Solution

The fecal solution can be administered via an upper GI (i.e., duodenal) or a lower GI (i.e., colonic) route. A nasogastric tube is not recommended due to risk of fecal aspiration if the recipient has gastric reflux or vomits. Colonic administration preferably occurs with the use of a colonoscope, although sigmoidoscopy and enemas have also been used in several studies. However, these approaches expose only part of the colon to the bacterial solution.

It is unclear which route is to be preferred. In CDI, both duodenal and colonic administration routes have provided excellent results (9, 12, 20). However, several systematic reviews and meta-analyses reported that colonoscopy achieved higher resolution rates of recurrent CDI and a similar safety profile compared to other routes of delivery (20–22). An individual patient data meta-analysis of FMT for CDI in nonrandomized trials showed failure rates of 5.6% and 17.9% after 1 and 3 months, respectively, in the upper GI group compared to 4.9% and 8.5% in the lower GI group (23). However, these results still need to be validated in a randomized controlled setting.

Another option is to apply the suspension by one or more enemas, especially in cases where gastroduodenoscopy or colonoscopy are contraindicated. Moreover, enema administration is widely available, does not require costly devices, and is less invasive than other routes. In the case of administration via enema, patients should be instructed to hold the infusate for at least 30 min and to remain supine to minimize the urge to defecate. The procedure could be repeated.

As the differences in efficacy are not sufficiently known, the choice between different administration modalities may depend on other factors. For example, in patients with GI motility disorders, the lower GI approach may be preferred, while in patients with toxic megacolon or severe colitis, the upper GI approach may be better suited due to the risk of colonic perforation.

Before administration, bowel preparation with laxatives may be considered, especially in the case of a lower GI approach. Bowel cleansing reduced the total bacterial load 31-fold on average (24) and may improve chances of successful engraftment of donor strains. We recommend using 1 to 2 liters of an osmotic laxative and to administer the bacterial solution at least 1 h after intake of the laxative. If a nasoduodenal tube is in

place, laxatives can be injected directly into the duodenum. Recipients may also orally ingest the laxative the night before FMT.

In some trials, proton pump inhibitors were given to recipients prior to administration of the bacterial solution. However, there is no evidence supporting the use of proton pump inhibitors in FMT, and thus we do not recommend it. In the case of CDI, antibiotics should not be given on the day of FMT, but pretreatment with antibiotics for 3 to 5 days prior to FMT can be considered.

Safety

When adhering to screening guidelines, FMT has been shown to be a relatively safe procedure, even in immunocompromised patients (25). To date, no cases of transmitted infectious diseases due to FMT have been reported. Minor short-term adverse events such as diarrhea, flatulence, abdominal discomfort, and cramping are common after FMT. Most of these adverse events are self-limiting and disappear within 2 days after FMT (9).

In the upper GI approach, there is a risk of fecal aspiration if the solution is administered in the stomach. One case of fatal aspiration pneumonia due to sedation during colonoscopy was published (26). Moreover, when using the lower GI approach, there is a risk of colonic perforation.

Regarding very-long-term risks (more than 5 years), little evidence is available (27). In theory, FMT could increase the risk of diseases associated with the gut microbiota, including obesity, inflammatory bowel disease (IBD), and colorectal cancer. Moreover, there is a theoretical possibility to transmit potentially harmful microbiota traits that cannot be apparent for decades. However, for recurrent CDI this does not really matter, as these patients are most often elderly and FMT could be a life-saving treatment. For other indications, long-term prospective studies are necessary to assess the risks. Moreover, as FMT has not undergone the traditional regulatory approval process of pharmaceutical products with sequential testing leading to large phase 3 trials assessing efficacy and safety prior to clinical utilization, the implementation of registry data collections should be encouraged to effectively deal with the issue of long-term monitoring of patients for adverse events. For example, the American Gastroenterological Association established a National Institutes of Health-funded registry to track patient outcomes associated with FMT (28).

FMT IN *C. DIFFICILE* INFECTION

CDI (formerly known as *C. difficile*-associated disease) is one of the most important health care-related infections. While *C. difficile* can be cultured from feces of 3% of healthy adults, in hospitalized patients colonization rates may be 20 to 30% (29). In the United States in 2001 to 2010, incidence rates of CDI were up to 8 per 1,000 discharges, with a mortality rate of up to 8.0% (30), which resulted in a financial impact of $3.2 billion/year (31).

CDI is driven mainly by production of toxins by *C. difficile*, although disease severity is not associated with fecal toxin concentrations (32). The clinical course of the disease is dependent on the host immune response and the virulence of the invading strain. The increasing prevalence and severity of CDI since the 2000s is most likely due to an increase in virulent strains, most notably ribotype 027, which is associated with higher mortality and transmissibility than other strains (31, 33). The colonic microbiota of patients suffering from CDI is deficient in members of *Firmicutes* and *Bacteroidetes*, whereas *Proteobacteria* species are enriched (34, 35).

Historically, the first-line treatment for patients with CDI has been metronidazole or vancomycin (recently, the more expensive fidaxomicin has also been approved for the treatment of CDI by the FDA). However, although most infections initially respond to this treatment, recurrence rates range from 20% after an initial episode to 60% after recurrent CDI (36, 37). The underlying mechanisms involved in recurrence are reexposure or reactivation of spores in patients who have an impaired immune response to infection and an impaired colonic epithelial barrier function.

Previously, recurrences were usually treated with an additional course of metronidazole or vancomycin. Starting with Eiseman in 1958 (8), more than 500 patient cases showing successful treatment with FMT have now been described. RCTs have confirmed the efficacy of FMT in recurrent CDI, with an overall cure rate of 85 to 90%, compared to a cure rate of 30% with standard therapy (9, 17).

Of particular interest is the *C. difficile* ribotype 027, also referred to as the North American pulsed-field type 1 and restriction endonuclease type BI or NAP1/BI/027 strain. This hypervirulent strain has spread globally in the past decades, from North America to Europe, Australia, and Southeast Asia, and is associated with regional and national outbreaks with high rates of disease recurrence and mortality (38–41). Large differences in prevalence exist between different regions and countries (42). In the 1990s, strains belonging to ribotype 027 were infrequently isolated from CDI patients. However, in a large prospective point-prevalence study examining stool samples from CDI patients in 482 hospitals across 20 European countries in 2012–2013, ribotype 027 was the most prevalent strain, accounting for 19% of cases (43). Most ribotype 027 strains were found to be localized mainly to four countries (Germany, Hungary, Poland, and Romania), highlighting national differences in prevalence.

The problem of *C. difficile* ribotype 027 is further increased because of its insensitivity to several antibiotics. For example, the strain has reduced sensitivity to both vancomycin and metronidazole and is resistant to moxifloxacin (44). Fidaxomicin, a high-cost drug that is effective against other strains, has poor activity against *C. difficile* ribotype 027 and may not be cost-effective (45, 46). Given these issues, FMT may be an especially effective treatment option for patients infected with this strain.

FMT is now recommended as one of the treatment options in recurrent CDI by both the European Society for Microbiology and Infectious Disease (ESCMID) and the American College of Gastroenterology (ACG) (46, 47). Moreover, given its efficacy in recurrent CDI, FMT has been tested in primary infection and immunocompromised patients (26, 48). More easily applicable therapies are also being investigated. Treatment with a frozen capsulized microbiota may be equally effective in CDI (17, 18, 49). Other research is focusing on mining for specific strains that are involved in protection against CDI. Thus, building on the success of FMT in CDI, further research may provide interesting new therapies that are more easily applicable and less invasive than current strategies. A recently published trial provided evidence that this strategy might be feasible (14). However, it has to be kept in mind that CDI is from a pathological viewpoint a relatively simple disease for which the causality of the gut microbiota is clear. Thus, while manipulation of the gut microbiota may be expected to be a successful treatment option in CDI, for other diseases this may not always be the case (Fig. 1).

FMT IN IBD

IBD encompasses several separate entities that include ulcerative colitis (UC) and Crohn's disease (CD). While both UC and CD are characterized by chronic relapsing inflammation of the bowel, there are important pathophysiological differences. UC generally affects the large intestine and is restricted to the epithelial lining of the gut, while CD can affect the entire gastrointestinal tract and a transmural pattern of inflammation is often seen. Nevertheless, there is overlap between the pathophysiology and clinical presentation, and a definitive distinction is not always possible.

Both UC and CD have been linked to gut microbiota dysbiosis. UC is characterized by a decrease in *Firmicutes* and *Bacteroidetes*, with an increase in *Proteobacteria* and *Actinobacteria* (50). However, it is unclear to what extent these shifts represent a cause or a consequence, as IBD is a complex disease involving genetic, dietary, immune system, and gut microbiota factors. Possibly, the interaction between the gut epithelium and the mucosal microbiota plays a larger role in the pathogenesis of the disease than the luminal microbiota. Indeed, so far, no intestinal bacterium has been found to be able to induce IBD. Moreover, FMT has rendered conflicting results in ulcerative colitis (51, 52). Nevertheless, animal models have shown a role for the gut microbiota in the pathogenesis of IBD, and the use of FMT in IBD is currently ongoing in several randomized studies, which will show whether and to what extent FMT can improve disease symptoms in (subsets of) patients with IBD. These studies will be pivotal in showing which bacterial strains should be developed as therapeutic targets for IBD.

The first report of infusion of donor feces for ulcerative colitis dates from 1989, when the patient-physician Bennet treated himself with multiple fecal enemas, resulting in long-term remission of his IBD flares (53). Since then, several FMT studies have been published with ranges of effects in patients with CD and UC. Importantly, the vast majority of trials on FMT in IBD are one-armed cohort studies or case series. In 2012, a meta-analysis of FMT found a 63% remission rate in UC patients, while 76% of IBD patients experienced a reduction in symptoms and 76% were able to stop taking drugs for their disease. Another meta-analysis of only cohort studies performed in 2014 found a clinical remission rate of 36% in IBD patients and 61% in CD patients. A subgroup analysis demonstrated a pooled estimate of clinical remission of 22% for UC (54). Of note, no RCTs were included in either of these meta-analyses.

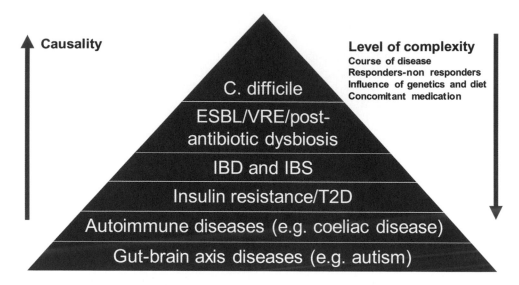

FIGURE 1 Causality of the gut microbiota in different diseases. The gut microbiota may have various levels of causality in diffent diseases. Diseases that have a more complex pathophysiology may respond less to fecal microbiota transplantation. ESBL, extended spectrum beta-lactamase producer; VRE, vancomycin-resistant enterococci; IBD, inflammatory bowel disease; IBS, irritable bowel syndrome; T2D, type 2 diabetes. Modified from *Molecular Metabolism* with permission of the publisher.

Two RCTs investigating the effect of FMT in UC patients have been performed so far. Moayyedi et al. (52) randomized 70 patients with active UC, defined as a Mayo Clinic score of ≥4 with an endoscopic Mayo score of ≥1 to receive allogenic FMT or placebo (water) via retention enema. Patients received 50 ml of fecal suspension from anonymous donors (all but one case) or a partner (one case) or water weekly for 6 weeks. Notably, the fecal suspension was either administered immediately (*n* = 16) or stored at −20°C and later thawed (*n* = 22). There was a significant difference in the primary endpoint of a full Mayo score of <3 and endoscopic Mayo score of 0 at 7 weeks after the first FMT, with nine patients (24%) in the FMT group achieving the endpoint versus two patients (5%) in the control group. FMT also resulted in a greater improvement in microbial diversity compared with placebo treatment.

Interestingly, the authors used only six donors to minimize variability of the intervention. Seven of nine patients in remission after FMT received fecal material from a single donor, while this donor was used in 18 cases. Three donors did not induce remission in any patient, although it is not described how many patients received FMT from these donors. The difference in treatment success between the best donor (7 of 18, 39%) and the other donors (2 of 20, 10%) was not statistically significant (*P* = 0.06). Thus, although there is a trend for superiority of one donor compared to the others, even fecal suspensions from this donor had various results in the patients.

In the other RCT, Rossen et al. (51) randomized 50 patients with mild to moderately active UC with a patient-reported simple clinical colitis activity index (SCCAI) score of ≥4 and ≤11 and an endoscopic Mayo score of ≥1 in a double-blind fashion to receive allogenic or autologous FMT. Patients received two duodenal FMTs of 500 ml fresh (≤6 h after production) fecal suspension 3 weeks apart after pretreatment with bowel lavage. Fifteen donors were used, of whom one was related to the recipient (partner).

In the intention-to-treat analysis, 7 of 23 patients (30.4%) who received allogenic FMT achieved the composite primary endpoint of a SCCAI score of ≤2 in combination with ≥1-point improvement on the combined Mayo endoscopic score of the sigmoid and rectum 12 weeks after the first FMT, compared to 5 of 25 (20.0%) in the autologous group. This difference was not significant (P = 0.51). In the per-protocol analysis, 7 of 17 allogenic FMT recipients (41.2%) compared to 5 of 25 controls (25.0%) achieved the primary endpoint (P = 0.29).

The authors could not identify "super-donors" or "poor donors." For example, one donor donated 12 times for eight patients, of whom four patients responded to treatment. Although microbial diversity as measured by the Shannon diversity index was not different between donors and patients at baseline, an improvement in diversity was seen in responders in both the allogenic FMT group (P = 0.06) and the autologous group (P = 0.01). Redundancy analysis showed that at 12 weeks, responders had a significantly higher microbiota composition similarity to that of their donors than did nonresponders.

These RCTs were rather different in their methodology, making it hard to interpret the different findings. Specifically, one study used weekly retention enema for 6 weeks, while the other used two duodenal infusions in 3 weeks. However, considering that neither study could identify a "superdonor," the response to FMT may be determined by engraftment of donor bacterial strains. Indeed, analyses of microbiota engraftment after FMT in metabolic syndrome patients revealed that same-donor recipients had various degrees of microbiota transfer, indicating differences in donor-recipient "compatibility" (55).

Regarding the effect of FMT on UC activity, a 2016 meta-analysis pooled the data from several nonrandomized cohort studies with these two RCTs and showed an overall clinical response rate of 65% and an overall clinical remission rate of 42% (56). However, it is important to note that the cohort studies were generally of very poor quality.

Thus, FMT offers promising therapeutic potential in UC, although more high-quality studies are needed. Of particular interest is determining the factors that influence response versus nonresponse.

Treating CD with FMT is more challenging than treating UC, as the former disease usually involves the small intestine rather than the large intestine. For example, FMT via enema does not reach the terminal ileum, the most frequently affected region in CD. Moreover, if multiple FMTs are needed, FMT via colonoscopy or duodenoscopy may not be feasible or well tolerated. Thus, the use of capsulized microbiota may be an interesting approach in this patient group. However, so far, no RCT investigating FMT in CD patients has been published.

Of note, use of FMT in IBD patients should be considered with caution, as in a small group of CD patients, adverse effects (transient fever, abdominal pains, bloating, and no clinical improvement with only transient effects on the host's fecal microbial composition) were reported upon three consecutive FMTs.

In conclusion, FMT is a promising therapy for IBD patients that may lead to major improvements in patient care. However, at present there is limited high-quality evidence, especially regarding CD. Moreover, there are some concerns regarding the safety of FMT in this vulnerable group of patients. Several randomized studies are ongoing to determine the safety, relevance, and best way of using FMT in this group. Until these trials have shown consistent results, clinicians should be cautious in recommending FMT to their IBD patients.

FMT IN METABOLIC DISEASE

Metabolic diseases, such as obesity, insulin resistance, metabolic syndrome, nonalcoholic fatty liver disease, and nonalcoholic steatohepatitis (NASH), constitute a major disease burden. For example, in 2014, more than 1.9 billion adults were overweight (body mass index [BMI] ≥ 25 kg/m²), of whom over 600 million were obese (BMI ≥ 30 kg/m²) (57). In the United States, one in three adults is obese (58). Obesity is associated with a wide range of pathologies, including cardiovascular disease, hypertension, type 2 diabetes mellitus (T2D), hyperlipidemia, stroke, several types of cancer, sleep apnea, liver and gallbladder disease, osteoarthritis, and gynecological problems (59). Thus, it is unsurprising that obesity and even overweight result in a significant increase in all-cause mortality (60).

Since the development of high-throughput next-generation sequencing techniques, there has been increasing interest in the role of the gut microbiota in metabolic diseases. As the gut microbiota is involved in the digestion and absorption of nutrients from the diet, direct energy absorption may be a major way in which the gut microbiota contributes to the development of obesity. Indeed, the gut microbiota converts indigestible fibers into energy-rich substrates such as short-chain fatty acids (SCFAs). Moreover, the gut microbiota promotes absorption of monosaccharides. Germfree mice remain significantly leaner than conventional mice, despite a higher food intake (61), while colonization of germfree mice increases total body fat content without changes in intake (62).

Several pathways are involved in signaling between the gut microbiota and the host and may regulate metabolic homeostasis. For example, SCFAs directly affect lipogenesis (63, 64), gut barrier function (65–67), gut motility (68), and immune responses (69–71). Moreover, the gut microbiota has been suggested to be involved in the secretion of several intestinal hormones that regulate metabolism. For example, SCFAs bind to G-protein-coupled receptor 41, mediating secretion of peptide YY, a hormone that reduces appetite (72, 73).

A third mechanism by which the gut microbiota is involved in the development of metabolic diseases is bacterial translocation. In this process, whole bacteria, bacterium-derived vesicles, or bacterial metabolites (such as lipopolysaccharide [LPS], a major component of the cell wall of Gram-negative bacteria that is highly immunogenic) translocate from the intestinal lumen into the systemic circulation and visceral adipose tissue. Indeed, both obesity and insulin resistance are associated with a low-grade inflammatory state characterized by endotoxemia (i.e., the presence of LPS in the plasma) (74). In particular, inflammation of visceral adipose tissue (which is in close proximity to the gut microbiota), which is characterized by infiltration of macrophages (75, 76) and increased production of cytokines (77), is a crucial driver in the development of insulin resistance.

While bacterial translocation is generally accepted to be a crucial factor in the development of insulin resistance in obesity, the exact mechanisms underlying bacterial translocation have not been elucidated. However, a high-fat diet seems to be an important trigger. For example, mice fed a high-fat diet for 4 weeks developed peripheral insulin resistance along with increased levels of circulating LPS and bacterial DNA, while a chronic infusion of LPS resulted in the same phenotype (74, 78). In humans, even a single high-fat meal has been shown to result in increases in LPS (79–81). The gut barrier dysfunction that leads to this "dietary endotoxemia" may be a direct consequence of the gut microbiota. For example, alterations in gut microbiota composition with subsequent translocation of bacterially derived antigens have been associated with nonalcoholic fatty liver disease and NASH (82–84).

So far, only one RCT studying the effect of fecal transplantation on insulin resistance has been performed (85). This trial showed an improvement of insulin sensitivity after lean-donor FMT. Interestingly, even in this small trial there was a clear distinction between responders and nonresponders, which was unrelated to the insulin sensitivity of the donor. An analysis of gut microbiota composition in patients included in several FMT studies showed an important diversity in donor bacterial engraftment (55). These results suggest that the effects of FMT may be dependent on donor-recipient compatibility and warrant further research.

The mechanisms underlying the favorable effects of FMT on insulin sensitivity are not yet clear. Future research should focus on the effect of FMT on bacterial translocation. Moreover, other methods of manipulation of the gut microbiota may be used. For example, vancomycin was shown to affect insulin sensitivity in humans (86), further suggesting an important causal role for the gut microbiota in the development of insulin resistance. Especially interesting in this regard is the role of gut microbiota manipulation on dietary bacterial translocation, which warrants further study.

Although the effect of FMT on insulin sensitivity is remarkable, it is unlikely to be used as a future therapy, as it is an invasive procedure. Moreover, gut microbiota composition has been shown to return to the original recipient composition, even when there is significant engraftment of donor bacteria (55). Instead, future research should aim to find specific causal agents involved in (the prevention of) bacterial translocation, ideally in human intervention studies.

FMT IN OTHER DISEASES

Irritable Bowel Syndrome

IBS is a chronic noninflammatory gastrointestinal disorder characterized by abdominal pain with diarrhea and/or constipation. In developed countries, the prevalence of IBS may be as high as 10 to 15% (87, 88). Given that IBS has a profound impact on quality of life and health care costs (89, 90), finding novel therapies is urgent.

Although the pathogenesis of IBS is not fully understood, there have been several associations with the gut microbiota. For example, IBS patients have a reduced variability of the gut microbiota compared to healthy controls (91). Moreover, IBS patients had lower levels of bifidobacteria and lactobacilli, while *Enterobacteriaceae* were more prevalent (92, 93). Other studies reported reduced populations of *Bacteroidetes* (94, 95) and lactobacilli and *Collinsella* (96) in IBS patients. Additionally, the microbiota of IBS patients may produce a lower amount of butyrate and higher amounts of sulfides and hydrogen than healthy microbiotas, which could promote IBS symptoms (20). Moreover, IBS patients have altered protein and carbohydrate energy metabolism within the gut (12) and increased amounts of acetic and propionic acids, which are associated with both the severity of abdominal pain and bloating symptoms (21).

A meta-analysis showed a positive effect of probiotics in IBS patients (97). However, high-quality data using the same probiotic in a randomized setting are scarce. Instead, FMT might offer a better alternative, as healthy donor feces represent a natural stable gut flora. So far, FMT has been used to treat IBS only in case series. One case series on FMT within this patient group showed that of 45 IBS patients with chronic, severe constipation who underwent FMT, a total of 60% obtained improved defecation and absence of bloating and abdominal pain during a follow-up of 9 to 19 months (98, 99). So far, no RCT evaluating FMT as a treatment option for IBS has been published. However, at the moment, one RCT is recruiting subjects (100). Thus, while there is no high-quality evidence so far, FMT may represent a viable therapeutic option for this patient group.

FMT in Intestinal Colonization by Multidrug-Resistant Pathogens

The increase in antimicrobial resistance, in part due to excessive use of antibiotics, is a major public health problem (101). Antimicrobial therapy for systemic disease, often given orally, has a major impact on the gut microbiota. A healthy gut microbiota may be able to prevent intestinal colonization by gut pathogens such as extended spectrum beta-lactamase (ESBL) producers. However, exposure to antibiotic leads to destruction of the gut microbiota, resulting in reduced colonization resistance.

FMT may offer a new way of treating intestinal colonization by multidrug-resistant pathogens. Indeed, animal studies have shown promising results (102, 103). For example, FMT resulted in decolonization of vancomycin-resistant enterococci (VRE) (104). In humans undergoing hematopoietic stem cell transplantation, patients who did not acquire VRE had higher levels of *Barnesiella* species in their feces samples than those who did (105). Thus, the composition of the gut microbiota may be important in maintaining colonization resistance. However, in humans, no prospective randomized intervention study has been performed on this subject. Our group did publish the first case report of a patient with an ESBL-producing *Escherichia coli*, which was eradicated by a single FMT (106). Moreover, five of five patients cleared methicillin-resistant *Staphylococcus aureus* (MRSA) after three jejunal administrations of FMT (107), while a study using RBX2660, an experimental microbiota suspension, for FMT in CDI patients showed that 8 of 11 VRE-positive patients became negative after treatment.

A search performed in December 2016 on www.clinicaltrials.gov revealed five trials that were under way to evaluate the effectivity of FMT against multidrug-resistant pathogens (NCT02312986, NCT02543866, NCT02461199, NCT02390622, NCT02472600). Thus, FMT offers a promising option in fighting colonization by multidrug-resistant pathogens, and important studies will be performed in the near future.

CONCLUSION

FMT has undergone a revival and is currently being tested as therapeutic agent in a variety of diseases. For example, a search performed in December 2016 on www.clinicaltrials.gov for intervention studies containing the terms "fecal" and "transplantation" revealed 103 active studies, of which 16 involved children aged 0 to 17 with a variety of indications. While there is no doubt about the efficacy of FMT in CDI, in other diseases the evidence is not as clear. In IBD and IBS, FMT has shown promising results that require further investigation. In particular, prospective RCTs are necessary to determine the effects of FMT in different patient groups.

Apart from CDI, IBD, and IBS, FMT may be useful in several other pathologies. While high-quality, placebo-controlled data so far are lacking, treatment by FMT could prove highly valuable in specific subsets of patients. Moreover, as there has been increasing interest in the relationship between gut microbiota and several autoimmune diseases, such as type 1 diabetes, idiopathic thrombocytopenic purpura (108), and even multiple sclerosis (109), FMT may even offer a future therapeutic strategy in these diseases. In conclusion, FMT is an exciting novel therapeutic option for a variety of diseases. However, high-quality evidence is lacking in most cases. Future therapy should resolve questions about the efficacy of FMT in diseases other than CDI.

CITATION

Bakker GJ, Nieuwdorp M. 2017. Fecal microbiota transplantation: therapeutic potential for a multitude of diseases beyond *Clostridium difficile*. Microbiol Spectrum 5(4):BAD-0008-2017.

REFERENCES

1. **Eckburg PB, Bik EM, Bernstein CN, Purdom E, Dethlefsen L, Sargent M, Gill SR, Nelson KE, Relman DA.** 2005. Diversity of the human intestinal microbial flora. *Science* **308:**1635–1638.
2. **Faith JJ, Guruge JL, Charbonneau M, Subramanian S, Seedorf H, Goodman AL,**

Clemente JC, Knight R, Heath AC, Leibel RL, Rosenbaum M, Gordon JI. 2013. The long-term stability of the human gut microbiota. *Science* **341:**1237439.

3. Jernberg C, Löfmark S, Edlund C, Jansson JK. 2010. Long-term impacts of antibiotic exposure on the human intestinal microbiota. *Microbiology* **156:**3216–3223.

4. Antonopoulos DA, Huse SM, Morrison HG, Schmidt TM, Sogin ML, Young VB. 2009. Reproducible community dynamics of the gastrointestinal microbiota following antibiotic perturbation. *Infect Immun* **77:**2367–2375.

5. Britton RA, Young VB. 2014. Role of the intestinal microbiota in resistance to colonization by *Clostridium difficile*. *Gastroenterology* **146:**1547–1553.

6. Zhang F, Luo W, Shi Y, Fan Z, Ji G. 2012. Should we standardize the 1,700-year-old fecal microbiota transplantation? *American J Gastroenterol* **107:**1755; author reply, **107:**1755–1756.

7. Lewin RA. 1999. *Merde: excursions in scientific, cultural, and socio-historical coprology*. Random House Inc, New York, NY.

8. Eiseman B, Silen W, Bascom GS, Kauvar AJ. 1958. Fecal enema as an adjunct in the treatment of pseudomembranous enterocolitis. *Surgery* **44:**854–859.

9. van Nood E, Vrieze A, Nieuwdorp M, Fuentes S, Zoetendal EG, de Vos WM, Visser CE, Kuijper EJ, Bartelsman JF, Tijssen JG, Speelman P, Dijkgraaf MG, Keller JJ. 2013. Duodenal infusion of donor feces for recurrent *Clostridium difficile*. *N Engl J Med* **368:**407–415.

10. Bakken JS, Borody T, Brandt LJ, Brill JV, Demarco DC, Franzos MA, Kelly C, Khoruts A, Louie T, Martinelli LP, Moore TA, Russell G, Surawicz C, Fecal Microbiota Transplantation Workgroup. 2011. Treating *Clostridium difficile* infection with fecal microbiota transplantation. *Clin Gastroenterol Hepatol* **9:**1044–1049.

11. König J, Siebenhaar A, Högenauer C, Arkkila P, Nieuwdorp M, Norén T, Ponsioen CY, Rosien U, Rossen NG, Satokari R, Stallmach A, de Vos W, Keller J, Brummer RJ. 2017. Consensus report: faecal microbiota transfer—clinical applications and procedures. *Aliment Pharmacol Ther* **45:**222–239.

12. Kassam Z, Lee CH, Hunt RH. 2014. Review of the emerging treatment of *Clostridium difficile* infection with fecal microbiota transplantation and insights into future challenges. *Clin Lab Med* **34:**787–798.

13. Gough E, Shaikh H, Manges AR. 2011. Systematic review of intestinal microbiota transplantation (fecal bacteriotherapy) for recurrent *Clostridium difficile* infection. *Clin Infect Dis* **53:**994–1002.

14. Khanna S, Pardi DS, Kelly CR, Kraft CS, Dhere T, Henn MR, Lombardo MJ, Vulic M, Ohsumi T, Winkler J, Pindar C, McGovern BH, Pomerantz RJ, Aunins JG, Cook DN, Hohmann EL. 2016. A novel microbiome therapeutic increases gut microbial diversity and prevents recurrent *Clostridium difficile* infection. *J Infect Dis* **214:**173–181.

15. Seres Therapeutics. 2016. *Seres Therapeutics announces interim results from SER-109 phase 2 ECOSPOR study in multiply recurrent* Clostridium difficile *infection*. http://ir.serestherapeutics.com/phoenix.zhtml?c=254006&p=irol-newsArticle&ID=2190006. Accessed 6 October 2016.

16. Ott SJ, Musfeldt M, Timmis KN, Hampe J, Wenderoth DF, Schreiber S. 2004. In vitro alterations of intestinal bacterial microbiota in fecal samples during storage. *Diagn Microbiol Infect Dis* **50:**237–245.

17. Youngster I, Sauk J, Pindar C, Wilson RG, Kaplan JL, Smith MB, Alm EJ, Gevers D, Russell GH, Hohmann EL. 2014. Fecal microbiota transplant for relapsing *Clostridium difficile* infection using a frozen inoculum from unrelated donors: a randomized, open-label, controlled pilot study. *Clin Infect Dis* **58:**1515–1522.

18. Lee CH, Steiner T, Petrof EO, Smieja M, Roscoe D, Nematallah A, Weese JS, Collins S, Moayyedi P, Crowther M, Ropeleski MJ, Jayaratne P, Higgins D, Li Y, Rau NV, Kim PT. 2016. Frozen vs fresh fecal microbiota transplantation and clinical resolution of diarrhea in patients with recurrent *Clostridium difficile* infection: a randomized clinical trial. *JAMA* **315:**142–149.

19. Costello SP, Tucker EC, La Brooy J, Schoeman MN, Andrews JM. 2016. Establishing a fecal microbiota transplant service for the treatment of *Clostridium difficile* infection. *Clin Infect Dis* **62:**908–914.

20. Cammarota G, Ianiro G, Gasbarrini A. 2014. Fecal microbiota transplantation for the treatment of *Clostridium difficile* infection: a systematic review. *J Clin Gastroenterol* **48:**693–702.

21. Kassam Z, Lee CH, Yuan Y, Hunt RH. 2013. Fecal microbiota transplantation for *Clostridium difficile* infection: systematic review and meta-analysis. *Am J Gastroenterol* **108:**500–508.

22. Drekonja D, Reich J, Gezahegn S, Greer N, Shaukat A, MacDonald R, Rutks I, Wilt TJ. 2015. Fecal microbiota transplantation for *Clostridium difficile* infection: a systematic review. *Ann Intern Med* **162:**630–638.

23. Furuya-Kanamori L, Doi SA, Paterson DL, Helms SK, Yakob L, McKenzie SJ, Garborg K,

Emanuelsson F, Stollman N, Kronman MP, Clark J, Huber CA, Riley TV, Clements AC. 2017. Upper versus lower gastrointestinal delivery for transplantation of fecal microbiota in recurrent or refractory *Clostridium difficile* infection: a collaborative analysis of individual patient data from 14 studies. *J Clin Gastroenterol* **51:**145–150.

24. **Jalanka J, Salonen A, Salojärvi J, Ritari J, Immonen O, Marciani L, Gowland P, Hoad C, Garsed K, Lam C, Palva A, Spiller RC, de Vos WM.** 2015. Effects of bowel cleansing on the intestinal microbiota. *Gut* **64:**1562–1568.

25. **Di Bella S, Gouliouris T, Petrosillo N.** 2015. Fecal microbiota transplantation (FMT) for *Clostridium difficile* infection: focus on immunocompromised patients. *J Infect Chemother* **21:**230–237.

26. **Kelly CR, Ihunnah C, Fischer M, Khoruts A, Surawicz C, Afzali A, Aroniadis O, Barto A, Borody T, Giovanelli A, Gordon S, Gluck M, Hohmann EL, Kao D, Kao JY, McQuillen DP, Mellow M, Rank KM, Rao K, Ray A, Schwartz MA, Singh N, Stollman N, Suskind DL, Vindigni SM, Youngster I, Brandt L.** 2014. Fecal microbiota transplant for treatment of *Clostridium difficile* infection in immunocompromised patients. *Am J Gastroenterol* **109:**1065–1071.

27. **Brandt LJ, Aroniadis OC, Mellow M, Kanatzar A, Kelly C, Park T, Stollman N, Rohlke F, Surawicz C.** 2012. Long-term follow-up of colonoscopic fecal microbiota transplant for recurrent *Clostridium difficile* infection. *Am J Gastroenterol* **107:**1079–1087.

28. **American Gastroenterological Association Center for Gut Microbiome Research & Education.** *Center establishes NIH-funded registry to track FMT.* http://www.gastro.org/about/initiatives/aga-center-for-gut-microbiome-research-education. Accessed 5 October 2016.

29. **Periman P.** 2002. Antibiotic-associated diarrhea. *N Engl J Med* **347:**145.

30. **Argamany JR, Aitken SL, Lee GC, Boyd NK, Reveles KR.** 2015. Regional and seasonal variation in *Clostridium difficile* infections among hospitalized patients in the United States, 2001–2010. *Am J Infect Control* **43:**435–440.

31. **Kuijper EJ, Coignard B, Tüll P, ESCMID Study Group for Clostridium difficile, EU Member States, European Centre for Disease Prevention and Control.** 2006. Emergence of *Clostridium difficile*-associated disease in North America and Europe. *Clin Microbiol Infect* **12** (Suppl 6)**:**2–18.

32. **Akerlund T, Svenungsson B, Lagergren A, Burman LG.** 2006. Correlation of disease severity with fecal toxin levels in patients with *Clostridium difficile*-associated diarrhea and distribution of PCR ribotypes and toxin yields in vitro of corresponding isolates. *J Clin Microbiol* **44:**353–358.

33. **Leffler DA, Lamont JT.** 2015. *Clostridium difficile* infection. *N Engl J Med* **372:**1539–1548.

34. **Antharam VC, Li EC, Ishmael A, Sharma A, Mai V, Rand KH, Wang GP.** 2013. Intestinal dysbiosis and depletion of butyrogenic bacteria in *Clostridium difficile* infection and nosocomial diarrhea. *J Clin Microbiol* **51:**2884–2892.

35. **Song Y, Garg S, Girotra M, Maddox C, von Rosenvinge EC, Dutta A, Dutta S, Fricke WF.** 2013. Microbiota dynamics in patients treated with fecal microbiota transplantation for recurrent *Clostridium difficile* infection. *PLoS One* **8:**e81330.

36. **Fekety R, McFarland LV, Surawicz CM, Greenberg RN, Elmer GW, Mulligan ME.** 1997. Recurrent *Clostridium difficile* diarrhea: characteristics of and risk factors for patients enrolled in a prospective, randomized, double-blinded trial. *Clin Infect Dis* **24:**324–333.

37. **McFarland LV, Surawicz CM, Rubin M, Fekety R, Elmer GW, Greenberg RN.** 1999. Recurrent *Clostridium difficile* disease: epidemiology and clinical characteristics. *Infect Control Hosp Epidemiol* **20:**43–50.

38. **He M, Miyajima F, Roberts P, Ellison L, Pickard DJ, Martin MJ, Connor TR, Harris SR, Fairley D, Bamford KB, D'Arc S, Brazier J, Brown D, Coia JE, Douce G, Gerding D, Kim HJ, Koh TH, Kato H, Senoh M, Louie T, Michell S, Butt E, Peacock SJ, Brown NM, Riley T, Songer G, Wilcox M, Pirmohamed M, Kuijper E, Hawkey P, Wren BW, Dougan G, Parkhill J, Lawley TD.** 2013. Emergence and global spread of epidemic healthcare associated *Clostridium difficile*. *Nat Genet* **45:**109–113.

39. **Rupnik M, Wilcox MH, Gerding DN.** 2009. *Clostridium difficile* infection: new developments in epidemiology and pathogenesis. *Nat Rev Microbiol* **7:**526–536.

40. **Valiente E, Cairns MD, Wren BW.** 2014. The *Clostridium difficile* PCR ribotype 027 lineage: a pathogen on the move. *Clin Microbiol Infect* **20:**396–404.

41. **Goorhuis A, Van der Kooi T, Vaessen N, Dekker FW, Van den Berg R, Harmanus C, van den Hof S, Notermans DW, Kuijper EJ.** 2007. Spread and epidemiology of *Clostridium difficile* polymerase chain reaction ribotype 027/toxinotype III in The Netherlands. *Clin Infect Dis* **45:**695–703.

42. **Rupnik M, Tambic Andrasevic A, Trajkovska Dokic E, Matas I, Jovanovic M, Pasic S, Kocuvan A, Janezic S.** 2016. Distribution of *Clostridium difficile* PCR ribotypes and high proportion of 027 and 176 in some hospitals in four South Eastern European countries. *Anaerobe* **42**:142–144.

43. **Davies KA, Ashwin H, Longshaw CM, Burns DA, Davis GL, Wilcox MH, EUCLID study group.** 2016. Diversity of *Clostridium difficile* PCR ribotypes in Europe: results from the European, multicentre, prospective, biannual, point-prevalence study of *Clostridium difficile* infection in hospitalised patients with diarrhoea (EUCLID), 2012 and 2013. *Euro Surveill* **21**:21.

44. **Adler A, Miller-Roll T, Bradenstein R, Block C, Mendelson B, Parizade M, Paitan Y, Schwartz D, Peled N, Carmeli Y, Schwaber MJ.** 2015. A national survey of the molecular epidemiology of *Clostridium difficile* in Israel: the dissemination of the ribotype 027 strain with reduced susceptibility to vancomycin and metronidazole. *Diagn Microbiol Infect Dis* **83**:21–24.

45. **Bartsch SM, Umscheid CA, Fishman N, Lee BY.** 2013. Is fidaxomicin worth the cost? An economic analysis. *Clin Infect Dis* **57**:555–561.

46. **Debast SB, Bauer MP, Kuijper EJ, European Society of Clinical Microbiology and Infectious Diseases.** 2014. European Society of Clinical Microbiology and Infectious Diseases: update of the treatment guidance document for *Clostridium difficile* infection. *Clin Microbiol Infect* **20**(Suppl 2):1–26.

47. **Surawicz CM, Brandt LJ, Binion DG, Ananthakrishnan AN, Curry SR, Gilligan PH, McFarland LV, Mellow M, Zuckerbraun BS.** 2013. Guidelines for diagnosis, treatment, and prevention of *Clostridium difficile* infections. *Am J Gastroenterol* **108**:478–498, quiz 499.

48. **Zainah H, Hassan M, Shiekh-Sroujieh L, Hassan S, Alangaden G, Ramesh M.** 2015. Intestinal microbiota transplantation, a simple and effective treatment for severe and refractory *Clostridium difficile* infection. *Dig Dis Sci* **60**:181–185.

49. **Youngster I, Russell GH, Pindar C, Ziv-Baran T, Sauk J, Hohmann EL.** 2014. Oral, capsulized, frozen fecal microbiota transplantation for relapsing Clostridium difficile infection. *JAMA* **312**:1772–1778.

50. **Frank DN, St Amand AL, Feldman RA, Boedeker EC, Harpaz N, Pace NR.** 2007. Molecular-phylogenetic characterization of microbial community imbalances in human inflammatory bowel diseases. *Proc Natl Acad Sci USA* **104**:13780–13785.

51. **Rossen NG, Fuentes S, van der Spek MJ, Tijssen JG, Hartman JH, Duflou A, Löwenberg M, van den Brink GR, Mathus-Vliegen EM, de Vos WM, Zoetendal EG, D'Haens GR, Ponsioen CY.** 2015. Findings from a randomized controlled trial of fecal transplantation for patients with ulcerative colitis. *Gastroenterology* **149**:110–118.e4.

52. **Moayyedi P, Surette MG, Kim PT, Libertucci J, Wolfe M, Onischi C, Armstrong D, Marshall JK, Kassam Z, Reinisch W, Lee CH.** 2015. Fecal microbiota transplantation induces remission in patients with active ulcerative colitis in a randomized controlled trial. *Gastroenterology* **149**: 102–109.e6.

53. **Bennet JD, Brinkman M.** 1989. Treatment of ulcerative colitis by implantation of normal colonic flora. *Lancet* **i**:164.

54. **Colman RJ, Rubin DT.** 2014. Fecal microbiota transplantation as therapy for inflammatory bowel disease: a systematic review and meta-analysis. *J Crohn's Colitis* **8**:1569–1581.

55. **Li SS, Zhu A, Benes V, Costea PI, Hercog R, Hildebrand F, Huerta-Cepas J, Nieuwdorp M, Salojärvi J, Voigt AY, Zeller G, Sunagawa S, de Vos WM, Bork P.** 2016. Durable coexistence of donor and recipient strains after fecal microbiota transplantation. *Science* **352**:586–589.

56. **Shi Y, Dong Y, Huang W, Zhu D, Mao H, Su P.** 2016. Fecal microbiota transplantation for ulcerative colitis: a systematic review and meta-analysis. *PLoS One* **11**:e0157259.

57. **World Health Organization.** 2016. *Obesity and overweight—fact sheet.* http://www.who.int/mediacentre/factsheets/fs311/en/. World Health Organization, Geneva, Switzerland.

58. **Flegal KM, Carroll MD, Ogden CL, Curtin LR.** 2010. Prevalence and trends in obesity among US adults, 1999–2008. *JAMA* **303**:235–241.

59. **Guh DP, Zhang W, Bansback N, Amarsi Z, Birmingham CL, Anis AH.** 2009. The incidence of co-morbidities related to obesity and overweight: a systematic review and meta-analysis. *BMC Public Health* **9**:88.

60. **Di Angelantonio E, et al, Global BMI Mortality Collaboration.** 2016. Body-mass index and all-cause mortality: individual-participant-data meta-analysis of 239 prospective studies in four continents. *Lancet* **388**:776–786.

61. **Bäckhed F, Manchester JK, Semenkovich CF, Gordon JI.** 2007. Mechanisms underlying the resistance to diet-induced obesity in germ-free mice. *Proc Natl Acad Sci USA* **104**: 979–984.

62. **Turnbaugh PJ, Ley RE, Mahowald MA, Magrini V, Mardis ER, Gordon JI.** 2006. An obesity-associated gut microbiome with increased capacity for energy harvest. *Nature* **444**:1027–1031.

63. Tremaroli V, Bäckhed F. 2012. Functional interactions between the gut microbiota and host metabolism. *Nature* **489:**242–249.

64. Bjursell M, Admyre T, Göransson M, Marley AE, Smith DM, Oscarsson J, Bohlooly-Y M. 2011. Improved glucose control and reduced body fat mass in free fatty acid receptor 2-deficient mice fed a high-fat diet. *Am J Physiol Endocrinol Metab* **300:**E211–E220.

65. Mariadason JM, Barkla DH, Gibson PR. 1997. Effect of short-chain fatty acids on paracellular permeability in Caco-2 intestinal epithelium model. *Am J Physiol* **272:**G705–G712.

66. Lewis K, Lutgendorff F, Phan V, Söderholm JD, Sherman PM, McKay DM. 2010. Enhanced translocation of bacteria across metabolically stressed epithelia is reduced by butyrate. *Inflamm Bowel Dis* **16:**1138–1148.

67. Kim MH, Kang SG, Park JH, Yanagisawa M, Kim CH. 2013. Short-chain fatty acids activate GPR41 and GPR43 on intestinal epithelial cells to promote inflammatory responses in mice. *Gastroenterology* **145:**396–406.e1-10.

68. Tazoe H, Otomo Y, Kaji I, Tanaka R, Karaki SI, Kuwahara A. 2008. Roles of short-chain fatty acids receptors, GPR41 and GPR43 on colonic functions. *J Physiol Pharmacol* **59** (Suppl 2):251–262.

69. Maslowski KM, Vieira AT, Ng A, Kranich J, Sierro F, Yu D, Schilter HC, Rolph MS, Mackay F, Artis D, Xavier RJ, Teixeira MM, Mackay CR. 2009. Regulation of inflammatory responses by gut microbiota and chemoattractant receptor GPR43. *Nature* **461:**1282–1286.

70. Segain JP, Raingeard de la Blétière D, Bourreille A, Leray V, Gervois N, Rosales C, Ferrier L, Bonnet C, Blottière HM, Galmiche JP. 2000. Butyrate inhibits inflammatory responses through NFkappaB inhibition: implications for Crohn's disease. *Gut* **47:** 397–403.

71. Tedelind S, Westberg F, Kjerrulf M, Vidal A. 2007. Anti-inflammatory properties of the short-chain fatty acids acetate and propionate: a study with relevance to inflammatory bowel disease. *World J Gastroenterol* **13:**2826–2832.

72. Samuel BS, Shaito A, Motoike T, Rey FE, Backhed F, Manchester JK, Hammer RE, Williams SC, Crowley J, Yanagisawa M, Gordon JI. 2008. Effects of the gut microbiota on host adiposity are modulated by the short-chain fatty-acid binding G protein-coupled receptor, Gpr41. *Proc Natl Acad Sci USA* **105:**16767–16772.

73. Grudell AB, Camilleri M. 2007. The role of peptide YY in integrative gut physiology and potential role in obesity. *Curr Opin Endocrinol Diabetes Obes* **14:**52–57.

74. Cani PD, Amar J, Iglesias MA, Poggi M, Knauf C, Bastelica D, Neyrinck AM, Fava F, Tuohy KM, Chabo C, Waget A, Delmée E, Cousin B, Sulpice T, Chamontin B, Ferrières J, Tanti JF, Gibson GR, Casteilla L, Delzenne NM, Alessi MC, Burcelin R. 2007. Metabolic endotoxemia initiates obesity and insulin resistance. *Diabetes* **56:**1761–1772.

75. Weisberg SP, McCann D, Desai M, Rosenbaum M, Leibel RL, Ferrante AW Jr. 2003. Obesity is associated with macrophage accumulation in adipose tissue. *J Clin Invest* **112:**1796–1808.

76. Weisberg SP, Hunter D, Huber R, Lemieux J, Slaymaker S, Vaddi K, Charo I, Leibel RL, Ferrante AW Jr. 2006. CCR2 modulates inflammatory and metabolic effects of high-fat feeding. *J Clin Invest* **116:**115–124.

77. Hotamisligil GS, Shargill NS, Spiegelman BM. 1993. Adipose expression of tumor necrosis factor-alpha: direct role in obesity-linked insulin resistance. *Science* **259:**87–91.

78. Amar J, Chabo C, Waget A, Klopp P, Vachoux C, Bermúdez-Humarán LG, Smirnova N, Bergé M, Sulpice T, Lahtinen S, Ouwehand A, Langella P, Rautonen N, Sansonetti PJ, Burcelin R. 2011. Intestinal mucosal adherence and translocation of commensal bacteria at the early onset of type 2 diabetes: molecular mechanisms and probiotic treatment. *EMBO Mol Med* **3:**559–572.

79. Laugerette F, Vors C, Géloën A, Chauvin MA, Soulage C, Lambert-Porcheron S, Peretti N, Alligier M, Burcelin R, Laville M, Vidal H, Michalski MC. 2011. Emulsified lipids increase endotoxemia: possible role in early postprandial low-grade inflammation. *J Nutr Biochem* **22:** 53–59.

80. Ghanim H, Abuaysheh S, Sia CL, Korzeniewski K, Chaudhuri A, Fernandez-Real JM, Dandona P. 2009. Increase in plasma endotoxin concentrations and the expression of Toll-like receptors and suppressor of cytokine signaling-3 in mononuclear cells after a high-fat, high-carbohydrate meal: implications for insulin resistance. *Diabetes Care* **32:**2281–2287.

81. Erridge C, Attina T, Spickett CM, Webb DJ. 2007. A high-fat meal induces low-grade endotoxemia: evidence of a novel mechanism of postprandial inflammation. *Am J Clin Nutr* **86:** 1286–1292.

82. Adachi Y, Moore LE, Bradford BU, Gao W, Thurman RG. 1995. Antibiotics prevent liver injury in rats following long-term exposure to ethanol. *Gastroenterology* **108:**218–224.

83. Verdam FJ, Rensen SS, Driessen A, Greve JW, Buurman WA. 2011. Novel evidence for chronic exposure to endotoxin in human non-

alcoholic steatohepatitis. *J Clin Gastroenterol* 45:149–152.

84. **Miele L, Valenza V, La Torre G, Montalto M, Cammarota G, Ricci R, Mascianà R, Forgione A, Gabrieli ML, Perotti G, Vecchio FM, Rapaccini G, Gasbarrini G, Day CP, Grieco A.** 2009. Increased intestinal permeability and tight junction alterations in nonalcoholic fatty liver disease. *Hepatology* 49: 1877–1887.

85. **Vrieze A, Van Nood E, Holleman F, Salojärvi J, Kootte RS, Bartelsman JF, Dallinga-Thie GM, Ackermans MT, Serlie MJ, Oozeer R, Derrien M, Druesne A, Van Hylckama Vlieg JE, Bloks VW, Groen AK, Heilig HG, Zoetendal EG, Stroes ES, de Vos WM, Hoekstra JB, Nieuwdorp M.** 2012. Transfer of intestinal microbiota from lean donors increases insulin sensitivity in individuals with metabolic syndrome. *Gastroenterology* 143:913–6.e7.

86. **Vrieze A, Out C, Fuentes S, Jonker L, Reuling I, Kootte RS, van Nood E, Holleman F, Knaapen M, Romijn JA, Soeters MR, Blaak EE, Dallinga-Thie GM, Reijnders D, Ackermans MT, Serlie MJ, Knop FK, Holst JJ, van der Ley C, Kema IP, Zoetendal EG, de Vos WM, Hoekstra JB, Stroes ES, Groen AK, Nieuwdorp M.** 2014. Impact of oral vancomycin on gut microbiota, bile acid metabolism, and insulin sensitivity. *J Hepatol* 60:824–831.

87. **Saito YA, Schoenfeld P, Locke GR III.** 2002. The epidemiology of irritable bowel syndrome in North America: a systematic review. *Am J Gastroenterol* 97:1910–1915.

88. **Lovell RM, Ford AC.** 2012. Global prevalence of and risk factors for irritable bowel syndrome: a meta-analysis. *Clin Gastroenterol Hepatol* 10:712–721.e4.

89. **Simrén M, Svedlund J, Posserud I, Björnsson ES, Abrahamsson H.** 2006. Health-related quality of life in patients attending a gastroenterology outpatient clinic: functional disorders versus organic diseases. *Clin Gastroenterol Hepatol* 4:187–195.

90. **Gralnek IM, Hays RD, Kilbourne A, Naliboff B, Mayer EA.** 2000. The impact of irritable bowel syndrome on health-related quality of life. *Gastroenterology* 119:654–660.

91. **Codling C, O'Mahony L, Shanahan F, Quigley EM, Marchesi JR.** 2010. A molecular analysis of fecal and mucosal bacterial communities in irritable bowel syndrome. *Dig Dis Sci* 55:392–397.

92. **Si JM, Yu YC, Fan YJ, Chen SJ.** 2004. Intestinal microecology and quality of life in irritable bowel syndrome patients. *World J Gastroenterol* 10:1802–1805.

93. **Balsari A, Ceccarelli A, Dubini F, Fesce E, Poli G.** 1982. The fecal microbial population in the irritable bowel syndrome. *Microbiologica* 5:185–194.

94. **Jeffery IB, O'Toole PW, Öhman L, Claesson MJ, Deane J, Quigley EM, Simrén M.** 2012. An irritable bowel syndrome subtype defined by species-specific alterations in faecal microbiota. *Gut* 61:997–1006.

95. **Rajilić-Stojanović M, Biagi E, Heilig HG, Kajander K, Kekkonen RA, Tims S, de Vos WM.** 2011. Global and deep molecular analysis of microbiota signatures in fecal samples from patients with irritable bowel syndrome. *Gastroenterology* 141:1792–1801.

96. **Kassinen A, Krogius-Kurikka L, Mäkivuokko H, Rinttilä T, Paulin L, Corander J, Malinen E, Apajalahti J, Palva A.** 2007. The fecal microbiota of irritable bowel syndrome patients differs significantly from that of healthy subjects. *Gastroenterology* 133:24–33.

97. **Ford AC, Quigley EM, Lacy BE, Lembo AJ, Saito YA, Schiller LR, Soffer EE, Spiegel BM, Moayyedi P.** 2014. Efficacy of prebiotics, probiotics, and synbiotics in irritable bowel syndrome and chronic idiopathic constipation: systematic review and meta-analysis. *Am J Gastroenterol* 109:1547–1561, quiz 1546, 1562.

98. **Vrieze A, de Groot PF, Kootte RS, Knaapen M, van Nood E, Nieuwdorp M.** 2013. Fecal transplant: a safe and sustainable clinical therapy for restoring intestinal microbial balance in human disease? *Best Pract Res Clin Gastroenterol* 27:127–137.

99. **Andrews PBT.** 1995. Bacteriotherapy for chronic constipation—a long term follow-up. *Gastroenterology* 108(Suppl 2):A563.

100. **National Clinical Trials.** 2014, updated March 2016. *Fecal microbiota transplantation in patients with irritable bowel syndrome.* https://clinicaltrials.gov/ct2/show/NCT02092402.

101. **Goossens H, Ferech M, Vander Stichele R, Elseviers M, ESAC Project Group.** 2005. Outpatient antibiotic use in Europe and association with resistance: a cross-national database study. *Lancet* 365:579–587.

102. **Vallance BA, Deng W, Jacobson K, Finlay BB.** 2003. Host susceptibility to the attaching and effacing bacterial pathogen *Citrobacter rodentium*. *Infect Immun* 71:3443–3453.

103. **Willing BP, Vacharaksa A, Croxen M, Thanachayanont T, Finlay BB.** 2011. Altering host resistance to infections through microbial transplantation. *PLoS One* 6:e26988.

104. **Ubeda C, Bucci V, Caballero S, Djukovic A, Toussaint NC, Equinda M, Lipuma L, Ling L,**

Gobourne A, No D, Taur Y, Jenq RR, van den Brink MR, Xavier JB, Pamer EG. 2013. Intestinal microbiota containing *Barnesiella* species cures vancomycin-resistant *Enterococcus faecium* colonization. *Infect Immun* **81:**965–973.

105. **Singh R, Nieuwdorp M, ten Berge IJ, Bemelman FJ, Geerlings SE.** 2014. The potential beneficial role of faecal microbiota transplantation in diseases other than *Clostridium difficile* infection. *Clin Microbiol Infect* **20:**1119–1125.

106. **Singh R, van Nood E, Nieuwdorp M, van Dam B, ten Berge IJ, Geerlings SE, Bemelman FJ.** 2014. Donor feces infusion for eradication of extended spectrum beta-lactamase producing *Escherichia coli* in a patient with end stage renal disease. *Clin Microbiol Infect* **20:**O977–O978.

107. **Wei Y, Gong J, Zhu W, Guo D, Gu L, Li N, Li J.** 2015. Fecal microbiota transplantation restores dysbiosis in patients with methicillin resistant *Staphylococcus aureus* enterocolitis. *BMC Infect Dis* **15:**265.

108. **Borody TJ, Campbell J, Torres M, Nowak A, Leis S.** 2011. Reversal of idiopathic thrombocytopenic purpura with fecal microbiota transplantation (FMT), abstr. *Am J Gastroenterol* **106:**S352.

109. **Borody TJ, Leis S, Campbell J, Torres M, Nowak A.** 2011. Fecal microbiota transplantation (FMT) in multiple sclerosis (MS), abstr P1111. American College of Gastroenterology and Postgraduate Course 2011, 28 October–2 November 2011, Washington, DC. http://www.fecalmicrobiotatransplant.com/2012/08/could-multiple-sclerosis-be-caused-by.html.

Enterococci and Their Interactions with the Intestinal Microbiome

13

KRISTA DUBIN[1,2] and ERIC G. PAMER[1,2,3]

BACKGROUND

The genus *Enterococcus* comprises over 50 species that can be found in diverse environments, from the soil to the gastrointestinal (GI) tract of animals and humans to the hospital environment (1, 2; http://www.bacterio.net/enterococcus.html). The first member of this Gram-positive genus was isolated in 1899 from a lethal case of endocarditis (3, 4). It was not until 1984 that enterococcal species were seen as genetically distinct from *Streptococcus* and assigned their own genus (3–5). Enterococci are Gram-positive facultative anaerobes that exist in chains or pairs and do not form spores. They grow optimally at 35°C, hydrolyze esculin in the presence of 40% bile salts, and are catalase negative (6, 7). Enterococcal species can be distinguished by phenotypic tests that rely on strains' ability to form acid in mannitol and sorbose broth and to hydrolyze arginine (8, 9).

Enterococci are found in the fecal content of insects, birds, reptiles, and mammals (2, 10). Named "entero" to denote their intestinal residence, *Enterococcus faecalis* and *Enterococcus faecium* were first isolated in the

[1]Immunology Program and Infectious Disease Service, Memorial Sloan-Kettering Cancer Center, New York, NY 10065; [2]Immunology and Microbial Pathogenesis Program, Weill Cornell Graduate School of Medical Sciences, New York, NY 10065; [3]Lucille Castori Center for Microbes, Inflammation, and Cancer, Memorial Sloan-Kettering Cancer Center, New York, NY 10065

Bugs as Drugs: Therapeutic Microbes for the Prevention and Treatment of Disease
Edited by Robert A. Britton and Patrice D. Cani
© 2016 American Society for Microbiology, Washington, DC
doi:10.1128/microbiolspec.BAD-0014-2016

early 1900s (11–13). Based on single nucleotide polymorphisms within 16S rRNA, enterococci are divided into seven evolutionarily distinct groups (14). *E. faecalis* is found in a host of different animals, suggesting that it was in evolutionary terms an early gut colonizer (14). In humans, *E. faecalis* and *E. faecium* are the most abundant species of this genus found in fecal content, accounting for up to 1% of the adult intestinal microbiota (15–19).

Enterococci have recently emerged as a prevalent multidrug-resistant health care-related pathogen. Since the late 1970s and 1980s, enterococcal species have developed increased resistance to several classes of antibiotics (14, 20, 21). Resistant enterococci densely colonize the gut following antibiotic treatment, which can deplete the GI tract of large swaths of protective commensals (22–24). Antibiotic use has increased the spread of drug-resistant enterococci in the hospital setting, leading to enterococci becoming one of the most common causes of hospital-associated infections (25).

Restoration of the intestinal microbiota to a healthy state is a new and developing approach to counter the continuing emergence of antibiotic-resistant microorganisms. However, manipulating the intestinal microbiome to prevent the spread of antibiotic-resistant bacterial strains, while also supporting the sensitive ecosystem of which enterococci are constituents, is a delicate task. It requires that we understand the relationship of enterococci to their natural intestinal habitat in the context of their dual life as commensals and health care-related pathogens. To do so, we discuss the road enterococci have traveled to become multidrug-resistant hospital-associated infectious agents that possess diversified genomes that allow them to survive in the postantibiotic intestinal niche. With that in mind, we can consider how best to manipulate or restore the enteric microbiota to benefit human health. In this article, we discuss the enterococci's (i) clinical importance, (ii) development of antibiotic resistance, (iii) diversity in genomic composition and habitats, and (iv) interaction with the intestinal microbiome that may help limit its infectious spread.

CLINICAL IMPORTANCE

Infections

Enterococci emerged as a leading hospital-associated pathogen in the late 1970s and 1980s (26). In the United States, enterococci cause roughly 66,000 infections each year (27). They are often cultured from mixed species infections of the pelvis, abdomen, and other soft tissues (28). Although the role that enterococci play in these infections is not often clear, they are frequently treated with antibiotics. Less commonly, enterococci can cause meningitis and septic arthritis in patients with comorbidities or who are immunocompromised (28).

Even more clinically important, enterococci are leading causes of hospital-associated bacteremia, endocarditis, and urinary tract infections (20, 26, 29). Enterococci are the second-most-common cause of health care-related bacteremia and are associated with an overall mortality of roughly 33% (25, 30). Enterococcal bacteremia is often preceded by dense colonization of the GI tract, from which enterococci can translocate into the bloodstream (23, 31). In addition, the loss of mucosal immunity and disruption of the GI barrier have been associated with enterococcal bacteremia; risk factors include mucositis, *Clostridium difficile* infection, and neutropenia (32–34).

Over 10% of infective endocarditis cases seen in North America are caused by enterococci, making it the second leading cause (35). Of the total cases of enterococcal endocarditis, more than 35% of infections are acquired in the hospital (36). Enterococci on damaged heart valves grow biofilms that grow into structures called vegetations. Prosthetic valves can also serve as a platform for enterococcal growth (36). As with bacteremia, enterococci that cause endocarditis are often former inhabitants of the GI or genitourinary tract that gained access to the bloodstream (37, 38). Over 10% of catheter-associated urinary tract infections are of enterococcal origin (29).

Transmission and Sources of Infectious Enterococci

Hospital-acquired enterococcal infections are of particular concern due to both their increasing prevalence and growing resistance to antibiotics. Enterococci can readily spread within hospital units (39–44). Transmission of enterococci in the clinical environment is aided by two key factors: the ability of enterococci to survive outside the GI tract and the potential for health care workers to inadvertently transfer bacteria to adjacent patients. Enterococcal species can survive for prolonged periods on hospital surfaces, such as medical devices and bed rails, creating fomites that are a major risk factor for further spread (45, 46). Enterococci are transferred from patient to patient via health care workers' hands (47, 48). Contaminated hands of medical staff can transfer vancomycin-resistant enterococci (VRE) to roughly 1 out of every 10 clean surfaces that the health care workers touch (49).

The GI tract is the major site colonized by VRE and thus is an important source of hospital-associated infections. Hospital contamination is increased when colonized patients become incontinent (50). The density of VRE in patients' fecal content is correlated with the number of VRE transmission events (47). For roughly every 10% increase in patients colonized with VRE, the risk of additional hospitalized individuals acquiring VRE rises by 40% (46). A critical mechanism by which hospitalized patients become densely colonized with VRE is antibiotic treatment; how antibiotics allow for VRE expansion is detailed in the last sections of this article. The majority of antibiotic regimens with antianaerobic activity result in high-burden intestinal VRE density (22). Metronidazole increases the risk for high-density VRE colonization by 3-fold in allogeneic hematopoietic stem cell transplant (allo-HSCT) patient cohorts (24). Other risk factors for colonization include the use of catheters in the bloodstream or urinary tract, prior surgery, length of hospital stay, and exposure to VRE-colonized patients (40, 47, 51–54).

Treatment

Severe cases of enterococcal infections, such as infections of heart valves, have relied on combination drug therapy (55, 56). Combined administration of penicillin and streptomycin (a beta-lactam and aminoglycoside, respectively) successfully cured 80% of enterococcal infective endocarditis cases, which previously had a mortality rate of between 20 and 50%, and became standard therapy by the 1950s (38, 57). Today, for infective endocarditis caused by ampicillin- and vancomycin-sensitive *E. faecalis* lacking high-level resistance to aminoglycosides, gentamicin is the preferred aminoglycoside used in combination with ampicillin. Ampicillin plus ceftriaxone is an alternative therapy for ampicillin-susceptible *E. faecalis*. This regimen has also been used to treat aminoglycoside-sensitive *E. faecalis* isolates, as it is associated with similar cure rates and less nephrotoxicity compared to ampicillin-gentamicin therapy (58, 59). Although *E. faecalis* isolates are intrinsically resistant to cephalosporins, the two beta-lactam antibiotics work synergistically by binding different penicillin-binding proteins (PBPs), the enzymes involved in bacterial cell wall synthesis (60). For ampicillin- and vancomycin-resistant isolates causing infective endocarditis, the majority of which are *E. faecium*, daptomycin or linezolid can be used, although clinical data about their efficacy are limited (61, 62).

There are few other examples of bactericidal synergy against enterococci, and novel antibiotic therapies are urgently needed for multidrug-resistant species (37). This clinical picture begs the question: how did commensal enterococci become such a challenging pathogen? The plasticity of the enterococcal genome is a key factor that has allowed the bacteria (i) to acquire traits that confer antibiotic resistance through mobile genetic elements, (ii) to diversify over time into lineages specifically adapted to the hospital environment, and (iii) to colonize the GI tract at greater densities following antibiotic exposure (37). We discuss each point in the following three sections.

DEVELOPMENT OF ANTIBIOTIC RESISTANCE

Roughly one-third of enterococcal infections in the United States are drug resistant, totaling 20,000 antibiotic-resistant cases per year, from which an estimated 1,300 patients succumb yearly (27). *E. faecalis* caused over 90% of clinical infections until the mid-1990s, at which point *E. faecium* became more clinically prevalent (63, 64). The rise of health care-related *E. faecium* strains has been attributed to the increased use of vancomycin and broad-spectrum antibiotics (20, 25, 37, 65). To date in the United States, *E. faecium* causes nearly a third of all enterococcal health care-related infections and constitutes over 75% of all health care-associated VRE strains (27, 29). The majority of *E. faecium* infections associated with medical equipment are vancomycin resistant and ampicillin resistant (80 to 87% and 90%, respectively) (25, 66).

VRE emerged in the mid-1980s, first in Europe among livestock and then in the United States in hospitals (67, 68). In the United States, glycopeptide resistance developed among hospital-adapted ampicillin-resistant isolates that were the predominant enterococci in hospital intestinal microbiota (21, 65). Vancomycin-resistant isolates have been associated with oral vancomycin used to treat antibiotic-associated diarrhea due to

C. difficile in hospitalized patients. Of note, administration of vancomycin intravenously is not correlated with the development of VRE infection (22, 24, 69). Vancomycin by this route results in low intestinal concentrations (70). In Europe, the issue of VRE was initially confined to animal husbandry. VRE was seen in livestock regularly exposed to antibiotics. Avoparcin, a growth-promoting antibiotic that also provides cross-resistance to vancomycin, is thought to have contributed to the rise of VRE (71–73). Avoparcin was subsequently banned from use in 1996, and the prevalence of VRE in animals decreased (74–76). However, VRE has made a recent appearance in European hospitals with isolates closely related to health care-associated strains found in the United States (77).

Enterococci harbor resistance through two means: (i) resistance that is encoded in the core genome of all enterococcal strains (intrinsic) and (ii) resistance that is passed among isolates on mobile genetic elements by horizontal transfer (acquired). Some of the mechanisms by which enterococci developed resistance to ampicillin, vancomycin, and daptomycin are briefly outlined in the following sections.

Antibiotic Resistance: Ampicillin

Beta-lactams, such as ampicillin, inhibit bacterial growth by modifying and thereby inactivating a group of enzymes called PBPs. PBPs cross-link side chains of peptidoglycan peptides during cell wall synthesis. Enterococcal strains harbor some intrinsic resistance to beta-lactams by producing PBP5, which is chromosomally encoded (78, 79). Given their low affinity to beta-lactam drugs, PBP5s can continue peptidoglycan synthesis as other PBPs are modified (80). Increased resistance to ampicillin is associated with mutations to the PBP5-encoding gene that further reduce the protein's affinity for beta-lactam antibiotics, such as mutations that result in amino acid substitutions near the active site (81–83). Resistance is further amplified when multiple mutations are present in the *pbp5* gene (83). Mutated alleles can be horizontally transferred to beta-lactam-susceptible strains *in vitro* (84). Altogether, the *pbp5* gene differs in nucleotide sequence by about 5% between sensitive and resistant strains (85). The acquisition of specific *pbp5* gene mutations contributed to the high-level ampicillin resistance that health care-related *E. faecium* isolates developed in the late 1970s and 1980s (21, 85, 86).

Antibiotic Resistance: Vancomycin

Glycopeptide antibiotics, such as vancomycin, prevent peptidoglycan cell wall synthesis by forming complexes with the D-ala-D-ala peptide terminus of peptidoglycan precursors, blocking enzymatic binding sites. Resistant isolates alter peptidoglycan precursors to form D-ala-D-lactate or D-ala-D-serine, with 1,000-fold to 7-fold lower drug-binding affinity, respectively (65, 87, 88). These modifications inhibit antibiotic binding while still allowing PBP enzymes to use these substrates to build a functional cell wall. In enterococci, nine gene clusters associated with resistance have been identified, with most being encoded on mobile elements (65). In response to glycopeptides, these resistance operons regulate the expression of a suite of enzymes that together create modified peptidoglycan precursors and remove those that are unaltered. The two major resistance operons are *vanA* and *vanB* (88). *vanA* gene loci are encoded on Tn*1546* or related transposons, conferring high-level resistance to vancomycin and teicoplanin. *vanB* gene clusters are found on Tn*5382*/Tn*1549*-type transposons either on plasmids or in the chromosome, providing moderate resistance to vancomycin only. Variants of these vancomycin-resistance gene loci are found worldwide (89).

Antibiotic Resistance: Daptomycin

Daptomycin is a recently introduced antibiotic for the treatment of multidrug-resistant enterococci; however, its bactericidal mechanism of action is not fully understood. It is thought to alter the cytoplasmic membrane and cause depolarization in a calcium-dependent manner, leading to a release of potassium ions from the cell and subsequent cell death (90, 91). For enterococci, the ability to resist daptomycin results in part from alterations in the composition of their cell membrane and envelope. Whole-genome sequencing of a pair of sequentially isolated vancomycin-resistant *E. faecalis* clones, the first daptomycin-sensitive and the second resistant, from a single patient's bloodstream identified in-frame deletions in three genes: *cls*, *gdpD*, and *liaF* (92). *cls* and *gdpD* encode proteins thought to play a role in phospholipid metabolism, and *liaF* is part of a regulatory system that coordinates the cell envelope response to antibiotics. Resequencing experiments found resistance-associated mutations that became fixed after only 2 weeks of *in vitro* serial passage with increasing concentrations of daptomycin (93). The transfer of the *cls* mutation to susceptible *E. faecalis* strains confers resistance to daptomycin (93). Comparative sequencing analyses were performed on five vancomycin-resistant *E. faecium* strain pairs, all initially susceptible and then later resistant to daptomycin, that colonized HSCT patients' GI tracts (94). These intestinal VRE isolates were exposed to systemic daptomycin as it was partially excreted into the gut, highlighting the capacity of the GI tract to serve as a reservoir for the development of antibiotic resistance, even at low antibiotic concentrations (94). Point mutations in the cardiolipin synthase-encoding gene *cls* were detected in four out of five of these isolate pairs.

Antibiotic Resistance: Genetics

In some enterococcal strains, such as vancomycin-resistant *E. faecalis* V583, acquired genetic elements make up 25% of the genome (95). There are two major types of plasmids in enterococci: pheromone-responsive and transposon-type. The pheromone-responsive plasmid pMG2200 encodes VanB-type vancomycin resistance (96). VanA-encoding pheromone-responsive plasmids can be transferred between *E. faecium* and *E. faecalis* (97). Large regions of the *E. faecalis* genome can be shuttled between isolates *in vitro* via conjugative plasmids, involving up to a quarter of the chromosome (98). Crossover between chromosomal and plasmid DNA can occur through insertion sequences (also known as IS elements). In *E. faecalis*, pheromone-responsive conjugative plasmids that contain IS256 copies can integrate into the chromosome of recipient strains *in vitro* and transfer chromosomal DNA from donor isolates, creating hybrid genomes (98). This plasticity of the enterococcal genome has important clinical implications. For example, the transfer of DNA among enterococci has led to multiple lineages of mutated *pbp5* genes conferring ampicillin resistance in hospital-associated strains (84, 85).

Transposons occur throughout the enterococcal genome and are of three types: conjugative, Tn3-family, and composite (flanking IS sequences). The *vanA* gene cluster is encoded by a Tn3-derivative transposon, Tn1546 (99). Tn916-family conjugative transposons include Tn5382 and Tn1549, which are the main genetic elements that contain the VanB resistance operon (100–102). The gene encoding PBP5 can also be transferred between enterococcal isolates with the Tn916-family conjugative transposon Tn5386 that carries the VanB cluster (103).

DIVERSITY IN GENOMIC COMPOSITION AND HABITATS

The genomic diversity seen among enterococcal strains has been well characterized by application of high-throughput whole-genome sequencing. The first enterococcal genome, published in 2002, belonged to *E. faecalis* V583 (95). Now, hundreds of completed or draft genomes are available (104). The GC content of enterococcal species can vary from 37 to 45%, and genome sizes can range from 2.7 to 3.6 Mb (105–107). Compared to commensal enterococcal strains, multidrug-resistant clinical isolates possess larger genomes, through the acquisition of foreign genetic material (107). Hospital-associated *E. faecalis* strains generally lack clustered regularly interspaced short palindromic repeat (CRISPR)-Cas systems that help block phage infections and cleave plasmid-encoded DNA (107, 108). In 48 *E. faecalis* strains, the absence of a CRISPR-Cas system was significantly correlated with resistance to two or more antibiotics (108). Multidrug-resistant *E. faecium* isolates are also generally CRISPR-Cas deficient, although this relationship has been demonstrated in smaller studies (108, 109). IS elements, such as IS16, drive genomic variation across isolates and likely aided hospital adaptation of enterococci as they transitioned from antibiotic sensitive to resistant (110–112). Additionally, recombination has been an important mechanism for generating diversity (89, 98, 113). By contrast, commensals are far less diverse; for example, *E. faecalis* OG1RF does not contain any laterally acquired mobile elements and harbors a CRISPR locus (114).

Population Genetics

Phylogenetic analyses have found considerable genomic differences between human commensal enterococci and endemic hospital strains. Health care-related strains are more closely related to animal isolates than human commensals (107, 115–117). Whole-genome sequencing of *E. faecium* isolates has revealed two major clades, one composed of community-derived isolates from healthy humans (clade B) and the other a complex cluster of animal-derived as well as hospital-associated strains (clade A). This split between clades occurred an estimated 3,000 years ago, which coincides roughly with the development of agriculture and animal domestication that conceivably separated animal and human commensals into distinct lineages (117). A second bifurcation occurred almost 75 years ago within clade A between modern health care-related strains and animal-derived isolates (117). Ampicillin-resistant strains are seen more frequently in pets than in healthy humans (118). Enterococcal strains of animal origin can act as a reservoir of antibiotic-resistance elements that can be shared with human isolates (119, 120). For example, *vanA* genes from animal-derived enterococci can be laterally transferred to human commensals in the gut (121, 122).

What is the evolutionary relationship between clinical enterococcal isolates? Numerous studies have employed multilocus sequence typing as a technique to resolve the enterococcal population structure (123). The process relies on sequencing amplified fragments of seven housekeeping genes (113, 124). Initial studies of *E. faecium* based on multilocus sequence typing found a distinct cluster of isolates that were enriched in hospitalized patients, named clonal complex 17 (89). *E. faecalis* isolates derived from the hospital environment also group together by multilocus sequence typing, namely into clonal complexes C2 and C9, which possess more resistance elements and pathogenicity island genes than other clusters (113, 125–127). However, clinical *E. faecium* isolates grouped in clonal complex 17 are not strictly clonal (111). In phylogenetic analyses that rely on the algorithm eBURST, spurious groupings can occur for species with high recombination rates, such as *E. faecium* (128). Analyses of *E. faecium* strains employing Bayesian models found three major hospital-associated lineages, indicating that health care-related isolates do not stem from a single ancestral strain (116). Rather, adaptive traits that characterize clinical isolates were likely acquired independently in different genetic backgrounds. Evidence that hospital-associated isolates derived from multiple lineages can also be seen by analyzing the sequence of a single resistance element. Specific amino acid changes in the PBP5 protein

are shared between isolates from different sequence types, and sequence variation was found within sequence types (85). These data indicate that antibiotic resistance developed on the background of multiple enterococcal strains that were poised for survival in the hospital setting.

Habitats

As previously stated, the GI tract is the primary habitat of enterococci. In animals, *E. faecalis*, *E. faecium*, *Enterococcus hirae*, and *Enterococcus durans* are the enterococcal species most commonly found in the gut microbiota (129). Comparisons of VRE in animals and humans have found strains to be host-specific (130). However, patient isolates have been detected in animals such as dogs and pigs, and as discussed above, hospital-adapted strains share a relatively recent close evolutionary relationship to animal isolates (76). While the GI tract represents the largest reservoir for enterococci, strains have also been found in the environment. It is thought that soil and water isolates are derived from fecal contamination (6, 131–133). Enterococci possess the ability to adapt to extraintestinal environments, as discussed with regard to hospitals. *E. faecalis* can survive in nutrient-poor environments, such as sterilized waste, for up to 12 days (134). Enterococci are frequently found in human sewage, particularly outside hospitals (135). Not surprisingly, enterococcal strains isolated from effluents are antibiotic resistant. Isolates cultured from sewage as early as the 1970s were resistant to tetracycline (136). In water, enterococci are used by the Environmental Protection Agency, in addition to total coliform bacteria, as a marker of fecal contamination, as the result of finding a correlation between swimmers' risk of GI infection and the number of enterococci cultured from the water site (137). In 2012, 24% of bodies of surface water in the United States were classified as impaired, a number of them due to enterococci (133).

In the human GI tract, enterococci live in the small and large intestine. Enterococcal strains represent roughly 1% of human fecal microbiota, with *E. faecalis* and *E. faecium* being the most common inhabitants (15–19). Average enterococci density in the GI tract is between 10^4 and 10^6 bacteria per gram wet weight, with *E. faecalis* found at a somewhat higher abundance than *E. faecium* (138, 139). However, in one study, *E. faecalis* was found in over 75% of fecal samples, while *E. faecium* was detected in 100% (140).

Intestinal commensals thrive in a finely tuned microbial ecology that has evolved over millennia, aiding in nutrient breakdown and the development of mucosal immunity (141, 142). Early-colonizing strains of commensal enterococci have been shown to contribute to colonic homeostasis through peroxisome proliferator-activated receptor-γ1-induced interleukin-10 and transforming growth factor-beta expression *in vitro* and can reduce the severity of infectious diarrhea in children (143–145). Perturbations to the intestinal microbiota disrupt this symbiotic relationship established with our microbial inhabitants, with important health consequences. Susceptibility to infections is the most well-documented pathology to result from changes in the microbiota, particularly in the context of antibiotic treatment, as detailed in the following section.

INTERACTIONS WITH THE INTESTINAL MICROBIOME

Colonization Resistance Mediated by the Intestinal Microbiota

The intestinal microbiota of healthy individuals is composed of a diverse consortium of bacteria (17, 146, 147). Individuals harbor a range of bacterial compositions, consisting of hundreds of microbial strains in the colon that mainly fall into the two major phyla: Gram-negative *Bacteroidetes* and Gram-positive *Firmicutes* (17, 148, 149). In addition to variations among individuals, differences in community structure are also found across body sites that exhibit different levels of stability over time, such as between the stable lower (fecal) and variable upper (oral) regions of the alimentary canal (150).

As previously noted, administration of broad-spectrum antibiotics allows drug-resistant strains such as VRE to expand dramatically in the gut by perturbing this sensitive microbial ecosystem (22–24, 151). VRE can expand to 99% of the intestinal lumen's microbiota in both antibiotic-treated mice and hospitalized patients (23). This overwhelming colonization is associated with translocation into the bloodstream and resulting VRE bacteremia (23, 24). In allo-HSCT patients, VRE colonization was found in over one-third of recipients, and these dominated patients had a 9-fold greater risk for VRE bacteremia (24). This risk persists over time; ampicillin administration leaves mice susceptible to VRE colonization for up to 4 weeks posttreatment, and VRE stably persists in the cecum for at least 60 days (23). In patients, resistant enterococci can persist for years after antibiotic exposure (152).

The concept of colonization resistance refers to the microbiota's ability to prevent the entry and growth of exogenous bacteria within its established, complex community (15, 153). Antibiotic treatment abrogates colonization resistance by depleting large swaths of intestinal commensal microorganisms, particularly anaerobic bacteria, that mediate this defense (15, 154–156).

Obligate anaerobes, such as members of the *Barnsiella* genus and *Clostridium* cluster XIVa, are highly correlated with intestinal VRE clearance following fecal microbial transplantation (156, 157). How obligate anaerobes provide a robust defense against invading VRE has not been fully elucidated. However, there are broad mechanisms that commensals can employ to exert colonization resistance and prevent infection: (i) indirect elimination that relies on stimulating innate mucosal immunity, (ii) continual maintenance of mucosal barrier integrity, and (iii) direct antagonism.

Indirect Inhibition through Innate Immune Defense

Intestinal microbes can stimulate innate receptors on immune cells and induce the production of antimicrobial peptides in other intestinal cell types. Paneth cells and intestinal epithelial cells produce RegIIIγ, a C-type lectin driven by Toll-like receptor (TLR) signaling with bactericidal activity against Gram-positive bacteria (158–160). Secreted RegIIIγ kills bacteria by binding to peptidoglycans of the bacterial cell wall and forming pores (161). Antibiotic treatment reduces expression of RegIIIγ and, in mice, increases susceptibility to VRE colonization and bacteremia (162). Oral administration of lipopolysaccharide mimics commensal microbial signals and restores RegIIIγ production, thereby increasing resistance to VRE (162). A signaling pathway driving RegIIIγ expression was delineated by administration of the bacterial TLR5 ligand, flagellin. Flagellin administered intravenously stimulates the CD103+ CD11b+ subset of dendritic cells to produce interleukin-23, which drives the interleukin-22-mediated production of RegIIIγ by intestinal epithelial cells (163). Commensals can thus work in concert with the mucosal immune system to suppress VRE outgrowth within the intestinal ecosystem.

Indirect Inhibition through Intestinal Barrier Maintenance

Intestinal microbes are separated from the mucosal epithelium and its distal lamina propria by mucus that coats the epithelial surface. The colonic epithelium is covered by a dense 50-μm-thick inner mucin layer composed primarily of Muc2 and a less dense outer stratum (164). Maintenance of a healthy epithelial barrier and intact gut physiology, such as gastric acid production, inhibits bacterial colonization of the GI tract (165). Goblet cells produce mucin, and secretion is stimulated by commensal bacteria in a MyD88-dependent manner (166–168).

Following antibiotic treatment, the mucin layer thins; without a robust physical barrier, intestinal microbes can directly access and potentially breach the epithelium (169). Both the density and composition of the mucus layers limit bacterial invasion. RegIIIγ is associated with mucin and reduces the density of intestinal bacteria near epithelial cells (170–172).

Compared to other antibiotic-resistant pathogens such as *Klebsiella pneumoniae*, VRE are spatially segregated from the intestinal mucus layer and adjacent epithelium even after antibiotic treatment with its notable mucin reduction (173). Visualization of the colonic lumen reveals that VRE do not infiltrate the inner mucin layer and, despite high luminal density, very few bacteria translocate to the mesenteric lymph nodes (173). Interestingly, cocolonization of mice with VRE and *K. pneumoniae*, which can more deeply penetrate the mucus coating, enables VRE to gain access to the mesenteric lymph nodes, possibly by *K. pneumoniae*-induced alterations to the mucin composition (173). Intact mucin production, which is in part regulated by commensal microbes, likely limits the invasive potential of intestinal enterococci.

Direct Inhibition by Anaerobic Commensals

In the first study of its kind for VRE, a defined consortium of commensals was identified as capable of restoring colonization resistance in mice (157). Antibiotic-treated mice were orally administered diluted doses of fecal microbiota from a colony of mice that had received ampicillin for over 15 years. Bacterial isolates in low-dose fractions that conferred resistance to VRE were identified, cultured, and administered in discrete combinations to mice maintained on ampicillin. Through a series of leave-one-out adoptive transfers, a minimum of four anaerobic isolates were found to successfully prevent and clear VRE from the gut: *Blautia producta*,

Clostridium bolteae, Bacteroides sartorii, and *Parabacteroides distasonis* (157). Of the four-commensal mixture, *B. producta* was shown *ex vivo* as the member that directly inhibits VRE growth, although the exact mechanism remains unknown. One possible mechanism of inhibition is through the production of toxic substances such as bacteriocins, which are small molecules with antimicrobial activity. *Lactococcus lactis* strains engineered to express bacteriocins significantly inhibited VRE growth *in vitro* (174). Oral administration of bacteriocin-producing *L. lactis* MM19 eliminated VRE at a faster rate from the gut of mice than mock treatment (175).

Direct Inhibition by Commensal Enterococci

Recent studies have examined the colonization dynamics between enterococcal commensals and health care-related isolates in the GI tract. While resistant isolates outcompete sensitive enterococci in the context of antibiotic pressure, intestinal colonization in patients declines following discharge (176). In *in vivo* competition assays that compared the colonization ability of *E. faecium* strains in antibiotic-treated mice, isolates from clade B (commensal-associated) outcompeted those from subclade A1 (hospital-derived) after 2 weeks (177).

Commensal enterococci have developed sophisticated defense mechanisms to eliminate exogenous enterococcal competitors from the gut. Bacteriocin-coding genes are commonly harbored on plasmids in enterococci. Commensal *E. faecalis* strains that express a pheromone-responsive conjugative plasmid encoding bacteriocin bac-21 outcompeted VRE lacking it (178). This plasmid, pPD1, is also quickly transferred to naive intestinal commensals by conjugation (178). Pheromones are secreted short lipoprotein signal peptide fragments that act as chemical messengers between bacteria and can mediate cell death. The multidrug-resistant *E. faecalis* isolate V583 harbors a plasmid called pTEF2 that renders it susceptible to a killing mechanism induced by commensal-derived pheromone cOB1 (179). Bacteriophages, or phages, are viruses that selectively infect and kill microbes. Given their selective killing, phages could be used therapeutically as a narrow-spectrum antimicrobial. *E. faecalis* strains that contain the bacteriophage φV1/7 in their genetic repertoire possess a growth advantage over related bacteria that lack it through phage-mediated lysis of competitors (180). In a mouse model of VRE bacteremia, intraperitoneal injection of ENB6 phage protected all mice when administered shortly after lethal VRE challenge and half of the mice when administered after the mice were moribund (181).

Enterococci as Probiotics

The benefits of using enterococci as probiotics have been controversial (182). Given the capacity of enterococcal isolates to share mobile virulence elements in the gut, there is concern about spreading antibiotic resistance if carried or obtained by probiotics. However, enterococcal strains such as *E. faecium* SF68 and *E. faecalis* Symbioflor have been marketed as probiotics for 2 decades without incident and with very few reported adverse events (182–184). Enterococcal probiotics have been shown to be effective in limiting GI infectious burden. A Cochrane meta-review of the literature found *E. faecium* SF68 to be an efficacious treatment of GI infections (184). Inoculation of *E. faecium* SF68 alone to adults and children with enteritis reduced the length of illness (182, 184–186). A probiotic mix containing *E. faecalis* as well as *Bacillus mesentericus* and *Clostridium butyricum* shortened the severity and duration of infectious diarrhea in children (145). In studies of diarrhea lasting 4 days or more, live *Lactobacillus casei* strain GG had a larger treatment effect size (0.59) than live *Enterococcus* SF68 (0.2), although the former had nearly twice as many participants enrolled in all trials (184).

Fecal Microbiota Transplantation and Probiotics as Treatment for VRE Colonization

Given the rise of antibiotic resistance, fecal microbiota transplantation (FMT) is an attractive alternative therapy to treat antibiotic-resistant pathogens and is an area of active research. FMT is remarkably successful at curing chronic, intractable *C. difficile* infection (187). A secondary analysis of a study involving patients with recurrent *C. difficile* infection showed that a human-derived FMT can reduce VRE colonization (188). However, the risk of unwittingly transmitting pathogenic microorganisms through FMTs is not insignificant, especially since many constituents of the microbiota have only recently been identified, if not characterized. This concern is particularly relevant to patients colonized with VRE, who are often immunocompromised. Researchers are actively exploring methods to perfect the acquisition of transferred bacteria and define critical members of FMTs that target infectious agents (189, 190).

To date, clinical trials studying the impact of probiotics on intestinal VRE carriage are limited. In a randomized study of 21 renal patients harboring VRE in their GI tract, ingestion of a yogurt supplemented with *Lactobacillus rhamnosus* GG reduced VRE density to the limit of detection in all patients receiving the probiotic (191). VRE burden decreased during a 3-week oral supplementation with *L. rhamnosus* GG in a randomized clinical trial of 61 children (192). This effect was not seen with 5-week administration of *L. rhamnosus* Lcr35 in a randomized study of nine patients (193). A 2-week course of *L. rhamnosus* GG administration in 11 patients with comorbidities also did not affect VRE colonization (194). Studies of enterococcal probiotics have failed to demonstrate their potential to limit drug-resistant enterococci colonization. In a prospective cohort study with over 500 hospitalized patients, a 10-strain mixture that contained *E. faecium* and numerous *Lactobacillus* isolates did not prevent ampicillin-resistant *E. faecium* acquisition (195).

The optimal design of probiotic consortia utilizes preclinical mouse models for candidate screening and follow-up mechanistic studies. Microbiome research relies on deep 16S rRNA gene and shotgun sequencing to profile bacterial communities of the gut and to predict candidate commensals that confer colonization resistance in time-series microbiota-reconstitution experiments. Ecological modeling of the microbiota using 16S sequencing data accurately predicted fluctuations in the composition of the microbiota following clindamycin administration and *C. difficile* colonization, and proposed the anaerobe *Coprobacillus* as a commensal capable of inhibiting enterococcal growth (196). *In vivo* adoptive transfer experiments allow investigators to further elucidate the mechanisms of colonization resistance provided by reconstituted commensals. In a mouse model of *C. difficile* infection, *Clostridium scindens* protected antibiotic-treated mice from *C. difficile* colonization by restoring secondary bile salt levels that inhibit the pathogen's growth (190). How these findings are best translated to treating at-risk patients is yet to be determined. In a promising phase 1b trial, orally administered capsules of 50 human-derived live *Firmicutes* spores prevented recurrent *C. difficile* infection, while the phase II clinical study found no efficacy (197, 198). A key question facing the translation of optimal bacterial combinations into patient therapy is what is required for a high transplantation efficacy. The study that defined a minimal consortium for VRE in mice highlights this challenge (157). Successful colonization of *B. producta* in ampicillin-treated mice required the adoptive transfer of three additional commensals. *B. sartorii* and *P. distasonis* inactivate ampicillin through the production of beta-lactamase, which was critical for ampicillin-sensitive isolates' survival in the GI tract, while *C. bolteae* supported *B. producta*'s engraftment through an unknown mechanism (157). Modulating the local gut environment through drug inactivation with probiotics is of particular importance for preventing VRE colonization in patients currently receiving antibiotics (199). Probiotic commensals can limit pathogen colonization in the gut by mitigating the disruptive effects of antibiotics to begin with. A *Bacteroides thetaiotaomicron* strain that produces a cephalosporinase has been shown to prevent intestinal VRE outgrowth by inactivating ceftriaxone and thus mitigating any significant changes to the microbiota (200).

Another open question is whether a protective microbial consortium should be tailored to individual patients, and if so, how to scale such a design. Given the falling costs of deep sequencing, profiling patients' microbiota may occur regularly in clinical practice. In the context of VRE, patients with different degrees of immune system impairment and treatment histories may benefit from personalized alterations to the minimally defined protective consortium. For example, patients who recently received antibiotics may be deficient in nutrients that resistance-mediating bacteria require to survive in the gut, necessitating additional isolates to support successful engraftment. Mouse models would not be a scalable approach to test these individual modifications. In this era of deep sequencing, we can potentially integrate diet, treatment regimens, and gut microbiome data to build machine-learning algorithms that can assess a patient's risk of VRE colonization and optimize probiotic combinations. Incorporating information on microbiome composition and function improved predictions of individuals' glycemic response following a meal and helped design dietary interventions for better glycemic control (201). Such data-driven approaches may help tailor preclinical findings to individual patients at scale to successfully mitigate their susceptibility to VRE colonization.

ACKNOWLEDGMENTS

This work was supported by the National Institutes of Health (NIH grant R01 AI42135), the National Cancer Institute (NCI grant P30 CA008748), and the Memorial Sloan Kettering Center for Microbes, Inflammation and Cancer (to E.G.P.). K.D. was supported by a Medical Scientist Training Program grant from the National Institute of General Medical Sciences, NIH (award T32GM007739 to the Weill Cornell/Rockefeller/Sloan Kettering Tri-Institutional MD-PhD Program).

CITATION

Dubin K, Pamer EG. 2017. Enterococci and their interactions with the intestinal microbiome. Microbiol Spectrum 5(6):BAD-0014-2016.

REFERENCES

1. **Euzeby JP.** 1997. List of bacterial names with standing in nomenclature: a folder available on the internet. *Int J Syst Bacteriol* **47:**590–592.
2. **Mundt JO.** 1963. Occurrence of enterococci in animals in a wild environment. *Appl Microbiol* **11:**136–140.
3. **MacCallum WG, Hastings TW.** 1899. A case of acute endocarditis caused by *Micrococcus zymogenes* (nov. spec.), with a description of the microorganism. *J Exp Med* **4:**521–534.
4. **Thiercelin ME, Jouhaud L.** 1899. Sur un diplocoque saprophyte de l'intestin susceptible de devenir pathogene. *CR Soc Biol* **5:**269–271.
5. **Schleifer KH, Kilpper-Bälz R.** 1984. Transfer of *Streptococcus faecalis* and *Streptococcus faecium* to the genus *Enterococcus* nom. Rev. as *Enterococcus faecalis* comb. nov. and *Enterococcus faecium* comb. nov. *Int J Syst Evol Microbiol* **34:**31–34.
6. **Sherman JM.** 1937. The streptococci. *Bacteriol Rev* **1:**3–97.
7. **Facklam RR.** 1973. Comparison of several laboratory media for presumptive identification of enterococci and group D streptococci. *Appl Microbiol* **26:**138–145.
8. **Facklam RR, Collins MD.** 1989. Identification of *Enterococcus* species isolated from human infections by a conventional test scheme. *J Clin Microbiol* **27:**731–734.
9. **Facklam RR, Carvalho MG, Teixeira LM.** 2002. History, taxonomy, biochemical characteristics, and antibiotic susceptibility testing of enterococci, p 1–54. *In* Gilmore MS, Clewell

DB, Courvalin P, Dunny GM, Murray BE, Rice LB (ed), *The Enterococci: Pathogenesis, Molecular Biology, and Antibiotic Resistance.* ASM Press, Washington, DC.

10. **Martin JD, Mundt JO.** 1972. Enterococci in insects. *Appl Microbiol* **24:**575–580.

11. **Thiercelin ME.** 1899. Morphologie et modes de reproduction de l'enterocoque. *C R Seances Soc Biol Fil* **11:**551–553.

12. **Andrewes FW, Horder TJ.** 1906. A study of streptococci pathogenic for man. *Lancet* **168:** 852–855.

13. **Orla-Jensen S.** 1919. The lactic acid bacteria. *Mem Acad R Soc Denmark Sci Ser* **85:**81–197.

14. **Gilmore MS, Lebreton F, van Schaik W.** 2013. Genomic transition of enterococci from gut commensals to leading causes of multidrug-resistant hospital infection in the antibiotic era. *Curr Opin Microbiol* **16:**10–16.

15. **Vollaard EJ, Clasener HA.** 1994. Colonization resistance. *Antimicrob Agents Chemother* **38:** 409–414.

16. **Sghir A, Gramet G, Suau A, Rochet V, Pochart P, Dore J.** 2000. Quantification of bacterial groups within human fecal flora by oligonucleotide probe hybridization. *Appl Environ Microbiol* **66:**2263–2266.

17. **Eckburg PB, Bik EM, Bernstein CN, Purdom E, Dethlefsen L, Sargent M, Gill SR, Nelson KE, Relman DA.** 2005. Diversity of the human intestinal microbial flora. *Science* **308:**1635–1638.

18. **Tendolkar PM, Baghdayan AS, Shankar N.** 2003. Pathogenic enterococci: new developments in the 21st century. *Cell Mol Life Sci* **60:**2622–2636.

19. **Lebreton F, Willems RJL, Gilmore MS.** 2014. Enterococcus diversity, origins in nature, and gut colonization. *In* Gilmore MS, et al. (ed), *Enterococci: From Commensals to Leading Causes of Drug Resistant Infection.* (Online.) Massachusetts Eye and Ear Infirmary, Boston, MA. https://www.ncbi.nlm.nih.gov/books/NBK190247/.

20. **Huycke MM, Sahm DF, Gilmore MS.** 1998. Multiple-drug resistant enterococci: the nature of the problem and an agenda for the future. *Emerg Infect Dis* **4:**239–249.

21. **Galloway-Peña JR, Nallapareddy SR, Arias CA, Eliopoulos GM, Murray BE.** 2009. Analysis of clonality and antibiotic resistance among early clinical isolates of *Enterococcus faecium* in the United States. *J Infect Dis* **200:** 1566–1573.

22. **Donskey CJ, Chowdhry TK, Hecker MT, Hoyen CK, Hanrahan JA, Hujer AM, Hutton-Thomas RA, Whalen CC, Bonomo RA, Rice LB.** 2000. Effect of antibiotic therapy on the density of vancomycin-resistant enterococci in the stool of colonized patients. *N Engl J Med* **343:**1925–1932.

23. **Ubeda C, Taur Y, Jenq RR, Equinda MJ, Son T, Samstein M, Viale A, Socci ND, van den Brink MR, Kamboj M, Pamer EG.** 2010. Vancomycin-resistant *Enterococcus* domination of intestinal microbiota is enabled by antibiotic treatment in mice and precedes bloodstream invasion in humans. *J Clin Invest* **120:**4332–4341.

24. **Taur Y, Xavier JB, Lipuma L, Ubeda C, Goldberg J, Gobourne A, Lee YJ, Dubin KA, Socci ND, Viale A, Perales MA, Jenq RR, van den Brink MR, Pamer EG.** 2012. Intestinal domination and the risk of bacteremia in patients undergoing allogeneic hematopoietic stem cell transplantation. *Clin Infect Dis* **55:** 905–914.

25. **Hidron AI, Edwards JR, Patel J, Horan TC, Sievert DM, Pollock DA, Fridkin SK, National Healthcare Safety Network Team, Participating National Healthcare Safety Network Facilities.** 2008. NHSN annual update: antimicrobial-resistant pathogens associated with healthcare-associated infections: annual summary of data reported to the National Healthcare Safety Network at the Centers for Disease Control and Prevention, 2006–2007. *Infect Control Hosp Epidemiol* **29:**996–1011.

26. **Jett BD, Huycke MM, Gilmore MS.** 1994. Virulence of enterococci. *Clin Microbiol Rev* **7:**462–478.

27. **CDC.** 2013. *Antibiotic resistance threats in the United States, 2013.* http://www.cdc.gov/drugresistance/threat-report-2013/.

28. **Agudelo Higuita NI, Huycke MM.** 2014. Enterococcal disease, epidemiology, and implications for treatment. *In* Gilmore MS, et al. (ed), *Enterococci: From Commensals to Leading Causes of Drug Resistant Infection.* (Online.) Massachusetts Eye and Ear Infirmary, Boston, MA. https://www.ncbi.nlm.nih.gov/books/NBK190429/.

29. **Weiner LM, Webb AK, Limbago B, Dudeck MA, Patel J, Kallen AJ, Edwards JR, Sievert DM.** 2016. Antimicrobial-resistant pathogens associated with healthcare-associated infections: summary of data reported to the National Healthcare Safety Network at the Centers for Disease Control and Prevention, 2011–2014. *Infect Control Hosp Epidemiol* **37:**1288–1301.

30. **Wisplinghoff H, Bischoff T, Tallent SM, Seifert H, Wenzel RP, Edmond MB.** 2004. Nosocomial bloodstream infections in US hospitals: analysis of 24,179 cases from a prospec-

tive nationwide surveillance study. *Clin Infect Dis* **39**:309–317.

31. **Berg RD.** 1999. Bacterial translocation from the gastrointestinal tract. *Adv Exp Med Biol* **473**:11–30.

32. **Kuehnert MJ, Jernigan JA, Pullen AL, Rimland D, Jarvis WR.** 1999. Association between mucositis severity and vancomycin-resistant enterococcal bloodstream infection in hospitalized cancer patients. *Infect Control Hosp Epidemiol* **20**:660–663.

33. **Roghmann MC, McCarter RJ Jr, Brewrink J, Cross AS, Morris JG Jr.** 1997. *Clostridium difficile* infection is a risk factor for bacteremia due to vancomycin-resistant enterococci (VRE) in VRE-colonized patients with acute leukemia. *Clin Infect Dis* **25**:1056–1059.

34. **Lautenbach E, Bilker WB, Brennan PJ.** 1999. Enterococcal bacteremia: risk factors for vancomycin resistance and predictors of mortality. *Infect Control Hosp Epidemiol* **20**:318–323.

35. **Murdoch DR, Corey GR, Hoen B, Miró JM, Fowler VG Jr, Bayer AS, Karchmer AW, Olaison L, Pappas PA, Moreillon P, Chambers ST, Chu VH, Falcó V, Holland DJ, Jones P, Klein JL, Raymond NJ, Read KM, Tripodi MF, Utili R, Wang A, Woods CW, Cabell CH, International Collaboration on Endocarditis-Prospective Cohort Study (ICE-PCS) Investigators.** 2009. Clinical presentation, etiology, and outcome of infective endocarditis in the 21st century: the International Collaboration on Endocarditis-Prospective Cohort Study. *Arch Intern Med* **169**:463–473.

36. **Anderson DJ, Murdoch DR, Sexton DJ, Reller LB, Stout JE, Cabell CH, Corey GR.** 2004. Risk factors for infective endocarditis in patients with enterococcal bacteremia: a case-control study. *Infection* **32**:72–77.

37. **Arias CA, Murray BE.** 2012. The rise of the *Enterococcus*: beyond vancomycin resistance. *Nat Rev Microbiol* **10**:266–278.

38. **Mandell GL, Kaye D, Levison ME, Hook EW.** 1970. Enterococcal endocarditis. An analysis of 38 patients observed at the New York Hospital-Cornell Medical Center. *Arch Intern Med* **125**:258–264.

39. **D'Agata EM, Green WK, Schulman G, Li H, Tang YW, Schaffner W.** 2001. Vancomycin-resistant enterococci among chronic hemodialysis patients: a prospective study of acquisition. *Clin Infect Dis* **32**:23–29.

40. **Boyce JM, Opal SM, Chow JW, Zervos MJ, Potter-Bynoe G, Sherman CB, Romulo RL, Fortna S, Medeiros AA.** 1994. Outbreak of multidrug-resistant *Enterococcus faecium* with transferable vanB class vancomycin resistance. *J Clin Microbiol* **32**:1148–1153.

41. **Boyce JM, Mermel LA, Zervos MJ, Rice LB, Potter-Bynoe G, Giorgio C, Medeiros AA.** 1995. Controlling vancomycin-resistant enterococci. *Infect Control Hosp Epidemiol* **16**:634–637.

42. **Handwerger S, Raucher B, Altarac D, Monka J, Marchione S, Singh KV, Murray BE, Wolff J, Walters B.** 1993. Nosocomial outbreak due to *Enterococcus faecium* highly resistant to vancomycin, penicillin, and gentamicin. *Clin Infect Dis* **16**:750–755.

43. **Cetinkaya Y, Falk P, Mayhall CG.** 2000. Vancomycin-resistant enterococci. *Clin Microbiol Rev* **13**:686–707.

44. **Howden BP, Holt KE, Lam MM, Seemann T, Ballard S, Coombs GW, Tong SY, Grayson ML, Johnson PD, Stinear TP.** 2013. Genomic insights to control the emergence of vancomycin-resistant enterococci. *MBio* **4**:e00412-13.

45. **Weinstein RA, Hota B.** 2004. Contamination, disinfection, and cross-colonization: are hospital surfaces reservoirs for nosocomial infection? *Clin Infect Dis* **39**:1182–1189.

46. **Drees M, Snydman DR, Schmid CH, Barefoot L, Hansjosten K, Vue PM, Cronin M, Nasraway SA, Golan Y.** 2008. Prior environmental contamination increases the risk of acquisition of vancomycin-resistant enterococci. *Clin Infect Dis* **46**:678–685.

47. **Austin DJ, Bonten MJ, Weinstein RA, Slaughter S, Anderson RM.** 1999. Vancomycin-resistant enterococci in intensive-care hospital settings: transmission dynamics, persistence, and the impact of infection control programs. *Proc Natl Acad Sci USA* **96**:6908–6913.

48. **Muto CA, Jernigan JA, Ostrowsky BE, Richet HM, Jarvis WR, Boyce JM, Farr BM, SHEA.** 2003. SHEA guideline for preventing nosocomial transmission of multidrug-resistant strains of *Staphylococcus aureus* and enterococcus. *Infect Control Hosp Epidemiol* **24**:362–386.

49. **Duckro AN, Blom DW, Lyle EA, Weinstein RA, Hayden MK.** 2005. Transfer of vancomycin-resistant enterococci via health care worker hands. *Arch Intern Med* **165**:302–307.

50. **Mayer RA, Geha RC, Helfand MS, Hoyen CK, Salata RA, Donskey CJ.** 2003. Role of fecal incontinence in contamination of the environment with vancomycin-resistant enterococci. *Am J Infect Control* **31**:221–225.

51. **Zervos MJ, Terpenning MS, Schaberg DR, Therasse PM, Medendorp SV, Kauffman CA.** 1987. High-level aminoglycoside-resistant enterococci. Colonization of nursing home and acute care hospital patients. *Arch Intern Med* **147**:1591–1594.

52. **Bonten MJ, Slaughter S, Ambergen AW, Hayden MK, van Voorhis J, Nathan C, Weinstein RA.** 1998. The role of "colonization pressure" in the spread of vancomycin-resistant enterococci: an important infection control variable. *Arch Intern Med* **158:**1127–1132.

53. **Tornieporth NG, Roberts RB, John J, Hafner A, Riley LW.** 1996. Risk factors associated with vancomycin-resistant *Enterococcus faecium* infection or colonization in 145 matched case patients and control patients. *Clin Infect Dis* **23:**767–772.

54. **Vergis EN, Hayden MK, Chow JW, Snydman DR, Zervos MJ, Linden PK, Wagener MM, Schmitt B, Muder RR.** 2001. Determinants of vancomycin resistance and mortality rates in enterococcal bacteremia: a prospective multicenter study. *Ann Intern Med* **135:**484–492.

55. **Jawetz E, Sonne M.** 1966. Penicillin-streptomycin treatment of enterococcal endocarditis. A re-evaluation. *N Engl J Med* **274:**710–715.

56. **Moellering RC Jr, Wennersten C, Weinberg AN.** 1971. Studies on antibiotic synergism against enterococci. I. Bacteriologic studies. *J Lab Clin Med* **77:**821–828.

57. **Murray BE.** 1990. The life and times of the *Enterococcus. Clin Microbiol Rev* **3:**46–65.

58. **Nigo M, Munita JM, Arias CA, Murray BE.** 2014. What's new in the treatment of enterococcal endocarditis? *Curr Infect Dis Rep* **16:**431.

59. **Munita JM, Arias CA, Murray BE.** 2013. Editorial commentary: *Enterococcus faecalis* infective endocarditis: is it time to abandon aminoglycosides? *Clin Infect Dis* **56:**1269–1272.

60. **Mainardi JL, Gutmann L, Acar JF, Goldstein FW.** 1995. Synergistic effect of amoxicillin and cefotaxime against *Enterococcus faecalis. Antimicrob Agents Chemother* **39:**1984–1987. (Erratum, **39:**2835.)

61. **Baddour LM, Wilson WR, Bayer AS, Fowler VG Jr, Tleyjeh IM, Rybak MJ, Barsic B, Lockhart PB, Gewitz MH, Levison ME, Bolger AF, Steckelberg JM, Baltimore RS, Fink AM, O'Gara P, Taubert KA, American Heart Association Committee on Rheumatic Fever, Endocarditis and Kawasaki Disease of the Council on Cardiovascular Disease in the Young, Council on Clinical Cardiology, Council on Cardiovascular Surgery and Anesthesia, and Stroke Council.** 2015. Infective endocarditis in adults: diagnosis, antimicrobial therapy, and management of complications: a scientific statement for healthcare professionals from the American Heart Association. *Circulation* **132:**1435–1486.

62. **O'Driscoll T, Crank CW.** 2015. Vancomycin-resistant enterococcal infections: epidemiology, clinical manifestations, and optimal management. *Infect Drug Resist* **8:**217–230.

63. **Treitman AN, Yarnold PR, Warren J, Noskin GA.** 2005. Emerging incidence of *Enterococcus faecium* among hospital isolates (1993 to 2002). *J Clin Microbiol* **43:**462–463.

64. **Top J, Willems R, Blok H, de Regt M, Jalink K, Troelstra A, Goorhuis B, Bonten M.** 2007. Ecological replacement of *Enterococcus faecalis* by multiresistant clonal complex 17 *Enterococcus faecium. Clin Microbiol Infect* **13:**316–319.

65. **Kristich CJ, Rice LB, Arias CA.** 2014. Enterococcal infection: treatment and antibiotic resistance. *In* Gilmore MS, et al. (ed), *Enterococci: From Commensals to Leading Causes of Drug Resistant Infection.* (Online.) Massachusetts Eye and Ear Infirmary, Boston, MA. http://www.ncbi.nlm.nih.gov/books/NBK190420/.

66. **Edelsberg J, Weycker D, Barron R, Li X, Wu H, Oster G, Badre S, Langeberg WJ, Weber DJ.** 2014. Prevalence of antibiotic resistance in US hospitals. *Diagn Microbiol Infect Dis* **78:**255–262.

67. **Leclercq R, Derlot E, Duval J, Courvalin P.** 1988. Plasmid-mediated resistance to vancomycin and teicoplanin in *Enterococcus faecium. N Engl J Med* **319:**157–161.

68. **Uttley AHC, George RC, Naidoo J, Woodford N, Johnson AP, Collins CH, Morrison D, Gilfillan AJ, Fitch LE, Heptonstall J.** 1989. High-level vancomycin-resistant enterococci causing hospital infections. *Epidemiol Infect* **103:**173–181.

69. **Carmeli Y, Eliopoulos GM, Samore MH.** 2002. Antecedent treatment with different antibiotic agents as a risk factor for vancomycin-resistant enterococcus. *Emerg Infect Dis* **8:**802–807.

70. **Currie BP, Lemos-Filho L.** 2004. Evidence for biliary excretion of vancomycin into stool during intravenous therapy: potential implications for rectal colonization with vancomycin-resistant enterococci. *Antimicrob Agents Chemother* **48:**4427–4429.

71. **Aarestrup FM.** 2000. Characterization of glycopeptide-resistant *Enterococcus faecium* (GRE) from broilers and pigs in Denmark: genetic evidence that persistence of GRE in pig herds is associated with coselection by resistance to macrolides. *J Clin Microbiol* **38:**2774–2777.

72. **Bates J.** 1997. Epidemiology of vancomycin-resistant enterococci in the community and the relevance of farm animals to human infection. *J Hosp Infect* **37:**89–101.

73. **Van Tyne D, Gilmore MS.** 2014. Friend turned foe: evolution of enterococcal virulence and antibiotic resistance. *Annu Rev Microbiol* **68:**337–356.

74. **Bager F, Aarestrup FM, Madsen M, Wegener HC.** 1999. Glycopeptide resistance in *Enterococcus faecium* from broilers and pigs following discontinued use of avoparcin. *Microb Drug Resist* **5:**53–56.

75. **Klare I, Badstübner D, Konstabel C, Böhme G, Claus H, Witte W.** 1999. Decreased incidence of VanA-type vancomycin-resistant enterococci isolated from poultry meat and from fecal samples of humans in the community after discontinuation of avoparcin usage in animal husbandry. *Microb Drug Resist* **5:**45–52.

76. **Hammerum AM.** 2012. Enterococci of animal origin and their significance for public health. *Clin Microbiol Infect* **18:**619–625.

77. **Werner G, Coque TM, Hammerum AM, Hope R, Hryniewicz W, Johnson A, Klare I, Kristinsson KG, Leclercq R, Lester CH, Lillie M, Novais C, Olsson-Liljequist B, Peixe LV, Sadowy E, Simonsen GS, Top J, Vuopio-Varkila J, Willems RJ, Witte W, Woodford N.** 2008. Emergence and spread of vancomycin resistance among enterococci in Europe. *Euro Surveill* **13:**19046. http://www.eurosurveillance.org/content/10.2807/ese.13.47.19046-en.

78. **Fontana R, Grossato A, Rossi L, Cheng YR, Satta G.** 1985. Transition from resistance to hypersusceptibility to beta-lactam antibiotics associated with loss of a low-affinity penicillin-binding protein in a *Streptococcus faecium* mutant highly resistant to penicillin. *Antimicrob Agents Chemother* **28:**678–683.

79. **Williamson R, le Bouguénec C, Gutmann L, Horaud T.** 1985. One or two low affinity penicillin-binding proteins may be responsible for the range of susceptibility of *Enterococcus faecium* to benzylpenicillin. *J Gen Microbiol* **131:**1933–1940.

80. **Fontana R, Cerini R, Longoni P, Grossato A, Canepari P.** 1983. Identification of a streptococcal penicillin-binding protein that reacts very slowly with penicillin. *J Bacteriol* **155:**1343–1350.

81. **Rybkine T, Mainardi JL, Sougakoff W, Collatz E, Gutmann L.** 1998. Penicillin-binding protein 5 sequence alterations in clinical isolates of *Enterococcus faecium* with different levels of β-lactam resistance. *J Infect Dis* **178:**159–163.

82. **Zorzi W, Zhou XY, Dardenne O, Lamotte J, Raze D, Pierre J, Gutmann L, Coyette J.** 1996. Structure of the low-affinity penicillin-binding protein 5 PBP5fm in wild-type and highly penicillin-resistant strains of *Enterococcus faecium*. *J Bacteriol* **178:**4948–4957.

83. **Rice LB, Bellais S, Carias LL, Hutton-Thomas R, Bonomo RA, Caspers P, Page MGP, Gutmann L.** 2004. Impact of specific *pbp5* mutations on expression of beta-lactam resistance in *Enterococcus faecium*. *Antimicrob Agents Chemother* **48:**3028–3032.

84. **Rice LB, Carias LL, Rudin S, Lakticová V, Wood A, Hutton-Thomas R.** 2005. *Enterococcus faecium* low-affinity pbp5 is a transferable determinant. *Antimicrob Agents Chemother* **49:**5007–5012.

85. **Galloway-Peña JR, Rice LB, Murray BE.** 2011. Analysis of PBP5 of early U.S. isolates of *Enterococcus faecium*: sequence variation alone does not explain increasing ampicillin resistance over time. *Antimicrob Agents Chemother* **55:**3272–3277.

86. **Grayson ML, Eliopoulos GM, Wennersten CB, Ruoff KL, De Girolami PC, Ferraro MJ, Moellering RC Jr.** 1991. Increasing resistance to beta-lactam antibiotics among clinical isolates of *Enterococcus faecium*: a 22-year review at one institution. *Antimicrob Agents Chemother* **35:**2180–2184.

87. **Arthur M, Courvalin P.** 1993. Genetics and mechanisms of glycopeptide resistance in enterococci. *Antimicrob Agents Chemother* **37:**1563–1571.

88. **Courvalin P.** 2006. Vancomycin resistance in Gram-positive cocci. *Clin Infect Dis* **42**(Suppl 1):S25–S34.

89. **Willems RJ, Top J, van Santen M, Robinson DA, Coque TM, Baquero F, Grundmann H, Bonten MJ.** 2005. Global spread of vancomycin-resistant *Enterococcus faecium* from distinct nosocomial genetic complex. *Emerg Infect Dis* **11:**821–828.

90. **Alborn WE Jr, Allen NE, Preston DA.** 1991. Daptomycin disrupts membrane potential in growing *Staphylococcus aureus*. *Antimicrob Agents Chemother* **35:**2282–2287.

91. **Silverman JA, Perlmutter NG, Shapiro HM.** 2003. Correlation of daptomycin bactericidal activity and membrane depolarization in *Staphylococcus aureus*. *Antimicrob Agents Chemother* **47:**2538–2544.

92. **Arias CA, Panesso D, McGrath DM, Qin X, Mojica MF, Miller C, Diaz L, Tran TT, Rincon S, Barbu EM, Reyes J, Roh JH, Lobos E, Sodergren E, Pasqualini R, Arap W, Quinn JP, Shamoo Y, Murray BE, Weinstock GM.** 2011. Genetic basis for *in vivo* daptomycin resistance in enterococci. *N Engl J Med* **365:**892–900.

93. **Palmer KL, Daniel A, Hardy C, Silverman J, Gilmore MS.** 2011. Genetic basis for daptomycin resistance in enterococci. *Antimicrob Agents Chemother* **55:**3345–3356.

94. **Lellek H, Franke GC, Ruckert C, Wolters M, Wolschke C, Christner M, Büttner H, Alawi M, Kröger N, Rohde H.** 2015. Emergence of

daptomycin non-susceptibility in colonizing vancomycin-resistant *Enterococcus faecium* isolates during daptomycin therapy. *Int J Med Microbiol* **305**:902–909.

95. **Paulsen IT, Banerjei L, Myers GSA, Nelson KER, Seshadri R, Read TD, Fouts DE, Eisen JA, Gill SR, Heidelberg JF, Tettelin H, Dodson RJ, Umayam L, Brinkac L, Beanan M, Daugherty S, DeBoy RT, Durkin S, Kolonay J, Madupu R, Nelson W, Vamathevan J, Tran B, Upton J, Hansen T, Shetty J, Khouri H, Utterback T, Radune D, Ketchum KA, Dougherty BA, Fraser CM.** 2003. Role of mobile DNA in the evolution of vancomycin-resistant *Enterococcus faecalis*. *Science* **299**:2071–2074.

96. **Zheng B, Tomita H, Inoue T, Ike Y.** 2009. Isolation of VanB-type *Enterococcus faecalis* strains from nosocomial infections: first report of the isolation and identification of the pheromone-responsive plasmids pMG2200, encoding VanB-type vancomycin resistance and a Bac41-type bacteriocin, and pMG2201, encoding erythromycin resistance and cytolysin (Hly/Bac). *Antimicrob Agents Chemother* **53**:735–747.

97. **Heaton MP, Discotto LF, Pucci MJ, Handwerger S.** 1996. Mobilization of vancomycin resistance by transposon-mediated fusion of a VanA plasmid with an *Enterococcus faecium* sex pheromone-response plasmid. *Gene* **171**:9–17.

98. **Manson JM, Hancock LE, Gilmore MS.** 2010. Mechanism of chromosomal transfer of *Enterococcus faecalis* pathogenicity island, capsule, antimicrobial resistance, and other traits. *Proc Natl Acad Sci USA* **107**:12269–12274.

99. **Arthur M, Molinas C, Depardieu F, Courvalin P.** 1993. Characterization of Tn1546, a Tn3-related transposon conferring glycopeptide resistance by synthesis of depsipeptide peptidoglycan precursors in *Enterococcus faecium* BM4147. *J Bacteriol* **175**:117–127.

100. **Carias LL, Rudin SD, Donskey CJ, Rice LB.** 1998. Genetic linkage and cotransfer of a novel, vanB-containing transposon (Tn5382) and a low-affinity penicillin-binding protein 5 gene in a clinical vancomycin-resistant *Enterococcus faecium* isolate. *J Bacteriol* **180**:4426–4434.

101. **Dahl KH, Lundblad EW, Rokenes TP, Olsvik O, Sundsfjord A.** 2000. Genetic linkage of the vanB2 gene cluster to Tn5382 in vancomycin-resistant enterococci and characterization of two novel insertion sequences. *Microbiology* **146**:1469–1479.

102. **Garnier F, Taourit S, Glaser P, Courvalin P, Galimand M.** 2000. Characterization of transposon Tn1549, conferring VanB-type resistance in *Enterococcus* spp. *Microbiology* **146**:1481–1489.

103. **Rice LB, Carias LL, Marshall S, Rudin SD, Hutton-Thomas R.** 2005. Tn5386, a novel Tn916-like mobile element in *Enterococcus faecium* D344R that interacts with Tn916 to yield a large genomic deletion. *J Bacteriol* **187**:6668–6677.

104. **Palmer KL, et al.** 2014. Enterococcal genomics. *In* Gilmore MS, et al. (ed), *Enterococci: From Commensals to Leading Causes of Drug Resistant Infection*. (Online.) Massachusetts Eye and Ear Infirmary, Boston, MA. https://www.ncbi.nlm.nih.gov/books/NBK190425/.

105. **van Schaik W, Willems RJL.** 2010. Genome-based insights into the evolution of enterococci. *Clin Microbiol Infect* **16**:527–532.

106. **Qin X, Galloway-Peña JR, Sillanpaa J, Roh JH, Nallapareddy SR, Chowdhury S, Bourgogne A, Choudhury T, Muzny DM, Buhay CJ, Ding Y, Dugan-Rocha S, Liu W, Kovar C, Sodergren E, Highlander S, Petrosino JF, Worley KC, Gibbs RA, Weinstock GM, Murray BE.** 2012. Complete genome sequence of *Enterococcus faecium* strain TX16 and comparative genomic analysis of *Enterococcus faecium* genomes. *BMC Microbiol* **12**:135.

107. **Palmer KL, Godfrey P, Griggs A, Kos VN, Zucker J, Desjardins C, Cerqueira G, Gevers D, Walker S, Wortman J, Feldgarden M, Haas B, Birren B, Gilmore MS.** 2012. Comparative genomics of enterococci: variation in *Enterococcus faecalis*, clade structure in *E. faecium*, and defining characteristics of *E. gallinarum* and *E. casseliflavus*. *MBio* **3**:e00318-11.

108. **Palmer KL, Gilmore MS.** 2010. Multidrug-resistant enterococci lack CRISPR-cas. *MBio* **1**:e00227-10.

109. **van Schaik W, Top J, Riley DR, Boekhorst J, Vrijenhoek JE, Schapendonk CM, Hendrickx AP, Nijman IJ, Bonten MJ, Tettelin H, Willems RJ.** 2010. Pyrosequencing-based comparative genome analysis of the nosocomial pathogen *Enterococcus faecium* and identification of a large transferable pathogenicity island. *BMC Genomics* **11**:239.

110. **Leavis HL, Willems RJL, van Wamel WJB, Schuren FH, Caspers MPM, Bonten MJM.** 2007. Insertion sequence-driven diversification creates a globally dispersed emerging multiresistant subspecies of *E. faecium*. *PLoS Pathog* **3**:e7.

111. **Willems RJ, van Schaik W.** 2009. Transition of *Enterococcus faecium* from commensal organism to nosocomial pathogen. *Future Microbiol* **4**:1125–1135.

112. **Werner G, Fleige C, Geringer U, van Schaik W, Klare I, Witte W.** 2011. IS element IS16 as a molecular screening tool to identify hospital-associated strains of *Enterococcus faecium*. *BMC Infect Dis* **11**:80.

113. **Ruiz-Garbajosa P, Bonten MJ, Robinson DA, Top J, Nallapareddy SR, Torres C, Coque TM, Cantón R, Baquero F, Murray BE, del Campo R, Willems RJ.** 2006. Multilocus sequence typing scheme for *Enterococcus faecalis* reveals hospital-adapted genetic complexes in a background of high rates of recombination. *J Clin Microbiol* **44**:2220–2228.

114. **Bourgogne A, Garsin DA, Qin X, Singh KV, Sillanpaa J, Yerrapragada S, Ding Y, Dugan-Rocha S, Buhay C, Shen H, Chen G, Williams G, Muzny D, Maadani A, Fox KA, Gioia J, Chen L, Shang Y, Arias CA, Nallapareddy SR, Zhao M, Prakash VP, Chowdhury S, Jiang H, Gibbs RA, Murray BE, Highlander SK, Weinstock GM.** 2008. Large scale variation in *Enterococcus faecalis* illustrated by the genome analysis of strain OG1RF. *Genome Biol* **9**: R110.

115. **Galloway-Peña J, Roh JH, Latorre M, Qin X, Murray BE.** 2012. Genomic and SNP analyses demonstrate a distant separation of the hospital and community-associated clades of *Enterococcus faecium*. *PLoS One* **7**:e30187.

116. **Willems RJL, Top J, van Schaik W, Leavis H, Bonten M, Sirén J, Hanage WP, Corander J.** 2012. Restricted gene flow among hospital subpopulations of *Enterococcus faecium*. *MBio* **3**:e00151-12.

117. **Lebreton F, van Schaik W, McGuire AM, Godfrey P, Griggs A, Mazumdar V, Corander J, Cheng L, Saif S, Young S, Zeng Q, Wortman J, Birren B, Willems RJ, Earl AM, Gilmore MS.** 2013. Emergence of epidemic multidrug-resistant *Enterococcus faecium* from animal and commensal strains. *MBio* **4**:e00534-13.

118. **de Regt MJA, van Schaik W, van Luit-Asbroek M, Dekker HAT, van Duijkeren E, Koning CJM, Bonten MJM, Willems RJL.** 2012. Hospital and community ampicillin-resistant *Enterococcus faecium* are evolutionarily closely linked but have diversified through niche adaptation. *PLoS One* **7**:e30319.

119. **Woodford N, Adebiyi AM, Palepou MF, Cookson BD.** 1998. Diversity of VanA glycopeptide resistance elements in enterococci from humans and nonhuman sources. *Antimicrob Agents Chemother* **42**:502–508.

120. **Willems RJ, Top J, van den Braak N, van Belkum A, Mevius DJ, Hendriks G, van Santen-Verheuvel M, van Embden JD.** 1999. Molecular diversity and evolutionary relationships of Tn1546-like elements in enterococci from humans and animals. *Antimicrob Agents Chemother* **43**:483–491.

121. **Lester CH, Frimodt-Møller N, Sørensen TL, Monnet DL, Hammerum AM.** 2006. *In vivo* transfer of the *vanA* resistance gene from an *Enterococcus faecium* isolate of animal origin to an *E. faecium* isolate of human origin in the intestines of human volunteers. *Antimicrob Agents Chemother* **50**:596–599.

122. **Kühn I, Iversen A, Finn M, Greko C, Burman LG, Blanch AR, Vilanova X, Manero A, Taylor H, Caplin J, Domínguez L, Herrero IA, Moreno MA, Möllby R.** 2005. Occurrence and relatedness of vancomycin-resistant enterococci in animals, humans, and the environment in different European regions. *Appl Environ Microbiol* **71**:5383–5390.

123. **Maiden MC, Bygraves JA, Feil E, Morelli G, Russell JE, Urwin R, Zhang Q, Zhou J, Zurth K, Caugant DA, Feavers IM, Achtman M, Spratt BG.** 1998. Multilocus sequence typing: a portable approach to the identification of clones within populations of pathogenic microorganisms. *Proc Natl Acad Sci USA* **95**:3140–3145.

124. **Homan WL, Tribe D, Poznanski S, Li M, Hogg G, Spalburg E, Van Embden JDA, Willems RJL.** 2002. Multilocus sequence typing scheme for *Enterococcus faecium*. *J Clin Microbiol* **40**: 1963–1971.

125. **Nallapareddy SR, Wenxiang H, Weinstock GM, Murray BE.** 2005. Molecular characterization of a widespread, pathogenic, and antibiotic resistance-receptive *Enterococcus faecalis* lineage and dissemination of its putative pathogenicity island. *J Bacteriol* **187**:5709–5718.

126. **Leavis HL, Bonten MJM, Willems RJL.** 2006. Identification of high-risk enterococcal clonal complexes: global dispersion and antibiotic resistance. *Curr Opin Microbiol* **9**:454–460.

127. **McBride SM, Fischetti VA, Leblanc DJ, Moellering RC Jr, Gilmore MS.** 2007. Genetic diversity among *Enterococcus faecalis*. *PLoS One* **2**:e582.

128. **Turner KME, Hanage WP, Fraser C, Connor TR, Spratt BG.** 2007. Assessing the reliability of eBURST using simulated populations with known ancestry. *BMC Microbiol* **7**:30.

129. **Devriese LA, Van de Kerckhove A, Kilpper-Bälz R, Schleifer KH.** 1987. Characterization and identification of *Enterococcus* species isolated from the intestines of animals. *Int J Syst Evol Microbiol* **37**:257–259.

130. **Willems RJL, Top J, van Den Braak N, van Belkum A, Endtz H, Mevius D, Stobberingh

E, van Den Bogaard A, van Embden JD. 2000. Host specificity of vancomycin-resistant *Enterococcus faecium. J Infect Dis* **182:**816–823.

131. **Ostrolenk M, Kramer N, Cleverdon RC.** 1947. Comparative studies of enterococci and *Escherichia coli* as indices of pollution. *J Bacteriol* **53:**197–203.

132. **Harwood VJ, Whitlock J, Withington V.** 2000. Classification of antibiotic resistance patterns of indicator bacteria by discriminant analysis: use in predicting the source of fecal contamination in subtropical waters. *Appl Environ Microbiol* **66:**3698–3704.

133. **Boehm AB, Sassoubre LM.** 2014. Enterococci as indicators of environmental fecal contamination. *In* Gilmore MS, et al. (ed), *Enterococci: From Commensals to Leading Causes of Drug Resistant Infection.* (Online.) Massachusetts Eye and Ear Infirmary, Boston, MA. https://www.ncbi.nlm.nih.gov/books/NBK190421/.

134. **Sinclair JL, Alexander M.** 1984. Role of resistance to starvation in bacterial survival in sewage and lake water. *Appl Environ Microbiol* **48:**410–415.

135. **Leclercq R, Oberlé K, Galopin S, Cattoir V, Budzinski H, Petit F.** 2013. Changes in enterococcal populations and related antibiotic resistance along a medical center-wastewater treatment plant-river continuum. *Appl Environ Microbiol* **79:**2428–2434.

136. **Van Embden JD, Engel HW, Van Klingeren B.** 1977. Drug resistance in group D streptococci of clinical and nonclinical origin: prevalence, transferability, and plasmid properties. *Antimicrob Agents Chemother* **11:**925–932.

137. **Wade TJ, Pai N, Eisenberg JNS, Colford JM Jr.** 2003. Do U.S. Environmental Protection Agency water quality guidelines for recreational waters prevent gastrointestinal illness? A systematic review and meta-analysis. *Environ Health Perspect* **111:**1102–1109.

138. **Chenoweth C, Schaberg D.** 1990. The epidemiology of enterococci. *Eur J Clin Microbiol Infect Dis* **9:**80–89.

139. **Noble CJ.** 1978. Carriage of group D streptococci in the human bowel. *J Clin Pathol* **31:**1182–1186.

140. **Layton BA, Walters SP, Lam LH, Boehm AB.** 2010. Enterococcus species distribution among human and animal hosts using multiplex PCR. *J Appl Microbiol* **109:**539–547.

141. **Hooper LV, Midtvedt T, Gordon JI.** 2002. How host-microbial interactions shape the nutrient environment of the mammalian intestine. *Annu Rev Nutr* **22:**283–307.

142. **Littman DR, Pamer EG.** 2011. Role of the commensal microbiota in normal and pathogenic host immune responses. *Cell Host Microbe* **10:**311–323.

143. **Are A, Aronsson L, Wang S, Greicius G, Lee YK, Gustafsson JA, Pettersson S, Arulampalam V.** 2008. Enterococcus faecalis from newborn babies regulate endogenous PPARγ activity and IL-10 levels in colonic epithelial cells. *Proc Natl Acad Sci USA* **105:**1943–1948.

144. **Wang S, Ng LH, Chow WL, Lee YK.** 2008. Infant intestinal *Enterococcus faecalis* downregulates inflammatory responses in human intestinal cell lines. *World J Gastroenterol* **14:**1067–1076.

145. **Chen CC, Kong MS, Lai MW, Chao HC, Chang KW, Chen SY, Huang YC, Chiu CH, Li WC, Lin PY, Chen CJ, Lin TY.** 2010. Probiotics have clinical, microbiologic, and immunologic efficacy in acute infectious diarrhea. *Pediatr Infect Dis J* **29:**135–138.

146. **Turnbaugh PJ, Ley RE, Hamady M, Fraser-Liggett CM, Knight R, Gordon JI.** 2007. The human microbiome project. *Nature* **449:**804–810.

147. **Huttenhower C, et al, Human Microbiome Project Consortium.** 2012. Structure, function and diversity of the healthy human microbiome. *Nature* **486:**207–214.

148. **Arumugam M, et al, MetaHIT Consortium.** 2011. Enterotypes of the human gut microbiome. *Nature* **473:**174–180.

149. **Koren O, Knights D, Gonzalez A, Waldron L, Segata N, Knight R, Huttenhower C, Ley RE.** 2013. A guide to enterotypes across the human body: meta analysis of microbial community structures in human microbiome datasets. *PLOS Comput Biol* **9:**e1002863.

150. **Ding T, Schloss PD.** 2014. Dynamics and associations of microbial community types across the human body. *Nature* **509:**357–360.

151. **Donskey CJ, Hanrahan JA, Hutton RA, Rice LB.** 1999. Effect of parenteral antibiotic administration on persistence of vancomycin-resistant *Enterococcus faecium* in the mouse gastrointestinal tract. *J Infect Dis* **180:**384–390.

152. **Sjölund M, Wreiber K, Andersson DI, Blaser MJ, Engstrand L.** 2003. Long-term persistence of resistant *Enterococcus* species after antibiotics to eradicate *Helicobacter pylori. Ann Intern Med* **139:**483–487.

153. **van der Waaij D, Berghuis-de Vries JM, Lekkerkerk-van der Wees.** 1971. Colonization resistance of the digestive tract in conventional and antibiotic-treated mice. *J Hyg (Lond)* **69:**405–411.

154. **Freter R.** 1955. The fatal enteric cholera infection in the guinea pig, achieved by inhibition of normal enteric flora. *J Infect Dis* **97:**57–65.

155. **Bohnhoff M, Miller CP, Martin WR.** 1964. Resistance of the mouse's intestinal tract to experimental *Salmonella* infection. *J Exp Med* **120:**817–828.

156. **Ubeda C, Bucci V, Caballero S, Djukovic A, Toussaint NC, Equinda M, Lipuma L, Ling L, Gobourne A, No D, Taur Y, Jenq RR, van den Brink MR, Xavier JB, Pamer EG.** 2013. Intestinal microbiota containing *Barnesiella* species cures vancomycin-resistant *Enterococcus faecium* colonization. *Infect Immun* **81:**965–973.

157. **Caballero S, Kim S, Carter RA, Leiner IM, Sušac B, Miller L, Kim GJ, Ling L, Pamer EG.** 2017. Cooperating commensals restore colonization resistance to vancomycin-resistant *Enterococcus faecium*. *Cell Host Microbe* **21:**592–602.e4.

158. **Cash HL, Whitham CV, Behrendt CL, Hooper LV.** 2006. Symbiotic bacteria direct expression of an intestinal bactericidal lectin. *Science* **313:**1126–1130.

159. **Brandl K, Plitas G, Schnabl B, DeMatteo RP, Pamer EG.** 2007. MyD88-mediated signals induce the bactericidal lectin RegIII γ and protect mice against intestinal *Listeria monocytogenes* infection. *J Exp Med* **204:**1891–1900.

160. **Vaishnava S, Behrendt CL, Ismail AS, Eckmann L, Hooper LV.** 2008. Paneth cells directly sense gut commensals and maintain homeostasis at the intestinal host-microbial interface. *Proc Natl Acad Sci USA* **105:**20858–20863.

161. **Mukherjee S, Zheng H, Derebe MG, Callenberg KM, Partch CL, Rollins D, Propheter DC, Rizo J, Grabe M, Jiang QX, Hooper LV.** 2014. Antibacterial membrane attack by a pore-forming intestinal C-type lectin. *Nature* **505:**103–107.

162. **Brandl K, Plitas G, Mihu CN, Ubeda C, Jia T, Fleisher M, Schnabl B, DeMatteo RP, Pamer EG.** 2008. Vancomycin-resistant enterococci exploit antibiotic-induced innate immune deficits. *Nature* **455:**804–807.

163. **Kinnebrew MA, Ubeda C, Zenewicz LA, Smith N, Flavell RA, Pamer EG.** 2010. Bacterial flagellin stimulates Toll-like receptor 5-dependent defense against vancomycin-resistant *Enterococcus* infection. *J Infect Dis* **201:**534–543.

164. **Godl K, Johansson MEV, Lidell ME, Mörgelin M, Karlsson H, Olson FJ, Gum JR Jr, Kim YS, Hansson GC.** 2002. The N terminus of the MUC2 mucin forms trimers that are held together within a trypsin-resistant core fragment. *J Biol Chem* **277:**47248–47256.

165. **Donskey CJ.** 2004. The role of the intestinal tract as a reservoir and source for transmission of nosocomial pathogens. *Clin Infect Dis* **39:**219–226.

166. **Johansson ME, Jakobsson HE, Holmén-Larsson J, Schütte A, Ermund A, Rodríguez-Piñeiro AM, Arike L, Wising C, Svensson F, Bäckhed F, Hansson GC.** 2015. Normalization of host intestinal mucus layers requires long-term microbial colonization. *Cell Host Microbe* **18:**582–592.

167. **Petersson J, Schreiber O, Hansson GC, Gendler SJ, Velcich A, Lundberg JO, Roos S, Holm L, Phillipson M.** 2011. Importance and regulation of the colonic mucus barrier in a mouse model of colitis. *Am J Physiol Gastrointest Liver Physiol* **300:**G327–G333.

168. **Frantz AL, Rogier EW, Weber CR, Shen L, Cohen DA, Fenton LA, Bruno MEC, Kaetzel CS.** 2012. Targeted deletion of MyD88 in intestinal epithelial cells results in compromised antibacterial immunity associated with downregulation of polymeric immunoglobulin receptor, mucin-2, and antibacterial peptides. *Mucosal Immunol* **5:**501–512.

169. **Wlodarska M, Willing B, Keeney KM, Menendez A, Bergstrom KS, Gill N, Russell SL, Vallance BA, Finlay BB.** 2011. Antibiotic treatment alters the colonic mucus layer and predisposes the host to exacerbated *Citrobacter rodentium*-induced colitis. *Infect Immun* **79:**1536–1545.

170. **Johansson MEV, Phillipson M, Petersson J, Velcich A, Holm L, Hansson GC.** 2008. The inner of the two Muc2 mucin-dependent mucus layers in colon is devoid of bacteria. *Proc Natl Acad Sci USA* **105:**15064–15069.

171. **Vaishnava S, Yamamoto M, Severson KM, Ruhn KA, Yu X, Koren O, Ley R, Wakeland EK, Hooper LV.** 2011. The antibacterial lectin RegIIIgamma promotes the spatial segregation of microbiota and host in the intestine. *Science* **334:**255–258.

172. **Loonen LMP, Stolte EH, Jaklofsky MTJ, Meijerink M, Dekker J, van Baarlen P, Wells JM.** 2014. REG3γ-deficient mice have altered mucus distribution and increased mucosal inflammatory responses to the microbiota and enteric pathogens in the ileum. *Mucosal Immunol* **7:**939–947.

173. **Caballero S, Carter R, Ke X, Sušac B, Leiner IM, Kim GJ, Miller L, Ling L, Manova K, Pamer EG.** 2015. Distinct but spatially overlapping intestinal niches for vancomycin-resistant *Enterococcus faecium* and carbapenem-resistant *Klebsiella pneumoniae*. *PLoS Pathog* **11:**e1005132.

174. **Borrero J, Chen Y, Dunny GM, Kaznessis YN.** 2015. Modified lactic acid bacteria detect and inhibit multiresistant enterococci. *ACS Synth Biol* **4:**299–306.

175. **Millette M, Cornut G, Dupont C, Shareck F, Archambault D, Lacroix M.** 2008. Capacity

of human nisin- and pediocin-producing lactic acid bacteria to reduce intestinal colonization by vancomycin-resistant enterococci. *Appl Environ Microbiol* **74:**1997–2003.

176. **Weisser M, Oostdijk EA, Willems RJL, Bonten MJM, Frei R, Elzi L, Halter J, Widmer AF, Top J.** 2012. Dynamics of ampicillin-resistant *Enterococcus faecium* clones colonizing hospitalized patients: data from a prospective observational study. *BMC Infect Dis* **12:**68.

177. **Montealegre MC, Singh KV, Murray BE.** 2016. Gastrointestinal tract colonization dynamics by different *Enterococcus faecium* clades. *J Infect Dis* **213:**1914–1922.

178. **Kommineni S, Bretl DJ, Lam V, Chakraborty R, Hayward M, Simpson P, Cao Y, Bousounis P, Kristich CJ, Salzman NH.** 2015. Bacteriocin production augments niche competition by enterococci in the mammalian gastrointestinal tract. *Nature* **526:**719–722.

179. **Gilmore MS, Rauch M, Ramsey MM, Himes PR, Varahan S, Manson JM, Lebreton F, Hancock LE.** 2015. Pheromone killing of multidrug-resistant *Enterococcus faecalis* V583 by native commensal strains. *Proc Natl Acad Sci USA* **112:**7273–7278.

180. **Duerkop BA, Clements CV, Rollins D, Rodrigues JLM, Hooper LV.** 2012. A composite bacteriophage alters colonization by an intestinal commensal bacterium. *Proc Natl Acad Sci USA* **109:**17621–17626.

181. **Biswas B, Adhya S, Washart P, Paul B, Trostel AN, Powell B, Carlton R, Merril CR.** 2002. Bacteriophage therapy rescues mice bacteremic from a clinical isolate of vancomycin-resistant *Enterococcus faecium. Infect Immun* **70:**204–210.

182. **Franz CM, Huch M, Abriouel H, Holzapfel W, Gálvez A.** 2011. Enterococci as probiotics and their implications in food safety. *Int J Food Microbiol* **151:**125–140.

183. **Domann E, Hain T, Ghai R, Billion A, Kuenne C, Zimmermann K, Chakraborty T.** 2007. Comparative genomic analysis for the presence of potential enterococcal virulence factors in the probiotic *Enterococcus faecalis* strain Symbioflor 1. *Int J Med Microbiol* **297:**533–539.

184. **Allen SJ, Martinez EG, Gregorio GV, Dans LF.** 2010. Probiotics for treating acute infectious diarrhoea. *Cochrane Database Syst Rev* (11):CD003048.

185. **Bellomo G, Mangiagle A, Nicastro L, Frigerio G.** 1980. A controlled double-blind study of SF68 strain as a new biological preparation for the treatment of diarrhoea in pediatrics. *Curr Ther Res* **28:**927–934.

186. **Buydens P, Debeuckelaere S.** 1996. Efficacy of SF 68 in the treatment of acute diarrhea. A placebo-controlled trial. *Scand J Gastroenterol* **31:**887–891.

187. **van Nood E, Vrieze A, Nieuwdorp M, Fuentes S, Zoetendal EG, de Vos WM, Visser CE, Kuijper EJ, Bartelsman JF, Tijssen JG, Speelman P, Dijkgraaf MG, Keller JJ.** 2013. Duodenal infusion of donor feces for recurrent *Clostridium difficile. N Engl J Med* **368:**407–415.

188. **Dubberke ER, Mullane KM, Gerding DN, Lee CH, Louie TJ, Guthertz H, Jones C.** 2016. Clearance of vancomycin-resistant *Enterococcus* concomitant with administration of a microbiota-based drug targeted at recurrent *Clostridium difficile* infection. *Open Forum Infect Dis* **3:**ofw133.

189. **Lahti L, Salojärvi J, Salonen A, Scheffer M, de Vos WM.** 2014. Tipping elements in the human intestinal ecosystem. *Nat Commun* **5:**4344.

190. **Buffie CG, Bucci V, Stein RR, McKenney PT, Ling L, Gobourne A, No D, Liu H, Kinnebrew M, Viale A, Littmann E, van den Brink MRM, Jenq RR, Taur Y, Sander C, Cross JR, Toussaint NC, Xavier JB, Pamer EG.** 2015. Precision microbiome reconstitution restores bile acid mediated resistance to *Clostridium difficile. Nature* **517:**205–208.

191. **Manley KJ, Fraenkel MB, Mayall BC, Power DA.** 2007. Probiotic treatment of vancomycin-resistant enterococci: a randomised controlled trial. *Med J Aust* **186:**454–457.

192. **Szachta P, Ignyś I, Cichy W.** 2011. An evaluation of the ability of the probiotic strain *Lactobacillus rhamnosus* GG to eliminate the gastrointestinal carrier state of vancomycin-resistant enterococci in colonized children. *J Clin Gastroenterol* **45:**872–877.

193. **Vidal M, Forestier C, Charbonnel N, Henard S, Rabaud C, Lesens O.** 2010. Probiotics and intestinal colonization by vancomycin-resistant enterococci in mice and humans. *J Clin Microbiol* **48:**2595–2598.

194. **Doron S, Hibberd PL, Goldin B, Thorpe C, McDermott L, Snydman DR.** 2015. Effect of *Lactobacillus rhamnosus* GG administration on vancomycin-resistant enterococcus colonization in adults with comorbidities. *Antimicrob Agents Chemother* **59:**4593–4599.

195. **de Regt MJA, Willems RJL, Hené RJ, Siersema PD, Verhaar HJJ, Hopmans TEM, Bonten MJM.** 2010. Effects of probiotics on acquisition and spread of multiresistant enterococci. *Antimicrob Agents Chemother* **54:**2801–2805.

196. **Stein RR, Bucci V, Toussaint NC, Buffie CG, Rätsch G, Pamer EG, Sander C, Xavier JB.** 2013. Ecological modeling from time-series inference: insight into dynamics and stability

of intestinal microbiota. *PLOS Comput Biol* **9:**
e1003388.

197. **Khanna S, Pardi DS, Kelly CR, Kraft CS,
Dhere T, Henn MR, Lombardo MJ, Vulic M,
Ohsumi T, Winkler J, Pindar C, McGovern
BH, Pomerantz RJ, Aunins JG, Cook DN,
Hohmann EL.** 2016. A novel microbiome
therapeutic increases gut microbial diversity
and prevents recurrent *Clostridium difficile*
infection. *J Infect Dis* **214:**173–181.

198. **Ratner M.** 2016. Seres's pioneering microbiome drug fails mid-stage trial. *Nat Biotechnol* **34:**1004–1005.

199. **Pamer EG.** 2014. Fecal microbiota transplantation: effectiveness, complexities, and linger-
ing concerns. *Mucosal Immunol* **7:**210–214.

200. **Stiefel U, Nerandzic MM, Pultz MJ, Donskey
CJ.** 2014. Gastrointestinal colonization with
a cephalosporinase-producing *Bacteroides*
species preserves colonization resistance
against vancomycin-resistant *Enterococcus* and
Clostridium difficile in cephalosporin-treated
mice. *Antimicrob Agents Chemother* **58:**4535–
4542.

201. **Zeevi D, Korem T, Zmora N, Israeli D, Rothschild
D, Weinberger A, Ben-Yacov O, Lador D, Avnit-
Sagi T, Lotan-Pompan M, Suez J, Mahdi
JA, Matot E, Malka G, Kosower N, Rein M,
Zilberman-Schapira G, Dohnalová L, Pevsner-
Fischer M, Bikovsky R, Halpern Z, Elinav E, Segal
E.** 2015. Personalized nutrition by prediction of
glycemic responses. *Cell* **163:**1079–1094.

D. NEXT-GENERATION MICROBIAL THERAPEUTICS: TOOLS AND REGULATION

Engineering Diagnostic and Therapeutic Gut Bacteria

14

BRIAN P. LANDRY[1] and JEFFREY J. TABOR[1,2]

INTRODUCTION AND BACKGROUND

Genetically engineered bacteria have the potential to diagnose and treat a wide range of diseases linked to the gastrointestinal tract, or gut. Such engineered microbes will be less expensive and invasive than current diagnostics and more effective and safe than current therapeutics. Recent advances in synthetic biology have dramatically improved the reliability with which bacteria can be engineered with the sensors, genetic circuits, and output (actuator) genes necessary for diagnostic and therapeutic functions. However, to deploy such bacteria *in vivo*, researchers must identify appropriate gut-adapted strains and consider performance metrics such as sensor detection thresholds, circuit computation speed, growth rate effects, and the evolutionary stability of engineered genetic systems. Other recent reviews have focused on engineering bacteria to target cancer (1, 2) or genetically modifying the endogenous gut microbiota *in situ* (3, 4). Here, we develop a standard approach for engineering "smart probiotics," which both diagnose and treat disease, as well as "diagnostic gut bacteria" and "drug factory probiotics," which perform only the former and latter function, respectively. We focus on the use of cutting-

[1]Department of Bioengineering, Rice University, Houston, TX 77030; [2]Department of Biosciences, Rice University, Houston, TX 77030

Bugs as Drugs: Therapeutic Microbes for the Prevention and Treatment of Disease
Edited by Robert A. Britton and Patrice D. Cani
© 2018 American Society for Microbiology, Washington, DC
doi:10.1128/microbiolspec.BAD-0020-2017

edge synthetic biology tools, gut-specific design considerations, and current and future engineering challenges.

Natural Probiotics

Natural probiotics are evolved organisms that are isolated, cultured, and consumed for a health benefit (5). Many bacterial strains have been developed as natural probiotics, most prominently those of the *Lactobacillus* and *Bifidobacterium* genera (6). These microbes have been used to treat *Clostridium* infection (7); inflammatory diseases such as obesity, diabetes, and inflammatory bowel disease (8); and neurological conditions such as anxiety, depression, and autism spectrum disorder (6), among other pathologies. Natural probiotics are known to exert beneficial effects by directly signaling with the human host through chemical or physical means or by altering the composition and metabolism of the gut microbiota (9). However, like all bacteria, natural probiotics have evolved complex gene regulatory networks that activate or silence therapeutic pathways in response to poorly understood intracellular and extracellular signals. Furthermore, the genetic and molecular mechanisms by which natural probiotics evolved to act are poorly understood (10). As a result, it has proven difficult to improve the efficacy of probiotic therapies, and natural probiotics have thus far yielded mixed success (11).

Smart Probiotics

An exciting alternative is to genetically engineer "smart probiotics": bacteria that sense the levels of one or more gut biomarkers, compute whether the profile of those biomarkers is diagnostic of disease, and respond by delivering a precise dose of one or more appropriate therapeutics (4, 12–14) (Fig. 1).

Smart probiotics offer benefits over traditional nonliving therapeutics (i.e., chemical or biologically produced [biologic] drugs) and natural probiotics. First, both smart and

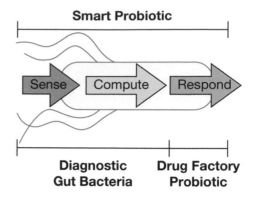

FIGURE 1 The three classes of engineered gut bacteria. Smart probiotics sense one or more biomarkers, compute that those biomarkers are present in a combination indicative of disease, and respond by delivering a precise dose of one or more appropriate therapeutics at the diseased tissue. Diagnostic gut bacteria sense one or more biomarkers, compute that those biomarkers are present in a combination indicative of disease, and produce a reporter which can be externally measured by a clinician. Drug factory probiotics constitutively produce a therapeutic within the body.

natural probiotics can deliver drugs locally to diseased tissues, resulting in increased efficacy and decreased side effects relative to systemic administration of traditional therapeutics. Second, bacteria produce drugs on-site, eliminating the need for expensive purification steps involved in chemical drug synthesis or fermenter-based biologic production. Third, due to the use of well-characterized engineered gene-regulatory networks, rather than poorly characterized evolved versions, therapeutic pathways can be activated far more reliably *in vivo* with smart as opposed to natural probiotics. Fourth, the genetic pathways resulting in the production of the therapeutic compounds are well-defined in smart probiotics. This feature is unlike natural probiotics, which may produce undefined mixtures of bioactive compounds whose effects are difficult to disentangle. Fifth, in stark contrast to their natural counterparts which are simply taken "as-is" from nature, smart probiotics are developed using iterative cycles of design, construction, testing, and learning, which enables continual performance improvements (Fig. 2). Finally, future advances in our understanding of the biology of gut-linked diseases will result in continued improvements in smart probiotic designs and expand the number of diseases that can be treated.

The foundation for smart probiotics was laid at the turn of the current century when Remaut and colleagues genetically modified the natural probiotic *Lactococcus lactis* to constitutively secrete the human anti-inflammatory cytokine protein interleukin-10 (IL-10) (Fig. 3A). We classify this IL-10-secreting *L. lactis* strain, and any bacterium engineered to constitutively produce a therapeutic within the body, as a "drug factory probiotic." Because drug factory probiotics perform only the "back end" delivery function, we consider them a simpler subclass of

smart probiotics (Fig. 1). As the authors intended, oral administration of the IL-10-secreting *L. lactis* reduces colon inflammation (colitis) by 50% in mice (15) (Fig. 3B). Furthermore, 10,000-fold lower IL-10 concentrations are required to achieve a therapeutic effect when delivered in the gastrointestinal tract by *L. lactis* compared to intraperitoneal administration (15). This increase in efficacy decreases the potential for unwanted immunosuppressive side effects. These benefits are clear examples of several of the advantages of smart probiotics.

The Remaut group later iterated on the IL-10-secreting *L. lactis* strain several times to improve its performance. One concern is uncontrolled growth of engineered bacteria within the gut. This may be detrimental to the health of the host or result in unintended escape into the environment and corresponding spread of synthetic DNA into natural

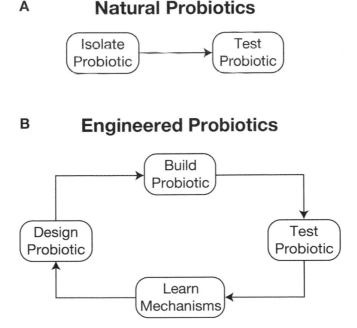

A   **Natural Probiotics**

Isolate Probiotic → Test Probiotic

B   **Engineered Probiotics**

Build Probiotic → Test Probiotic → Learn Mechanisms → Design Probiotic → Build Probiotic

FIGURE 2 A comparison of the development process for natural and engineered probiotics. (A) Natural probiotics are isolated and then tested for efficacy without an ability to methodically improve their capabilities. (B) In contrast, engineered probiotics undergo a design-build-test-learn cycle which allows for continual probiotic improvement and knowledge gain with each iteration.

A   Drug Factory Probiotic:
IL-10 Treatment of Inflammation

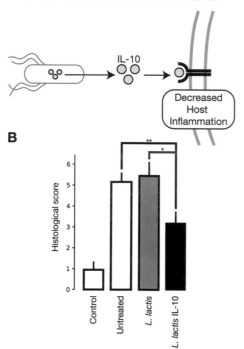

C   Diagnostic Gut Bacteria:
Host Inflammation

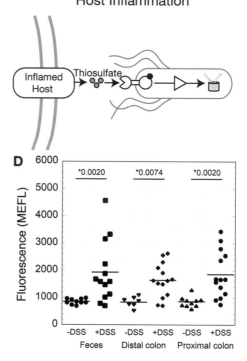

E   Diagnostic Gut Bacteria:
Diet Administered Antibiotic

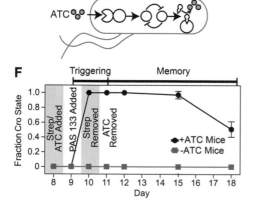

G   Diagnostic Gut Bacteria:
Diet Administered Sugar

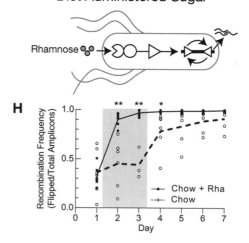

populations. To overcome this problem, the authors introduced a genomic mutation resulting in thymidine auxotrophy, making their drug factory probiotic dependent on thymidine added to laboratory growth media for survival. Indeed, this biocontainment strategy greatly decreases survival in the porcine gut (16). Additionally, a phase I clinical trial for treatment of Crohn's disease revealed that this second-generation IL-10-secreting *L. lactis* does not generate systemic or long-term side effects and that the biocontainment strategy functions as intended in humans (17). However, a subsequent phase IIA trial failed to demonstrate statistically significant beneficial effects in humans. Unfortunately, the reasons for this failure are unknown (18). Nonetheless, to improve efficacy, the strain has since been re-engineered to secrete single-chain antibodies that bind tumor necrosis factor alpha (TNFα) (i.e., anti-TNFα nanobodies), preventing its ability to stimulate inflammation (19). Clinical trials using the anti-TNFα nanobody-secreting *L. lactis* to treat inflammatory bowel disease are now being pursued (20; https://www.dna.com/Technologies/ActoBiotics).

Undoubtedly inspired by the *L. lactis* work, other groups have since engineered drug factory probiotics to treat colitis (17, 19, 21–28), diabetes (29–32), obesity (33), and numerous pathogen infections (34–38). These efforts are all based on traditional genetic engineering approaches wherein a heterologous genetic pathway is simply introduced into a gut-relevant bacterial host. On the other hand, exciting advances are being made by incorporating modern synthetic biology technologies into smart probiotic designs.

Synthetic Biology

Synthetic biology is a new engineering discipline wherein living organisms are genetically programmed to carry out unnatural behaviors, with applications in medicine, agriculture, energy, manufacturing, and fundamental biology research, among other enterprises (14, 39–41). In contrast to traditional genetic engineering approaches, synthetic biologists program cellular behaviors using the "sense-compute-respond" paradigm adapted from electrical engineering (42) (Fig. 4). Here,

FIGURE 3 Examples of current engineered gut bacteria. (A) A drug factory probiotic was made by engineering *L. lactis* to constitutively produce IL-10. IL-10 is secreted by the bacteria and then bound by the IL-10 receptor in the gut, resulting in downregulation of host inflammation. **(B)** DSS was used to induce inflammation in mice, and disease pathology was measured with histological scores. Treatment with the IL-10 drug factory probiotic was found to decrease symptoms by 50% compared to untreated mice or mice administered the natural probiotic *L. lactis*. **(C)** A diagnostic gut bacterium was created by engineering *E. coli* Nissle to sense thiosulfate, which is produced in the gut during inflammation. The thiosulfate is sensed by the ttrSR TCS, which activates expression of the fluorescent protein sfGFP. **(D)** sfGFP fluorescence of bacteria isolated from the feces and distal and proximal colon was measured and found to be significantly increased in mice experiencing inflammation in each location. Panel adapted from *Mol Syst Biol* (55) with permission of the publisher. **(E)** *E. coli* NGF-1 was modified to express the ATC sensor TetR, which controlled expression of the cro TF. The cro TF is one component of the lambda phage cro/cI toggle switch. ATC altered the start of the switch to become cro-dominant, and therefore produce LacZ protein, which produces a blue pigment. **(F)** The ATC-sensing diagnostic gut bacteria were administered to mice which were administered ATC via drinking water. Temporary administration of ATC was found to activate LacZ production, and the memory was retained for up to 1 week. Panel adapted from *Proceedings of the National Academy of Sciences* (56) with permission of the publisher. **(G)** The native RhaR rhamnose sensor in *B. thetaiotaomicron* was used to control expression of the Int12 recombinase, which permanently inverts a barcode segment of DNA in the genome. **(H)** The rhamnose diagnostic gut bacteria switched the state of the barcode as detected via qPCR when administered rhamnose in drinking water. However, even without administration of rhamnose, the sensor toggled states, due to either leaky recombination or residual rhamnose in the plant-based chow. Panel reprinted from *Cell Systems* (51) with permission of the publisher.

organisms are engineered to express genetically encoded sensors, such as signal transduction pathways, that detect specific chemical or physical inputs inside or outside the cell. Sensors convert chemical or physical inputs into biological outputs such as gene transcription. These biological outputs, in turn, serve as inputs into engineered genetic circuits, to which the sensors are linked (43, 44). Genetic circuits are networks of interacting regulatory molecules, such as transcription factors (TFs) and their target promoters, that perform computations such as multi-input logic or memory. Finally, the circuits control the activity of actuator genes, such as metabolic pathways or secreted proteins, which program the cell to change its own state or the state of its environment. Importantly, sensors, circuits, and actuators (i.e., devices) are designed to be modular, such that they function in the same manner in different genetic, organismal, or environmental contexts. This modularity enables a large number of new designs to be rapidly imagined, constructed, and tested, while increasing predictability and improving performance.

Genetically Encoded Sensors

Bacteria have evolved thousands of genetically encoded sensors, many of which can be repurposed to diagnose disease. These fall into two major categories: one-component systems (OCSs) and two-component systems (TCSs).

OCSs, cytoplasmic TFs that directly interact with and are allosterically modulated by chemical and physical inputs, are the largest class of bacterial sensors (45) and have been used for gut-relevant sensing applications. In *in vitro* work, synthetic biologists have utilized OCSs that respond to acyl-homoserine lactone quorum-sensing autoinducers to program *Escherichia coli* to monitor communication between pathogenic *Pseudomonas aeruginosa* on solid agar (46) and in biofilms (47). In an *ex vivo* study, NorR, an OCS activated by nitric oxide, was used to detect the presence of inflammatory signaling in an epithelial cell coculture of intestinal explants (48). Finally, various orally administered gut-adapted bacteria have been used to sense dietary lactose (49), xylan (50), and rhamnose (51), as well as fucose produced by the

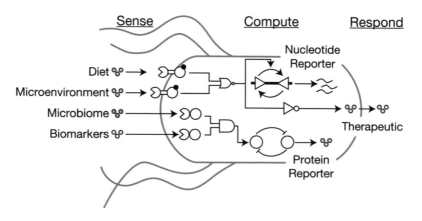

FIGURE 4 An outline of the types of sense, compute, and respond behavior an engineered gut bacterium can exhibit. Chemicals from a variety of sources within the gut may be of interest to a smart bacterium, including the host diet, compounds produced locally by the host in the bacterium's microenvironment, signals from other components of the microbiome, and general biomarkers of host disease. Computation is performed with a variety of logic gates and memory elements. The bacterium actuates a response with a therapeutic molecule in the case of a smart probiotic, or by producing a nucleotide or protein-based reporter for a diagnostic gut bacterium.

gut microbiota (52) in the mouse gastrointestinal tract. Though they will surely play a major role in future diagnostic efforts, OCSs are limited by the fact that they cannot sense disease biomarkers that are not transported across the membrane or do not induce secondary chemical or physical changes inside the cell.

TCSs are the largest family of signal transduction pathways in biology (53, 54) and the primary means by which bacteria sense extracellular stimuli. TCSs are composed of a membrane-bound or cytoplasmic sensor histidine kinase (SK) and a cytoplasmic response regulator protein. In the presence of a specific stimulus, the SK phosphorylates the response regulator, which then binds DNA and activates or represses transcription from one or more output promoters.

In recent work, we hypothesized that thiosulfate ($S_2O_3^{2-}$) could serve as a novel biomarker of colitis and set out to engineer a gut-adapted bacterium to sense it in mouse models. However, no genetically encoded thiosulfate sensor had previously been reported. Therefore, we developed a combined computational and experimental approach to discover the first known biological thiosulfate sensor, a TCS from the marine bacterium *Shewanella halifaxensis* (55). We expressed this TCS, which we named ThsSR, in the natural probiotic *E. coli* Nissle 1917 (also known as Nissle), and encoded the reporter gene superfolder green fluorescent protein (*sfgfp*) as the output (Fig. 3C). We then orally administered the thiosulfate-sensing Nissle strain to control mice and mice administered the colitis-inducing compound dextran sodium sulfate (DSS) and performed flow cytometry on bacteria sampled from the colon and feces 6 hours later. As hypothesized, we observed that ThsSR is activated in mice with, but not without, colitis (Fig. 3D). Furthermore, the greater the extent of inflammation, the greater the ThsSR activity, suggesting that thiosulfate may be a novel colitis biomarker (55).

Importantly, our flow cytometry method enables identification and analysis of sensor strains without eliminating the native gut bacteria via broad-spectrum antibiotic treatment or germ-free methods. This feature enables minimally invasive measurements of biomarkers in native gut pathways and could generate more physiologically relevant results that are more likely to translate to clinical conditions. We are now investigating whether thiosulfate is a colitis biomarker in humans and whether our engineered bacterium could be advanced as a clinical diagnostic.

Our thiosulfate-sensing Nissle strain is an early example of a "diagnostic gut bacterium." This class of engineered gut bacteria utilize sensors, or sensors linked to genetic circuits (discussed below), to diagnose a gut-linked disease via expression of a reporter gene (Fig. 2).

Genetic Circuits

Genetic circuits can be inserted between sensors and reporter genes to increase the quality, accuracy, or duration of diagnostic gut bacterial readouts. In a pioneering proof-of-principle study, Silver and coworkers used the *E. coli* tetracycline repressor (TetR) to express the phage λ transcriptional repressor cro, which in turn flipped the cI/cro transcriptional toggle switch from a cI- to a cro-dominant state in the presence of the tetracycline derivative anhydrotetracycline (aTc) (Fig. 3E). In this design, the cI-repressible promoter P_r is used to drive expression of the reporter gene *lacZ*, which is detected via production of a blue pigment indicator in X-gal agar plate growth media. First, the group transformed the mouse gut-derived *E. coli* strain NGF-1 with this sensor-circuit device. The device was integrated into the genome of NGF-1 to enable long-term evolutionary stability. Then they pretreated mice with the antibiotic streptomycin to clear the native gut flora, and orally administered the aTc-sensing NGF-1 strain to the mice, enabling long-term colonization (i.e., persistent growth in the gut without repeated oral administration). Once colonized, the engineered

NGF-1 strain reports exposure to aTc supplied in drinking water by flipping to the cro-dominant state, which is detected by plating the fecal matter on X-gal-containing media (56). Impressively, the aTc sensor device remains activated for over 1 week after exposure to aTc due to the stability of the λ genetic switch (Fig. 3F).

Tetrathionate ($S_4O_6^{2-}$), the oxidative dimer of thiosulfate, has also been implicated as a colitis biomarker (57, 58). Recently, the Silver group modified their aTc-sensing gut bacterium to function as a tetrathionate sensor by replacing *tetR* with the tetrathionate-sensing *Salmonella enterica* serovar Typhimurium TCS *ttrSR* (59, 60). The tetrathionate-sensing NGF-1 was orally administered to mice pretreated with streptomycin, resulting in stable levels of engineered bacteria in the feces after 6 months. Impressively, DNA sequencing and functional screening of fecal isolates showed that the tetrathionate sensor device had not lost the ability to respond to tetrathionate. For diagnosis, the strain was then administered to control mice and the *Salmonella* infection and IL-10 mouse models of colitis. A significant portion of the sensor bacteria switched to the activated cro-dominant state in the colitis compared to control mice. However, activation only occurred in an average of 1% and 5% of bacteria for the *Salmonella* and IL-10 models, respectively, compared to 100% activation of the sensor *in vitro*, with some diseased mice not giving rise to any activated colonies. This limitation demonstrates the need for further design-build-test-learn cycles to improve the performance of these diagnostic gut bacteria.

Additionally, though thiosulfate and tetrathionate are both anaerobic electron acceptors for bacterial respiration, tetrathionate is preferred and may be rapidly consumed by the gut microbiota. This fact may have contributed to the low tetrathionate signal observed by Silver and coworkers. Indeed, we did not observe colitis-dependent activation of a different tetrathionate-sensing TCS in DSS-treated mice with a native microbiota

(55). Taken together, these results suggest that tetrathionate may not be an ideal colitis biomarker.

Recombinases that invert promoter-containing DNA segments (61) or engineered barcode sequences (62) are an alternative circuit design for long-term memory in diagnostic gut bacteria. In a recent study by Lu, Voigt, and coworkers, a recombinase was used to invert a genomic DNA barcode in the human commensal *Bacteroides thetaiotaomicron* to remember exposure to diet-derived rhamnose in the mouse gut (51) (Fig. 3D). However, appreciable background recombination was observed in this study, highlighting the need for future engineering cycles to improve performance. Ultimately, though, all of these early studies clearly demonstrate the exciting potential of diagnostic gut bacteria, particularly as more biomarkers are identified and bacterial sensors developed.

Genetically Encoded Therapeutic Actuators

Drug factory probiotic design efforts have generated over 25 genetically encoded therapeutic actuators targeting diverse diseases (Table 1). A major class is bacterially secreted human proteins that augment human signaling networks. These include IL-10 (15) and anti-TNFα nanobodies (19), which treat colitis, and glycolipoprotein-1 (63), which treats diabetes. A second important class is bacterial proteins that augment human signaling networks. Examples of this class include the Toll-like receptor 2 stimulator LcrV protein from *Yersinia pseudotuberculosis* (25) and the superoxide dismutase SodA protein from *L. lactis* (22), both of which decrease symptoms of colitis. A final class is genetic pathways that produce therapeutic metabolites. For example, expression of At1g78690, an *N*-acyltransferase, led to production of *N*-acylphosphatidylethanolamines (NAPEs), which reduced food intake and obesity in mice (30). In another example, expression of the *Propionibacterium acnes* linoleic acid isomerase coPAI led to production of conjugated linoleic acid, which altered fatty acid composition and decreased body fat (33). The synthetic biology approach described above will enable integration of these and other therapeutic actuators into smart probiotics to increase their therapeutic efficacy and decrease associated side effects.

ENGINEERING SMART PROBIOTICS

When setting out to construct a smart probiotic, one must make a series of basic design decisions. These include selecting a chassis organism and gut disease biomarkers, identifying the computations that need to be performed, and determining the appropriate therapeutic response. A toolkit of chassis organisms and genetic parts has been developed to accomplish these goals. Furthermore, synthetic biology techniques are available for developing new chassis and parts when current options are insufficient. Finally, deploying smart probiotics within the complex and dynamic gut environment presents additional challenges that require further design considerations.

Chassis Selection

The criteria for selecting smart probiotic chassis partially diverge from those used when selecting natural probiotics. Similar to natural probiotics, one must consider the ability of the chassis to survive transit through the gastrointestinal tract, colonize particular macroscopic or microscopic geographical locations within the gut, and reach desired densities therein. On the other hand, the amenability of the chassis to DNA transformation, the availability of tools to modify its genome, and the repertoire of sensors, genetic circuits, and actuators compatible with it are also essential to consider.

Previous studies have established a number of "off-the-shelf" chassis with different properties. Multiple strains of the Gram-negative facultative anaerobe *E. coli*, the traditional workhorse of synthetic biology, have been deployed in mice for different purposes. These include laboratory strains (35, 37, 52, 64), Nissle (34, 38, 55), and NGF-1 (56, 60, 65). The Gram-negative anaerobe *B. thetaiotaomicron* has recently been developed as a new smart probiotic chassis (51). This bacterium belongs to the phylum *Bacteroidetes*, which is one of the two dominant phyla in human stool (66). Gram-positive facultative anaerobe alternatives include *Lactobacillus casei* (23, 26–28, 34), *Lactobacillus gasseri* (24, 32), *Lactobacillus paracasei* (33, 36), *Lactobacillus plantarum* (22), and *L. lactis* (15, 17, 19, 22–28, 31, 32, 34, 67–69). Many of these lactic acid bacteria, along with *Bacteroides xylanisolvens*, a relative of *B. thetaiotaomicron*, have Generally Recognized As Safe recognition by the U.S. Food and Drug Administration (70), facilitating their use in humans.

Colonization

The ability of an organism to colonize a specific biogeographical gut location may be necessary for effective diagnosis or treatment of disease. For example, when targeting a patient with ulcerative colitis, which impacts the large intestine, it may be beneficial for the organism to colonize the large intestine (71). On the other hand, if treating the related Crohn's disease, wherein pathology extends from the mouth to anus (71), colonization of the small intestine may also improve the therapeutic effects. Members of the *Bacteroidaceae* family, which are found in higher numbers in the colon, may be better suited for the former disease, whereas members of the *Lactobacillaceae* family, which are found in both the small intestine and colon, may be better suited for the latter (72). Furthermore, specific genetic determinants within a species can result in different colonization capabilities (72), which opens the door for engineering chassis bacteria with specific colonization patterns.

TABLE 1 Examples of engineered gut bacteria[a]

Type	Disease targeted	Compound sensed	Therapeutic produced	Chassis	In vivo	Reference(s)
Drug factory probiotic	Autoimmune diseases		Ovalbumin	*L. lactis*	X	67
	Cholera		Chimeric lipopolysaccharide	*E. coli* E56b	X	37
	Cholera		CAI-1	*E. coli* Nissle 1917	X	38
	Celiac		DQ8 gliadin epitope	*L. lactis*	X	68
	Colitis		IL-10	*L. lactis*	X	15, 17
	Colitis		Trefoil factors	*L. lactis*	X	21
	Colitis		DNA for TGF-β1	*E. coli* BM2710	X	64
	Colitis		SOD	*L. plantarum*	X	22
	Colitis		SOD	*L. lactis*	X	22
	Colitis		Manganese-dependent catalase	*L. casei*	X	23
	Colitis		SOD	*L. gasseri*	X	24
	Colitis		LcrV	*L. lactis*	X	25
	Colitis		Anti-TNFα nanobodies	*L. lactis*	X	19
	Colitis		SOD	*L. casei*	X	26
	Colitis		SOD	*L. casei*	X	27
	Colitis		CAT	*L. casei*	X	27
	Colitis		Elafin	*L. casei*	X	28
	Colitis		Elafin	*L. lactis*	X	28
	Colitis		IL-10	*L. lactis*	X	29
	Diabetes		NAPEs	*E. coli* Nissle 1917	X	30
	Diabetes		Glutamic acid decarboxylase	*L. lactis*	X	31
	Diabetes		IL-10	*L. lactis*	X	31
	Diabetes		GLP-1	*L. gasseri*	X	32

Category	Condition	Input	Output	Strain		Reference
	E. coli		Lactoferrin	L. casei	X	34
	E. coli		Chimeric lipopolysaccharide	E. coli E56b	X	35
	Listeria monocytogenes		Listeria adhesion protein	L. paracasei	X	36
	Obesity		Conjugated linoleic acid	L. paracasei	X	33
Diagnostic gut bacteria	Citrobacter rodentium	Fucose		E. coli BW25113	X	52
	Colitis	NO		E. coli		48
	Colitis	Tetrathionate		E. coli NGF-1	X	60
	Colitis	Tetrathionate		E. coli Nissle 1917	X	55
	Colitis	Thiosulfate		E. coli Nissle 1917	X	55
	Diet sensor	Lactose		Streptococcus thermophilus	X	49
	Diet sensor	ATC		E. coli NGF-1	X	56
	Diet sensor	Arabinogalactan		B. thetaiotaomicron	X	51
	Diet sensor	IPTG		B. thetaiotaomicron	X	51
	Diet sensor	Rhamnose		B. thetaiotaomicron	X	51
Smart probiotic	Colitis	Xylan	IL-2	B. ovatus		156
	Colitis	Xylan	Keratinocyte growth factor-2	B. ovatus	X	50
	Colitis	Xylan	TGF-β1	B. ovatus	X	157
	Diabetes	Nisin	Insulin	L. lactis		158
	Diabetes	Glucose	GLP-1	E. coli Nissle 1917		63
	Diabetes	Glucose	PDX-1	E. coli Nissle 1917		63
	Pseudomonas aeruginosa	3OC12HSL	E7 lysis	E. coli		47
	P. aeruginosa	3OC12HSL	Bacteriocin	E. coli MG1655		46

[a]Abbreviations: CAT, catalase; GLP-1, glucagon-like peptide 1; IPTG, isopropyl-β-D-thiogalactopyranoside; NAPE, N-acylphosphatidylethanolamine; PDX-1, pancreatic and duodenal homeobox gene 1; SOD, superoxide dismutase; TGF, transforming growth factor.

Alternatively, when engineering diagnostic gut bacteria, it may be beneficial to have bacteria that do not colonize the gut. For example, our thiosulfate-sensing Nissle strain (55) survives passage through the gut but does not appear to colonize or reach high numbers when the native gut microbiota is intact (73). These features result in minimal perturbations to the native gut microbiota relative to other strains which may outcompete native flora for specific niches and thereby alter gut microbiota or host physiology. For example, alterations to gut microbiota can lead to the highly undesirable side effects of inflammation (74) or opportunistic pathogen infection (75).

Genetic Tractability

The capacity to perform genetic modifications that yield desired outcomes is fundamental for smart probiotic design but varies widely between gut bacterial chassis. Genetic tractability requires tools for reliable DNA transformation, control of gene expression, and posttranslational control of protein processes such as secretion. A wide array of sensors, circuit components, and actuators are also needed and will be covered in depth in later sections.

E. coli has an unrivaled genetic toolbox, which we will use to exemplify the parts required to engineer smart probiotics. DNA transformation can be accomplished via chemical or electrical disruption of the membrane, phage-mediated transduction, or conjugation from another bacterium. To persist, the transferred DNA requires self-replicating elements (76) or genomic integration (77). Selectable markers such as antibiotic resistance genes are important for obtaining and maintaining transformants in the laboratory but do not appear to be required for retention of plasmid DNAs in short-term *in vivo* experiments (55, 73). The transcription rate of sensor, circuit, or actuator mRNAs can be precisely controlled using well-characterized constitutive promoter libraries (78, 79) or chemically inducible promoters (80, 81).

Termination of transcription is important to prevent unwanted cross-talk between different transcribed elements on a contiguous piece of engineered DNA. Previous work has generated large libraries of well-characterized transcription terminators, many of them very efficient (82, 83). The mRNA translation rate is commonly used to control the protein expression level. The translation rate of a target gene can easily be tuned in *E. coli* by computational design of custom ribosome binding site (RBS) sequences via the RBS calculator (84–86) or through the use of the more modular "bicistronic design" RBSs developed by Endy, Arkin, and coworkers (79). Translated *E. coli* proteins can be functionalized with tags that facilitate their secretion from the cell (87) or rapid degradation (88). These *E. coli* parts have primarily been characterized in laboratory strains. However, recent work demonstrated that a complex circuit could be transferred from a laboratory strain to a native gut isolate while maintaining complete functionality (56) despite possible differences in individual part performance between strains.

When using a chassis other than *E. coli*, many of the aforementioned tools will be unavailable or poorly developed. Thus, techniques to rapidly generate reliable new genetic tools in non-*E. coli* chassis are needed. This goal was recently demonstrated by Lu, Voigt, and colleagues in *B. thetaiotaomicron* (51). To transform this less tractable organism, a conjugative plasmid containing the genetic construct was assembled in *E. coli* and subsequently transferred to *B. thetaiotaomicron* via conjugation. Once transformed, the plasmid expressed an integrase (89) that catalyzed its integration into a fixed site in the genome. The authors then designed a library of synthetic promoters resulting in a 20-fold range of reporter gene expression levels by inserting a 26-bp DNA sequence in different regions of the native housekeeping sigma factor's promoter, P_{BT1311}. They also developed three carbohydrate-inducible promoters by taking advantage of natively expressed proteins and a synthetic IPTG-inducible promoter from *E. coli*. To vary translation strength, they modified the native RBS of the 50S ribosomal protein gene *rpiL** by targeting conserved positions, resulting in a 1,000-fold range of gene expression levels.

Several parts have been developed for *Lactobacilli* as well (90). These include nisin- (91), peptide pheromone SppIP- (92), IPTG-, and xylose- (93) inducible promoters and constitutive promoter libraries (94). A range of replicative plasmids (90) also exist, as do single-stranded DNA recombineering techniques to generate point mutations in chromosomal DNA (95, 96). However, the current lack of a consensus organism in this genus will require many of these parts to be recharacterized in the specific species selected as a chassis.

Sensor Design

The simplest way to engineer a smart probiotic sensor entails expressing nonnative output genes (e.g., reporters, genetic circuit components) from endogenous chemical or physical input-responsive promoters with no additional engineering of the chassis (49, 51, 52). Though convenient, this approach can produce false negatives or positives due to the poorly understood and complex gene regulatory networks that control the activity of endogenous promoters. This method can be improved upon by knocking out the sensor genes that control the promoter of interest and expressing codon-altered versions of their open reading frames under nonnative promoters, RBSs, and so on. This process, termed genetic refactoring (97–100), can break the key connections in the native control networks, making sensor performance more reliable. However, sensor proteins may still be subject to posttranslational regulation, which can interfere with their function. An even more reliable approach is to port sensors from unrelated organisms into the chassis of interest (55, 101, 102) and optimize

their genetic encoding and expression levels for optimal sensor performance (103).

Sensor portability

In many instances, sensors of targeted disease biomarkers have not evolved in the chassis of interest. Thus, sensors often need to be ported between organisms. The successful transfer of LacI (51, 93) and TetR homologs (104, 105) between evolutionarily distant organisms demonstrates the portability of OCSs. OCS portability is improved by the fact that a single protein performs both the sensing and transcriptional control functions.

This feature stands in contrast to TCSs, which have different sensing and effecting proteins, resulting in the need to perform a two-dimensional gene expression optimization (55, 102, 103). SKs are often membrane bound, which could compromise TCS functionality when transported between organisms with drastically different membrane structures. Additionally, SKs often require poorly characterized accessory sensor proteins that allosterically modulate the SK in the presence of the input. If known, such accessory proteins must also be expressed and optimized in the new chassis. If unknown, the TCS will fail to function if the chassis lacks them. Thus, despite their benefits in sensing diverse extracellular signals, TCSs are sometimes more difficult to engineer than OCSs.

Sensor performance characteristics

Most synthetic biological sensors have been characterized in bench experiments where the growth media, growth phase, density, and other factors that influence the function of synthetic genetic systems are controlled. However, chemical, microbial, and host biological aspects of the gut are poorly understood, spatially heterogeneous, and vary over time in a single individual or between individuals. Gut environment variations impact the growth and physiology of engineered gut bacteria and may therefore introduce variability in sensor performance.

One way to overcome sensor variability is to increase the dynamic range (i.e., the ratio of sensor output in the maximally versus minimally active states) (106). A larger dynamic range allows for more distinguishable bits of information to pass through a sensor, resulting in more accurate measurements of the input. Sensor dynamic range can be increased by optimizing the expression level of sensor proteins or the sequence of sensor output promoters to eliminate cryptic constitutive transcriptional start sites that increase leakiness (103). Additionally, TCSs utilize phosphorylation/dephosphorylation cycles that make them more robust than OCSs to fluctuations in the expression levels of sensor proteins (107). This benefit may make TCSs more reliable sensors than OCSs in the gut.

The threshold sensitivity of a sensor to its input is an important and often overlooked factor that is fundamental to gut performance. Clinically relevant biomarker levels are likely to fall within specific ranges, and sensors must match these ranges to successfully diagnose a patient. Few studies have examined general methods of tuning the threshold sensitivities of sensors (108), and much work remains to address this problem. Additionally, many biological sensors are sensitive to only a small range of input concentrations and do not respond outside of that range, which makes them ill suited for quantifying a wide range of biomarker levels. Recent techniques enable the expansion of the range over which a sensor is sensitive, making it capable of measuring a broad range of input concentrations (109).

Sensor outlook

Currently, only a tiny fraction of evolved bacterial sensors have been characterized. Furthermore, it is likely that off-the-shelf sensors will not be available for new disease biomarkers identified in forthcoming gut metabolomic or similar studies. To develop new sensors, new OCS and TCS sensor genes can be easily identified via bioinformatic analyses (45, 54). However, their inputs can seldom be predicted, and there are few efficient methods for discovering them experimentally. In some cases, sensor domain homology can be utilized to predict the class of inputs (110, 111), or the local genomic context can be analyzed to identify nearby metabolic clusters which may be linked to the sense compound (55). Alternatively, the transcriptome response of a natural gut microbiome can be probed for sensors that are upregulated in a diseased state, which often indicates activation of the sensor (112). This may allow identification of sensors for a particular disease without prior knowledge of the compound that is being detected. These sensors can then be refactored and characterized in a defined environment to determine the specific disease biomarker sensed. Future advances in synthetic biology methods which allow many OCSs and TCSs to be screened for responses to inputs in high throughput should greatly increase the number of available sensors (Fig. 5A).

Genetic Logic Circuits

Genetic logic circuits can be used to increase the accuracy of smart probiotic diagnoses. For example, dietary nitrate is quickly consumed by the microbiota in the proximal gut (113), whereas nitrate produced due to inflammatory diseases can be found within the colon (114). Therefore, if nitrate was detected at the same time as a large intestine biomarker, then colitis would be likely, and it may be appropriate to secrete an anti-inflammatory compound. However, if nitrate was sensed alongside a small intestine biomarker, it would likely be of dietary origin rather than due to inflammation and should therefore be ignored. To execute such higher-order sensing, smart probiotics require multiple sensors and genetic logic circuits capable of integrating the biological inputs from those sensors simultaneously.

Parts to implement logic

TFs are proteins that bind DNA operator sites to activate or repress transcription from

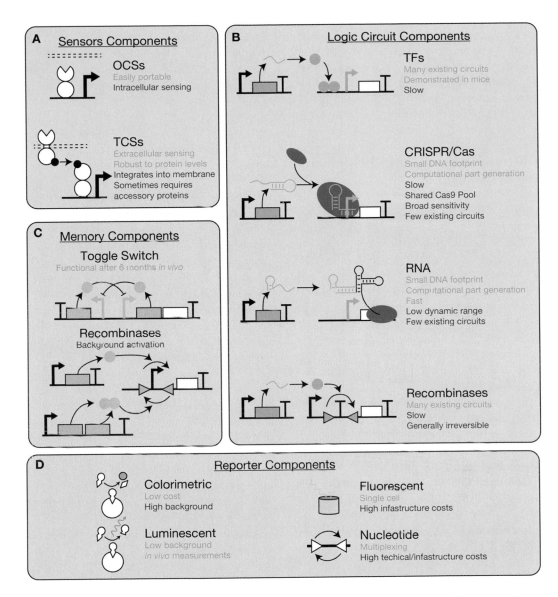

FIGURE 5 The different components used to construct an engineered gut bacterium. The pros and cons of each component are listed in green and red text, respectively. (A) Sensors can be selected from OCSs or TCSs. (B) Logic circuits can be constructed using TFs, CRISPR/Cas repressors, RNA-based sRNA transcriptional activators, or serine recombinases. (C) Genetic memory can take the form of a toggle switch or recombined DNA. (D) The state of a circuit can be assayed using colorimetric, luminescent, fluorescent, or nucleotide reporters.

promoters. TFs are the primary means by which synthetic biologists engineer logic. Several TF-based part families have been engineered and used to construct a remarkable range of genetic logic circuits.

Recently, Voigt and colleagues engineered a library of over 10 orthogonal homologs of the TetR transcriptional repressor (104). Here, orthogonality refers to the fact that each TetR homolog represses only its target promoter, and not the promoter of any other TetR homolog in the library. Each orthogonal TetR/promoter pair comprises a simple transcriptional "inverter" circuit wherein high expression of a TetR homolog from an upstream (input) promoter results in low transcription from the corresponding repressible (output) promoter (104). In follow-up work, the group used the library to construct a series of NOR logic circuits, which are active only in the absence of two different TetR homologs. The group then wrote a new *in silico* program for automated genetic logic circuit design (named Cello, for cellular logic). Cello was used to computationally design the DNA sequences encoding 52 different genetic logic circuits, many that perform complicated operations typically associated with electronic systems. Initially, 94% of their genetic circuits failed due to undefined interactions between neighboring promoters and the genes they transcribed (115). To overcome this challenge, the group standardized the 15 bp upstream of the promoter with a random DNA sequence to remove variable effects of the upstream sequence. They also placed a ribozyme between the promoter and RBS which cleaves off any mRNA nucleotides encoded by the promoter to prevent the promoter from influencing translation initiation from the RBS (116). When these genetic parts were added alongside restrictions on the physical ordering of genetic parts along a DNA sequence to further reduce context-dependent performance changes, the success rate increased to a remarkable 71% (115). The vast majority of logical operations that one may want to engineer into an *E. coli* smart probiotic could now be implemented using this approach.

The CRISPR (clustered regularly interspaced short palindromic repeats) interference (CRISPRi) TF-design technology offers several benefits for genetic logic circuit design. In CRISPRi, a nuclease-deficient *Streptococcus pyogenes* Cas9 protein (dCas9) binds to an engineered guide RNA, which drives it to bind and repress virtually any promoter in

a sequence-specific manner (117). Voigt and coworkers also engineered an orthogonal library of transcriptional inverters using CRISPRi. In particular, they designed a series of synthetic promoters with divergent spacer regions between the -35 and -10 elements, and cognate small guide RNAs (sgRNAs) that target each promoter sequence specifically. These inverters were then combined to create NOR (output is on only when no inputs are present), OR (output is on when any of multiple inputs are present), and AND (output is on only when all inputs are present) logic using one, two, and four interacting gRNAs, respectively (118). Unlike the TetR work, where the operator sites of most repressor homologs had to be discovered via arduous high-throughput protein/DNA binding array methods, these CRISPRi logic gates could be designed largely using Watson-Crick base-pairing rules. Indeed, dozens or hundreds of CRISPRi circuits can be easily engineered due to this feature (119). CRISPRi circuits are also promising because each sgRNA is on the order of 60 bp, resulting in a small and therefore inexpensive, simple to assemble, and possibly more evolutionarily stable DNA footprint. However, each sgRNA competes for a single pool of Cas9, creating a point of possible retroactivity and thus circuit failure (14). Retroactivity occurs when the activity of downstream components of a circuit alters the performance of upstream components in an unexpected fashion (120). Lastly, sgRNA-regulated promoters, when compared to traditional TF-regulated promoters, are sensitive over a broader range of regulator concentrations, resulting in a less digital-like response. This broad sensitivity can result in propagation of variability or stochastic noise through the genetic circuit, which can also cause circuits to fail (121).

RNA molecules can also be used to engineer transcriptional logic circuits. This class of designs was originally demonstrated by Arkin and coworkers, who utilized the copy number control mechanism of the pT181 plasmid to engineer an antisense RNA that promotes the formation of a transcriptional terminator on a target RNA, preventing downstream transcription. Orthogonal regulatory RNAs were created and used to construct a NOR gate and a three-step cascade (122). Lucks and coworkers built upon this work by inverting the effect of the antisense RNA through the addition of an anti-anti-terminator RNA sequence and creating the first sRNA transcriptional activators (123), which have been employed to create a two-input AND gate (123) and a three-step cascade (124). The ability to computationally generate novel regulatory RNAs (124), combined with their small size, facilitates the creation of circuits containing a large number of nodes. However, this has yet to be demonstrated and is possibly hampered by the low dynamic range frequently observed with RNA-based regulation.

Finally, serine recombinases, proteins that bind DNA at specific sequences and invert or excise intervening DNA (125), have been used to orient transcriptional control elements on DNA to control the flow of RNA polymerase. These have enabled circuits that can count to 3 (126), form a large number of two-input Boolean logic gates (61, 127), and create state machines that remember both the presence and order of input signals (128). However, it can be difficult to balance the expression levels of all circuit components, particularly when reversible serine recombinases are used (129).

Computation speed

The gut environment changes rapidly in space and time, and noncolonizing bacteria pass through the mouse gastrointestinal tract in several hours (55, 65, 73, 130). Moreover, colonizing bacteria face temporal changes in response to diet, exercise, and biogeographic position. Current transcriptional circuits exhibit dynamics that are likely to be too slow for many diagnostic and therapeutic applications. In particular, changes in stable protein concentrations are limited by the rate of dilution due to cell growth, and it may take many doublings to dilute or produce enough pro-

tein to traverse the sensitive region of a downstream node in a logic circuit (131). Circuits containing four (115) and nine TFs (132) have both been shown to take 5 hours to compute a final state. Recombinase circuits are even slower; a single inversion step has been measured to take 2 (62), 3 (127), and 6 hours (132), whereas two-part gates were found to take 8 (62) and 9 hours (127) to fully respond. A single CRISPRi inverter has been shown to have a 10- to 90-minute delay and take 4 to 5 hours to switch between on and off states when controlling a stable protein (117, 118). Furthermore, genetic circuits transiently produce incorrect outputs (115), which could lead to improper diagnoses and therapeutic responses by smart probiotics.

The response times of transcriptional logic circuits can be accelerated by adding degradation tags to TF components (133). However, this approach can generate a new problem where TF components compete for a finite supply of degradation machinery (134) and therefore create a potential point of retroactivity. This problem could be overcome by engineered orthogonal degradation systems (135), though this work is still at early stages. Unlike proteins, RNA is naturally labile, and RNA-based circuits should therefore compute solutions more quickly. *In vivo* rates of RNA circuits have not been measured, but *in vitro* work suggests they could be as low as 5 minutes for each computational step (136).

Robustness to environmental variability

A smart probiotic will experience a highly variable environment as its traverses the host from the mouth through the gut, but its circuits must function consistently to diagnose and treat disease reliably (137, 138). Growth rate is likely to change depending on factors such as gut location and variations in diet. These growth rate changes can dramatically alter circuit performance, particularly with stable proteins whose steady-state levels are linked to protein dilution. This challenge can be addressed by integrating feedback mechanisms such as negative autoregulation into computational nodes to compensate for growth effects (139, 140). Fluctuations in circuit performance appear particularly problematic for recombinase-based circuits because most implement irreversible computations. Temporary environments during administration or transit through the gut could prematurely result in permanent computation, giving false results. This may be addressable with reversible recombination (129), but this technique has not been explored in detail.

Long-term functionality

In some cases, it may be beneficial for smart probiotic circuits to function for long periods of time in the gut. To accomplish this goal, colonizing smart probiotics need to compete with the native microbiota while maintaining the ability to compute new treatments in response to alterations in disease state. If an engineered genetic circuit decreases the growth rate of the smart probiotic chassis, it could cripple the ability of the engineered organism to compete with the native gut microbiota. Such toxicity can occur with virtually all engineered genetic systems and has been reported in CRISPRi (118), TetR homolog (104, 115), and recombinase (62) circuits. Additionally, irreversible recombinase computation is particularly ill suited for long-term computation since it can only compute a response once and cannot respond to a changing environment. The only long-term study of computational circuit persistence showed that the genomic λ-derived toggle switch constructed using protein-based TFs (Fig. 3F) is capable of surviving for 6 months in an antibiotic pretreated mouse gut without losing functionality, highlighting the stability of this design strategy (60).

Logic circuit outlook

Given current technologies, we believe that the most promising method for engineering genetic logic into smart probiotics is to use TetR-based TFs (Fig. 5B). Benefits include the availability of a large library of parts and the ability to design complex circuits in an automated fashion. Additionally, there are no significant drawbacks such as the toxicity associated with CRISPRi circuits since nontoxic TetR homologs have been identified. Furthermore, TetR-based circuits are reversible (albeit slow), unlike most recombinase-based systems.

An interesting unexplored alternative is to replicate the computation observed in posttranslational networks such as phosphorelays (141). Bacteria have been shown to contain multistep histidine kinase phosphorelays which can integrate signals from different sensors with AND logic (142). The protein components of these phosphorelays have evolved in a highly modular nature (53), suggesting that they may be generally engineerable (143, 144). Such a network would provide fast posttranslational computation that may also be robust to changes in protein levels resulting from the complex gut environment (107).

Memory Circuits

For diagnostic gut bacteria to report the state of diseases within the gut after passage in feces, they require the ability to remember previous exposure to disease biomarkers. The two current approaches used to form memory in the gut are TF-based toggle switches (56, 60) and recombinases (51) (Fig. 5C).

Toggle switches

In a foundational paper in the field of synthetic biology, Collins and colleagues engineered a genetic toggle switch composed of two mutually repressing TFs, each of which prevented the other from being transcribed. They demonstrated that this circuit can remember exposure to different environmental signals even after the signals are removed (145, 146). This work was inspired by the λ cI/cro toggle switch that controls the bacteriophage's decision to stay in a lysogenic state or to switch to a lytic state after transduction of its host (147). The previously discussed aTc-sensing (Fig. 3E) (56) and tetrathionate-sensing (60) diagnostic gut bacteria utilized the λ toggle switch "as-is" to implement memory within the gut.

Recombinases

Recent work has focused on the use of recombinases as a form of memory (51, 62, 129), in addition to their capability as logic circuit components. Recombinases have been used to record the presence of lactose (148) and rhamnose (51) within the gut. However, in both cases large amounts of background activation of the system were observed, limiting the time window in which there were identifiable differences between treatment and control mice (Fig. 3H) (51, 148). This may result from the fact that recording of the memory is irreversible, causing low levels of noisy recombination that accumulate false-positive outcomes over time. To address the irreversibility of recombination, Endy and colleagues expressed an excisionase, which reverses the recombination event, restoring DNA to its original sequence. After exhaustive tuning of expression levels, they created a strain which was able to toggle its memory between exposure to two different inducers for over seven cycles of induction (129).

Memory circuits outlook

The toggle switch has demonstrated clear superiority in its ability to accurately record a memory for a long period of time in the gut. However, if future diagnostic gut bacteria require memory of many different signals, the large number of available recombinase modules (62) may make them an attractive alternative. Additionally, future diagnosis may seek to report many different levels of exposure compared to the binary nature of the previously discussed memory elements. An interesting alternative is the use of retrons, which perform 6-bp modifications of DNA sequences at a much lower rate than serine recombinases. This has enabled continuous integration of both signal amplitude and duration over many days at a population level (149) and may be useful for diagnosis of diseases with highly dynamic biomarkers.

Genetic Actuators: Reporters

A range of reporter genes allow for measurement of sensor or genetic circuit outputs (Fig. 5D).

Colorimetric reporters

Colorimetric reporters have a long history of use in biotechnology, most prominently through the enzymatic activity of the *lacZ* gene on X-gal, producing a blue pigment (150), which has been employed in diagnostic gut bacteria (Fig. 3E) (56). Colorimetric assays are an attractive reporter system since they are low cost and do not require special instrumentation. When applied in a clinical setting, fecal coloration could enable simple in-home readouts of the state of engineered bacteria exiting the gut, but this approach may be limited by high background fecal pigmentation.

Luminescent reporters

Luminescent reporter genes, such as bacterial luciferase, typically yield increased sensitivity over colorimetric reporters due to very low background luminescence in fecal samples (151). Luminescence requires the addition of a luciferin substrate or its metabolic production by the bacteria themselves. Numerous luciferases are available, and each has different brightness, luciferin requirements, and output wavelengths. All luciferases require a luminometer instrument for measurement, making them less convenient than colorimetric reporters. However, high signal-to-background makes luminescent reporters desirable for clinical diagnostic gut bacteria.

Fluorescent reporters

Fluorescent measurement of bacteria from the gut allows single cell data to be collected from bacterial populations via flow cytometry (55, 65) or microscopy (52). Such analyses can be valuable in the research setting to detect more complex population-level changes such as bimodality, which are likely to occur in the complex gut environment. Single cell measurements can also be critical for troubleshooting engineered circuit performance (115). However, fluorescent reporter genes are less suited to clinical applications due to large expensive instruments and processing requirements, including a postgut aerobic incubation to allow for the oxygen-dependent maturation of the fluorophores (55).

Nucleic acid reporters

Direct sequencing of nucleic acid changes resulting from engineered bacterial recombination (51) may be the most promising diagnostic modality. A unique challenge of characterization of bacteria in the gut is the extreme cost of a single replicate compared to test tube experiments. Sequencing of barcoded DNA allows for measurement of entire libraries of bacteria in a single heterogeneous culture (152). This approach could be applied to single mice to test thousands of candidate synthetic probiotic sensors in parallel. Similarly, it would allow for the clinical use of many different probiotic diagnostics, enabling multiplexing of diagnostic gut bacteria. This approach has higher technical and infrastructure costs than other reporter methods, but these are likely to decrease in the future, making this a very promising avenue of investigation.

EXPERIMENTAL VALIDATION

Testing engineered gut bacteria in animal models or human trials is slow and expensive. Thus, it is prudent to validate and debug smart probiotic prototypes in a series of increasingly complex *in vitro* environments before final *in vivo* environments.

Defined Media

Defined media are useful for testing well-defined hypotheses on the performance of synthetic sensing, computing, or responding components. Questions about specific components may include what compounds a sensor binds or what levels of actuator can be produced. Broader system-wide questions

include the following: Does expression of the synthetic system affect growth rates of the chassis (i.e., toxicity)? How do the expression levels of system proteins affect probiotic performance? and How does the growth rate of the chassis affect circuit performance? The high throughput and low cost of defined media allow for in-depth interrogation of these parameters. In addition, their relevance to more complex models may be improved by the development of standard defined media which replicate the gut environment through the inclusion of more complex carbohydrate and protein sources, as well as the use of anaerobic chambers.

Bioreactors

The effect of the microbiome can be incorporated by using *in vitro* bioreactors which utilize defined media seeded with murine or human microbiome samples (137, 153). The presence of a microbiome allows for testing of interactions between the synthetic probiotic constituents or by-products of the microbiota. This involves sensing by-products of the microbiome or affecting the constituents of the microbiome. Additionally, it provides a competitive environment where basic stability questions of the synthetic constructs can be preliminarily investigated. There exists a range of microbiome bioreactors which may be suited for different chassis organisms. It will be important to standardize the use of particular models and verify that they reflect *in vivo* performance for specific chassis organisms by comparing parameters such as growth rate and protein production levels.

Mouse Models

As with other therapeutics, mouse models are the most effective method for testing the performance of synthetic probiotics at diagnosing and treating disease. Probiotic bacteria can be integrated into existing murine disease models to demonstrate either sensing of relevant compounds (55, 60) or alleviation of disease markers (15). In addition to testing direct interaction of the synthetic system with the host, this can demonstrate the effect of the complex gut environment on the synthetic system (51, 55, 56, 60). Additionally, it can allow for investigation of differential effects due to different environments spatially throughout the gut.

A range of microbiome models are used in mouse studies, including native, antibiotic-treated, gnotobiotic, and exogenous microbiomes. Many strains of bacteria, including most *E. coli* used in engineered gut bacteria, have difficulty competing against the native microbiota, so antibiotic treatment is used to facilitate colonization with antibiotic-resistant engineered gut bacteria. Likewise, gnotobiotic mice, which are raised in germ-free conditions and do not contain a gut microbiome, are easily colonized. However, large-scale perturbations of the gut environment may confound the study of gut-related diseases. For example, the commonly used colitis model, DSS treatment of mice, has been observed to be ineffective when conducted in the absence of a microbiome (154). Gnotobiotic mice can also be colonized with an exogenous microbiome either in the form of a defined consortium (155) or transplanted from human microbiome samples. The benefits and drawbacks of each of these models in testing engineered gut bacteria are largely unknown, making the best course of action replicating the methods traditionally used in the disease model which is being studied to allow comparison of the treatment effectiveness to more traditional therapeutic methods. Finally, pigs, whose gastrointestinal tract closely resembles that of humans, have been used to test the performance and biosafety of engineered probiotics prior to proceeding to human trials (16).

OUTLOOK

The application of tools developed by synthetic biologists to engineered gut bacteria

will result in a step change in their efficacy and complexity. The *ad hoc* genetic implementations of drug factory probiotics over the past 2 decades will be improved through the use of well-characterized, high-performance expression systems in a wide variety of chassis organisms. This will enable higher expression of therapeutic compounds in more gut-relevant probiotic organisms, increasing their therapeutic efficacy.

Initial diagnostic gut bacteria (55, 60) will be improved upon by discovering more disease-relevant sensors and by studying their localized activation *in vivo*. New sensors can be generated using bioinformatic mining of microbiome data sets coupled with high-throughput library screening in mouse models using nucleotide-based reporters. Study of the biogeographic activation of disease-relevant sensors will determine the specifics of disease activity. In addition to their clinical applications, diagnostic gut bacteria will serve as scientific tools to locally measure specific metabolites within gut models.

These advances in engineering gut bacteria will enable the creation of the first smart probiotics capable of sensing and treating human disease within the gut. The engineering design-build-test cycle will allow for continual integration of knowledge gained from the study of host-microbiome interactions, natural probiotics, and synthetic biology to iteratively build upon existing smart probiotics. This will result in the bacteria being capable of sensing multiple disease states and localized environmental signals, computing a desired course of treatment, and administering this treatment from within the human gut. Localized diagnosis and treatment will make smart bacteria more effective and safer therapeutics.

DEFINITIONS

Actuator: A molecule which changes the bacterial cell state or the state of its environment, such as metabolic enzymes or secreted signaling proteins.

Biological output: A bacterially produced molecule such as an RNA, transcription factor, or therapeutic molecule.

Cellular memory: The ability of a cell to maintain a response to a sensed input after removal of that input.

Chassis: A bacterial species used to host a synthetic DNA to create an engineered gut bacterium.

Chemical or physical inputs: The signals that an engineered bacterium detects to compute an appropriate response. Examples include traditional inducers, disease biomarkers, and quorum-signaling molecules.

Colonization: The ability of bacterial species to survive in an environment for an extended period of time without repeated oral administration.

Device: A biological system composed of one or more components which performs a specific well-defined task with inputs and outputs; this can include sensors, genetic circuits, or actuators.

Diagnostic gut bacteria: Bacteria that sense one or more biomarkers, compute that those biomarkers are present in a combination indicative of disease, and produce a reporter which can be externally measured by a clinician.

Drug factory probiotic: Bacteria engineered to constitutively produce a therapeutic molecule within the body.

Genetic circuit: A network of interacting regulatory molecules, such as transcription factors and their target promoters, that perform computations such as multi-input logic or memory to convert a chemical or physical input into a biological output.

One-component system (OCS): Cytoplasmic transcription factors that directly interact with and are allosterically modulated by chemical and physical inputs.

Retroactivity: The effect of downstream circuit component activity on the performance of upstream circuit components.

Sensor: A genetically encoded molecule, often an RNA or protein, that converts a chemical or physical input into a change in a biological signal such as kinase activity or transcription rate.

Smart probiotic: Bacteria that sense one or more biomarkers, compute that those biomarkers are present in a combination indicative of disease, and respond by delivering a precise dose of one or more appropriate therapeutics at the diseased tissue.

Two-component system (TCS): A bacterial sensing network composed of a membrane-bound or cytoplasmic sensor histidine kinase which senses a chemical or physical input and regulates a cytoplasmic response regulator that controls promoter activity.

ACKNOWLEDGMENTS

B.L. is supported by the Department of Defense, Air Force Office of Scientific Research, National Defense Science and Engineering Graduate (NDSEG) Fellowship, 32 CFR 168a. Smart probiotic research in the Tabor laboratory is supported by the Office of Naval Research Young Investigator (N00014-14-1-0487) and NSF CAREER (1553317) programs and the Welch Foundation (C-1856).

CITATION

Landry BP, Tabor JJ. 2017. Engineering diagnostic and therapeutic gut bacteria. Microbiol Spectrum 5(5):BAD-0020-2017.

REFERENCES

1. **Hosseinidoust Z, Mostaghaci B, Yasa O, Park B-W, Singh AV, Sitti M.** 2016. Bioengineered and biohybrid bacteria-based systems for drug delivery. *Adv Drug Deliv Rev* **106**(Pt A):27–44.

2. **Chien T, Doshi A, Danino T.** 2017. Advances in bacteria cancer therapies using synthetic biology. *Curr Opin Syst Biol* **5**:1–8.

3. **Sheth RU, Cabral V, Chen SP, Wang HH.** 2016. Manipulating bacterial communities by *in situ* microbiome engineering. *Trends Genet* **32:**189–200.

4. **Mimee M, Citorik RJ, Lu TK.** 2016. Microbiome therapeutics: advances and challenges. *Adv Drug Deliv Rev* **105**(Pt A):44–54.

5. **WHO.** 2006. *Probiotics in Food: Health and Nutritional Properties and Guidelines for Evaluation.* Food and Agriculture Organization of the UN, London, Ontario, Canada. http://www.fao.org/food/food-safety-quality/a-z-index/probiotics/en/

6. **Wang H, Lee I-S, Braun C, Enck P.** 2016. Effect of probiotics on central nervous system functions in animals and humans: a systematic review. *J Neurogastroenterol Motil* **22:**589–605.

7. **Choi HH, Cho Y-S.** 2016. Fecal microbiota transplantation: current applications, effectiveness, and future perspectives. *Clin Endosc* **49:**257–265.

8. **Bron PA, Kleerebezem M, Brummer R-J, Cani PD, Mercenier A, MacDonald TT, Garcia-Ródenas CL, Wells JM.** 2017. Can probiotics modulate human disease by impacting intestinal barrier function? *Br J Nutr* **117:**93–107.

9. **Bermudez-Brito M, Plaza-Díaz J, Muñoz-Quezada S, Gómez-Llorente C, Gil A.** 2012. Probiotic mechanisms of action. *Ann Nutr Metab* **61:**160–174.

10. **Sarkar A, Mandal S.** 2016. Bifidobacteria: insight into clinical outcomes and mechanisms of its probiotic action. *Microbiol Res* **192:**159–171.

11. **Rogers NJ, Mousa SA.** 2012. The shortcomings of clinical trials assessing the efficacy of probiotics in irritable bowel syndrome. *J Altern Complement Med* **18:**112–119.

12. **Holmes E, Kinross J, Gibson GR, Burcelin R, Jia W, Pettersson S, Nicholson JK.** 2012. Therapeutic modulation of microbiota-host metabolic interactions. *Sci Transl Med* **4:**137rv6.

13. **Claesen J, Fischbach MA.** 2015. Synthetic microbes as drug delivery systems. *ACS Synth Biol* **4:**358–364.

14. **Brophy JAN, Voigt CA.** 2014. Principles of genetic circuit design. *Nat Methods* **11:**508–520.

15. **Steidler L, Hans W, Schotte L, Neirynck S, Obermeier F, Falk W, Fiers W, Remaut E.** 2000. Treatment of murine colitis by *Lactococcus lactis* secreting interleukin-10. *Science* **289:**1352–1355.

16. **Steidler L, Neirynck S, Huyghebaert N, Snoeck V, Vermeire A, Goddeeris B, Cox E,** Remon JP, Remaut E. 2003. Biological containment of genetically modified *Lactococcus lactis* for intestinal delivery of human interleukin 10. *Nat Biotechnol* **21:**785–789.

17. **Braat H, Rottiers P, Hommes DW, Huyghebaert N, Remaut E, Remon JP, van Deventer SJH, Neirynck S, Peppelenbosch MP, Steidler L.** 2006. A phase I trial with transgenic bacteria expressing interleukin-10 in Crohn's disease. *Clin Gastroenterol Hepatol* **4:**754–759.

18. **Bermúdez-Humarán LG, Aubry C, Motta J-PP, Deraison C, Steidler L, Vergnolle N, Chatel J-MM, Langella P.** 2013. Engineering lactococci and lactobacilli for human health. *Curr Opin Microbiol* **16:**278–283.

19. **Vandenbroucke K, de Haard H, Beirnaert E, Dreier T, Lauwereys M, Huyck L, Van Huysse J, Demetter P, Steidler L, Remaut E, Cuvelier C, Rottiers P.** 2010. Orally administered *L. lactis* secreting an anti-TNF nanobody demonstrate efficacy in chronic colitis. *Mucosal Immunol* **3:**49–56.

20. **Intrexon Corporation.** 2016. *ActoBiotics® platform: a novel class of oral biotherapeutics.* https://www.dna.com/.

21. **Vandenbroucke K, Hans W, Van Huysse J, Neirynck S, Demetter P, Remaut E, Rottiers P, Steidler L.** 2004. Active delivery of trefoil factors by genetically modified *Lactococcus lactis* prevents and heals acute colitis in mice. *Gastroenterology* **127:**502–513.

22. **Han W, Mercenier A, Ait-Belgnaoui A, Pavan S, Lamine F, van Swam II, Kleerebezem M, Salvador-Cartier C, Hisbergues M, Bueno L, Theodorou V, Fioramonti J.** 2006. Improvement of an experimental colitis in rats by lactic acid bacteria producing superoxide dismutase. *Inflamm Bowel Dis* **12:**1044–1052.

23. **Rochat T, Bermúdez-Humarán L, Gratadoux J-J, Fourage C, Hoebler C, Corthier G, Langella P.** 2007. Anti-inflammatory effects of *Lactobacillus casei* BL23 producing or not a manganese-dependant catalase on DSS-induced colitis in mice. *Microb Cell Fact* **6:**22.

24. **Carroll IM, Andrus JM, Bruno-Bárcena JM, Klaenhammer TR, Hassan HM, Threadgill DS.** 2007. Anti-inflammatory properties of *Lactobacillus gasseri* expressing manganese superoxide dismutase using the interleukin 10-deficient mouse model of colitis. *Am J Physiol Gastrointest Liver Physiol* **293:**G729–G738.

25. **Foligne B, Dessein R, Marceau M, Poiret S, Chamaillard M, Pot B, Simonet M, Daniel C.** 2007. Prevention and treatment of colitis with *Lactococcus lactis* secreting the immunomodulatory *Yersinia* LcrV protein. *Gastroenterology* **133:**862–874.

26. **Watterlot L, Rochat T, Sokol H, Cherbuy C, Bouloufa I, Lefèvre F, Gratadoux JJ, Honvo-Hueto E, Chilmonczyk S, Blugeon S, Corthier G, Langella P, Bermúdez-Humarán LG.** 2010. Intragastric administration of a superoxide dismutase-producing recombinant Lactobacillus casei BL23 strain attenuates DSS colitis in mice. *Int J Food Microbiol* **144:**35–41.

27. **LeBlanc JG, del Carmen S, Miyoshi A, Azevedo V, Sesma F, Langella P, Bermúdez-Humarán LG, Watterlot L, Perdigon G, de Moreno de LeBlanc A.** 2011. Use of superoxide dismutase and catalase producing lactic acid bacteria in TNBS induced Crohn's disease in mice. *J Biotechnol* **151:**287–293.

28. **Motta J-P, Bermúdez-Humarán LG, Deraison C, Martin L, Rolland C, Rousset P, Boue J, Dietrich G, Chapman K, Kharrat P, Vinel J-P, Alric L, Mas E, Sallenave J-M, Langella P, Vergnolle N.** 2012. Food-grade bacteria expressing elafin protect against inflammation and restore colon homeostasis. *Sci Transl Med* **4:**158ra144.

29. **Takiishi T, Korf H, Van Belle TL, Robert S, Grieco FA, Caluwaerts S, Galleri L, Spagnuolo I, Steidler L, Van Huynegem K, Demetter P, Wasserfall C, Atkinson MA, Dotta F, Rottiers P, Gysemans C, Mathieu C.** 2012. Reversal of autoimmune diabetes by restoration of antigen-specific tolerance using genetically modified *Lactococcus lactis* in mice. *J Clin Invest* **122:** 1717–1725.

30. **Chen Z, Guo L, Zhang Y, Walzem RL, Pendergast JS, Printz RL, Morris LC, Matafonova E, Stien X, Kang L, Coulon D, McGuinness OP, Niswender KD, Davies SS.** 2014. Incorporation of therapeutically modified bacteria into gut microbiota inhibits obesity. *J Clin Invest* **124:**3391–3406.

31. **Robert S, Gysemans C, Takiishi T, Korf H, Spagnuolo I, Sebastiani G, Van Huynegem K, Steidler L, Caluwaerts S, Demetter P, Wasserfall CH, Atkinson MA, Dotta F, Rottiers P, Van Belle TL, Mathieu C.** 2014. Oral delivery of glutamic acid decarboxylase (GAD)-65 and IL10 by *Lactococcus lactis* reverses diabetes in recent-onset NOD mice. *Diabetes* **63:**2876–2887.

32. **Duan FF, Liu JH, March JC.** 2015. Engineered commensal bacteria reprogram intestinal cells into glucose-responsive insulin-secreting cells for the treatment of diabetes. *Diabetes* **64:**1794–1803.

33. **Rosberg-Cody E, Stanton C, O'Mahony L, Wall R, Shanahan F, Quigley EM, Fitzgerald GF, Ross RP.** 2011. Recombinant lactobacilli expressing linoleic acid isomerase can modu-late the fatty acid composition of host adipose tissue in mice. *Microbiology* **157:**609–615.

34. **Chen H-L, Lai Y-W, Chen C-S, Chu T-W, Lin W, Yen C-C, Lin M-F, Tu M-Y, Chen C-M.** 2010. Probiotic *Lactobacillus casei* expressing human lactoferrin elevates antibacterial activity in the gastrointestinal tract. *Biometals* **23:**543–554.

35. **Paton AW, Jennings MP, Morona R, Wang H, Focareta A, Roddam LF, Paton JC.** 2005. Recombinant probiotics for treatment and prevention of enterotoxigenic *Escherichia coli* diarrhea. *Gastroenterology* **128:**1219–1228.

36. **Koo OK, Amalaradjou MAR, Bhunia AK.** 2012. Recombinant probiotic expressing *Listeria* adhesion protein attenuates *Listeria monocytogenes* virulence *in vitro*. *PLoS One* **7:** e29277.

37. **Focareta A, Paton JC, Morona R, Cook J, Paton AW.** 2006. A recombinant probiotic for treatment and prevention of cholera. *Gastroenterology* **130:**1688–1695.

38. **Duan F, March JC.** 2010. Engineered bacterial communication prevents *Vibrio cholerae* virulence in an infant mouse model. *Proc Natl Acad Sci USA* **107:**11260–11264.

39. **Gordley RM, Bugaj LJ, Lim WA.** 2016. Modular engineering of cellular signaling proteins and networks. *Curr Opin Struct Biol* **39:**106–114.

40. **Smanski MJ, Zhou H, Claesen J, Shen B, Fischbach MA, Voigt CA.** 2016. Synthetic biology to access and expand nature's chemical diversity. *Nat Rev Microbiol* **14:**135–149.

41. **Dobrin A, Saxena P, Fussenegger M.** 2016. Synthetic biology: applying biological circuits beyond novel therapies. *Integr Biol* **8:** 409–430.

42. **Tabor JJ, Groban ES, Voigt CA.** 2009. Performance characteristics for sensors and circuits used to program *E. coli*, p 401–439. *In* Lee SY (ed), *Systems Biology and Biotechnology of* Escherichia coli. Springer, Dordrecht, The Netherlands.

43. **Olson EJ, Hartsough LA, Landry BP, Shroff R, Tabor JJ.** 2014. Characterizing bacterial gene circuit dynamics with optically programmed gene expression signals. *Nat Methods* **11:**449–455.

44. **Castillo-Hair SM, Igoshin OA, Tabor JJ.** 2015. How to train your microbe: methods for dynamically characterizing gene networks. *Curr Opin Microbiol* **24:**113–123.

45. **Ulrich LE, Koonin EV, Zhulin IB.** 2005. One-component systems dominate signal transduction in prokaryotes. *Trends Microbiol* **13:**52–56.

46. **Gupta S, Bram EE, Weiss R.** 2013. Genetically programmable pathogen sense and destroy. *ACS Synth Biol* **2:**715–723.

47. **Saeidi N, Wong CK, Lo T-MT-M, Nguyen HX, Ling H, Leong SSJ, Poh CL, Chang MW.** 2011. Engineering microbes to sense and eradicate *Pseudomonas aeruginosa*, a human pathogen. *Mol Syst Biol* 7:521.

48. **Archer EJ, Robinson AB, Süel GM.** 2012. Engineered *E. coli* that detect and respond to gut inflammation through nitric oxide sensing. *ACS Synth Biol* 1:451–457.

49. **Drouault S, Anba J, Corthier G.** 2002. *Streptococcus thermophilus* is able to produce a β-galactosidase active during its transit in the digestive tract of germ-free mice. *Appl Environ Microbiol* 68:938–941.

50. **Hamady ZZR, Scott N, Farrar MD, Lodge JPA, Holland KT, Whitehead T, Carding SR.** 2010. Xylan-regulated delivery of human keratinocyte growth factor-2 to the inflamed colon by the human anaerobic commensal bacterium *Bacteroides ovatus*. *Gut* 59:461 469.

51. **Mimee M, Tucker AC, Voigt CA, Lu TK.** 2015. Programming a human commensal bacterium, *Bacteroides thetaiotaomicron*, to sense and respond to stimuli in the murine gut microbiota. *Cell Syst* 1:62–71. (Erratum, https://doi.org/10.1016/J.CELS.2016.03.007.)

52. **Pickard JM, Maurice CF, Kinnebrew MA, Abt MC, Schenten D, Golovkina TV, Bogatyrev SR, Ismagilov RF, Pamer EG, Turnbaugh PJ, Chervonsky AV.** 2014. Rapid fucosylation of intestinal epithelium sustains host-commensal symbiosis in sickness. *Nature* 514:638–641.

53. **Gao R, Stock AM.** 2009. Biological insights from structures of two-component proteins. *Annu Rev Microbiol* 63:133–154.

54. **Galperin MY.** 2010. Diversity of structure and function of response regulator output domains. *Curr Opin Microbiol* 13:150–159.

55. **Daeffler KN-M, Galley JD, Sheth RU, Ortiz-Velez LC, Bibb CO, Shroyer NF, Britton RA, Tabor JJ.** 2017. Engineering bacterial thiosulfate and tetrathionate sensors for detecting gut inflammation. *Mol Syst Biol* 13:923.

56. **Kotula JW, Kerns SJ, Shaket LA, Siraj L, Collins JJ, Way JC, Silver PA.** 2014. Programmable bacteria detect and record an environmental signal in the mammalian gut. *Proc Natl Acad Sci USA* 111:4838–4843.

57. **Winter SE, Thiennimitr P, Winter MG, Butler BP, Huseby DL, Crawford RW, Russell JM, Bevins CL, Adams LG, Tsolis RM, Roth JR, Bäumler AJ.** 2010. Gut inflammation provides a respiratory electron acceptor for *Salmonella*. *Nature* 467:426–429.

58. **Winter SE, Lopez CA, Bäumler AJ.** 2013. The dynamics of gut-associated microbial communities during inflammation. *EMBO Rep* 14:319–327.

59. **Hensel M, Hinsley AP, Nikolaus T, Sawers G, Berks BC.** 1999. The genetic basis of tetrathionate respiration in *Salmonella typhimurium*. *Mol Microbiol* 32:275–287.

60. **Riglar DT, Giessen TW, Baym M, Kerns SJ, Niederhuber MJ, Bronson RT, Kotula JW, Gerber GK, Way JC, Silver PA.** 2017. Engineered bacteria can function in the mammalian gut long-term as live diagnostics of inflammation. *Nat Biotechnol* 35:653–658.

61. **Siuti P, Yazbek J, Lu TK.** 2013. Synthetic circuits integrating logic and memory in living cells. *Nat Biotechnol* 31:448–452.

62. **Yang L, Nielsen AAK, Fernandez-Rodriguez J, McClune CJ, Laub MT, Lu TK, Voigt CA.** 2014. Permanent genetic memory with >1-byte capacity. *Nat Methods* 11:1261–1266.

63. **Duan F, Curtis KL, March JC.** 2008. Secretion of insulinotropic proteins by commensal bacteria: rewiring the gut to treat diabetes. *Appl Environ Microbiol* 74:7437–7438.

64. **Castagliuolo I, Beggiao E, Brun P, Barzon L, Goussard S, Manganelli R, Grillot-Courvalin C, Palù G.** 2005. Engineered *E. coli* delivers therapeutic genes to the colonic mucosa. *Gene Ther* 12:1070–1078.

65. **Myhrvold C, Kotula JW, Hicks WM, Conway NJ, Silver PA.** 2015. A distributed cell division counter reveals growth dynamics in the gut microbiota. *Nat Commun* 6:10039.

66. **Huttenhower C, et al, Human Microbiome Project Consortium.** 2012. Structure, function and diversity of the healthy human microbiome. *Nature* 486:207–214.

67. **Huibregtse IL, Snoeck V, de Creus A, Braat H, De Jong EC, Van Deventer SJH, Rottiers P.** 2007. Induction of ovalbumin-specific tolerance by oral administration of *Lactococcus lactis* secreting ovalbumin. *Gastroenterology* 133:517–528.

68. **Huibregtse IL, Marietta EV, Rashtak S, Koning F, Rottiers P, David CS, van Deventer SJH, Murray JA.** 2009. Induction of antigen-specific tolerance by oral administration of *Lactococcus lactis* delivered immunodominant DQ8-restricted gliadin peptide in sensitized nonobese diabetic Abo Dq8 transgenic mice. *J Immunol* 183:2390–2396.

69. **Caluwaerts S, Vandenbroucke K, Steidler L, Neirynck S, Vanhoenacker P, Corveleyn S, Watkins B, Sonis S, Coulie B, Rottiers P.** 2010. AG013, a mouth rinse formulation of *Lactococcus lactis* secreting human trefoil factor 1, provides a safe and efficacious therapeutic tool for treating oral mucositis. *Oral Oncol* 46:564–570.

70. **Pontes DS, de Azevedo MSP, Chatel J-M, Langella P, Azevedo V, Miyoshi A.** 2011. *Lactococcus lactis* as a live vector: heterologous protein production and DNA delivery systems. *Protein Expr Purif* **79:**165–175.

71. **Conrad K, Roggenbuck D, Laass MW.** 2014. Diagnosis and classification of ulcerative colitis. *Autoimmun Rev* **13:**463–466.

72. **Donaldson GP, Lee SM, Mazmanian SK.** 2016. Gut biogeography of the bacterial microbiota. *Nat Rev Microbiol* **14:**20–32.

73. **Schultz M, Watzl S, Oelschlaeger TA, Rath HC, Göttl C, Lehn N, Schölmerich J, Linde HJ.** 2005. Green fluorescent protein for detection of the probiotic microorganism *Escherichia coli* strain Nissle 1917 (EcN) *in vivo*. *J Microbiol Methods* **61:**389–398.

74. **Spees AM, Wangdi T, Lopez CA, Kingsbury DD, Xavier MN, Winter SE, Tsolis RM, Bäumler AJ.** 2013. Streptomycin-induced inflammation enhances *Escherichia coli* gut colonization through nitrate respiration. *MBio* **4:**e00430-13.

75. **Kamada N, Chen GY, Inohara N, Núñez G.** 2013. Control of pathogens and pathobionts by the gut microbiota. *Nat Immunol* **14:**685–690.

76. **Shetty RP, Endy D, Knight TF Jr.** 2008. Engineering BioBrick vectors from BioBrick parts. *J Biol Eng* **2:**5.

77. **St-Pierre F, Cui L, Priest DG, Endy D, Dodd IB, Shearwin KE.** 2013. One-step cloning and chromosomal integration of DNA. *ACS Synth Biol* **2:**537–541.

78. **Kelly JR, Rubin AJ, Davis JH, Ajo-Franklin CM, Cumbers J, Czar MJ, de Mora K, Glieberman AL, Monie DD, Endy D.** 2009. Measuring the activity of BioBrick promoters using an *in vivo* reference standard. *J Biol Eng* **3:**4.

79. **Mutalik VK, Guimaraes JC, Cambray G, Lam C, Christoffersen MJ, Mai Q-A, Tran AB, Paull M, Keasling JD, Arkin AP, Endy D.** 2013. Precise and reliable gene expression via standard transcription and translation initiation elements. *Nat Methods* **10:**354–360.

80. **Lutz R, Bujard H.** 1997. Independent and tight regulation of transcriptional units in *Escherichia coli* via the LacR/O, the TetR/O and AraC/I1-I2 regulatory elements. *Nucleic Acids Res* **25:**1203–1210.

81. **Cox RS III, Surette MG, Elowitz MB.** 2007. Programming gene expression with combinatorial promoters. *Mol Syst Biol* **3:**145.

82. **Chen Y-J, Liu P, Nielsen AAK, Brophy JAN, Clancy K, Peterson T, Voigt CA.** 2013. Characterization of 582 natural and synthetic terminators and quantification of their design constraints. *Nat Methods* **10:**659–664.

83. **Cambray G, Guimaraes JC, Mutalik VK, Lam C, Mai Q-A, Thimmaiah T, Carothers JM, Arkin AP, Endy D.** 2013. Measurement and modeling of intrinsic transcription terminators. *Nucleic Acids Res* **41:**5139–5148.

84. **Salis HM, Mirsky EA, Voigt CA.** 2009. Automated design of synthetic ribosome binding sites to control protein expression. *Nat Biotechnol* **27:**946–950.

85. **Espah Borujeni A, Channarasappa AS, Salis HM.** 2014. Translation rate is controlled by coupled trade-offs between site accessibility, selective RNA unfolding and sliding at upstream standby sites. *Nucleic Acids Res* **42:**2646–2659.

86. **Farasat I, Kushwaha M, Collens J, Easterbrook M, Guido M, Salis HM.** 2014. Efficient search, mapping, and optimization of multi-protein genetic systems in diverse bacteria. *Mol Syst Biol* **10:**731.

87. **Yoon SH, Kim SK, Kim JF.** 2010. Secretory production of recombinant proteins in *Escherichia coli*. *Recent Pat Biotechnol* **4:**23–29.

88. **Andersen JB, Sternberg C, Poulsen LK, Bjørn SP, Givskov M, Molin S.** 1998. New unstable variants of green fluorescent protein for studies of transient gene expression in bacteria. *Appl Environ Microbiol* **64:**2240–2246.

89. **Wang J, Shoemaker NB, Wang GR, Salyers AA.** 2000. Characterization of a *Bacteroides* mobilizable transposon, NBU2, which carries a functional lincomycin resistance gene. *J Bacteriol* **182:**3559–3571.

90. **Bosma EF, Forster J, Nielsen AT.** 2017. Lactobacilli and pediococci as versatile cell factories: evaluation of strain properties and genetic tools. *Biotechnol Adv* **35:**419–442.

91. **Mierau I, Kleerebezem M.** 2005. 10 years of the nisin-controlled gene expression system (NICE) in *Lactococcus lactis*. *Appl Microbiol Biotechnol* **68:**705–717.

92. **Karlskås IL, Maudal K, Axelsson L, Rud I, Eijsink VGH, Mathiesen G.** 2014. Heterologous protein secretion in lactobacilli with modified pSIP vectors. *PLoS One* **9:**e91125.

93. **Heiss S, Hörmann A, Tauer C, Sonnleitner M, Egger E, Grabherr R, Heinl S.** 2016. Evaluation of novel inducible promoter/repressor systems for recombinant protein expression in *Lactobacillus plantarum*. *Microb Cell Fact* **15:**50.

94. **Rud I, Jensen PR, Naterstad K, Axelsson L.** 2006. A synthetic promoter library for constitutive gene expression in *Lactobacillus plantarum*. *Microbiology* **152:**1011–1019.

95. **van Pijkeren JP, Britton RA.** 2014. Precision genome engineering in lactic acid bacteria. *Microb Cell Fact* **13**(Suppl 1):S10.

96. **Oh JH, van Pijkeren JP.** 2014. CRISPR-Cas9-assisted recombineering in *Lactobacillus reuteri. Nucleic Acids Res* **42**:e131.

97. **Chan LY, Kosuri S, Endy D.** 2005. Refactoring bacteriophage T7. *Mol Syst Biol* **1**:2005.0018.

98. **Temme K, Zhao D, Voigt CA.** 2012. Refactoring the nitrogen fixation gene cluster from *Klebsiella oxytoca. Proc Natl Acad Sci USA* **109**: 7085–7090.

99. **Zhou H, Vonk B, Roubos JA, Bovenberg RAL, Voigt CA.** 2015. Algorithmic co-optimization of genetic constructs and growth conditions: application to 6-ACA, a potential nylon-6 precursor. *Nucleic Acids Res* **43**:10560–10570.

100. **Burén S, Young EM, Sweeny EA, Lopez-Torrejón G, Veldhuizen M, Voigt CA, Rubio LM.** 2017. Formation of nitrogenase NifDK tetramers in the mitochondria of *Saccharomyces cerevisiae. ACS Synth Biol* **6**:1043–1055.

101. **Tabor JJ, Levskaya A, Voigt CA.** 2011. Multichromatic control of gene expression in *Escherichia coli. J Mol Biol* **405**:315–324.

102. **Ramakrishnan P, Tabor JJ.** 2016. Repurposing synechocystis PCC6803 UirS-UirR as a UV-violet/green photoreversible transcriptional regulatory tool in *E. coli. ACS Synth Biol* **5**:733–740.

103. **Schmidl SR, Sheth RU, Wu A, Tabor JJ.** 2014. Refactoring and optimization of light-switchable *Escherichia coli* two-component systems. *ACS Synth Biol* **3**:820–831.

104. **Stanton BC, Nielsen AAK, Tamsir A, Clancy K, Peterson T, Voigt CA.** 2014. Genomic mining of prokaryotic repressors for orthogonal logic gates. *Nat Chem Biol* **10**:99–105.

105. **Stanton BC, Siciliano V, Ghodasara A, Wroblewska L, Clancy K, Trefzer AC, Chesnut JD, Weiss R, Voigt CA.** 2014. Systematic transfer of prokaryotic sensors and circuits to mammalian cells. *ACS Synth Biol* **3**:880–891.

106. **Beal J.** 2015. Signal-to-noise ratio measures efficacy of biological computing devices and circuits. *Front Bioeng Biotechnol* **3**:93.

107. **Shinar G, Milo R, Martínez MR, Alon U.** 2007. Input output robustness in simple bacterial signaling systems. *Proc Natl Acad Sci USA* **104**:19931–19935.

108. **Rubens JR, Selvaggio G, Lu TK.** 2016. Synthetic mixed-signal computation in living cells. *Nat Commun* **7**:11658.

109. **Daniel R, Rubens JR, Sarpeshkar R, Lu TK.** 2013. Synthetic analog computation in living cells. *Nature* **497**:619–623.

110. **Rockwell NC, Martin SS, Lagarias JC.** 2012. Red/green cyanobacteriochromes: sensors of color and power. *Biochemistry* **51**:9667–9677.

111. **Rockwell NC, Martin SS, Lagarias JC.** 2016. Identification of cyanobacteriochromes detecting far-red light. *Biochemistry* **55**:3907–3919.

112. **Hermsen R, Erickson DW, Hwa T.** 2011. Speed, sensitivity, and bistability in auto-activating signaling circuits. *PLOS Comput Biol* **7**: e1002265.

113. **Lundberg JO, Govoni M.** 2004. Inorganic nitrate is a possible source for systemic generation of nitric oxide. *Free Radic Biol Med* **37**:395–400.

114. **Winter SE, Winter MG, Xavier MN, Thiennimitr P, Poon V, Keestra AM, Laughlin RC, Gomez G, Wu J, Lawhon SD, Popova IE, Parikh SJ, Adams LG, Tsolis RM, Stewart VJ, Bäumler AJ.** 2013. Host-derived nitrate boosts growth of *E. coli* in the inflamed gut. *Science* **339**:708–711.

115. **Nielsen AAK, Der BS, Shin J, Vaidyanathan P, Paralanov V, Strychalski EA, Ross D, Densmore D, Voigt CA.** 2016. Genetic circuit design automation. *Science* **352**:aac7341.

116. **Lou C, Stanton B, Chen Y-J, Munsky B, Voigt CA.** 2012. Ribozyme-based insulator parts buffer synthetic circuits from genetic context. *Nat Biotechnol* **30**:1137–1142.

117. **Qi LS, Larson MH, Gilbert LA, Doudna JA, Weissman JS, Arkin AP, Lim WA.** 2013. Repurposing CRISPR as an RNA-guided platform for sequence-specific control of gene expression. *Cell* **152**:1173–1183.

118. **Nielsen AA, Voigt CA.** 2014. Multi-input CRISPR/Cas genetic circuits that interface host regulatory networks. *Mol Syst Biol* **10**:763.

119. **Gander MW, Vrana JD, Voje WE, Carothers JM, Klavins E.** 2017. Digital logic circuits in yeast with CRISPR-dCas9 NOR gates. *Nat Commun* **8**:15459.

120. **Del Vecchio D.** 2015. Modularity, context-dependence, and insulation in engineered biological circuits. *Trends Biotechnol* **33**:111–119.

121. **Bradley RW, Buck M, Wang B.** 2016. Recognizing and engineering digital-like logic gates and switches in gene regulatory networks. *Curr Opin Microbiol* **33**:74–82.

122. **Lucks JB, Qi L, Mutalik VK, Wang D, Arkin AP.** 2011. Versatile RNA-sensing transcriptional regulators for engineering genetic networks. *Proc Natl Acad Sci USA* **108**:8617–8622.

123. **Chappell J, Takahashi MK, Lucks JB.** 2015. Creating small transcription activating RNAs. *Nat Chem Biol* **11**:214–220.

124. **Westbrook AM, Lucks JB.** 2017. Achieving large dynamic range control of gene expression with a compact RNA transcription-translation regulator. *Nucleic Acids Res* **45**:5614–5624.

125. **Argos P, et al.** 1986. The integrase family of site-specific recombinases: regional similarities and global diversity. *EMBO J* **5**:433–440.

126. **Friedland AE, Lu TK, Wang X, Shi D, Church G, Collins JJ.** 2009. Synthetic gene networks that count. *Science* **324**:1199–1202.

127. **Bonnet J, Yin P, Ortiz ME, Subsoontorn P, Endy D.** 2013. Amplifying genetic logic gates. *Science* **340**:599–603.

128. **Roquet N, Soleimany AP, Ferris AC, Aaronson S, Lu TK.** 2016. Synthetic recombinase-based state machines in living cells. *Science* **353**: aad8559.

129. **Bonnet J, Subsoontorn P, Endy D.** 2012. Rewritable digital data storage in live cells via engineered control of recombination directionality. *Proc Natl Acad Sci USA* **109**:8884–8889.

130. **Daniel C, Poiret S, Dennin V, Boutillier D, Pot B.** 2013. Bioluminescence imaging study of spatial and temporal persistence of *Lactobacillus plantarum* and *Lactococcus lactis* in living mice. *Appl Environ Microbiol* **79**:1086–1094.

131. **Alon U.** 2006. *An Introduction to Systems Biology: Design Principles of Biological Circuits.* CRC Press, Boca Raton, FL.

132. **Moon TS, Lou C, Tamsir A, Stanton BC, Voigt CA.** 2012. Genetic programs constructed from layered logic gates in single cells. *Nature* **491**:249–253.

133. **Prindle A, Selimkhanov J, Li H, Razinkov I, Tsimring LS, Hasty J.** 2014. Rapid and tunable post-translational coupling of genetic circuits. *Nature* **508**:387–391.

134. **Cookson NA, Mather WH, Danino T, Mondragón-Palomino O, Williams RJ, Tsimring LS, Hasty J.** 2011. Queueing up for enzymatic processing: correlated signaling through coupled degradation. *Mol Syst Biol* **7**:561.

135. **Cameron DE, Collins JJ.** 2014. Tunable protein degradation in bacteria. *Nat Biotechnol* **32**:1276–1281.

136. **Takahashi MK, Chappell J, Hayes CA, Sun ZZ, Kim J, Singhal V, Spring KJ, Al-Khabouri S, Fall CP, Noireaux V, Murray RM, Lucks JB.** 2015. Rapidly characterizing the fast dynamics of RNA genetic circuitry with cell-free transcription-translation (TX-TL) systems. *ACS Synth Biol* **4**:503–515.

137. **Moser F, Broers NJ, Hartmans S, Tamsir A, Kerkman R, Roubos JA, Bovenberg R, Voigt CA.** 2012. Genetic circuit performance under conditions relevant for industrial bioreactors. *ACS Synth Biol* **1**:555–564.

138. **Tropini C, Earle KA, Huang KC, Sonnenburg JL.** 2017. The gut microbiome: connecting spatial organization to function. *Cell Host Microbe* **21**:433–442.

139. **Klumpp S, Hwa T.** 2014. Bacterial growth: global effects on gene expression, growth feedback and proteome partition. *Curr Opin Biotechnol* **28**:96–102.

140. **Shopera T, He L, Oyetunde T, Tang YJ, Moon TS.** 2017. Decoupling resource-coupled gene expression in living cells. *ACS Synth Biol* **6**:1596–1604.

141. **Salvado B, Vilaprinyo E, Sorribas A, Alves R.** 2015. A survey of HK, HPt, and RR domains and their organization in two-component systems and phosphorelay proteins of organisms with fully sequenced genomes. *PeerJ* **3**:e1183.

142. **Long T, Tu KC, Wang Y, Mehta P, Ong NP, Bassler BL, Wingreen NS.** 2009. Quantifying the integration of quorum-sensing signals with single-cell resolution. *PLoS Biol* **7**:e1000068.

143. **Walthers D, Tran VK, Kenney LJ.** 2003. Interdomain linkers of homologous response regulators determine their mechanism of action. *J Bacteriol* **185**:317–324.

144. **Nakajima M, Ferri S, Rögner M, Sode K.** 2016. Construction of a miniaturized chromatic acclimation sensor from cyanobacteria with reversed response to a light signal. *Sci Rep* **6**:37595.

145. **Gardner TS, Cantor CR, Collins JJ.** 2000. Construction of a genetic toggle switch in *Escherichia coli*. *Nature* **403**:339–342.

146. **Kobayashi H, Kaern M, Araki M, Chung K, Gardner TS, Cantor CR, Collins JJ.** 2004. Programmable cells: interfacing natural and engineered gene networks. *Proc Natl Acad Sci USA* **101**:8414–8419.

147. **Ptashne M.** 2004. *A Genetic Switch Phage Lambda Revisited.* Cold Spring Harbor Laboratory Press, Cold Spring Harbor, NY.

148. **Junjua M, Galia W, Gaci N, Uriot O, Genay M, Bachmann H, Kleerebezem M, Dary A, Roussel Y.** 2014. Development of the recombinase-based *in vivo* expression technology in *Streptococcus thermophilus* and validation using the lactose operon promoter. *J Appl Microbiol* **116**: 620–631.

149. **Farzadfard F, Lu TK.** 2014. Genomically encoded analog memory with precise *in vivo* DNA writing in living cell populations. *Science* **346**:1256272.

150. **Horwitz JP, Chua J, Curby RJ, Tomson AJ, Darooge MA, Fisher BE, Mauricio J, Klundt I.** 1964. Substrates for cytochemical demonstration of enzyme activity. I. Some substituted 3-indolyl-β-D-glycopyranosides. *J Med Chem* **7**:574–575.

151. **Corthier G, Delorme C, Ehrlich SD, Renault P.** 1998. Use of luciferase genes as biosensors

to study bacterial physiology in the digestive tract. *Appl Environ Microbiol* **64:**2721–2722.

152. **Kosuri S, Goodman DB, Cambray G, Mutalik VK, Gao Y, Arkin AP, Endy D, Church GM.** 2013. Composability of regulatory sequences controlling transcription and translation in *Escherichia coli. Proc Natl Acad Sci USA* **110:** 14024–14029.

153. **Auchtung JM, Robinson CD, Farrell K, Britton RA.** 2016. Minibioreactor arrays (MBRAs) as a tool for studying *C. difficile* physiology in the presence of a complex community. *Methods Mol Biol* **1476:**235–258.

154. **Chassaing B, Aitken JD, Malleshappa M, Vijay-Kumar M.** 2014. Dextran sulfate sodium (DSS)-induced colitis in mice. *Curr Protoc Immunol* **104:**Unit 15.25.

155. **Bucci V, Tzen B, Li N, Simmons M, Tanoue T, Bogart E, Deng L, Yeliseyev V, Delaney ML, Liu Q, Olle B, Stein RR, Honda K, Bry L, Gerber GK.** 2016. MDSINE: Microbial

Dynamical Systems INference Engine for microbiome time-series analyses. *Genome Biol* **17:**121.

156. **Farrar MD, Whitehead TR, Lan J, Dilger P, Thorpe R, Holland KT, Carding SR.** 2005. Engineering of the gut commensal bacterium *Bacteroides ovatus* to produce and secrete biologically active murine interleukin-2 in response to xylan. *J Appl Microbiol* **98:**1191–1197.

157. **Hamady ZZR, Scott N, Farrar MD, Wadhwa M, Dilger P, Whitehead TR, Thorpe R, Holland KT, Lodge JPA, Carding SR.** 2011. Treatment of colitis with a commensal gut bacterium engineered to secrete human TGF-β1 under the control of dietary xylan I. *Inflamm Bowel Dis* **17:**1925–1935.

158. **Ng DTW, Sarkar CA.** 2011. Nisin-inducible secretion of a biologically active single-chain insulin analog by *Lactococcus lactis* NZ9000. *Biotechnol Bioeng* **108:**1987–1996.

Use of Traditional and Genetically Modified Probiotics in Human Health: What Does the Future Hold?

15

LUIS G. BERMÚDEZ-HUMARÁN[1] and PHILIPPE LANGELLA[1]

INTRODUCTION

Advances in recombinant technology (e.g., genetic engineering) and in the understanding of the human immune system have led to prodigious advances in the development of novel delivery systems for mucosal administration (1, 2). The administration of therapeutic molecules through mucosal routes offers several important advantages over conventional strategies (i.e., systemic injection) such as reduction of secondary effects, easy administration, and the possibility to modulate both systemic and mucosal immune responses (3). Moreover, it is important for molecules of health interest that exert their effects at mucosal surfaces, the gastrointestinal tract (GIT), for example, to be delivered directly to the appropriate site. Nonetheless, a major disadvantage of the mucosal route of administration is that the actual amount of protein to be administered needs to be large due to the very small quantities of protein that survive degradation at mucosal surfaces such as the GIT (1, 3).

It is becoming increasingly apparent that alternative approaches to conventional mucosal delivery systems (e.g., inert systems such as liposomes or nanoparticles and live attenuated bacterial or viral vectors) are required to control diseases in humans in the 21st century. The design of novel approaches combining genetic engineering and probiotic bacteria that allow precise

[1]Micalis Institute, INRA, AgroParisTech, Université Paris-Saclay, 78350 Jouy-en-Josas, France
Bugs as Drugs: Therapeutic Microbes for the Prevention and Treatment of Disease
Edited by Robert A. Britton and Patrice D. Cani
© 2018 American Society for Microbiology, Washington, DC
doi:10.1128/microbiolspec.BAD-0016-2016

targeting of molecules of health interest to the mucosa can represent an attractive alternative to attenuated pathogenic vectors (1, 4). Hence, the generation and use of such genetically modified probiotics (GMPs), expressing therapeutic molecules, can offer the opportunity to further investigate their effects for food, nutrition, environment, and health.

PROBIOTICS AND HUMAN HEALTH

The word "probiotic" is derived from Greek and means "for life" and was introduced in 1953 by Werner Kollath. Probiotics are defined as "live microorganisms that, when administered in adequate amounts, confer a health benefit on the host" (reference 5, p 11). The probiotic concept was born in the beginning of the 20th century (1906) when Henry Tissier (a French pediatrician at the Pasteur Institute, Paris) reported clinical benefits in treating diarrhea in children with bifidobacteria (initially called *Bacillus bifidus communis*), a dominant genus in the gut microbiota of breast-fed babies (6). The claimed effect was a displacement of pathogenic bacteria by bifidobacteria (6). Then, Elie Metchnikoff (a Russian microbiologist who received the Nobel Prize in Physiology or Medicine in 1908) issued the following hypothesis: the longevity of Bulgarians is associated with their high consumption of fermented foods, and particularly with the live lactic acid bacteria (LAB) they contain (6). Two major concepts arose from his observations: (i) live bacteria that interact with humans can have beneficial effects, and (ii) these bacteria and their host have developed sophisticated cross-talk strategies which allow them to combine efforts to maintain or restore host health. Finally, in 1965, Lilly and Stilwell proposed the use of probiotics to enhance intestinal health (6).

Today, numerous bacteria are used as probiotics, and the most common strains belong to *Bifidobacterium* and *Lactobacillus* spp. Some species of these genera are natural inhabitants of the GIT, where they favorably influence intestinal microbiota homeostasis by inhibiting growth of harmful bacteria, maintaining a good epithelial barrier homeostasis, and promoting efficient food digestion, among other beneficial effects (7). However, commercial abuse of the term "probiotic" has become a major issue, with many products exploiting the term without meeting the requisite criteria. Moreover, probiotic products have received the legitimate attention of regulatory authorities that have an interest in protecting consumers from misleading claims. So far, the only approved probiotic claim by the European Food Safety Authority (EFSA) currently relates to improved lactose digestion through the action of the yogurt starters *Lactobacillus delbrueckii* subsp. *bulgaricus* and *Streptococcus salivarius* subsp. *thermophilus* (8). Indeed, many people who have congenital lactase (the enzyme that degrades lactose) deficiency do not tolerate this sugar (which is abundant in milk products). Clinical manifestations include diarrhea, abdominal colic, and flatulence. Interestingly, these symptoms appear with milk ingestion but are basically absent when yogurt is ingested. Thus, the EFSA has approved a health claim for *L. delbrueckii* subsp. *bulgaricus* and *S. salivarius* subsp. *thermophilus* in helping lactose digestion (8). This claim has been accepted because the mode of action is clearly understood and is due to the bacterial production of β-galactosidase, which degrades lactose in both the yogurt and in the gut. However, with the advances of the technology and the "omics" era (e.g., metagenomics, metabolomics, proteomics, etc.), as well as with the establishment of well-controlled pre- and clinical trials, novel probiotic claims (other than lactose digestion) will certainly be approved in the next few years. In the following paragraphs, we will briefly describe some beneficial effects of different probiotic strains to treat human diseases, particularly gastrointestinal disorders.

An important use of probiotics is the protection against pathogens. Indeed, probiotics might function as a physical barrier, impeding the colonization of the GIT by pathogenic bacteria. The most notable results have been obtained with some species of lactobacilli and bifidobacteria, which have been found to be particularly effective in treating diarrhea in newborns (9). Modulation of host immunity and promotion of host defense are the other most commonly supported benefits of probiotic consumption (7). The probiotic preparation VSL#3, which contains a mixture of eight bacteria, including lactobacilli and bifidobacteria species, has been shown to display anti-inflammatory properties, as well as protective effects in a murine model of intestinal inflammation (10). In this context, human clinical trial results have confirmed various therapeutic effects of such selected strains of probiotics in inflammatory bowel diseases (IBDs), notably VSL#3 in pouchitis patients (11), *Escherichia coli* Nissle 1917 in ulcerative colitis patients (12), and *Lactobacillus salivarius* UCC4331 and *Bifidobacterium infantis* 35624 strains in irritable bowel syndrome (IBS) (13). Oral administration of a strain of *Lactobacillus plantarum* to interleukin (IL) 10 knockout mice attenuates the severity of the spontaneous colitis in these mice (14). Recent studies in preclinical murine models have also shown that *Lactobacillus casei* BL23 can stimulate systemic immunity and protect against intestinal inflammation (20) as well as colorectal cancer (15). *Bifidobacterium animalis* subsp. *lactis* CNCM I-2494, a probiotic strain with a long background of use in fermented dairy products (16), was able to restore gut barrier permeability in gut inflammation (17). Finally, *L. casei* has been found to be capable of stimulating an immune response in children who take an oral vaccine against rotavirus, which causes acute diarrhea in infants and young children in developing countries (18).

Probiotics can also act by reducing oxidative stress, which is characterized by an uncontrolled increase in the concentration of reactive oxidative species in the GIT, a phenomenon frequently observed in IBD patients

(19). Hence, some studies have shown the potential effect of different probiotic strains in the treatment of IBD using a variety of animal models (20–22). Also, *Lactobacillus rhamnosus* CNCM I-3690, selected for its antioxidant properties *in vitro* (23), has shown anti-inflammatory activities in a colitis murine model as well as protective effects to induced barrier hyperpermeability in mice (24).

Altogether, these results confirm the potential of probiotics to regulate the host immune system and suggest complex crosstalk between the host and bacteria.

USE OF GMPs TO PREVENT AND TO TREAT HUMAN DISEASES

Considering the need to develop novel effective strategies for the delivery of therapeutic molecules at mucosal surfaces, Gram-positive LAB have emerged as attractive vehicles for the oral, intranasal, vaginal, and rectal delivery of such molecules at the end of the 20th century. Indeed, the potential of these bacteria to act as live mucosal vehicles, in particular, food-grade *Lactococcus lactis* strains, has been intensively investigated in the past 2 decades (25). Strikingly, these GM lactococci have been successfully used as vectors to deliver functional proteins at the mucosal level in preclinical studies using murine models, reproducing different human pathologies such as IBD, IBS, obesity, diabetes, and cancer (1). Since probiotic therapy is mainly focused on modulation of host immunity and promotion of host defense (see above), we can assume that GMPs are potential attractive candidates to deliver molecules of therapeutic interest to mucosal surfaces to prevent and to treat human diseases. Interestingly, the administration of such GMPs would allow a significant reduction in the treatments' costs, a reduction of secondary effects, easy administration, and the possibility to modulate both systemic and mucosal immune responses. Oral administration is definitely the most common and convenient route of drug administration because of its simplicity, noninvasive nature, and low discomfort levels for patients. In addition, this route displays efficient therapeutic effects for certain disorders of the GIT such as IBD or IBS.

As previously stated, *L. lactis* has been the LAB most widely genetically engineered for the production and delivery of therapeutic molecules thus far. In addition, phase I and II clinical trials using GM strains of *L. lactis* secreting either IL-10 (26) or TTF (27) to treat Crohn's disease and mucositis patients, respectively, have opened up new horizons in the use of GMPs in humans. Unfortunately, despite all the considerable and impressive work done using *L. lactis* as a live delivery vector, this bacterium has some drawbacks because of its very short survival time in the GIT and its lack of intrinsic immune-modulatory properties in contrast to lactobacilli which can persist longer in the GIT and possess interesting immune-modulatory properties such as anti-inflammatory activities (20, 28); these properties could enhance the anti-inflammatory potential of a GM strain in the context of IBD therapy, or pro-inflammatory activities, an interesting feature that could be exploited in the context of vaccination against a pathogen (e.g., adjuvant effect) (28). Thus, two other genera which have been subjected to recent investigations for heterologous expression of proteins of medical interest are *Bifidobacterium* and *Lactobacillus* spp. Indeed, the use of GM lactobacilli or bifidobacteria to produce and deliver recombinant proteins is an interesting and growing field of research, since these genera present several advantages compared to *L. lactis* when used as live mucosal vehicles, such as an increased persistence in the GIT and the immune-modulatory properties of some strains.

As mentioned previously, IBD is frequently associated with oxidative stress and epithelial damage; hence, GMPs delivering antioxidant enzymes can be an attractive preventive and therapeutic tool. Therefore, one strategy to

prevent and treat intestinal inflammation is the use of GMPs to deliver antioxidant enzymes such as catalase, glutathione peroxidase, glutathione reductase, glutathione-S-transferase, or superoxide dismutase (SOD), which may be able to reduce reactive oxidative species concentrations in the GIT. A GM strain of *Lactobacillus gasseri* that produces SOD has been shown to exhibit anti-inflammatory effects in an IL-10-deficient mouse colitis model (29). In addition, GM strains of *L. casei* BL23 that produce either SOD or a manganese-dependent catalase were shown to display protective effects against reactive oxidative species and intestinal inflammation in mice (20, 30). Another well-designed study demonstrated that a mix of two GM strains of *Streptococcus thermophilus* CRL807 (a bacterium previously used as a starter to prepare a yogurt) with anti-inflammatory and anticancer properties, producing either catalase or SOD enzymes, displays higher anti-inflammatory effects than the wild-type counterpart strain in a murine model of colitis (31).

Recent studies have shown the important role of proteases and their endogenous inhibitors in the pathology of IBD (32). In this context, oral administration of a GM strain of *L. casei* BL23 that produces elafin, an endogenous protease inhibitor found in the human gut (33), prevents inflammation, accelerates mucosal healing, and restores colon homeostasis in different colitis models in mice (33). These encouraging results suggest that there may be a potential clinical application of GMP delivering elafin for IBD prevention and treatment in the future.

Bifidobacterium is another genus recently exploited as a GMP for drug delivery. The preliminary studies reporting the use of GM *Bifidobacterium* spp. to deliver drugs were by intravenous or systemic administration, rather than oral administration, to treat solid tumors in different animal models (34). The use of these methods was undoubtedly due to the ability of this genus to migrate from vascularized sites toward the tumors. This selective migration was attributed to the preference of *Bifidobacterium* spp. for anaerobic sites such as the hypoxic microenvironment found in solid tumors (34). It was not until a few years ago that the ability of a GM *Bifidobacterium longum* strain to deliver an anti-inflammatory molecule (i.e., IL-10 cytokine) was evaluated after oral administration in inflamed mice (35, 36). More recently, a study showed that oral administration with a GM *B. longum* strain expressing alpha-melanocyte-stimulating hormone (α-MSH) is efficient to treat colitis in mice (46). These results suggest an alternative approach to treat IBD by using GMP as a live vector to deliver α-MSH.

IS THERE A NEED FOR THE USE OF GMPs IN HUMANS?

The case of the anti-inflammatory IL-10 for the treatment of IBD, a common denominator for diseases such as Crohn's disease and ulcerative colitis, is illustrative of the real need for the use of GMP in humans. IBD is a damaging chronic intestinal inflammation caused by a breach of tolerance for intestinal microbiota. IBD requires lifelong medication, having both fundamental medical as well as economic consequences. To make IBD treatment work, it is crucial to develop cheap and easy-to-administer therapeutics that are devoid of side effects. IL-10 was initially considered a good candidate for such IBD therapy. However, when IL-10 is applied by injection, side effects are induced that impede long-term use at elevated concentrations (37). The use of GM *L. lactis* for localized IL-10 synthesis may circumvent these fundamental obstacles. Delivery at the intestine of IL-10 by GM *L. lactis* treats or prevents IBD in mice (26).

In the same vein, intravenous administration with anti-tumor necrosis factor alpha (TNF-α) antibodies (e.g., infliximab, a human-murine chimeric monoclonal antibody that blocks the action of TNF-α) proved to be a breakthrough for IBD patients. However, although repetitive administrations of these antibodies can be effective, the treatment is costly, and it can be complicated by loss of response and associated with side effects (38, 39). Because several of these undesirable outcomes are associated with systemic application (i.e., intravenous injection), they might be solved by the use of a GM microorganism for local delivery of anti-TNF-α antibodies (40) (as for IL-10 cytokine).

Altogether, these studies show the interest in the use of GM *L. lactis* strains for local delivery of therapeutic molecules, and although there is no scientific evidence to support that these GM microorganisms are dangerous for human administration, it is indispensable to clearly demonstrate that it is safe to use such GMP strains.

CONCLUSIONS AND PERSPECTIVES

The results obtained in a phase I clinical trial conducted with a recombinant strain of *L. lactis* that produces IL-10 cytokine (see above and reference 41) revealed not only that the containment strategy used to construct this recombinant strain was safe and effective, but that local delivery of IL-10 to mucosal surfaces by a GM organism is also feasible in humans (42). Moreover, a phase IIa clinical trial in patients suffering from Crohn's disease confirmed that the main primary endpoints of the study using this GM *L. lactis* strain expressing human IL-10 (named AG011) were achieved: safety and tolerability of the recombinant strain, environmental containment of the GM organism, and assessment of biomarkers associated with the strain. Unfortunately, concerning the endpoints of the evolution of the disease, the clinical results did not reveal a statistically significant difference in mucosal healing compared to the placebo group. Thus, we can envisage how ongoing work in different areas will help to improve the use of GM strains on human health, such as the use of more persistent LAB species (e.g., lactobacilli), the expression system to increase the quantities of the molecule delivered *in situ*, and the use of combinations of recombinant strains producing different types of therapeutic molecules (for review see reference 1). Such strategies should be tested in human clinical trials. Hence, a new phase Ib clinical trial using a GM strain of *L. lactis* expressing another therapeutic molecule, the human trefoil factor 1 (27), named AG013, showed that this GM organism was safe and well tolerated in patients with oral mucositis, an important inflammation and ulceration of the membranes covering the oral cavity, throat, and esophagus and among the most commonly reported adverse events associated with cancer chemotherapy. Strikingly, preliminary data demonstrated positive efficacy of this GM strain of *L. lactis* against oral mucositis in 25 patients compared to placebo (43).

In addition, a few challenges remain before potentially using GMP that expresses human elafin (e.g., recombinant lactobacilli strains) (33, 44) in clinical studies (P. Langella, personal communication). Certainly, elafin has been shown to be safe when delivered to humans (45), and GMPs have also been shown to be safe when given orally to humans (42). However, the safety of elafin-expressing GMP in humans remains to be tested, and a human clinical trial to address safety concerns will be necessary.

There is currently a large body of data in preclinical models to support the potential use of GM microorganisms as new therapies for human diseases (in particular, IBD). However, there is still a long way to go to reach the market for human use since important safety and regulatory issues still need to be addressed in depth.

CITATION

Bermúdez-Humarán LG, Langella P. 2017. Use of traditional and genetically modified probiotics in human health: what does the future hold? Microbiol Spectrum 5(5):BAD-0016-2016.

REFERENCES

1. **Bermúdez-Humarán LG, Aubry C, Motta JP, Deraison C, Steidler L, Vergnolle N, Chatel JM, Langella P.** 2013. Engineering lactococci and lactobacilli for human health. *Curr Opin Microbiol* **16:**278–283.
2. **Davitt CJ, Lavelle EC.** 2015. Delivery strategies to enhance oral vaccination against enteric infections. *Adv Drug Deliv Rev* **91:**52–69.
3. **Holmgren J, Czerkinsky C.** 2005. Mucosal immunity and vaccines. *Nat Med* **11**(Suppl): S45–S53.
4. **Bermúdez-Humarán LG, Kharrat P, Chatel JM, Langella P.** 2011. Lactococci and lactobacilli as mucosal delivery vectors for therapeutic proteins and DNA vaccines. *Microb Cell Fact* **10**(Suppl 1)**:**S4.
5. **Food and Agriculture Organization of the United Nations.** 2002. *Joint FAO/WHO Working Group report on drafting guidelines for the evaluation of probiotics in food.* Food and Agriculture Organization, London, Canada.
6. **Lilly DM, Stillwell RH.** 1965. Probiotics: growth-promoting factors produced by microorganisms. *Science* **147:**747–748.
7. **Martín R, Miquel S, Ulmer J, Kechaou N, Langella P, Bermúdez-Humarán LG.** 2013. Role of commensal and probiotic bacteria in human health: a focus on inflammatory bowel disease. *Microb Cell Fact* **12:**71.
8. **Hill C, Guarner F, Reid G, Gibson GR, Merenstein DJ, Pot B, Morelli L, Canani RB, Flint HJ, Salminen S, Calder PC, Sanders ME.** 2014. Expert consensus document. The International Scientific Association for Probiotics and Prebiotics consensus statement on the scope and appropriate use of the term probiotic. *Nat Rev Gastroenterol Hepatol* **11:**506–514.
9. **Hempel S, Newberry SJ, Maher AR, Wang Z, Miles JNV, Shanman R, Johnsen B, Shekelle PG.** 2012. Probiotics for the prevention and treatment of antibiotic-associated diarrhea: a systematic review and meta-analysis. *JAMA* **307:**1959–1969.
10. **Jijon H, Backer J, Diaz H, Yeung H, Thiel D, McKaigney C, De Simone C, Madsen K.** 2004. DNA from probiotic bacteria modulates murine and human epithelial and immune function. *Gastroenterology* **126:**1358–1373.
11. **Gionchetti P, Rizzello F, Venturi A, Brigidi P, Matteuzzi D, Bazzocchi G, Poggioli G, Miglioli M, Campieri M.** 2000. Oral bacteriotherapy

as maintenance treatment in patients with chronic pouchitis: a double-blind, placebo-controlled trial. *Gastroenterology* 119:305–309.

12. **Kruis W, Fric P, Pokrotnieks J, Lukás M, Fixa B, Kascák M, Kamm MA, Weismueller J, Beglinger C, Stolte M, Wolff C, Schulze J.** 2004. Maintaining remission of ulcerative colitis with the probiotic *Escherichia coli* Nissle 1917 is as effective as with standard mesalazine. *Gut* 53:1617–1623.

13. **O'Mahony L, McCarthy J, Kelly P, Hurley G, Luo F, Chen K, O'Sullivan GC, Kiely B, Collins JK, Shanahan F, Quigley EMM.** 2005. *Lactobacillus* and *Bifidobacterium* in irritable bowel syndrome: symptom responses and relationship to cytokine profiles. *Gastroenterology* 128:541–551.

14. **Schultz M, Veltkamp C, Dieleman LA, Grenther WB, Wyrick PB, Tonkonogy SL, Sartor RB.** 2002. *Lactobacillus plantarum* 299V in the treatment and prevention of spontaneous colitis in interleukin-10-deficient mice. *Inflamm Bowel Dis* 8:71–80.

15. **Lenoir M, Del Carmen S, Cortes-Perez NG, Lozano-Ojalvo D, Munoz-Provencio D, Chain F, Langella P, de Moreno de LeBlanc A, LeBlanc JG, Bermudez-Humaran LG.** 2016. *Lactobacillus casei* BL23 regulates Treg and Th17 T-cell populations and reduces DMH-associated colorectal cancer. *J Gastroenterol* 51:862–873.

16. **Rochet V, Rigottier-Gois L, Ledaire A, Andrieux C, Sutren M, Rabot S, Mogenet A, Bresson JL, Cools S, Picard C, Goupil-Feuillerat N, Doré J.** 2008. Survival of *Bifidobacterium animalis* DN-173 010 in the faecal microbiota after administration in lyophilised form or in fermented product: a randomised study in healthy adults. *J Mol Microbiol Biotechnol* 14:128–136.

17. **Martín R, Laval L, Chain F, Miquel S, Natividad J, Cherbuy C, Sokol H, Verdu EF, van Hylckama Vlieg J, Bermudez-Humaran LG, Smokvina T, Langella P.** 2016. *Bifidobacterium animalis* ssp. *lactis* CNCM-I2494 restores gut barrier permeability in chronically low-grade inflamed mice. *Front Microbiol* 7:608.

18. **Isolauri E, Joensuu J, Suomalainen H, Luomala M, Vesikari T.** 1995. Improved immunogenicity of oral D x RRV reassortant rotavirus vaccine by *Lactobacillus casei* GG. *Vaccine* 13:310–312.

19. **Bhattacharyya A, Chattopadhyay R, Mitra S, Crowe SE.** 2014. Oxidative stress: an essential factor in the pathogenesis of gastrointestinal mucosal diseases. *Physiol Rev* 94:329–354.

20. **Rochat T, Bermúdez-Humarán L, Gratadoux JJ, Fourage C, Hoebler C, Corthier G, Langella P.** 2007. Anti-inflammatory effects of *Lactobacillus casei* BL23 producing or not a manganese-

dependant catalase on DSS-induced colitis in mice. *Microb Cell Fact* 6:22.

21. **Santos Rocha C, Lakhdari O, Blottière HM, Blugeon S, Sokol H, Bermúdez-Humarán LG, Azevedo V, Miyoshi A, Doré J, Langella P, Maguin E, van de Guchte M.** 2012. Anti-inflammatory properties of dairy lactobacilli. *Inflamm Bowel Dis* 18:657–666.

22. **Torres-Maravilla E, Lenoir M, Mayorga-Reyes L, Allain T, Sokol H, Langella P, Sánchez-Pardo ME, Bermúdez-Humarán LG.** 2016. Identification of novel anti-inflammatory probiotic strains isolated from pulque. *Appl Microbiol Biotechnol* 100:385–396.

23. **Grompone G, Martorell P, Llopis S, González N, Genovés S, Mulet AP, Fernández-Calero T, Tiscornia I, Bollati-Fogolín M, Chambaud I, Foligné B, Montserrat A, Ramón D.** 2012. Anti-inflammatory *Lactobacillus rhamnosus* CNCM I-3690 strain protects against oxidative stress and increases lifespan in *Caenorhabditis elegans*. *PLoS One* 7:e52493.

24. **Laval L, Martin R, Natividad JN, Chain F, Miquel S, Descléc de Maredsous C, Capronnier S, Sokol H, Verdu EF, van Hylckama Vlieg JE, Bermúdez-Humarán LG, Smokvina T, Langella P.** 2015. *Lactobacillus rhamnosus* CNCM I-3690 and the commensal bacterium *Faecalibacterium prausnitzii* A2-165 exhibit similar protective effects to induced barrier hyper-permeability in mice. *Gut Microbes* 6:1–9.

25. **Bermúdez-Humarán LG.** 2009. *Lactococcus lactis* as a live vector for mucosal delivery of therapeutic proteins. *Hum Vaccin* 5:264–267.

26. **Steidler L, Hans W, Schotte L, Neirynck S, Obermeier F, Falk W, Fiers W, Remaut E.** 2000. Treatment of murine colitis by *Lactococcus lactis* secreting interleukin-10. *Science* 289:1352–1355.

27. **Caluwaerts S, Vandenbroucke K, Steidler L, Neirynck S, Vanhoenacker P, Corveleyn S, Watkins B, Sonis S, Coulie B, Rottiers P.** 2010. AG013, a mouth rinse formulation of *Lactococcus lactis* secreting human trefoil factor 1, provides a safe and efficacious therapeutic tool for treating oral mucositis. *Oral Oncol* 46:564–570.

28. **Kechaou N, Chain F, Gratadoux JJ, Blugeon S, Bertho N, Chevalier C, Le Goffic R, Courau S, Molimard P, Chatel JM, Langella P, Bermúdez-Humarán LG.** 2013. Identification of one novel candidate probiotic *Lactobacillus plantarum* strain active against influenza virus infection in mice by a large-scale screening. *Appl Environ Microbiol* 79:1491–1499.

29. **Carroll IM, Andrus JM, Bruno-Bárcena JM, Klaenhammer TR, Hassan HM, Threadgill DS.** 2007. Anti-inflammatory properties of *Lactoba-*

cillus gasseri expressing manganese superoxide dismutase using the interleukin 10-deficient mouse model of colitis. *Am J Physiol Gastrointest Liver Physiol* **293:**G729–G738.

30. **Watterlot L, Rochat T, Sokol H, Cherbuy C, Bouloufa I, Lefèvre F, Gratadoux JJ, Honvo-Hueto E, Chilmonczyk S, Blugeon S, Corthier G, Langella P, Bermúdez-Humarán LG.** 2010. Intragastric administration of a superoxide dismutase-producing recombinant *Lactobacillus casei* BL23 strain attenuates DSS colitis in mice. *Int J Food Microbiol* **144:**35–41.

31. **del Carmen S, de Moreno de LeBlanc A, Martin R, Chain F, Langella P, Bermúdez-Humarán LG, LeBlanc JG.** 2014. Genetically engineered immunomodulatory *Streptococcus thermophilus* strains producing antioxidant enzymes exhibit enhanced anti-inflammatory activities. *Appl Environ Microbiol* **80:**869–877.

32. **Motta JP, Magne L, Descamps D, Rolland C, Squarzoni-Dale C, Rousset P, Martin L, Cenac N, Balloy V, Huerre M, Fröhlich LF, Jenne D, Wartelle J, Belaaouaj A, Mas E, Vinel JP, Alric L, Chignard M, Vergnolle N, Sallenave JM.** 2011. Modifying the protease, antiprotease pattern by elafin overexpression protects mice from colitis. *Gastroenterology* **140:**1272–1282.

33. **Motta JP, Bermúdez-Humarán LG, Deraison C, Martin L, Rolland C, Rousset P, Boue J, Dietrich G, Chapman K, Kharrat P, Vinel JP, Alric L, Mas E, Sallenave JM, Langella P, Vergnolle N.** 2012. Food-grade bacteria expressing elafin protect against inflammation and restore colon homeostasis. *Sci Transl Med* **4:**158ra144.

34. **Kimura NT, Taniguchi S, Aoki K, Baba T.** 1980. Selective localization and growth of *Bifidobacterium bifidum* in mouse tumors following intravenous administration. *Cancer Res* **40:**2061–2068.

35. **Yao J, Wang JY, Lai MG, Li YX, Zhu HM, Shi RY, Mo J, Xun AY, Jia CH, Feng JL, Wang LS, Zeng WS, Liu L.** 2011. Treatment of mice with dextran sulfate sodium-induced colitis with human interleukin 10 secreted by transformed *Bifidobacterium longum*. *Mol Pharm* **8:**488–497.

36. **Zhang D, Wei C, Yao J, Cai X, Wang L.** 2015. Interleukin-10 gene-carrying bifidobacteria ameliorate murine ulcerative colitis by regulating regulatory T cell/T helper 17 cell pathway. *Exp Biol Med (Maywood)* **240:**1622–1629.

37. **Herfarth H, Schölmerich J.** 2002. IL-10 therapy in Crohn's disease: at the crossroads. *Gut* **50:**146–147.

38. **West RL, Zelinkova Z, Wolbink GJ, Kuipers EJ, Stokkers PC, van der Woude CJ.** 2008. Immunogenicity negatively influences the outcome of adalimumab treatment in Crohn's disease. *Aliment Pharmacol Ther* **28:**1122–1126.

39. **Pascual-Salcedo D, Plasencia C, Ramiro S, Nuño L, Bonilla G, Nagore D, Ruiz Del Agua A, Martínez A, Aarden L, Martín-Mola E, Balsa A.** 2011. Influence of immunogenicity on the efficacy of long-term treatment with infliximab in rheumatoid arthritis. *Rheumatology (Oxford)* **50:**1445–1452.

40. **Vandenbroucke K, de Haard H, Beirnaert E, Dreier T, Lauwereys M, Huyck L, Van Huysse J, Demetter P, Steidler L, Remaut E, Cuvelier C, Rottiers P.** 2010. Orally administered *L. lactis* secreting an anti-TNF nanobody demonstrate efficacy in chronic colitis. *Mucosal Immunol* **3:**49–56.

41. **Steidler L, Neirynck S, Huyghebaert N, Snoeck V, Vermeire A, Goddeeris B, Cox E, Remon JP, Remaut E.** 2003. Biological containment of genetically modified *Lactococcus lactis* for intestinal delivery of human interleukin 10. *Nat Biotechnol* **21:**785–789.

42. **Braat H, Rottiers P, Hommes DW, Huyghebaert N, Remaut E, Remon JP, van Deventer SJ, Neirynck S, Peppelenbosch MP, Steidler L.** 2006. A phase I trial with transgenic bacteria expressing interleukin-10 in Crohn's disease. *Clin Gastroenterol Hepatol* **4:**754–759.

43. **Limaye SA, Haddad RI, Cilli F, Sonis ST, Colevas AD, Brennan MT, Hu KS, Murphy BA.** 2013. Phase 1b, multicenter, single blinded, placebo-controlled, sequential dose escalation study to assess the safety and tolerability of topically applied AG013 in subjects with locally advanced head and neck cancer receiving induction chemotherapy. *Cancer* **119:**4268–4276.

44. **Bermúdez-Humarán LG, Motta JP, Aubry C, Kharrat P, Rous-Martin L, Sallenave JM, Deraison C, Vergnolle N, Langella P.** 2015. Serine protease inhibitors protect better than IL-10 and TGF-β anti-inflammatory cytokines against mouse colitis when delivered by recombinant lactococci. *Microb Cell Fact* **14:**26.

45. **Shaw L, Wiedow O.** 2011. Therapeutic potential of human elafin. *Biochem Soc Trans* **39:**1450–1454.

46. **Wei P, Yang Y, Ding Q, Li X, Sun H, Liu Z, Huang J, Gong Y.** 2016. Oral delivery of *Bifidobacterium longum* expressing α-melanocyte-stimulating hormone to combat ulcerative colitis. *J Med Microbiol* **65:**160–168.

Genetic Tools for the Enhancement of Probiotic Properties

16

LAURA ORTIZ-VELEZ[1] and ROBERT BRITTON[1]

INTRODUCTION

With renewed interest in the human microbiome and its role in human health, unique opportunities for using microbes as therapeutics have recently emerged. These opportunities range from the traditional probiotics to the engineering of intestinal mutualistic bacteria to deliver therapeutic proteins (1–3). However, a more in-depth understanding of how intestinal microbes impact human health and how they function in the complex, dynamic environment of the gastrointestinal tract (GIT) requires advancements in genetic tools for nonmodel strains.

Lactic acid bacteria (LAB) are a heterogeneous group of bacteria characterized by their ability to produce lactic acid as a fermentation product, including genera such as *Lactococcus*, *Lactobacillus*, and *Streptococcus* (4). These microorganisms have been explored as therapeutic delivery systems since many members of this group have a proven safety profile and several tools have been developed to manipulate their genomes (1, 2, 5). Although most of the genetic work was originally done with *Lactococcus lactis*, engineering of species from the *Lactobacillus* genera has gained ground since they are more adapted for survival in the GIT (6–8). Significant progress in genetic tool development for lactobacilli during the past decade has paved

[1]Molecular Virology and Microbiology, Baylor College of Medicine, Houston, TX 77030

Bugs as Drugs: Therapeutic Microbes for the Prevention and Treatment of Disease

Edited by Robert A. Britton and Patrice D. Cani

© 2018 American Society for Microbiology, Washington, DC

doi:10.1128/microbiolspec.BAD-0018-2016

the way for important discoveries concerning how these bacteria metabolize bile acids and interact with the immune system and their use for the development of therapeutic delivery vehicles (7, 9–12).

In this article we will review the development of genetic tools for lactobacilli and highlight some of the more recent advancements that are allowing for precision genome engineering of probiotics. Finally, we will finish with a discussion of the development of genetic tools for the delivery of therapeutics to the human gut.

DEVELOPMENT OF GENETIC TOOLS FOR THE MANIPULATION OF LACTOBACILLI

The development of strategies to genetically manipulate LAB dates back to the 1970s when the first studies of *L. lactis* plasmids began, which was facilitated by the development of recombinant DNA technology in the 1980s (13, 14). *L. lactis* was the genetic workhorse of the LAB field, with a wide variety of gene knockout/editing technologies and regulated expression systems being developed over the past 30 years. We refer the reader to excellent, detailed reviews of the various tools for *L. lactis* and will focus our discussion on the tools developed for the genus *Lactobacillus*, with references to tools borrowed from *L. lactis* (15–21).

Traditional Chromosomal Integration Strategies

Several methods have been explored to achieve stable integration of sequences in lactobacilli such as the use of insertion sequence (IS) elements, phage-integration systems, and homologous recombination-based systems. The use of IS elements to manipulate lactobacillus genomes was initially established by Walker and Klaenhammer, who constructed suicide vectors harboring the IS*1223* element from *Lactobacillus johnsonii* that successfully promoted insertion of sequences into *Lacto-*

bacillus acidophilus, *Lactobacillus gasseri*, and *L. johnsonii* genomes (22). Similarly, phage-based integration systems have been developed using a phage-encoded integrase (*int*) and regions on the phage (*attP*) that promote site-specific recombination at homologous specific chromosomal locations (*attB*). Raya et al. developed this system by constructing an insertional vector which uses elements from the Φadh phage from *L. gasseri* to introduce sequences into the chromosome of this strain (23). Similarly, an integration vector based on the temperate phage mv4 from *Lactobacillus delbrueckii* subsp. *bulgaricus* has been constructed to integrate sequences into the tRNA(Ser) gene from *Lactobacillus plantarum* LP80 (24). Although these systems based on IS elements and phages are available, their employment is restricted by the presence and distribution of the IS and *att* sequences in the genome.

Homologous recombination-based systems have traditionally been employed in bacteria, including lactobacilli, to achieve chromosomal insertions, deletions, and gene replacements (25, 26). In general, these systems employ suicide vectors (unable to replicate in the host) that contain sequences of identity to the location in the bacterial genome to be modified. The homologous regions promote crossover events to mediate genomic integration of either the complete vector (in the case of a single crossover) or exclusively the sequences flanked by the homologous regions (in the case of double-crossover events). An important requirement of using these systems is the establishment of efficient transformation protocols since they primarily rely on the recombination frequency of the bacterium, which is normally fairly low (27, 28).

Most recombination systems designed to integrate DNA into LAB chromosomes are based on the use of nonreplicative suicide vectors, which contain an antibiotic marker and homologous sequences to the insertion site (25, 26). The inability to replicate in the cell requires the integration of the plasmid into the chromosome to maintain antibiotic resistance. Because many lactobacilli are poorly transformable, it was necessary to use strategies that allowed for conditional replication of plasmids (28, 29). Initial experiments performed in *L. plantarum* using conditionally replicating plasmids allowed the stable integration of the α-amylase, endoglucanase, and levanase genes either by single-crossover (30) or by double-crossover events (29, 31).

Russell and Klaenhammer developed a widely applicable system to achieve site-specific chromosomal integration and disruption of genes in several *Lactobacillus* species, such as the β-galactosidase gene (*lacL*) in *L. acidophilus* NCFM as well as the β-glucuronidase gene (*gusA*) in *L. gasseri* ADH (32). This system is based on the use of conditionally replicating pORI vectors, which are derived from the broad-host-range lactococcal pWV01 vector and have been successfully employed in *L. lactis* for genome engineering (32, 33). These vectors contain an origin of replication but lack an essential replication protein, RepA. Therefore RepA must be provided in *trans* by the host to allow propagation of the vector.

The transformation of the nonreplicating pORI constructs with homologous sequences to the targeted genomic region should facilitate chromosomal integration. However, due to the low transformation efficiency of some lactobacillus species, a temperature-sensitive vector (helper plasmid) that supplies the RepA protein in *trans* is used to initially mediate replication and establishment of the pORI plasmid into the cell prior to the recombination of the homologous regions present in the plasmid (32). Shifting the strain to the non-permissive temperature for the helper vector causes the plasmid to be lost, and RepA is no longer able to assist the pORI plasmid to replicate. Thus, the only way to maintain antibiotic resistance is for the plasmid to recombine with homologous regions located in the chromosome (32).

The pORI system has been successfully adapted to many species of lactobacilli and has brought genetics to a number of systems that had no alternatives. However, the lack of additional plasmids that have novel replication origins has meant that performing simple tasks such as complementation has not been possible. Because single-crossover insertion of plasmids can recombine out of the chromosome, selective pressure needs to be maintained to ensure that the mutant is stable. Such mutants are not good candidates for *in vivo* experiments, because it is difficult to maintain such selective pressure *in vivo*. Finally, multiple plasmids can recombine into each other, which can create instability and alterations in phenotypes. Therefore, alternatives to single-crossover or efficient double-crossover genetics have been pursued.

Cre-*lox*-Based System for Double-Crossover Integration

The marginal efficiency of classical double-crossover integration systems has led to the exploration of other methodologies such as the Cre-*lox* system to increase the rate at which marker-free gene replacements are achieved (26, 34, 35). This system employs the recombinase Cre to mediate site-specific recombination between its recognition sites, denominated *loxP* sites. The orientation of the recognition sites dictates the end result of the recombination, generating deletions when the sites have the same direction or inversions in the case of opposite directions. Lambert et al. adapted the Cre-*lox* recombination system to the traditional homologous recombination strategies in lactobacillus to create a toolbox that allows multiple chromosomal deletions with selectable marker removal (26). Gene replacements are constructed in several steps. Initially, a gene-specific mutagenesis vector is generated by molecular cloning, which harbors sequences with homology to the targeted insertion site and the *lox66*-P_{32}-*cat*-*lox71* cassette. This cassette contains two asymmetric *loxP* sites (*lox66* and *lox71*) and the P_{32}-*cat* gene that allows for the constitutive expression of the chloramphenicol (CM)-resistance marker. The vector itself contains an erythromycin (EM)-resistance gene; thus, single crossovers are selected based on double resistance to both antibiotics, whereas double crossovers are detected because of their resistance to CM and sensitivity to EM. Once the *lox66*-P$_{32}$-*cat*-*lox71* cassette is integrated into the targeted gene by a double crossover, a plasmid that allows transient expression of the recombinase Cre is transformed into the cells, mediating recombination of the *lox* sites and excision of the *cat* marker. Recombination between *lox66* and *lox71* generates one *loxP* site with a wild-type (WT) sequence and another one with two mutated inverted repeats (*lox72*). Cre-mediated recombination between these residual sites (*loxP* WT and *lox72*) is 8-fold lower than Cre-mediated recombination between *lox66* and *lox71* (36). Therefore, the probability of having recombination events in untargeted *loxP* sites after Cre-mediated chromosomal integration is considerably reduced. Consequently, several rounds of the Cre-*lox* system can be performed in the same strain to achieve multiple gene deletions. This system has allowed for successful knockouts of several genes in *L. plantarum*, including the α-galactosidase (*melA*), the bile salt hydrolase (*bsh1*), and the alanine racemase gene (*alr*), as well as the two 1,3-propanediol dehydrogenase genes from *Lactobacillus reuteri* DSM 20016 (26, 37, 38).

The Uracil-Phosphoribosyltransferase (*upp*)-Based Counterselection Gene Replacement System

The *upp*-based counterselection system has been used in many bacterial systems (39–41). As a strategy to create an efficient chromosomal integration system in lactobacilli, Goh et al. used the uracil-phosphoribosyltransferase enzyme as a counterselection marker to screen for recombinants that have undergone a double crossover with pORI-based plasmids (42). The uracil-phosphoribosyl-

transferase enzyme metabolizes the uracil analogue 5-fluorouracil to produce toxic metabolites that result in cell death. This system employs an *L. acidophilus* NCFM strain in which the *upp* gene has been deleted; therefore, it is able to grow in the presence of 5-fluorouracil. The strain is then transformed with a pORI-based counterselectable integration vector containing the *upp* selection marker, the EM antibiotic gene, and homologous sequences to the insertion site. This strain also harbors an unstable helper plasmid that provides RepA in *trans* and has a CM selection marker; thus, cells that have undergone single crossovers can be easily selected based on their resistance to EM and sensitivity to CM. Transformants with double crossovers are detected based on their sensitivity to EM and their ability to grow in the presence of 5-fluorouracil. The system has been used to efficiently disrupt the lipoteichoic acid synthesis gene (*ltaS*) in *L. gasseri* ATCC 33323 and the S-layer-associated gene (*slpX*) from *L. acidophilus* NCFM and to mediate free marker integration of *gusA* into the same strain (25, 42, 43).

Alanine Racemase as a Food-Grade Selection Marker

Alanine racemase (*alr*) has been explored as an alternative marker to the traditional antibiotic-resistance genes to produce a food-grade selection system for *L. plantarum* (37, 44–46). The alanine racemase enzyme catalyzes the conversion of D-alanine to L-alanine; thus, disruption of this gene generates an auxotrophic mutant for L-alanine. Based on this requirement, a plasmid expressing the *alr* gene into the Δ*alr* null mutant should be maintained in the cell without the need for antibiotic selection. The *alr*-based system was originally developed by Bron et al. and subsequently modified by Nguyen to generate food-grade expression systems using derivatives from the pSIP vectors and evaluating the expression of β-galactosidase in *L. plantarum* WCFS1 (37, 44).

Emerging Technologies for Genome Manipulation of LAB

Genome manipulation of lactobacilli is being transformed by the development of precision genome engineering tools that speed up our ability to edit bacterial genomes, such as recombination-mediated genetic engineering (recombineering) and CRISPR (clustered regularly interspaced short palindromic repeats)-Cas-based engineering (47–49). Recombineering technology has increased mutation efficiencies to such a degree that, in many cases, genome editing can be achieved without the need for antibiotic selection. Recombineering was initially developed to edit the *Escherichia coli* chromosome, maximizing the ability to manipulate its genome without the necessity of restriction enzymes or antibiotic selection (50). Recently, recombineering was successfully established in *L. reuteri* and *L. lactis* using single-stranded DNA (ssDNA) as a substrate to generate targeted mutations (48). Meanwhile, double-stranded DNA (dsDNA) recombineering was developed to achieve efficient marker-free gene replacements in *L. plantarum* (47).

Cas9 targeting of bacterial genomes was initially established for *Streptococcus pneumoniae* and *E. coli* by Wenyan et al., and since then it has enhanced genome editing due to its high degree of target specificity in bacteria (51). CRISPR-Cas has also been used in bacteria to increase recombineering efficiencies by facilitating integration or deletions of large pieces of DNA from the genome.

Recombineering for Genome Engineering in LAB

Recombineering has emerged as a relatively simple methodology that enables efficient genome editing of bacterial and eukaryotic genomes (52–54). This tool accomplishes chromosomal manipulation by promoting homologous recombination between an extra chromosomal source of dsDNA and the genome, minimizing or abolishing the employ-

ment of restriction enzymes traditionally used with molecular cloning techniques. Recombineering stands out over other genetic tools to manipulate LAB genomes because it allows precise insertions of point mutations into the chromosome at an efficient rate in a high throughput fashion without the necessity of any selective marker (48).

Recombineering was developed based on the activity of the λ phage red system, which comprises the Gam, Exo, and Beta proteins. The Gam protein promotes suppression of host nucleases, and Exo is an exonuclease that modifies dsDNA to mediate genome editing. The Beta recombinase is an ssDNA binding protein that promotes annealing and recombination of the genome with a dsDNA substrate that has homology to the location in the chromosome being edited (55). Yang et al. generated an efficient dsDNA recombineering tool to remodel the *L. plantarum* WCFS1 genome by employing homologs of an exonuclease (*lp_0642*), a possible host-nuclease inhibitor (*lp_0640*), and a previously described ssDNA binding protein (*lp_0641*) from the prophage P1 of this strain (47) (Fig. 1). Combination of this tool with the *loxP*/Cre system enabled efficient disruption of the glucosamine-6-phosphate isomerase gene (*gnp*) and the replacement of the D lactate dehydrogenase (*ldhD*) gene by the *gusA* gene in *L. plantarum* WCFS1 (47). Unlike ssDNA recombineering, dsDNA recombineering allows genomic manipulation of large DNA fragments, since long dsDNA substrates can be integrated into the genome (up to 4.7 kb in *L. plantarum*) (47).

Oligonucleotide-Mediated Recombineering for Precision Genome Editing

ssDNA recombineering is a variation of the original recombineering strategy that allows the use of single-stranded oligonucleotides as a substrate rather than dsDNA (48, 56) (Fig. 2). In this scenario, only expression of the ssDNA binding protein Beta from λ phage

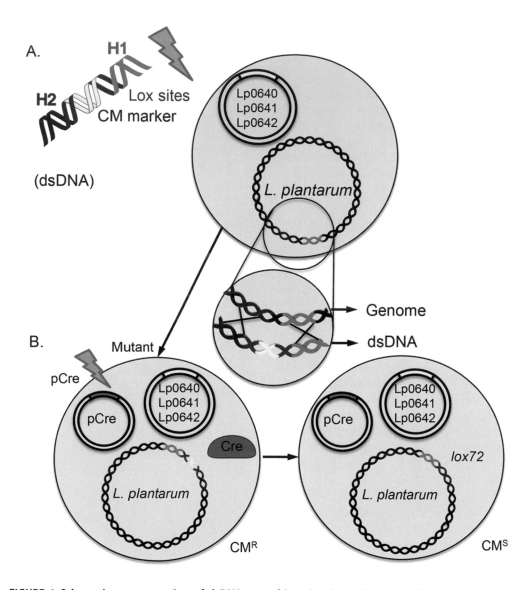

FIGURE 1 Schematic representation of dsDNA recombineering in *L. plantarum*. (A) A piece of dsDNA harboring the *lox66-cat-lox71* cassette (*lox66* and *lox71* sites, red; Cat/CM marker, yellow) and regions with homology to the genomic insertion site (H1, green; H2, blue) is transformed into *L. plantarum* expressing an exonuclease (Lp0642), a possible host nuclease inhibitor (Lp0640), and an ssDNA binding protein (Lp0641). **(B)** Once the dsDNA fragments are integrated into the genome, which renders the cells resistant to CM (CM^r), bacteria are transformed with a plasmid that induces the expression of the recombinase Cre to recombine the *loxP* sites. This recombination deletes the CM marker contained inside the *lox* sites, rendering the cells CM-sensitive and leaving a modified *loxP* site (*lox72*).

or the RecT recombinase from the Rac prophage is required (55, 56). These recombinases and functional homologs mediate the incorporation of an oligonucleotide that contains the desired mutation to be incor-

porated into the genome. Screening of the recombinant cells is facilitated by a variation of the traditional PCR, called the mismatch amplification mutation assay-PCR (MAMA-PCR), in which one of the oligomers spe-

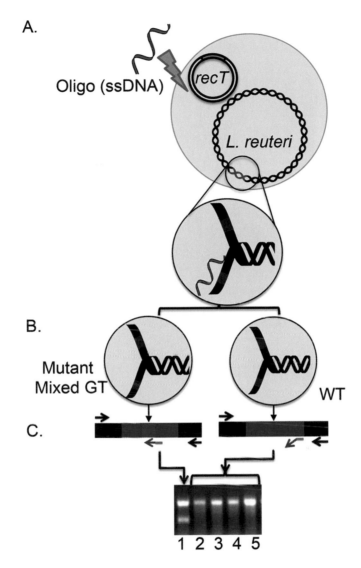

FIGURE 2 Schematic representation of ssDNA recombineering in *L. reuteri*. (A) An oligomer harboring the mutation (red) and regions with homology to the genomic insertion site (blue) is transformed into cells expressing RecT. **(B)** The oligomer is incorporated into the lagging strand being synthesized at the DNA replication fork, generating a mutant with a mixed genotype (GT). **(C)** Screening of the mutant is done by MAMA-PCR, using two oligomers that amplify from a WT sequence (black) and a third oligomer (red-blue) that only amplifies when the mutation is incorporated. Thus, two amplicons are generated in the case of the mutant (lane 1), whereas only one amplicon is generated in the case of the WT (lanes 2 to 5). After the mixed genotype is identified, single colony purification is done to isolate cells containing only the mutation (pure genotype).

cifically anneals to the targeted mutation, producing amplification of DNA only when the desired mutation is incorporated (48, 57). Screening can also be carried out by PCR followed by restriction digestion or Sanger se-

quencing. Oligonucleotide-mediated recombineering was successfully established in LAB by van Pijkeren and Britton, achieving chromosomal recombineering efficiencies of up to 19% in *L. reuteri* and *L. lactis* (48, 58). Several parameters that can be explored to adapt or improve this technology to other LAB have been described (58).

As an example of how recombineering can be used to modify the active site of an enzyme, van Pijkeren and Britton used this technology to create a vancomycin-sensitive derivative of *L. reuteri* by altering Ddl ligase (48). The enzyme Ddl ligase forms a dipeptide of two alanines that is then used to form the muramyl peptide involved in peptidoglycan construction (59). The glycopeptide vancomycin binds to the terminal alanine present in these muramyl peptides, inhibiting peptidoglycan biogenesis (60). Many lactobacilli, including *L. reuteri,* encode a Ddl ligase that creates an Ala-lactate depsipeptide rather than the Ala-Ala dipeptide, which renders these strains naturally resistant to high concentrations of vancomycin (61). Elegant work from the Walsh laboratory has shown that a single amino acid change in the active site of the Ddl ligase from *E. coli* is sufficient to alter activity of this enzyme from a dipeptide ligase to a depsipeptide ligase (62, 63). Van Pijkeren and Britton were able to identify the active site of the Ddl ligase from *L. reuteri* using structural modeling and overlays of the Ddl ligase from *E. coli* and *L. reuteri.* Normally, *L. reuteri* is resistant to a >512 µg/ml concentration of vancomycin. Recombineering was employed to modify the active site of the Ddl ligase in *L. reuteri* and to alter its substrate specificity toward the Ala-Ala dipeptide. This generated a strain sensitive to vancomycin (MIC = 1.5 µg/ml) that may have an important safety value in future engineered strains of *L. reuteri.*

Combining Cas9 Genome Editing with ssDNA Recombineering To Edit Genomes with Low Recombineering Efficiency

Although ssDNA recombineering has the potential to be applied to a wide variety of lactobacilli, the genome editing activity varies dramatically between species and even within

strains of the same species. When recombineering frequency drops below 0.3%, the ability to screen for mutations without the need for selection becomes untenable. We have shown that ssDNA recombineering works in a number of bacterial species, but the efficiency is sufficiently low that recovering unselected mutations is almost impossible (48).

The adaptation of CRISPR-Cas systems to specifically target specific sites within genomes presents an opportunity to enhance the ability to perform ssDNA recombineering in bacteria (51, 64). CRISPR-Cas systems have been characterized as defense systems against incoming foreign DNA, with "memory" of past invasions captured by spacer sequences that match plasmids or phages. The biology and biochemistry of CRISPR-Cas systems are beyond the scope of this article, and the reader is referred to recent reviews on this subject (51, 65–69). We will focus on the class II CRISPR systems that have been engineered for precision genome engineering of eukaryotic and bacterial genomes.

The major players of class II CRISPR-Cas systems relevant for bacterial genome engineering are the nuclease Cas9 and guide RNAs (gRNAs). Cas9 is an RNA-directed DNA endonuclease that enables precision targeting of DNA cleavage within a genome, while the gRNAs specifically define where Cas9 will cleave. Like other class II CRISPR systems, Cas9 also requires a *trans*-activating small RNA (tracrRNA) to direct target cleavage. By expressing tracrRNA and gRNAs that match the sequence to be targeted, along with a proper protospacer adjacent motif, one can direct Cas9 to make a double-strand break nearly anywhere in the genome (49, 51) (Fig. 3). In eukaryotes, nonhomologous end-joining results in mutations in the site of the genome being targeted, which has allowed Cas9 genome editing to be used to build genome-wide loss of function libraries in human and animal cell lines (70, 71). In bacteria, these double-strand breaks are repaired efficiently and almost never result in mutations of the gene (72). This efficient repair of these breaks is

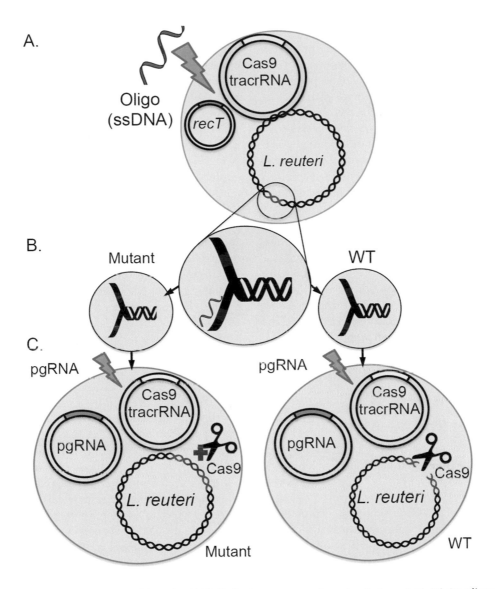

FIGURE 3 Overview of recombineering/CRISPR-Cas9 genome engineering in *L. reuteri*. (A) An oligomer harboring the mutation (red) and regions with homology to the genomic insertion site (blue) is transformed into *L. reuteri* expressing RecT, Cas9, and its tracrRNA. (B) The oligomer targets the lagging strains and is incorporated into one of the DNA strands at the replication fork. When cells divide, a mixed population of WT and mutant cells is generated. (C) A plasmid expressing guide RNA (pgRNA) that targets the WT sequence is introduced into the cell. Cas9 is directed by the gRNA to cleave DNA of cells that did not incorporate the mutations (WT), whereas cells that incorporate the mutation are void of cleavage (mutant).

what allows ssDNA recombineering to be combined with Cas9 to edit genomes in bacteria that have lower recombineering efficiencies (51, 64).

To combine ssDNA recombineering and Cas9 editing in LAB, a bacterial strain is transformed with a plasmid containing RecT and a second plasmid containing Cas9 along with tracrRNA. Next, an oligonucleotide that would generate a mutation in the genome is transformed into the cell. Rather than screening for the mutation in unselected colonies by MAMA-PCR or restriction digest, the surviving colonies are transformed with a plasmid that contains a gRNA that directs Cas9 to target the WT sequence of the genome. Cells that have not incorporated the oligonucleotide into the genome will have a perfect match to the gRNA and will be rendered nonviable due to the constant action of Cas9 on the genome. Thus, only mutants will be recovered after Cas9 editing, eliminating the need for screening for mutations. As proof of concept, the ability to enhance ssDNA recombineering has been demonstrated in both *E. coli* and *L. reuteri* (49, 51, 73). However, both *E. coli* and *L. reuteri* are efficient at ssDNA recombineering, so it remains to be seen if this can be applied to bacteria where ssDNA recombineering is not as efficient.

Inducible Gene Expression

The ability to control gene expression by manipulating the environment in which bacteria are growing dates back to early, groundbreaking research on the *lac* operon by Jacob and Monod (74). Inducible gene expression is very useful for exploring expression of proteins whose effects on the host producing it are not known and/or are likely to be toxic. Additionally, these promoters allow researchers to switch expression of the desired gene from off to on, offering stringent control over the expression of the gene. Many inducible promoters have already been employed with success to control gene expression in LAB, including promoters activated by lactose (*placA*), zinc (*pzn*), xylose (*pxylT*), pH shifts (*p170*), phage attack, and temperature (*pL/pR*) stress, as well as the promoter from the stress-induced controlled expression system (75–81).

One of the most widely and successfully inducible promoters used in LAB, particularly *L. lactis*, is the *nisin* inducible promoter (*pnisA*) from the *nisin*-controlled expression system (82–84). This quorum-sensing-based system was developed about 2 decades ago using elements from the bacteriocin *nisin* operon from *L. lactis*, which comprises the *nisin*-inducible promoter (*pnisA*), the histidine kinase (NisK), and the response regulator (NisR). NisK and NisR form the two-component system that turns on gene expression from *pnisA* in the presence of *nisin*. The *nisin*-controlled expression system has been adapted for gene expression purposes in other LAB such as *Streptococcus thermophilus*, *Streptococcus agalactiae*, *S. pneumoniae*, *L. reuteri*, and *Enterococcus faecalis*, among others (83, 85, 86). The simplicity and adaptability of these vectors have facilitated and promoted the use of LAB, not only in their traditional roles in food production and preservation, but also as delivery vehicles for various groups of proteins, including antigens, antibodies, and cytokines. Although the *nisin*-controlled expression system has been successful in several LAB, the system has not been functionally adapted to many *Lactobacillus* species (83, 85).

Another set of inducible promoters that have been particularly successful in lactobacilli are the promoters from the pSIP group of expression vectors, constructed by Sørvig and colleagues (87). The pSIP expression systems were developed using genetic elements from a two-component system involved in the synthesis of sakacin A (pSIP300 series) and sakacin P (pSIP400 series) bacteriocins in *Lactobacillus sakei*. Among the pSIP vectors, pSIP411 has achieved the highest level of controllable expression in several *Lactobacillus* strains (88, 89). For this reason, pSIP411 has become one of the most widely used expression systems in lactobacilli. This vector has served to induce the production of proteins such as β-glucuronidase, aminopeptidase, β-galactosidase, and green fluorescent protein in several lactobacilli strains including *L. reuteri*, *L. plantarum*, and *L. gasseri* (37, 87–90). Karlskås et al. modified the system to generate a secretion system that promotes extracellular delivery of the staphylococcal nuclease A (*nucA*) from various *Lactobacillus* species (89). Similarly, Nguyen generated a stable food-grade expression system based on the pSIP vectors by replacing the antibiotic marker of the vector for the *upp* counterselection marker (37). The use of the *upp* marker in an *upp* knockout background allows the selection of cells that harbor the pSIP constructs, without the need of antibiotics.

Impact of New Genetic Technologies on the Safety and Efficacy of Probiotic Bacteria

The use of bacteria as biotherapeutics holds much promise as we move forward from probiotics as dietary supplements to scientifically backed prevention and treatment of disease with bacteria. Bacteria as therapeutics have challenges not associated with inert small-molecule drugs, including the fact they can and will evolve over time. In addition, with precision genome engineering tools becoming available for bacteria that have positive impacts on health, it will be possible to make subtle alterations in the genome to optimize the safety and efficacy of these strains. Thus, the line between genetically modified organisms (GMOs) and "naturally" occurring mutants that are not considered GMOs is now challenging to discern. With recombineering technology, it is possible to engineer a mutation into a bacterial genome that, when finished, would be impossible to tell apart from a mutation arising spontaneously. While the latter would not be considered a GMO, in reality there is no difference between the safety of the two strains, and the fact that one mutation arose spontaneously and the other was engineered is the only true difference. To fully realize the potential of probiotics in the prevention and treatment of human disease, it will be necessary to hold a vigorous debate regarding the implications of precision genetic editing technology in therapeutic bacteria.

ENGINEERED PROBIOTICS FOR THE HETEROLOGOUS EXPRESSION OF THERAPEUTIC PROTEINS

In addition to being used as traditional probiotics, lactobacilli also have been investigated as delivery systems for therapeutic proteins (21). Synthetic biology, next-generation sequencing, and improved genome-editing technology have made it possible to explore novel ways of engineering microbes to produce therapeutic proteins and compounds to improve human health. While many lactobacilli and *L. lactis* have been engineered to secrete human proteins, relatively few have been tested in humans (1, 18, 21, 91). The successful use of interleukin-10-secreting *L. lactis* for the treatment of colitis in mice has been described and led to the testing of interleukin-10-producing *L. lactis* for the treatment of inflammatory bowel disease in humans (92). Although interleukin-10-producing *L. lactis* did not ultimately show efficacy in inflammatory bowel disease patients, quite a bit was learned about the use of microbial platforms for the delivery of therapeutic proteins. Below we discuss some of the challenges scientists face in making functional and secreting functional therapeutic proteins in LAB. For a more thorough literature review of the use of *L. lactis* and lactobacilli as biotherapeutic delivery vehicles, we refer the reader elsewhere (11, 19–21, 91, 93).

Conceptual Challenges

One of the biggest hurdles scientists face in developing therapeutic delivery systems is engineering organisms that have evolved to live in the intestinal environment rather than lab-adapted strains that are conditioned to grow on laboratory media. Lactobacilli offer an attractive avenue for such platforms, because many strains isolated from humans have long been used in probiotic preparations, and the necessary tools are being developed. Many *Lactobacillus* species have also been vetted for their survivability in animal and human intestinal tracts, indicating that several strains have the ability to traverse the complex environments of the intestine and remain viable to be able to deliver proteins to sites of pathology (4, 94). This is a key limitation of platforms such as *L. lactis*, which despite a plethora of strong genetic tools for protein expression and secretion, lacks the ability to survive in the human GIT. This is because *L. lactis* is involved in milk fermentation and has an optimum growth temperature of 30°C, an environment that is far from the harsh environment of the intestinal tract, and this has limited the utility of *L. lactis* in humans.

Now that genetic tools for human-associated lactobacilli are becoming more readily available, combined with emerging concepts from synthetic and systems biology, the time is right for engineering precision therapeutic delivery vehicles for humans. We propose a number of criteria that we consider key to generating an ideal delivery vehicle. The organism must:

1. Survive in the intestinal tract
2. Have a remarkable safety profile
3. Deliver the therapeutic payload only when in the presence of pathology
4. Turn off the therapeutic payload when pathology is resolved
5. Self-destruct upon or before exiting the body
6. Have stable integration into the chromosome to prevent horizontal gene transfer
7. Be unable to stably colonize the intestine
8. Have a stable system that will deliver a reliable output
9. Remain viable and functional when grown in an industrial format for dissemination to patients

We propose these criteria as a guideline that will lead to the generation of therapeutic microorganisms with minimal safety concerns and efficacious therapeutic activity. These criteria will be especially important for the delivery of proteins that may induce deleterious effects when released for prolonged times, such as is the case of several therapeutic targets including cytokines and hormones that stimulate cell growth and could potentially promote cancer when administered constantly. Nonetheless, there will be scenarios in which the application of these guidelines will be redefined depending on the therapeutic goal. For instance, when the delivery of proteins for long periods is needed, such as for treatment of chronic gastrointestinal diseases, the use of microorganisms that colonize the GIT might be more beneficial than organisms that transiently inhabit the intestinal tract. In these special cases, it will be necessary to have strategies to promote biocontainment as well as to control the colonization of the GMO to reinforce the safety of the system.

Technical Challenges

The engineering of nonmodel organisms for clinical applications generates a clear series of technical challenges in that very little is known about genetic manipulation, gene expression, and protein secretion in these organisms. Although the speed at which genome engineering strategies are developed is increasing, it still requires a huge investment of time and effort to be applied to nontraditional microorganisms. This creates a requirement for tools that can be easily transferred and adapted to a large number of nonmodel microbes that have a good profile for employment in therapeutic purposes. Similarly, the application of synthetic biology approaches to identify libraries of promoters and ribosome binding sites with different strengths ranging from low to high expression is necessary to begin building gene expression tools that will be employed *in vivo*. Efficient protein secretion or delivery strategies are also required. For instance, a systems-style approach was demonstrated with the intestinal bacterium *Bacteroides thetaiotaomicron*, which has been studied for over 25 years for its impact on intestinal physiology. Mimee et al.

identified a series of gene expression modules that allowed for a 4-order-of-magnitude dynamic range of expression and showed expression of a luciferase reporter gene in the GIT (95). For the case of *Lactobacillus*, Rud developed a synthetic promoter library for constitutive gene expression, achieving up to 4 logs of gene expression in *L. plantarum* (96). Similar approaches are under way for use in other *Lactobacillus* species such as *L. reuteri* in which promoter and ribosomal binding site libraries have been developed, achieving similar dynamic ranges (Ortiz-Velez and Britton, unpublished results).

Safety Considerations

A major challenge for using engineered probiotics in humans is the fact they are GMOs and in many cases will be expressing proteins derived from humans. Therefore, the utmost care must be taken to ensure that these organisms are not released into the environment, where they could be adsorbed by another person or possibly transfer the therapeutic cassette to another bacterium. Another concern is the deleterious effect that genome manipulation as well as population numbers of a nontraditional microorganism might have on microbiome functioning and overall human health. Proper and rigorous characterization of the safety of these GMOs should help to prevent the occurrence of this type of issue.

CONCLUSIONS

LAB, particularly *Lactobacillus* species, are microorganisms with great potential as therapeutic delivery systems due to their remarkable safety profile and ability to survive in the human GIT. Interest in manipulating these microorganisms for industrial and therapeutic purposes has enabled the development of several tools that facilitate and expedite editing of their genomes. Engineered LAB have evidenced the potential that these organisms may have as probiotics or therapeutic delivery systems. Although there is a long way to go until we can efficiently and reliably engineer nonmodel gut microorganisms, it is important to start having discussions about the generation and implications of the use of GMOs in human health care. These types of initiatives will facilitate and hasten the application of these novel therapeutic options in humans in a safe manner.

CITATION

Ortiz-Velez L, Britton R. 2017. Genetic tools for the enhancement of probiotic properties. *Microbiol Spectrum* 5(5):BAD-0018-2016.

REFERENCES

1. **Steidler L, Hans W, Schotte L, Neirynck S, Obermeier F, Falk W, Fiers W, Remaut E.** 2000. Treatment of murine colitis by *Lactococcus lactis* secreting interleukin-10. *Science* **289:** 1352–1355.

2. **Motta J-P, Bermudez-Humaran LG, Deraison C, Martin L, Rolland C, Rousset P, Boue J, Dietrich G, Chapman K, Kharrat P, Vinel J-P, Alric L, Mas E, Sallenave J-M, Langella P, Vergnolle N.** 2012. Food-grade bacteria expressing elafin protect against inflammation and restore colon homeostasis. *Sci Transl Med* **4:** 158ra144–158ra144.

3. **Vanderhoof JA, Whitney DB, Antonson DL, Hanner TL, Lupo JV, Young RJ.** 1999. *Lactobacillus* GG in the prevention of antibiotic-associated diarrhea in children. *J Pediatr* **135:** 564–568.

4. **Stiles ME, Holzapfel WH.** 1997. Lactic acid bacteria of foods and their current taxonomy. *Int J Food Microbiol* **36:**1–29.

5. **Steidler L, Neirynck S, Huyghebaert N, Snoeck V, Vermeire A, Goddeeris B, Cox E, Remon JP, Remaut E.** 2003. Biological containment of genetically modified *Lactococcus lactis* for intestinal delivery of human interleukin 10. *Nat Biotechnol* **21:**785–789.

6. **de Moreno de LeBlanc A, Del Carmen S, Chatel JM, Miyoshi A, Azevedo V, Langella P, Bermúdez-Humarán LG, LeBlanc JG.** 2015. Current review of genetically modified lactic acid bacteria for the prevention and treatment of colitis using murine models. *Gastroenterol Res Pract* **2015:**146972.

7. Liu X, Lagenaur LA, Simpson DA, Essenmacher KP, Frazier-Parker CL, Liu Y, Tsai D, Rao SS, Hamer DH, Parks TP, Lee PP, Xu Q. 2006. Engineered vaginal lactobacillus strain for mucosal delivery of the human immunodeficiency virus inhibitor cyanovirin-N. *Antimicrob Agents Chemother* 50:3250–3259.

8. Seegers JFML. 2002. Lactobacilli as live vaccine delivery vectors: progress and prospects. *Trends Biotechnol* 20:508–515.

9. Wells JM. 2011. Immunomodulatory mechanisms of lactobacilli. *Microb Cell Fact* 10 (Suppl 1):S17.

10. Whitehead K, Versalovic J, Roos S, Britton RA. 2008. Genomic and genetic characterization of the bile stress response of probiotic *Lactobacillus reuteri* ATCC 55730. *Appl Environ Microbiol* 74: 1812–1819.

11. Daniel C, Roussel Y, Kleerebezem M, Pot B. 2011. Recombinant lactic acid bacteria as mucosal biotherapeutic agents. *Trends Biotechnol* 29:499–508.

12. Bermúdez-Humarán LG, Aubry C, Motta JP, Deraison C, Steidler L, Vergnolle N, Chatel JM, Langella P. 2013. Engineering lactococci and lactobacilli for human health. *Curr Opin Microbiol* 16:278–283.

13. Kok J, van der Vossen JMBM, Venema G. 1984. Construction of plasmid cloning vectors for lactic streptococci which also replicate in *Bacillus subtilis* and *Escherichia coli*. *Appl Environ Microbiol* 48:726–731.

14. Weisblum B, Graham MY, Gryczan T, Dubnau D. 1979. Plasmid copy number control: isolation and characterization of high-copy-number mutants of plasmid pE194. *J Bacteriol* 137:635–643.

15. Morello E, Bermúdez-Humarán LG, Llull D, Solé V, Miraglio N, Langella P, Poquet I. 2008. *Lactococcus lactis*, an efficient cell factory for recombinant protein production and secretion. *J Mol Microbiol Biotechnol* 14:48–58.

16. Le Loir Y, Azevedo V, Oliveira SC, Freitas DA, Miyoshi A, Bermúdez-Humarán LG, Nouaille S, Ribeiro LA, Leclercq S, Gabriel JE, Guimaraes VD, Oliveira MN, Charlier C, Gautier M, Langella P. 2005. Protein secretion in *Lactococcus lactis*: an efficient way to increase the overall heterologous protein production. *Microb Cell Fact* 4:2.

17. Bermúdez-Humarán LG. 2009. *Lactococcus lactis* as a live vector for mucosal delivery of therapeutic proteins. *Hum Vaccin* 5:264–267.

18. Wyszyńska A, Kobierecka P, Bardowski J, Jagusztyn-Krynicka EK. 2015. Lactic acid bacteria: 20 years exploring their potential as live vectors for mucosal vaccination. *Appl*

Microbiol Biotechnol 99:2967–2977. (Erratum, 99:4531. doi:10.1007/s00253-015-6569-2.)

19. Cano-Garrido O, Seras-Franzoso J, Garcia-Fruitós E. 2015. Lactic acid bacteria: reviewing the potential of a promising delivery live vector for biomedical purposes. *Microb Cell Fact* 14:137.

20. LeBlanc JG, Aubry C, Cortes-Perez NG, de Moreno de LeBlanc A, Vergnolle N, Langella P, Azevedo V, Chatel JM, Miyoshi A, Bermúdez-Humarán LG. 2013. Mucosal targeting of therapeutic molecules using genetically modified lactic acid bacteria: an update. *FEMS Microbiol Lett* 344:1–9.

21. Wells JM, Mercenier A. 2008. Mucosal delivery of therapeutic and prophylactic molecules using lactic acid bacteria. *Nat Rev Microbiol* 6: 349–362.

22. Walker DC, Klaenhammer TR. 1994. Isolation of a novel IS3 group insertion element and construction of an integration vector for *Lactobacillus* spp. *J Bacteriol* 176:5330–5340.

23. Raya RR, Fremaux C, De Antoni GL, Klaenhammer TR. 1992. Site-specific integration of the temperate bacteriophage phi adh into the *Lactobacillus gasseri* chromosome and molecular characterization of the phage (attP) and bacterial (attB) attachment sites. *J Bacteriol* 174:5584–5592.

24. Dupont L, Boizet-Bonhoure B, Coddeville M, Auvray F, Ritzenthaler P. 1995. Characterization of genetic elements required for site-specific integration of *Lactobacillus delbrueckii* subsp. *bulgaricus* bacteriophage mv4 and construction of an integration-proficient vector for *Lactobacillus plantarum*. *J Bacteriol* 177:586–595.

25. Douglas GL, Klaenhammer TR. 2011. Directed chromosomal integration and expression of the reporter gene gusA3 in *Lactobacillus acidophilus* NCFM. *Appl Environ Microbiol* 77:7365–7371.

26. Lambert JM, Bongers RS, Kleerebezem M. 2007. Cre-lox-based system for multiple gene deletions and selectable-marker removal in *Lactobacillus plantarum*. *Appl Environ Microbiol* 73:1126–1135.

27. Vos M, Didelot X. 2009. A comparison of homologous recombination rates in bacteria and archaea. *ISME J* 3:199–208.

28. Klaenhammer TR. 1995. Genetics of intestinal lactobacilli. *Int Dairy J* 5:1019–1058.

29. Hols P, Ferain T, Garmyn D, Bernard N, Delcour J. 1994. Use of homologous expression-secretion signals and vector-free stable chromosomal integration in engineering of *Lactobacillus plantarum* for alpha-amylase and levanase expression. *Appl Environ Microbiol* 60:1401–1413.

30. Scheirlinck T, Mahillon J, Joos H, Dhaese P, Michiels F. 1989. Integration and expression

of alpha-amylase and endoglucanase genes in the *Lactobacillus plantarum* chromosome. *Appl Environ Microbiol* **55**:2130–2137.

31. **Fitzsimons A, Hols P, Jore J, Leer RJ, O'Connell M, Delcour J.** 1994. Development of an amylolytic *Lactobacillus plantarum* silage strain expressing the *Lactobacillus amylovorus* alpha-amylase gene. *Appl Environ Microbiol* **60**:3529–3535.

32. **Russell WM, Klaenhammer TR.** 2001. Efficient system for directed integration into the *Lactobacillus acidophilus* and *Lactobacillus gasseri* chromosomes via homologous recombination. *Appl Environ Microbiol* **67**:4361–4364.

33. **Law J, Buist G, Haandrikman A, Kok J, Venema G, Leenhouts K.** 1995. A system to generate chromosomal mutations in *Lactococcus lactis* which allows fast analysis of targeted genes. *J Bacteriol* **177**:7011–7018.

34. **Sauer B.** 1987. Functional expression of the cre-lox site-specific recombination system in the yeast *Saccharomyces cerevisiae*. *Mol Cell Biol* **7**:2087–2096.

35. **Sauer B, Henderson N.** 1988. Site-specific DNA recombination in mammalian cells by the Cre recombinase of bacteriophage P1. *Proc Natl Acad Sci USA* **85**:5166–5170.

36. **Albert H, Dale EC, Lee E, Ow DW.** 1995. Site specific integration of DNA into wild-type and mutant lox sites placed in the plant genome. *Plant J* **7**:649–659.

37. **Nguyen TT, Mathiesen G, Fredriksen L, Kittl R, Nguyen TH, Eijsink VGH, Haltrich D, Peterbauer CK.** 2011. A food-grade system for inducible gene expression in *Lactobacillus plantarum* using an alanine racemase-encoding selection marker. *J Agric Food Chem* **59**:5617–5624.

38. **Stevens MJA, Vollenweider S, Meile L, Lacroix C.** 2011. 1,3-Propanediol dehydrogenases in *Lactobacillus reuteri*: impact on central metabolism and 3-hydroxypropionaldehyde production. *Microb Cell Fact* **10**:61.

39. **Croux C, Nguyen N-P-T, Lee J, Raynaud C, Saint-Prix F, Gonzalez-Pajuelo M, Meynial-Salles I, Soucaille P.** 2016. Construction of a restriction-less, marker-less mutant useful for functional genomic and metabolic engineering of the biofuel producer *Clostridium acetobutylicum*. *Biotechnol Biofuels* **9**:23.

40. **Wang Y, Zhang C, Gong T, Zuo Z, Zhao F, Fan X, Yang C, Song C.** 2015. An *upp*-based markerless gene replacement method for genome reduction and metabolic pathway engineering in *Pseudomonas mendocina* NK-01 and *Pseudomonas putida* KT2440. *J Microbiol Methods* **113**:27–33.

41. **Shi T, Wang G, Wang Z, Fu J, Chen T, Zhao X.** 2013. Establishment of a markerless mutation delivery system in *Bacillus subtilis* stimulated by a double-strand break in the chromosome. *PLoS One* **8**:e81370.

42. **Goh YJ, Azcárate-Peril MA, O'Flaherty S, Durmaz E, Valence F, Jardin J, Lortal S, Klaenhammer TR.** 2009. Development and application of a *upp*-based counterselective gene replacement system for the study of the S-layer protein SlpX of *Lactobacillus acidophilus* NCFM. *Appl Environ Microbiol* **75**:3093–3105.

43. **Selle K, Goh YJ, O'Flaherty S, Klaenhammer TR.** 2014. Development of an integration mutagenesis system in *Lactobacillus gasseri*. *Gut Microbes* **5**:326–332.

44. **Bron PA, Benchimol MG, Lambert J, Palumbo E, Deghorain M, Delcour J, De Vos WM, Kleerebezem M, Hols P.** 2002. Use of the *alr* gene as a food-grade selection marker in lactic acid bacteria. *Appl Environ Microbiol* **68**:5663–5670.

45. **Palumbo E, Favier CF, Deghorain M, Cocconcelli PS, Grangette C, Mercenier A, Vaughan EE, Hols P.** 2004. Knockout of the alanine racemase gene in *Lactobacillus plantarum* results in septation defects and cell wall perforation. *FEMS Microbiol Lett* **233**:131–138.

46. **Hols P, Defrenne C, Ferain T, Derzelle S, Delplace B, Delcour J.** 1997. The alanine racemase gene is essential for growth of *Lactobacillus plantarum*. *J Bacteriol* **179**:3804–3807.

47. **Yang P, Wang J, Qi Q.** 2015. Prophage recombinases-mediated genome engineering in *Lactobacillus plantarum*. *Microb Cell Fact* **14**:154.

48. **van Pijkeren J-P, Britton RA.** 2012. High efficiency recombineering in lactic acid bacteria. *Nucleic Acids Res* **40**:e76.

49. **Oh J-H, van Pijkeren J-P.** 2014. CRISPR-Cas9-assisted recombineering in *Lactobacillus reuteri*. *Nucleic Acids Res* **42**:e131.

50. **Yang XW, Model P, Heintz N.** 1997. Homologous recombination based modification in *Escherichia coli* and germline transmission in transgenic mice of a bacterial artificial chromosome. *Nat Biotechnol* **15**:859–865.

51. **Jiang W, Bikard D, Cox D, Zhang F, Marraffini LA.** 2013. RNA-guided editing of bacterial genomes using CRISPR-Cas systems. *Nat Biotechnol* **31**:233–239.

52. **Court DL, Sawitzke JA, Thomason LC.** 2002. Genetic engineering using homologous recombination. *Annu Rev Genet* **36**:361–388.

53. **Sharan SK, Thomason LC, Kuznetsov SG, Court DL.** 2009. Recombineering: a homologous recombination-based method of genetic engineering. *Nat Protoc* **4**:206–223.

54. **Montiel D, Kang H-S, Chang F-Y, Charlop-Powers Z, Brady SF.** 2015. Yeast homologous recombination-based promoter engineering for the activation of silent natural product biosynthetic gene clusters. *Proc Natl Acad Sci USA* **112:** 8953–8958.

55. **Mosberg JA, Lajoie MJ, Church GM.** 2010. Lambda red recombineering in *Escherichia coli* occurs through a fully single-stranded intermediate. *Genetics* **186:**791–799.

56. **Yu D, Sawitzke JA, Ellis H, Court DL.** 2003. Recombineering with overlapping single-stranded DNA oligonucleotides: testing a recombination intermediate. *Proc Natl Acad Sci USA* **100:**7207–7212.

57. **Cha RS, Zarbl H, Keohavong P, Thilly WG.** 1992. Mismatch amplification mutation assay (MAMA): application to the c-H-ras gene. *PCR Methods Appl* **2:**14–20.

58. **van Pijkeren JP, Neoh KM, Sirias D, Findley AS, Britton RA.** 2012. Exploring optimization parameters to increase ssDNA recombineering in *Lactococcus lactis* and *Lactobacillus reuteri.* *Bioengineered* **3:**209–217.

59. **al-Bar OA, O'Connor CD, Giles IG, Akhtar M.** 1992. D-alanine: D-alanine ligase of *Escherichia coli*: expression, purification and inhibitory studies on the cloned enzyme. *Biochem J* **282:**747–752.

60. **Kahne D, Leimkuhler C, Lu W, Walsh C.** 2005. Glycopeptide and lipoglycopeptide antibiotics. *Chem Rev* **105:**425–448.

61. **Chapot-Chartier M-P, Kulakauskas S.** 2014. Cell wall structure and function in lactic acid bacteria. *Microb Cell Fact* **13**(Suppl 1)**:**S9.

62. **Park IS, Lin CH, Walsh CT.** 1996. Gain of D-alanyl-D-lactate or D-lactyl-D-alanine synthetase activities in three active-site mutants of the *Escherichia coli* D-alanyl-D-alanine ligase B. *Biochemistry* **35:**10464–10471.

63. **Il-Park IS, Walsh CT.** 1997. D-Alanyl-D-lactate and D-alanyl-D-alanine synthesis by D-alanyl-D-alanine ligase from vancomycin-resistant *Leuconostoc mesenteroides*: effects of a phenylalanine 261 to tyrosine mutation. *J Biol Chem* **272:**9210–9214.

64. **Wang HH, Isaacs FJ, Carr PA, Sun ZZ, Xu G, Forest CR, Church GM.** 2009. Programming cells by multiplex genome engineering and accelerated evolution. *Nature* **460:**894–898.

65. **Terns MP, Terns RM.** 2011. CRISPR-based adaptive immune systems. *Curr Opin Microbiol* **14:**321–327.

66. **Doudna JA, Charpentier E.** 2014. The new frontier of genome engineering with CRISPR-Cas9. *Science* **346:**1258096.

67. **Ran FA, Hsu PD, Wright J, Agarwala V, Scott DA, Zhang F.** 2013. Genome engineering using the CRISPR-Cas9 system. *Nat Protoc* **8:**2281–2308.

68. **Hsu PD, Lander ES, Zhang F.** 2014. Development and applications of CRISPR-Cas9 for genome engineering. *Cell* **157:**1262–1278.

69. **Marraffini LA.** 2015. CRISPR-Cas immunity in prokaryotes. *Nature* **526:**55–61.

70. **Mao Z, Bozzella M, Seluanov A, Gorbunova V.** 2008. DNA repair by nonhomologous end joining and homologous recombination during cell cycle in human cells. *Cell Cycle* **7:**2902–2906.

71. **Mali P, Yang L, Esvelt KM, Aach J, Guell M, DiCarlo JE, Norville JE, Church GM.** 2013. RNA-guided human genome engineering via Cas9. *Science* **339:**823–826.

72. **Brissett NC, Doherty AJ.** 2009. Repairing DNA double-strand breaks by the prokaryotic non-homologous end-joining pathway. *Biochem Soc Trans* **37:**539–545.

73. **Reisch CR, Prather KLJ.** 2015. The no-SCAR (Scarless Cas9 Assisted Recombineering) system for genome editing in *Escherichia coli*. *Sci Rep* **5:**15096.

74. **Jacob F, Monod J.** 1961. Genetic regulatory mechanisms in the synthesis of proteins. *J Mol Biol* **3:**318–356.

75. **Eaton TJ, Shearman CA, Gasson MJ.** 1993. The use of bacterial luciferase genes as reporter genes in *Lactococcus*: regulation of the *Lactococcus lactis* subsp. *lactis* lactose genes. *J Gen Microbiol* **139:**1495–1501.

76. **Llull D, Poquet I.** 2004. New expression system tightly controlled by zinc availability in *Lactococcus lactis*. *Appl Environ Microbiol* **70:**5398–5406.

77. **Miyoshi A, Jamet E, Commissaire J, Renault P, Langella P, Azevedo V.** 2004. A xylose-inducible expression system for *Lactococcus lactis*. *FEMS Microbiol Lett* **239:**205–212.

78. **Madsen SM, Arnau J, Vrang A, Givskov M, Israelsen H.** 1999. Molecular characterization of the pH-inducible and growth phase-dependent promoter P170 of *Lactococcus lactis*. *Mol Microbiol* **32:**75–87.

79. **Kok J.** 1996. Inducible gene expression and environmentally regulated genes in lactic acid bacteria. *Antonie van Leeuwenhoek* **70:**129–145.

80. **Benbouziane B, Ribelles P, Aubry C, Martin R, Kharrat P, Riazi A, Langella P, Bermúdez-Humarán LG.** 2013. Development of a stress-inducible controlled expression (SICE) system in *Lactococcus lactis* for the production and delivery of therapeutic molecules at mucosal surfaces. *J Biotechnol* **168:**120–129.

81. **O'Sullivan DJ, Walker SA, West SG, Klaenhammer TR.** 1996. Development of an expression strategy using a lytic phage to trigger explosive plasmid amplification and gene expression. *Biotechnology (N Y)* **14:**82–87.

82. **de Ruyter PG, Kuipers OP, de Vos WM.** 1996. Controlled gene expression systems for *Lactococcus lactis* with the food-grade inducer nisin. *Appl Environ Microbiol* **62:**3662–3667.

83. **Eichenbaum Z, Federle MJ, Marra D, de Vos WM, Kuipers OP, Kleerebezem M, Scott JR.** 1998. Use of the lactococcal nisA promoter to regulate gene expression in Gram-positive bacteria: comparison of induction level and promoter strength. *Appl Environ Microbiol* **64:** 2763–2769.

84. **Mierau I, Kleerebezem M.** 2005. 10 years of the nisin-controlled gene expression system (NICE) in *Lactococcus lactis*. *Appl Microbiol Biotechnol* **68:**705–717.

85. **Wu C-M, Lin C-F, Chang Y-C, Chung T-C.** 2006. Construction and characterization of nisin-controlled expression vectors for use in *Lactobacillus reuteri*. *Biosci Biotechnol Biochem* **70:**757–767.

86. **Piard JC, Hautefort I, Fischetti VA, Ehrlich SD, Fons M, Gruss A.** 1997. Cell wall anchoring of the *Streptococcus pyogenes* M6 protein in various lactic acid bacteria. *J Bacteriol* **179:**3068–3072.

87. **Sørvig E, Mathiesen G, Naterstad K, Eijsink VGH, Axelsson L.** 2005. High-level, inducible gene expression in *Lactobacillus sakei* and *Lactobacillus plantarum* using versatile expression vectors. *Microbiology* **151:**2439–2449.

88. **Tauer C, Heinl S, Egger E, Heiss S, Grabherr R.** 2014. Tuning constitutive recombinant gene expression in *Lactobacillus plantarum*. *Microb Cell Fact* **13:**150.

89. **Karlskås IL, Maudal K, Axelsson L, Rud I, Eijsink VGH, Mathiesen G.** 2014. Heterologous protein secretion in *Lactobacilli* with modified pSIP vectors. *PLoS One* **9:**e91125.

90. **Karimi S, Ahl D, Vågesjö E, Holm L, Phillipson M, Jonsson H, Roos S.** 2016. *In vivo* and *in vitro* detection of luminescent and fluorescent *Lactobacillus reuteri* and application of red fluorescent mCherry for assessing plasmid persistence. *PLoS One* **11:**e0151969.

91. **Berlec A, Ravnikar M, Štrukelj B.** 2012. Lactic acid bacteria as oral delivery systems for biomolecules. *Pharmazie* **67:**891–898.

92. **Braat H, Rottiers P, Hommes DW, Huyghebaert N, Remaut E, Remon JP, van Deventer SJH, Neirynck S, Peppelenbosch MP, Steidler L.** 2006. A phase I trial with transgenic bacteria expressing interleukin-10 in Crohn's disease. *Clin Gastroenterol Hepatol* **4:**754–759.

93. **Bermúdez-Humarán LG, Kharrat P, Chatel J-M, Langella P.** 2011. Lactococci and lactobacilli as mucosal delivery vectors for therapeutic proteins and DNA vaccines. *Microb Cell Fact* **10**(Suppl 1):S4.

94. **Oh PL, Benson AK, Peterson DA, Patil PB, Moriyama EN, Roos S, Walter J.** 2010. Diversification of the gut symbiont *Lactobacillus reuteri* as a result of host-driven evolution. *ISME J* **4:**377–387.

95. **Mimee M, Tucker AC, Voigt CA, Lu TK.** 2015. Programming a human commensal bacterium, *Bacteroides thetaiotaomicron*, to sense and respond to stimuli in the murine gut microbiota. *Cell Syst* **1:**62–71.

96. **Rud I, Jensen PR, Naterstad K, Axelsson L.** 2006. A synthetic promoter library for constitutive gene expression in *Lactobacillus plantarum*. *Microbiology* **152:**1011–1019.

Genome Editing of Food-Grade Lactobacilli To Develop Therapeutic Probiotics

17

JAN-PETER VAN PIJKEREN[1] and RODOLPHE BARRANGOU[2]

INTRODUCTION

For thousands of years, lactic acid bacteria (LAB) have been interwoven with our food supply. The earliest evidence of milk use dates back to 7,000 years BCE (1), while cheeses were produced as early as 6,000 years BCE (2). Advances in our understanding of the microbial world in the past couple of centuries have enabled microbiology-based food manufacturing on an industrial scale. Not only are LAB used to ferment dairy products, but they are also applied to pickle vegetables, to cure meats, and to produce alcoholic beverages such as wine and sake (3, 4). This long history of safe consumption led to the consideration that many LAB strains are Generally Recognized As Safe (GRAS). As early as 1906, LAB were linked to the promotion of human health. The Russian Nobel laureate Élie Metchnikoff hypothesized that ingestion of yogurt prolonged life in Eastern European populations by reducing "putrefying" [sic] bacteria. His linkage of the perceived longevity of the Eastern European populations with consumption of fermented dairy products (5) made him the grandfather of modern probiotics. Probiotics are defined as "live microorganisms, which when administrated in adequate amounts, confer a health benefit to the host" (6). Metchnikoff's probiotic theory of life

[1]Department of Food Science, University of Wisconsin-Madison, Madison, WI 53706; [2]Department of Food, Bioprocessing, and Nutrition Sciences, North Carolina State University, Raleigh, NC 27695
Bugs as Drugs: Therapeutic Microbes for the Prevention and Treatment of Disease
Edited by Robert A. Britton and Patrice D. Cani
© 2018 American Society for Microbiology, Washington, DC
doi:10.1128/microbiolspec.BAD-0013-2016

prolongation was never directly tested, and researchers reported in 1924 that LAB present in yogurt, specifically *Lactobacillus bulgaricus*, most likely do not reduce "putrifying" bacteria in the intestine because *L. bulgaricus* did not survive gastrointestinal (GI) transit (7). Other groups challenged this finding. Elli et al. demonstrated that both *Streptococcus thermophilus* and *L. bulgaricus* were present in human feces after yogurt ingestion (8).

Regardless, Metchnikoff's theory was born that bacteria could be health-promoting through modifying the composition of the bacterial population that inhabits our intestine. In 2017, this translates into the use of (tailored) probiotics to modify the gut microbiota to promote human health. Today we can engineer LAB in general, and recent advances have made it possible to engineer select probiotic strains in a high-throughput manner. Also, we have an increased appreciation and understanding of the role of the gut microbiota in health and disease. Thus, the contemporary application of tailored probiotics to promote human health brings Metchnikoff's theory a step closer to reality. In this article, we discuss emerging applications of LAB to promote human health. Specifically, we focus on lactobacilli as tailored probiotics. We will highlight the potential of clustered regularly interspaced short palindromic repeats (CRISPRs) and the CRISPR-associated enzyme (Cas) as a broadly applicable molecular tool to engineer probiotics. Also, we will discuss the potential of engineered probiotics to deliver engineered bacteriophages harnessing user-defined CRISPRs to selectively kill target pathogens. Such approaches open new avenues to modulate the microbiome composition and function and to alter microbial populations by both the removal of select pathogens and the addition of probiotic bacteria.

LACTOBACILLUS STRAIN SELECTION

The application of LAB as bacterial therapeutics was first demonstrated by Steidler et al. (9). The cheese bacterium *Lactococcus lactis* MG1363 was engineered to secrete murine interleukin-10 (IL-10). Oral administration of the recombinant lactic acid bacterium significantly reduced intestinal inflammation in two mouse models of disease. The authors demonstrated (i) the presence of murine IL-10 in the colon of IL10$^{-/-}$ mice and (ii) that *de novo* synthesis of murine IL-10 by recombinant *L. lactis* during GI transit resulted in amelioration of intestinal inflammation. Subsequently, the *L. lactis* workhorse has been exploited to deliver a variety of recombinant proteins (10, 11) and DNA (12–14) and has paved the way to harness other microbes as delivery vehicles. As these studies clearly demonstrate that *L. lactis* can be a successful delivery vehicle, what rationale supports the development of a therapeutic delivery platform using a microbe other than *L. lactis*? One argument arises from the fact that *L. lactis* is a microbe that originates from a plant environment and has adapted to thrive in milk, not in humans (15). Because the optimal growth temperature of *L. lactis* is 30°C, some researchers may choose to select a strain that thrives at 37°C. A higher *in vivo* metabolic rate is predicted to yield increased therapeutic protein delivery, which may be desirable. Also, the efficiency of survival following GI transit can be a selection criterion. Several strains have been identified, including some lactobacilli, that better survive the conditions encountered during GI transit compared to *L. lactis* (16, 17).

Selection of strains that thrive at 37°C and can withstand the harsh *in vivo* conditions can thus be a key criterion. In addition, some research groups have exploited natural health-promoting strains, such as *Escherichia coli* Nissle 1917. Although not within the focus of this chapter, *E. coli* Nissle 1917 is notable as the only probiotic *E. coli* in use for over a century and is now being developed as a therapeutic delivery platform (18–20). A clear advantage is that researchers can tap into the most comprehensive genetic toolbox available for bacteria. *E. coli* Nissle 1917 is one of the few Gram-negative probiotics, in contrast to the plethora of Gram-positive probiotics that are widely represented by lactobacilli. While lactobacilli are being exploited as delivery vehicles, strain selection will be key for successful design of tailored probiotics.

Leveraging *Lactobacillus*'s Genetic Diversity for Strain Selection

Lactobacillus is an extraordinary, diverse genus that contains over 200 distinct species and is the largest genus within the LAB (21). Lactobacilli are found in a wide variety of environmental niches, including plants and animals, and several species are commonly found in the GI tract of mammals (22). Many strains can withstand the harsh conditions encountered during GI transit, i.e., stomach acids and bile acids, which makes select undomesticated lactobacilli strains attractive delivery vehicles (23 26). It is important to emphasize the use of undomesticated strains because prolonged *in vitro* incubation will lead to adaptation to the new environment, and some traits may be lost, e.g., traits required to thrive *in vivo*. For example, *E. coli* K-12 has lost its ability to thrive *in vivo* because it has been cultured for nearly a century under laboratory conditions (27, 28). Analogously, a *Lactobacillus* strain that was isolated from the intestine 50 years ago and cultured *in vitro* since, may therefore not be the best choice for use as an *in vivo* delivery vehicle.

This broad genetic diversity, even between strains of the same species, also contributes to variation in the efficiency of genome editing. The van Pijkeren laboratory demonstrated that different *Lactobacillus reuteri* strains yield transformation efficiencies that differ as much as 100-fold (unpublished data). Also, single-stranded DNA recombineering (SSDR) procedures, optimized for *L. reuteri* ATCC PTA 6475, have not yielded recombinants in *L. reuteri* DSM 17938 (unpublished data). The lack of recombinants in *L. reuteri* DSM 17938 is not linked to differences in transformation efficiencies. Therefore, the intraspecies vari-

ation in *L. reuteri* is enough to cause major differences in the genome editing ability.

That strain-to-strain differences impact the ability to engineer bacterial genomes is not unique to lactobacilli. For example, "wild" isolates from *E. coli* were found to be more resistant to genome editing than *E. coli* K-12 (29). Thus, differences between strains are obvious and need to be taken into consideration when developing a strain as a therapeutic delivery vehicle.

Probiotic Features: a Closer Look at Strain-Level Differences

One common misconception is that all members of the genus *Lactobacillus*, or a particular *Lactobacillus* species, are probiotic. Probiotic characteristics are typically strain-dependent. A major contributing factor is the aforementioned extraordinary genetic diversity, which is also prevalent at the intraspecies level. Comparative and functional genomics have revealed several examples that demonstrate probiotic strain specificity. The two examples that we highlight here are *Lactobacillus salivarius* and *L. reuteri*.

L. salivarius UCC118 is a candidate probiotic microbe for which several probiotic features have been validated by *in vivo* animal trials, including anti-inflammatory properties and production of an antimicrobial peptide (30–35). A screen among 88 lactobacilli, which included 35 *L. salivarius* strains, revealed that the isolate *L. salivarius* CCUG 47825 bound fibrinogen at levels comparable to the Gram-positive pathogen *Staphylococcus aureus* (36). This is an undesirable characteristic because the interaction between a fibrinogen-binding protein and blood platelets can lead to platelet aggregation (37). Although strain UCC118 lacks the gene encoding the fibrinogen-binding protein, this gene is present but not expressed in several *L. salivarius* strains. Thus, selection of a candidate delivery strain requires genome-mining strategies to eliminate strains encoding potential undesirable gene products. In addition, not all strains of the same species share probiotic characteristics. For example, the antimicrobial product reuterin and the anti-inflammatory product histamine, the latter coded by the *hdc* gene cluster, are mostly specific to a single clade of *L. reuteri* strains (38–41). In addition to proper strain selection, availability or development of a genetic toolbox will be key to developing tailored probiotics.

LACTOBACILLUS GENOME EDITING

One approach to enhance health-promoting properties is the ability to transform cells with exogenous DNA to genetically modify and engineer their genome. Depending on the type of application and the organism of choice, such engineering can be the first hurdle in the development of a LAB therapeutic. Several tools have been developed, but their application can be strain-dependent. Our discussion will not cover genetic engineering tools comprehensively, but we will briefly highlight some tools that have been developed and applied to lactobacilli. These include Cre-lox (42), bacteriophage integrases (43), introns (44), and two-plasmid integration systems (45, 46). To create DNA insertions or deletions following Campbell-like integration, the *upp*-encoded uracil phosphoribosyltransferase can be used in some strains to identify cells in which the second homologous recombination event occurred (47). Such tools have been very valuable to the LAB research community, but high-throughput engineering approaches to make subtle mutations in a LAB genome have been limited until more recently.

The Britton laboratory developed SSDR in *L. lactis*, *L. reuteri*, and *Lactobacillus plantarum* (48). The procedure was optimized for use in *L. reuteri* and *L. lactis*, while proof of concept was demonstrated in *L. plantarum*. SSDR allows the user to create single-nucleotide changes in the chromosome without the need for antibiotic selection. Only an oligonucleo-

tide is needed to generate the desired mutation(s) in the chromosome, and no cloning is required. SSDR can also be applied to make small deletions (<250 bp) in the chromosome which also do not require selection. The design and application of SSDR were recently reviewed by the same authors (49). The van Pijkeren laboratory combined SSDR with CRISPR-Cas selection in *L. reuteri* (50). CRISPR-Cas further advanced the applicability of SSDR. Low-efficiency mutants are enriched in the population following CRISPR-Cas-mediated killing of the wild-type cells. Now, mutant genotypes can be identified that previously were not possible. For example, an oligonucleotide can be used to generate 1-kb deletions or to perform targeted codon mutagenesis.

The next section will discuss CRISPR and the CRISPR-Cas protein (51) because the CRISPR-Cas technology has driven the genome editing revolution. Indeed, we believe that LAB, and lactobacilli in particular, have an untapped potential to exploit CRISPR-Cas for genetic engineering purposes (21).

CRISPR-Cas Systems

CRISPR-Cas constitutes the adaptive immune system of bacteria to protect against invasive elements such as bacteriophages and plasmids (52). Entry of the foreign DNA into the bacterial cell results in incorporation of small DNA fragments into the CRISPR locus as novel spacers integrated between CRISPR repeats (52). The CRISPR locus is transcribed and processed, yielding small CRISPR RNAs (crRNAs) that guide Cas effector nuclease toward complementary target sequences (53, 54). Subsequent exposure to foreign DNA for which the cell has a complementary crRNA results in the formation of a DNA-RNA duplex in a sequence-specific manner. The crRNA thus guides Cas nucleases to cleave the foreign double-stranded DNA, yielding sequence-specific targeting (55, 56). Next, the invasive DNA is degraded by host nucleases, which interrupts and prevents replication of the targeted DNA (57).

There are two classes and six main types of CRISPR-Cas systems, which both provide DNA-encoded and RNA-mediated targeting of nucleic acid in a sequence-specific manner (51) (Fig. 1). Of all CRISPR-Cas systems, the type II system is the most streamlined. Type II systems hinge upon only four *cas* genes, namely *cas1*, *cas2*, *cas9*, and *csn2/cas4*, and a dual crRNA:tracrRNA (58) complex that guides the Cas9 nuclease to generate a double-stranded break for sequence-specific cleavage of DNA (55, 56). In eukaryotes, upon genesis of a double-stranded break, the endogenous DNA repair machinery patches back the two cleaved DNA ends using non-homologous end-joining or replaces the native sequence by homology-directed repair using either a similar sequence within the genome (either another allele or a homologous sequence) or a provided template. Non-homologous end-joining-based repair typically yields random single nucleotide polymorphisms and short indels, whereas homology-directed repair enables precise modification of DNA sequences. Commonly, the sequence altered by the repair machinery is construed as an "edited" version of the wild-type sequence—hence the CRISPR-enabled genome editing

craze leading to its widespread use in genetic engineering (59).

Since the first proof of concept in 2013 that the human genome can be edited using Cas9, a plethora of CRISPR-based technologies have been developed to alter the genome, the transcriptome, and the epigenome (60). Scientists around the globe implemented CRISPR-Cas in different scientific fields of study, with applications for bacteria, archaea, eukarya, and even viruses. In addition to the broad adoption of these technologies in plants and mammals, the microbiology community has started to harness these CRISPR-based tools for organisms that are widely used in medicine, biotechnology, and agriculture (61, 62). We believe there is potential for the implementation of that technology in GRAS LAB for the development of engineered biotherapeutic agents (63).

The CRISPR literature is too extensive to discuss in depth. Therefore, we suggest a few of the many reviews that discuss the biology and genetics of CRISPR-Cas systems (64, 65), as well as CRISPR-based technologies and their applications in genome editing and beyond (66, 67). Here, our intent is to focus on microbial applications in general, and specifically on genome editing for enhanced health-promoting abilities.

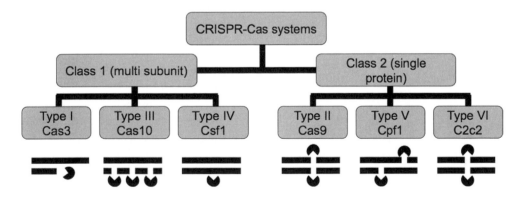

FIGURE 1 CRISPR-Cas systems. Two primary classes of CRISPR-Cas systems have been established, based on the nature of the effector proteins that direct targeting: either multisubunit complexes (class 1) or single effector proteins (class 2). Each major type of effector protein drives select cleavage of target nucleic acid, generating single-strand exonucleolytic cleavage (type I), shredding (type III), unknown (type IV), blunt cleavage (types II and VI), or sticky-end dual nicking (type V).

CRISPR-Cas Genome Editing in Lactobacilli

After CRISPR-Cas was discovered in 2007 (52), different groups started to use it in 2013 as a genome editing machine (61, 62). At the time of writing this review, CRISPR-Cas-based genetic engineering in lactobacilli has only been applied in *L. reuteri* (50). A recent extensive comparative genomics study revealed that CRISPR-Cas systems are widely distributed in the genus *Lactobacillus*. The authors of this work suggested that this may be due to phage predation, horizontal gene transfer, and the extensive genome remodeling, which collectively contribute to this genus's genetic diversity (21, 68, 69). Whereas CRISPR-Cas systems are present in approximately 46% of the total bacterial genomes present in CRISPR databases, the genus *Lactobacillus* encodes CRISPR-Cas systems in nearly 63% of the sequenced genomes (21). The wealth of CRISPR-Cas systems in lactobacilli provides researchers with the opportunity to use native Cas enzymes, combined with user-defined CRISPR arrays, to select for (low-efficiency) recombinant genotypes (70). This naturally encoded resource expands the genetic engineering potential of a group of organisms that has been historically challenging to engineer, including probiotic strains. We expect that the CRISPR toolbox, combined with technologies such as SSDR, will simplify and accelerate development of next-generation probiotics (50, 71).

LACTOBACILLI AS THE CHASSIS FOR TAILORED PROBIOTICS

Editing Native Genes To Alter the Probiotic Immune-Modulatory Profile

One approach to enhancing probiotic properties is to modify native genes that contribute to immunomodulation. Although an overall mechanistic understanding of probiotic features is still mostly lacking, the bacterial outer cell surface plays key roles in probiotic-host interactions (72). The outer cell surface of Gram-positive bacteria consists of a thick peptidoglycan layer that contains polymers of phosphate-alditol groups in addition to proteins and polysaccharides. The polymers of phosphate-alditol groups are also known as teichoic acids (TAs). TAs can be linked to the peptidoglycan (cell wall TAs) or to the membrane via glycolipids (lipoteichoic acids [LTAs]) (73, 74). The presence of TAs seems to be conserved in lactobacilli, though some species, including *Lactobacillus casei*, *Lactobacillus rhamnosus*, *Lactobacillus fermentum*, and *L. reuteri*, do not produce cell wall TAs (75). The established role of TAs in immunomodulation offers a potential target for improving probiotic efficiency. For example, TAs act on mammalian Toll-like receptors that stimulate dendritic cells and subsequently lead to cytokine responses (76, 77). Also, TAs can impact the adhesion of bacteria to host cells (78). Thus, alteration of such cell wall components by genome engineering approaches could further enhance the probiotic profile of a strain. Whereas purified LTAs of *L. plantarum* WCFS1 elicited a proinflammatory response, integration of a suicide knockout vector in the gene responsible for D-alanylation of TAs shifted the immunomodulatory profile to anti-inflammatory. Moreover, the genetically modified strain provided enhanced protection in a murine colitis model (79). This elegant work and that of others (80–83) not only shed light on *Lactobacillus*-mediated immunomodulation, but also provides an exciting opportunity to explore this pathway to enhance probiotic features.

Chronic inflammation in the colon can lead to development of colon cancer. Engineered probiotics with an improved anti-inflammatory profile may be useful to prevent colon cancer. An example is a derivative of *Lactobacillus acidophilus* NCFM, which did not produce LTAs following deletion of the gene encoding a phosphoglycerol transferase (84). This mutant was generated by a two-plasmid system (45), which is an adaptation from the pVE6007/pORI19 system (85). Mice prone to developing polyps in the colon due to a mutation in the adenomatous polyposis coli (*Apc*) gene developed significantly fewer polyps in the colon and ileum when administered the engineered probiotic lacking LTAs compared to the probiotic wild-type strain. The authors demonstrated that the wild-type and recombinant probiotic differentially modulated T-regulatory cells, which are known to play a fundamental role in the development of cancer.

In addition to modification of TAs, lactobacilli surface proteins—including cell wall-anchored proteins—also play a key role in immunomodulation; this topic has been extensively reviewed by others (86–88).

Increased understanding of the cell wall architecture of select probiotics will provide us with novel opportunities to tailor its structure for enhanced immune-modulatory properties. Basic human intervention studies with these tailored probiotics are much needed before we can fully embrace the potential of such engineered probiotics. Elegant gnotobiotic mouse models are available to characterize the interplay among (tailored) probiotics, the gut microbiota (89, 90), and the murine immune system. However, the very simple question remains: can a strong anti-inflammatory immune response observed in mice, after exposure to a human-derived tailored probiotic, be replicated in human subjects exposed to the same tailored probiotic?

Lactobacilli as Antimicrobial Production Factories To Alter the Microbiota

For decades, LAB have been exploited as microbial production factories for a wide array of proteins and metabolites (91–95). For *in vivo* applications, lactobacilli can be attractive vehicles to transport and deliver select molecules in the GI tract; however, strains need to be selected carefully. First, a strain must be able to survive passage through the GI tract. Second, one needs to be able to engineer the genome. Lactobacilli with these characteristics may function as robust mother-ships to transport and deliver therapeutics, including select antimicrobial molecules, in the GI tract. In this section we will describe the potential of lactobacilli as delivery vehicles of antimicrobial compounds to selectively alter the composition of the GI microbial community. Such lactobacilli-mediated therapies may serve as complementary or even alternative strategies to antibiotic treatment to combat antibiotic resistance, a major health threat in 21st century medicine.

Increased understanding of both the pathogenic nature of select microbes and the fundamental role of the GI microbiota in maintaining or promoting human health (96) has created a conundrum in health care. As of today, antibiotics are the primary line of treatment to eradicate bacterial pathogens. Yet application of broad-spectrum antibiotics typically results in major perturbations of the GI microbiota (97). These perturbations, especially in early life, have been correlated with long-lasting metabolic changes leading to undesirable outcomes such as obesity and allergic asthma (98, 99). Immunocompromised and elderly individuals are at increased risk of developing antibiotic-associated colitis and diarrhea (100). Also, historical overuse of antibiotics in both agriculture and health care has selected for microbes with antibiotic resistance (101). Efforts to identify novel antimicrobials, in both industrial and academic settings, have been mostly futile. A major hurdle in the identification and development of novel antimicrobials is the requirement of the molecule to effectively penetrate the bacterial cell wall for subsequent activity (102). As an alternative to the development of novel antimicrobials, expanding the natural probiotic potential with native, or bacteriophage-derived, antimicrobials may offer a supplemental or alternative strategy to antibiotics. Next, we will discuss the application of probiotic-derived natural antimicrobials and bacteriophage-derived endolysins, i.e., "enzybiotics" to antimicrobial treatments (103).

Enhancing Native Antimicrobial Activity

LAB are well known for their extensive heterogenic repertoire of antimicrobial compounds, including bacteriocins (104). Bacteriocins are small ribosomally synthesized peptides that can inhibit or kill other bacteria. The functional diversity of this family of antimicrobials is large, as illustrated by the fact that bacteriocins can collectively target a wide array of Gram-negative and Gram-positive bacteria (105). Although several bacteriocin-containing products have been developed for commercial purposes, clinicians have not yet widely explored the application of bacteriocins to target pathogens.

Although narrow-spectrum bacteriocins would be preferred, broad-spectrum bacteriocins may be useful to alleviate a bacterial infection of unknown source. Bacteriocin-mediated impact on the gut microbiota composition can be substantial, as demonstrated by Abp118, a broad-spectrum bacteriocin produced by L. salivarius UCC118 (106). The microbiota of mice and pigs were compared between groups that were administered L. salivarius wild-type or L. salivarius Δabp118. The authors confirmed that the presence of the bacteriocin-producing lactobacilli alters the gut microbiota composition; however, there were no significant changes in the microbial diversity. Nevertheless, this study and that of others (107) demonstrated that a bacteriocin-producing probiotic can eradicate select members of the gut microbiota, providing a rationale to engineer bacteriocins for enhanced efficacy. One example is the most extensively characterized bacteriocin, nisin, which is produced by select L. lactis strains and streptococci. Here, we will focus on NisA, one of the six natural nisin variants. Members of the Hill laboratory subjected nisA to site-directed and saturation mutagenesis, and recovered mutants with enhanced activity against Gram-positive and Gram-negative pathogens (108, 109). These examples clearly demonstrate the value of "classical" genetic approaches for generating probiotics with improved function. The above-described methodology was based on modification of a plasmid-encoded nisin by PCR. Recent technological developments now enable codon saturation mutagenesis in the chromosome of select lactobacilli. For example, the van Pijkeren laboratory combined SSDR with CRISPR-Cas selection in L. reuteri to perform one-step codon saturation mutagenesis (50). A single transformation of an oligonucleotide containing the NNK motif (N= A/T/G/C and K= G/T) yielded a pool of recombinants in which a single codon was modified to encode all 20 amino acids. These approaches could be multiplexed to accelerate the discovery of probiotics with enhanced antimicrobial activity.

As an alternative to codon mutagenesis to identify novel antimicrobial variants, genetic engineering approaches can also be applied to improve the production of the antimicrobial. Improved production was previously achieved for reuterin, also known as 3-hydroxypropionaldehyde (3-HPA) (110). Select L. reuteri strains produce reuterin as an intermediate during glycerol fermentation to yield 1,3-propanediol (111). Reuterin has broad-spectrum activity (38, 112, 113). The gene cluster responsible for 1,3-propanediol production (and thus reuterin) is the propanediol utilization (pdu) operon. By SSDR, six bases were modified in the promoter region driving expression of the pdu operon. The recombinant strain produced more reuterin (114), resulting in 3-fold-increased killing efficacy of E. coli compared to the wild-type strain (110). Also, deletion of the gene encoding 1,3-propanediol reductase, which is responsible for the conversion of reuterin to 1,3-propanediol, yielded approximately 4-fold more reuterin compared to the wild-type (115). Therefore, a double mutant derivative in which increased expression of the pdu operon is combined with deletion of the 1,3-propanediol reductase gene has the potential to yield a tailored probiotic with superior in vivo killing activity. As with any mutation that is either naturally acquired or engineered, it remains to be seen if the new genotype impacts *in vivo* fitness.

Enzybiotics

Bacteriophages are known to be the most ubiquitous form of life on planet Earth. In the GI tract alone, ~10^{15} bacteriophages are predicted to be present. Except for filamentous bacteriophages, which the host excretes (116, 117), other bacteriophages require host lysis to release progeny phage. Two proteins play a key role in degrading the bacterial cell wall: holins and lysins (118). During bacteriophage replication, biologically active lysins are present in the cytosol but require expression of a membrane protein, holin, to release the virions from the cell. When holin levels are optimal, the lysin can access the peptidoglycan layer for cleavage that leads to bacterial cell lysis (119). So far, five main groups of lysins have been identified that can be distinguished from one another based on their cleavage specificity for the different bonds within the peptidoglycan (Fig. 2) (120). Structurally, lysins can consist of a single catalytic domain, which is typical for lysins derived from bacteriophages targeting Gram-negative bacteria (121). Bacteriophages targeting Gram-positive bacteria typically encode lysins that contain multiple domains: an N-terminal catalytic domain and a C-terminal cell wall-binding domain (122, 123). Few lysins have been identified with three domains (124).

Since their discovery over a century ago, bacteriophages have been exploited to kill select microbes via their production of holins and/or endolysins. Historically, bacteriophage therapy was mainly focused in Eastern Europe, whereas the wide application of antibiotics was preferred in the United States (125). The advantages of chemically synthesized molecules over biologically manufactured viruses include ease and consistency. However, the emerging and rapidly expanding threat of antibiotic resistance has led to a revival of the use of bacteriophages in therapy, though clinical success—specifically to

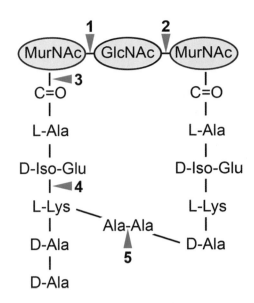

FIGURE 2 Endolysin target sites within the Gram-positive peptidoglycan matrix. A simplified overview of the peptidoglycan matrix in which the target sites of the five bacteriophage-derived endolysins are indicated with green arrows. The arrows refer to the following endolysin types: (1) muramidase, also referred to as lysozyme, (2) glucosaminidase, (3) amidase, (4) γ-endopeptidase, and (5) endopeptidase. The figure is adapted from reference 120.

target GI microbes—has so far been limited. Successful application of bacteriophage therapy to target microbes in the gut requires the bacteriophage to maintain biological activity following exposure to stomach acids and bile acids, which has proven to be problematic in general (126).

One approach that may hold promise is to use lactobacilli to deliver bacteriophage lysins *in situ* to kill the bacterial target. The basis for this approach is that (i) many lactobacilli are able to efficiently survive passage through the GI tract (23–26), (ii) the cell wall-binding domain determines a narrow host range (127, 128), which makes them suitable for heterologous expression, and (iii) various *in vitro* and *in vivo* studies have demonstrated that heterologously expressed lysins can kill select Gram-positive bacteria (129–132). Some studies have reported that lysins can also be effective against Gram-negative bacteria despite the presence of an outer cell membrane (133, 134). Various databases provide a valuable resource to select lysins for heterologous expression. For example, EnzyBase2 contains over 2,000 enzybiotics encompassing 1,800 enzybiotics derived from natural resources (bacteriophages) and approximately 200 synthetic enzybiotics (135). Also, the PHAST (PHAge Search Tool) database provides a wealth of information on bacteriophage genomes, both complete and remnant, that allows users to search for bacteriophage-derived endolysins for heterologous expression (136). Though theoretically promising, these resources have not been fully explored.

The application of enzybiotics may be suitable for *Clostridium difficile* infections. *C. difficile* is the leading cause of nosocomial antibiotic-associated diarrhea, and a major contributing factor to *C. difficile* disease is antibiotics. Antibiotics cause a significant disruption of patients' GI microbiota, which allows *C. difficile* to quickly expand and results in toxin-induced diarrhea, among other clinical manifestations (137). In up to 30% of people previously treated for a *C. difficile* infection, every future antibiotic treatment will trigger another episode of *C. difficile* expansion, mostly instigated by hypervirulent strains. The emerging hypervirulent phenotype (138), identification of strains that are resistant to fluoroquinolones (139), and the realistic prospect that acquired antibiotic resistance will go beyond the documented fluoroquinolone resistance (140, 141) collectively create the potential for a *C. difficile* epidemic. A highly successful remedy for recurrent *C. difficile* infections is a fecal microbial transplant. Although FMT has a success rate of ~90%, it has become evident in the last decade that a variety of diseases are linked to differences in the gut microbiota composition (142), including obesity (143, 144), and widespread fecal microbial transplant application should be approached with caution. This is supported by a recent report describing the

case of a woman who received a fecal microbial transplant and subsequently rapidly gained 37 pounds and became obese (145). Thus, more subtle and specific approaches to treating *C. difficile* are much needed. Therefore, approaches to eradicate *C. difficile* using approaches that do not disturb the microbiota, such as *in situ* delivery of enzybiotics, have the potential to become alternative treatment strategies. Successful expression of the *C. difficile* enzybiotic CD27L has been demonstrated in *L. lactis* (146), but proof of concept in mouse models of *C. difficile* infection is thus far lacking.

CRISPR-Based Antimicrobials

Though the biological purpose of CRISPR-Cas is to serve as an immune system against invasive nucleic acids in bacteria and archaea, they can be repurposed for other applications, including as programmable antimicrobials (147) (Fig. 3). Indeed, what renders CRISPR machines desirable for genome editing in eukaryotes makes them lethal antimicrobials in prokaryotes (148). The rationale for CRISPR-Cas lethality in bacteria is that many bacteria lack (efficient) nonhomologous end-joining systems (149). Therefore, self-targeting CRISPR spacers are highly lethal and are selected against during accidental acquisition of spacers from the host chromosome (150). This is a tremendous opportunity for the repurposing of endogenous or exogenous CRISPR-Cas systems for self-targeting in bacteria, as programmable and specific antimicrobials (147). Proof of concept has been generated *in vivo* and *in vitro*, using both type I and type II CRISPR-Cas systems and harnessing both native and heterologous Cas nucleases (147, 151, 152).

However, the primary challenge is *in situ* delivery, especially in the GI tract. We envision that there is a significant potential for using engineered probiotic bacteria as "Trojan horses" for the local delivery of engineered bacteriophage that carry a

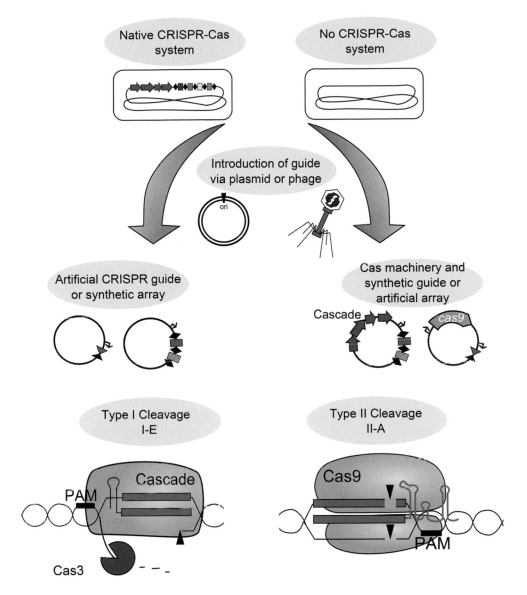

FIGURE 3 Repurposing CRISPR-Cas systems as antimicrobials. If endogenous CRISPR-Cas systems are natively present in the target organism (left), they can be repurposed and redirected toward self-targeting by delivering either CRISPR guide RNAs or synthetic CRISPR arrays that contain a self-targeting spacer that contains sequences homologous to those of the host chromosome. Alternatively, for organisms in which no CRISPR-Cas systems are universally present, or active (right), both the CRISPR arrays (or guide RNAs) and the Cas machinery (Cas effector nucleases such as Cascade or Cas9) can be delivered via plasmids or phages. Various types of CRISPR-Cas systems can be harnessed for lethal self-targeting (bottom), encompassing both class 1 and class 2 systems, exemplified by the type I-E system, hinging on the Cas3 exonuclease for extensive shredding of a DNA strand (bottom left), or by the type II-A system, hinging on the Cas9 endonuclease for genesis of double-stranded DNA breaks (bottom right).

CRISPR-cassette for self-targeting in pathogenic bacteria. One approach would be to engineer a hybrid between a plasmid and a bacteriophage to yield a phasmid for heterogenic bacteriophage production in the probiotic bacteria (Fig. 4). The generation of a phasmid was demonstrated 3 decades ago by fusion of the *E. coli* bacteriophage P2 with plasmid pBR322 (153). Replication of the phasmid could be established from either the plasmid replication proteins or from the bacteriophage replication proteins. Functional virions were produced by both replication methods. With the development of high-throughput assembling technologies, such as Gibson assembly (154), building synthetic DNA fragments such as phasmids, containing double-stranded DNA bacteriophage DNA, is a realistic approach. The CRISPR array, specific for the pathogen to be targeted, can be embedded in the bacteriophage genome for packaging, analogous to what has been described previously (151, 152). Once the phasmid is established in the probiotic, virions are produced in the cytosol. To release the virions *in situ*, a promoter that is activated upon exposure to an *in vivo* environmental cue (i.e., bile) can be fused to a probiotic-specific holin to lyse the engineered probiotic (155). Not only does efficient lysis result in therapeutic delivery, but it is also key to establishing biological containment. The released virions inject the DNA in the target pathogen to deliver the CRISPR array, which yields strain-specific killing when combined with the native Cas proteins. An advantage of the CRISPR approach is that CRISPR-Cas kills bacteria without lysis, which limits the release of toxins upon killing.

Without a doubt, the production of biologically active virions, aside from the potential hurdle to establish a large phasmid in the *Lactobacillus* cell, will be challenging, yet its potential to target pathogens in a strain-specific manner is unprecedented. Our vision is that the technological advances that have been made in the past decade, especially in the field of synthetic biology, combined with a growing research community studying lactobacilli, will inevitably lead to engineered probiotics that can modify the gut microbiota in a strain-specific manner.

FUTURE PERSPECTIVES

Overall, the examples we have provided illustrate how food-grade bacteria in general, and probiotic lactobacilli in particular, can be used to promote human health. As long as the scientific community continues to expand the genetic toolboxes for LAB, we envision that LAB will provide great potential to modulate the microbiota. In particular, the application of CRISPR-based technologies has the potential to eradicate target microbes in a strain-specific manner.

Advancing this field must include considerations of the ancillary forces and dimensions that drive and enable technological advances, such as intellectual property, regulatory processes, and consumer acceptance. The ongoing CRISPR intellectual property battles are somewhat hindering the adoption of this technology for food, agricultural, and clinical applications, given the lack of clarity around freedom to operate. Furthermore, regulatory approvals are still pending in some cases, and regulatory processes are unclear and/or yet to be defined in others. Lastly, consumer acceptance of genetically modified organisms remains a challenge that extends beyond the scientific dialogue, and much progress remains to be achieved. Nonetheless, the momentum of the ongoing microbiology renaissance remains strong, fueled by CRISPR technological advances and our increasing awareness of the microbiome.

ACKNOWLEDGMENTS

The van Pijkeren laboratory is grateful for support from BioGaia AB (Stockholm, Sweden); the UW-Madison Food Research Institute; the UW-Madison Institute of Clinical and Translational Research funded by the

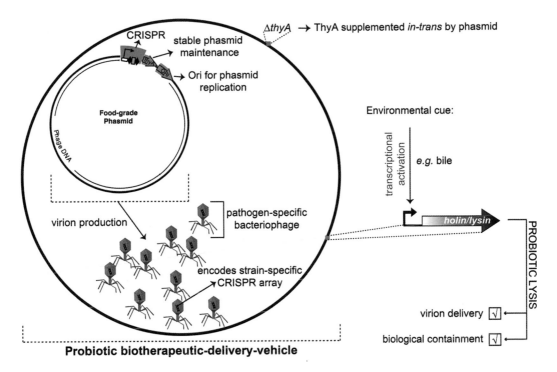

FIGURE 4 Probiotic dual-delivery system of CRISPR-coding bacteriophages. Conceptual overview of an engineered probiotic encoding phasmid-derived virions that harbor a CRISPR array to target pathogens upon release from the probiotic delivery host. Amplicons of a pathogen-derived double-stranded DNA bacteriophage are fused with a plasmid origin of replication (ORI), a probiotic auxotrophic marker, and a CRISPR cassette. The phasmid-encoded auxotrophic marker, when deleted from the bacterial chromosome, yields stable phasmid replication. The phasmid will reproduce virions, which encode engineered CRISPR arrays, in the cytosol of the cell. Release of the engineered virions can be achieved by placing a gene encoding a holin and/or endolysin protein, which is known to lyse the probiotic, under the control of a promoter that is activated upon sensing environmental cues, i.e., bile salts, in the small intestine. These already have been identified in bacteria (156), which can be adapted for use in probiotics. Successful lysis achieves both biological containment and delivery of the engineered virions *in situ*. When the virions attach to the target pathogen, DNA will be injected. Delivery of the user-defined CRISPR array will, combined with native Cas enzymes, result in strain-specific killing of the pathogen.

National Center for Advancing Translational Science award UL1TR000427; the National Institute of Allergy and Infectious Diseases of the National Institutes of Health under award number 1R21AI121662; the National Institute of Food and Agriculture, U.S. Department of Agriculture, Hatch award number MSN185615; and the American Cancer Society under award number IRG-15-213-51.

The authors thank Laura Hogan (UW-Madison Institute of Clinical and Translational Research) for copyediting our manuscript.

ACKNOWLEDGMENTS

R.B. and J.P.V.P. are inventors on several patents related to various uses of CRISPR-Cas systems, and J.P.V.P. is an inventor on patents related to probiotic delivery systems. R.B. is a board member of Caribou Biosciences, a founder and advisor of Intellia Therapeutics, and a founder and advisor of Locus Biosciences, companies that are involved in the commercialization of CRISPR applications.

CITATION

van Pijkeren J-P, Barrangou R. 2017. Genome editing of food-grade lactobacilli to develop therapeutic probiotics. Microbiol Spectrum 5(4):BAD-0013-2016.

REFERENCE

1. **Evershed RP, Payne S, Sherratt AG, Copley MS, Coolidge J, Urem-Kotsu D, Kotsakis K, Ozdoğan M, Ozdoğan AE, Nieuwenhuyse O, Akkermans PMMG, Bailey D, Andeescu R-R, Campbell S, Farid S, Hodder I, Yalman N, Ozbaşaran M, Biçakci E, Garfinkel Y, Levy T, Burton MM.** 2008. Earliest date for milk use in the Near East and southeastern Europe linked to cattle herding. *Nature* **455:**528–531.
2. **Salque M, Bogucki PI, Pyzel J, Sobkowiak-Tabaka I, Grygiel R, Szmyt M, Evershed RP.** 2013. Earliest evidence for cheese making in the sixth millennium BC in northern Europe. *Nature* **493:**522–525.
3. **Das D, Goyal A.** 2012. Lactic acid bacteria in food industry, p 757–772. *In Microorganisms in Sustainable Agriculture and Biotechnology.* Springer Netherlands, Dordrecht, The Netherlands.
4. **König H, Fröhlich J.** 2009. Lactic acid bacteria, p 3–29. *In* König H, Fröhlich J, Unden G (ed), *Biology of Microorganisms on Grapes, in Must and in Wine.* Springer, Heidelberg, Germany.
5. **Metchnikoff E.** 1910. *The Prolongation of Life. Optimistic Studies.* G.P. Putnam's Sons, New York, NY.
6. **Hill C, Guarner F, Reid G, Gibson GR, Merenstein DJ, Pot B, Morelli L, Canani RB, Flint HJ, Salminen S, Calder PC, Sanders ME.** 2014. Expert consensus document. The International Scientific Association for Probiotics and Prebiotics consensus statement on the scope and appropriate use of the term probiotic. *Nat Rev Gastroenterol Hepatol* **11:**506–514.
7. **Kulp WL, Rettger LF.** 1924. Comparative study of *Lactobacillus acidophilus* and *Lactobacillus bulgaricus. J Bacteriol* **9:**357–395.
8. **Elli M, Callegari ML, Ferrari S, Bessi E, Cattivelli D, Soldi S, Morelli L, Goupil Feuillerat N, Antoine JM.** 2006. Survival of yogurt bacteria in the human gut. *Appl Environ Microbiol* **72:**5113–5117.
9. **Steidler L, Hans W, Schotte L, Neirynck S, Obermeier F, Falk W, Fiers W, Remaut E.** 2000. Treatment of murine colitis by *Lactococcus lactis* secreting interleukin-10. *Science* **289:**1352–1355.
10. **Bahey-El-Din M, Gahan CGM, Griffin BT.** 2010. *Lactococcus lactis* as a cell factory for delivery of therapeutic proteins. *Curr Gene Ther* **10:**34–45.
11. **Robert S, Steidler L.** 2014. Recombinant *Lactococcus lactis* can make the difference in antigen-specific immune tolerance induction, the type 1 diabetes case. *Microb Cell Fact* **13** (Suppl 1):S11.
12. **Guimarães V, Innocentin S, Chatel J-M, Lefèvre F, Langella P, Azevedo V, Miyoshi A.** 2009. A new plasmid vector for DNA delivery using lactococci. *Genet Vaccines Ther* **7:**4.
13. **Chatel J-M, Pothelune L, Ah-Leung S, Corthier G, Wal J-M, Langella P.** 2008. *In vivo* transfer of plasmid from food-grade transiting lactococci to murine epithelial cells. *Gene Ther* **15:**1184–1190.
14. **de Azevedo M, Karczewski J, Lefévre F, Azevedo V, Miyoshi A, Wells JM, Langella P, Chatel J-M.** 2012. *In vitro* and *in vivo* characterization of DNA delivery using recombinant *Lactococcus lactis* expressing a mutated form of *L. monocytogenes* internalin A. *BMC Microbiol* **12:**299.
15. **Cavanagh D, Fitzgerald GF, McAuliffe O.** 2015. From field to fermentation: the origins of *Lactococcus lactis* and its domestication to the dairy environment. *Food Microbiol* **47:**45–61.
16. **Daniel C, Poiret S, Dennin V, Boutillier D, Pot B.** 2013. Bioluminescence imaging study of spatial and temporal persistence of *Lactobacillus plantarum* and *Lactococcus lactis* in living mice. *Appl Environ Microbiol* **79:**1086–1094.
17. **Vesa T, Pochart P, Marteau P.** 2000. Pharmacokinetics of *Lactobacillus plantarum* NCIMB 8826, *Lactobacillus fermentum* KLD, and *Lactococcus lactis* MG 1363 in the human gastrointestinal tract. *Aliment Pharmacol Ther* **14:**823–828.
18. **Ou B, Yang Y, Tham WL, Chen L, Guo J, Zhu G.** 2016. Genetic engineering of probiotic *Escherichia coli* Nissle 1917 for clinical application. *Appl Microbiol Biotechnol* **100:**8693–8699.
19. **Sonnenborn U.** 2016. *Escherichia coli* strain Nissle 1917--from bench to bedside and back: history of a special *Escherichia coli* strain with probiotic properties. *FEMS Microbiol Lett* **363:** fnw212.
20. **Wassenaar TM.** 2016. Insights from 100 years of research with probiotic *E. coli. Eur J Microbiol Immunol (Bp)* **6:**147–161.
21. **Sun Z, Harris HMB, McCann A, Guo C, Argimón S, Zhang W, Yang X, Jeffery IB, Cooney JC, Kagawa TF, Liu W, Song Y, Salvetti**

E, Wrobel A, Rasinkangas P, Parkhill J, Rea MC, O'Sullivan O, Ritari J, Douillard FP, Paul Ross R, Yang R, Briner AE, Felis GE, de Vos WM, Barrangou R, Klaenhammer TR, Caufield PW, Cui Y, Zhang H, O'Toole PW. 2015. Expanding the biotechnology potential of lactobacilli through comparative genomics of 213 strains and associated genera. *Nat Commun* **6:**8322.

22. **Giraffa G.** 2014. Overview of the ecology and biodiversity of the LAB, p 45–54. *In* Holzapfel WH, Wood BJB (ed), *Lactic Acid Bacteria.* John Wiley & Sons, Chichester, United Kingdom.

23. **Oozeer R, Leplingard A, Mater DDG, Mogenet A, Michelin R, Seksek I, Marteau P, Doré J, Bresson J-L, Corthier G.** 2006. Survival of *Lactobacillus casei* in the human digestive tract after consumption of fermented milk. *Appl Environ Microbiol* **72:**5615–5617.

24. **Frese SA, Hutkins RW, Walter J.** 2012. Comparison of the colonization ability of autochthonous and allochthonous strains of lactobacilli in the human gastrointestinal tract. *Adv Microbiol* **2:**399–409.

25. **Pitino I, Randazzo CL, Mandalari G, Lo Curto A, Faulks RM, Le Marc Y, Bisignano C, Caggia C, Wickham MSJ.** 2010. Survival of *Lactobacillus rhamnosus* strains in the upper gastrointestinal tract. *Food Microbiol* **27:**1121–1127.

26. **de Vries MC, Vaughan EE, Kleerebezem M, de Vos WM.** 2006. *Lactobacillus plantarum*: survival, functional and potential probiotic properties in the human intestinal tract. *Int Dairy J* **16:**1018–1028.

27. **Fux CA, Shirtliff M, Stoodley P, Costerton JW.** 2005. Can laboratory reference strains mirror "real-world" pathogenesis? *Trends Microbiol* **13:**58–63.

28. **Eydallin G, Ryall B, Maharjan R, Ferenci T.** 2014. The nature of laboratory domestication changes in freshly isolated *Escherichia coli* strains. *Environ Microbiol* **16:**813–828.

29. **Derous V, Deboeck F, Hernalsteens J-P, De Greve H.** 2011. Reproducible gene targeting in recalcitrant *Escherichia coli* isolates. *BMC Res Notes* **4:**213.

30. **O'Hara AM, O'Regan P, Fanning A, O'Mahony C, Macsharry J, Lyons A, Bienenstock J, O'Mahony L, Shanahan F.** 2006. Functional modulation of human intestinal epithelial cell responses by *Bifidobacterium infantis* and *Lactobacillus salivarius. Immunology* **118:**202–215.

31. **O'Callaghan J, Buttó LF, MacSharry J, Nally K, O'Toole PW.** 2012. Influence of adhesion and bacteriocin production by *Lactobacillus salivarius* on the intestinal epithelial cell transcriptional response. *Appl Environ Microbiol* **78:**5196–5203.

32. **Ryan KA, O'Hara AM, van Pijkeren J-P, Douillard FP, O'Toole PW.** 2009. *Lactobacillus salivarius* modulates cytokine induction and virulence factor gene expression in *Helicobacter pylori. J Med Microbiol* **58:**996–1005.

33. **O'Shea EF, O'Connor PM, Raftis EJ, O'Toole PW, Stanton C, Cotter PD, Ross RP, Hill C.** 2011. Production of multiple bacteriocins from a single locus by gastrointestinal strains of *Lactobacillus salivarius. J Bacteriol* **193:**6973–6982.

34. **Miyauchi E, O'Callaghan J, Buttó LF, Hurley G, Melgar S, Tanabe S, Shanahan F, Nally K, O'Toole PW.** 2012. Mechanism of protection of transepithelial barrier function by *Lactobacillus salivarius*: strain dependence and attenuation by bacteriocin production. *Am J Physiol Gastrointest Liver Physiol* **303:**G1029–G1041.

35. **Corr SC, Li Y, Riedel CU, O'Toole PW, Hill C, Gahan CGM.** 2007. Bacteriocin production as a mechanism for the antiinfective activity of *Lactobacillus salivarius* UCC118. *Proc Natl Acad Sci USA* **104:**7617–7621.

36. **Collins J, van Pijkeren J-P, Svensson L, Claesson MJ, Sturme M, Li Y, Cooney JC, van Sinderen D, Walker AW, Parkhill J, Shannon O, O'Toole PW.** 2012. Fibrinogen-binding and platelet-aggregation activities of a *Lactobacillus salivarius* septicaemia isolate are mediated by a novel fibrinogen-binding protein. *Mol Microbiol* **85:**862–877.

37. **Fitzgerald JR, Foster TJ, Cox D.** 2006. The interaction of bacterial pathogens with platelets. *Nat Rev Microbiol* **4:**445–457.

38. **Spinler JK, Taweechotipatr M, Rognerud CL, Ou CN, Tumwasorn S, Versalovic J.** 2008. Human-derived probiotic *Lactobacillus reuteri* demonstrate antimicrobial activities targeting diverse enteric bacterial pathogens. *Anaerobe* **14:**166–171.

39. **Spinler JK, Sontakke A, Hollister EB, Venable SF, Oh PL, Balderas MA, Saulnier DMA, Mistretta T-A, Devaraj S, Walter J, Versalovic J, Highlander SK.** 2014. From prediction to function using evolutionary genomics: human-specific ecotypes of *Lactobacillus reuteri* have diverse probiotic functions. *Genome Biol Evol* **6:**1772–1789.

40. **Hemarajata P, Gao C, Pflughoeft KJ, Thomas CM, Saulnier DM, Spinler JK, Versalovic J.** 2013. *Lactobacillus reuteri*-specific immunoregulatory gene rsiR modulates histamine production and immunomodulation by *Lactobacillus reuteri. J Bacteriol* **195:**5567–5576.

41. **Thomas CM, Hong T, van Pijkeren J-P, Hemarajata P, Trinh DV, Hu W, Britton RA, Kalkum M, Versalovic J.** 2012. Histamine derived from probiotic *Lactobacillus reuteri*

suppresses TNF via modulation of PKA and ERK signaling. *PLoS One* **7**:e31951.

42. **Lambert JM, Bongers RS, Kleerebezem M.** 2007. Cre-lox-based system for multiple gene deletions and selectable-marker removal in *Lactobacillus plantarum*. *Appl Environ Microbiol* **73**:1126–1135.

43. **Auvray F, Coddeville M, Ritzenthaler P, Dupont L.** 1997. Plasmid integration in a wide range of bacteria mediated by the integrase of *Lactobacillus delbrueckii* bacteriophage mv4. *J Bacteriol* **179**:1837–1845.

44. **Sasikumar P, Paul E, Gomathi S, Abhishek A, Sasikumar S, Selvam GS.** 2016. Mobile group II intron based gene targeting in *Lactobacillus plantarum* WCFS1. *J Basic Microbiol* **56**:1107–1116.

45. **Russell WM, Klaenhammer TR.** 2001. Efficient system for directed integration into the *Lactobacillus acidophilus* and *Lactobacillus gasseri* chromosomes via homologous recombination. *Appl Environ Microbiol* **67**:4361–4364.

46. **van Pijkeren J-P, Canchaya C, Ryan KA, Li Y, Claesson MJ, Sheil B, Steidler L, O'Mahony L, Fitzgerald GF, van Sinderen D, O'Toole PW.** 2006. Comparative and functional analysis of sortase-dependent proteins in the predicted secretome of *Lactobacillus salivarius* UCC118. *Appl Environ Microbiol* **72**:4143–4153.

47. **Goh Y-J, Azcárate-Peril MA, O'Flaherty S, Durmaz E, Valence F, Jardin J, Lortal S, Klaenhammer TR.** 2009. Development and application of a upp-based counterselective gene replacement system for the study of the S-layer protein SlpX of *Lactobacillus acidophilus* NCFM. *Appl Environ Microbiol* **75**:3093–3105.

48. **van Pijkeren J-P, Britton RA.** 2012. High efficiency recombineering in lactic acid bacteria. *Nucleic Acids Res* **40**:e76.

49. **van Pijkeren J-P, Britton RA.** 2014. Precision genome engineering in lactic acid bacteria. *Microb Cell Fact* **13**(Suppl 1):S10.

50. **Oh J-H, van Pijkeren J-P.** 2014. CRISPR-Cas9-assisted recombineering in *Lactobacillus reuteri*. *Nucleic Acids Res* **42**:e131.

51. **Makarova KS, Wolf YI, Alkhnbashi OS, Costa F, Shah SA, Saunders SJ, Barrangou R, Brouns SJJ, Charpentier E, Haft DH, Horvath P, Moineau S, Mojica FJM, Terns RM, Terns MP, White MF, Yakunin AF, Garrett RA, van der Oost J, Backofen R, Koonin EV.** 2015. An updated evolutionary classification of CRISPR-Cas systems. *Nat Rev Microbiol* **13**:722–736.

52. **Barrangou R, Fremaux C, Deveau H, Richards M, Boyaval P, Moineau S, Romero DA,** Horvath P. 2007. CRISPR provides acquired resistance against viruses in prokaryotes. *Science* **315**:1709–1712.

53. **Brouns SJJ, Jore MM, Lundgren M, Westra ER, Slijkhuis RJH, Snijders APL, Dickman MJ, Makarova KS, Koonin EV, van der Oost J.** 2008. Small CRISPR RNAs guide antiviral defense in prokaryotes. *Science* **321**:960–964.

54. **Marraffini LA, Sontheimer EJ.** 2010. CRISPR interference: RNA-directed adaptive immunity in bacteria and archaea. *Nat Rev Genet* **11**:181–190.

55. **Garneau JE, Dupuis M-È, Villion M, Romero DA, Barrangou R, Boyaval P, Fremaux C, Horvath P, Magadán AH, Moineau S.** 2010. The CRISPR/Cas bacterial immune system cleaves bacteriophage and plasmid DNA. *Nature* **468**:67–71.

56. **Gasiunas G, Barrangou R, Horvath P, Siksnys V.** 2012. Cas9-crRNA ribonucleoprotein complex mediates specific DNA cleavage for adaptive immunity in bacteria. *Proc Natl Acad Sci USA* **109**:E2579–E2586.

57. **Barrangou R.** 2015. Diversity of CRISPR-Cas immune systems and molecular machines. *Genome Biol* **16**:247.

58. **Deltcheva E, Chylinski K, Sharma CM, Gonzales K, Chao Y, Pirzada ZA, Eckert MR, Vogel J, Charpentier E.** 2011. CRISPR RNA maturation by trans-encoded small RNA and host factor RNase III. *Nature* **471**:602–607.

59. **Pennisi E.** 2013. The CRISPR craze. *Science* **341**:833–836.

60. **Hilton IB, D'Ippolito AM, Vockley CM, Thakore PI, Crawford GE, Reddy TE, Gersbach CA.** 2015. Epigenome editing by a CRISPR-Cas9-based acetyltransferase activates genes from promoters and enhancers. *Nat Biotechnol* **33**:510–517.

61. **Mali P, Yang L, Esvelt KM, Aach J, Guell M, DiCarlo JE, Norville JE, Church GM.** 2013. RNA-guided human genome engineering via Cas9. *Science* **339**:823–826.

62. **Cong L, Ran FA, Cox D, Lin S, Barretto R, Habib N, Hsu PD, Wu X, Jiang W, Marraffini LA, Zhang F.** 2013. Multiplex genome engineering using CRISPR/Cas systems. *Science* **339**:819–823.

63. **Selle K, Barrangou R.** 2015. Harnessing CRISPR-Cas systems for bacterial genome editing. *Trends Microbiol* **23**:225–232.

64. **Barrangou R, Marraffini LA.** 2014. CRISPR-Cas systems: prokaryotes upgrade to adaptive immunity. *Mol Cell* **54**:234–244.

65. **Sontheimer EJ, Barrangou R.** 2015. The bacterial origins of the CRISPR genome-editing revolution. *Hum Gene Ther* **26**:413–424.

66. Hsu PD, Lander ES, Zhang F. 2014. Development and applications of CRISPR-Cas9 for genome engineering. *Cell* **157**:1262–1278.

67. Sander JD, Joung JK. 2014. CRISPR-Cas systems for editing, regulating and targeting genomes. *Nat Biotechnol* **32**:347–355.

68. Makarova K, Slesarev A, Wolf Y, Sorokin A, Mirkin B, Koonin E, Pavlov A, Pavlova N, Karamychev V, Polouchine N, Shakhova V, Grigoriev I, Lou Y, Rohksar D, Lucas S, Huang K, Goodstein DM, Hawkins T, Plengvidhya V, Welker D, Hughes J, Goh Y, Benson A, Baldwin K, Lee J-H, Díaz-Muñiz I, Dosti B, Smeianov V, Wechter W, Barabote R, Lorca G, Altermann E, Barrangou R, Ganesan B, Xie Y, Rawsthorne H, Tamir D, Parker C, Breidt F, Broadbent J, Hutkins R, O'Sullivan D, Steele J, Unlu G, Saier M, Klaenhammer T, Richardson P, Kozyavkin S, Weimer B, Mills D. 2006. Comparative genomics of the lactic acid bacteria. *Proc Natl Acad Sci USA* **103**:15611–15616.

69. Canchaya C, Claesson MJ, Fitzgerald GF, van Sinderen D, O'Toole PW. 2006. Diversity of the genus *Lactobacillus* revealed by comparative genomics of five species. *Microbiology* **152**:3185–3196.

70. Selle K, Klaenhammer TR, Barrangou R. 2015. CRISPR-based screening of genomic island excision events in bacteria. *Proc Natl Acad Sci USA* **112**:8076–8081.

71. Barrangou R, van Pijkeren J-P. 2016. Exploiting CRISPR-Cas immune systems for genome editing in bacteria. *Curr Opin Biotechnol* **37**:61–68.

72. Kleerebezem M, Hols P, Bernard E, Rolain T, Zhou M, Siezen RJ, Bron PA. 2010. The extracellular biology of the lactobacilli. *FEMS Microbiol Rev* **34**:199–230.

73. Brown L, Wolf JM, Prados-Rosales R, Casadevall A. 2015. Through the wall: extracellular vesicles in Gram-positive bacteria, mycobacteria and fungi. *Nat Rev Microbiol* **13**:620–630.

74. Brown S, Santa Maria JP Jr, Walker S. 2013. Wall teichoic acids of Gram-positive bacteria. *Annu Rev Microbiol* **67**:313–336.

75. Chapot-Chartier M-P, Kulakauskas S. 2014. Cell wall structure and function in lactic acid bacteria. *Microb Cell Fact* **13**(Suppl 1):S9.

76. Matsuguchi T, Takagi A, Matsuzaki T, Nagaoka M, Ishikawa K, Yokokura T, Yoshikai Y. 2003. Lipoteichoic acids from *Lactobacillus* strains elicit strong tumor necrosis factor alpha-inducing activities in macrophages through Toll-like receptor 2. *Clin Diagn Lab Immunol* **10**:259–266.

77. Dessing MC, Schouten M, Draing C, Levi M, von Aulock S, van der Poll T. 2008. Role played by Toll-like receptors 2 and 4 in lipoteichoic acid-induced lung inflammation and coagulation. *J Infect Dis* **197**:245–252.

78. Walter J, Loach DM, Alqumber M, Rockel C, Hermann C, Pfitzenmaier M, Tannock GW. 2007. D-alanyl ester depletion of teichoic acids in *Lactobacillus reuteri* 100-23 results in impaired colonization of the mouse gastrointestinal tract. *Environ Microbiol* **9**:1750–1760.

79. Grangette C, Nutten S, Palumbo E, Morath S, Hermann C, Dewulf J, Pot B, Hartung T, Hols P, Mercenier A. 2005. Enhanced antiinflammatory capacity of a *Lactobacillus plantarum* mutant synthesizing modified teichoic acids. *Proc Natl Acad Sci USA* **102**:10321–10326.

80. Kaji R, Kiyoshima-Shibata J, Nagaoka M, Nanno M, Shida K. 2010. Bacterial teichoic acids reverse predominant IL-12 production induced by certain *Lactobacillus* strains into predominant IL-10 production via TLR2-dependent ERK activation in macrophages. *J Immunol* **184**:3505–3513.

81. Duncker SC, Wang L, Hols P, Bienenstock J. 2008. The D-alanine content of lipoteichoic acid is crucial for *Lactobacillus plantarum*-mediated protection from visceral pain perception in a rat colorectal distension model. *Neurogastroenterol Motil* **20**:843–850.

82. Smelt MJ, de Haan BJ, Bron PA, van Swam I, Meijerink M, Wells JM, Kleerebezem M, Faas MM, de Vos P. 2013. The impact of *Lactobacillus plantarum* WCFS1 teichoic acid D-alanylation on the generation of effector and regulatory T-cells in healthy mice. *PLoS One* **8**:e63099.

83. Korhonen R, Kosonen O, Korpela R, Moilanen E. 2004. The expression of COX2 protein induced by *Lactobacillus rhamnosus* GG, endotoxin and lipoteichoic acid in T84 epithelial cells. *Lett Appl Microbiol* **39**:19–24.

84. Khazaie K, Zadeh M, Khan MW, Bere P, Gounari F, Dennis K, Blatner NR, Owen JL, Klaenhammer TR, Mohamadzadeh M. 2012. Abating colon cancer polyposis by *Lactobacillus acidophilus* deficient in lipoteichoic acid. *Proc Natl Acad Sci USA* **109**:10462–10467.

85. Law J, Buist G, Haandrikman A, Kok J, Venema G, Leenhouts K. 1995. A system to generate chromosomal mutations in *Lactococcus lactis* which allows fast analysis of targeted genes. *J Bacteriol* **177**:7011–7018.

86. Bron PA, Tomita S, Mercenier A, Kleerebezem M. 2013. Cell surface-associated compounds of probiotic lactobacilli sustain the strain-specificity dogma. *Curr Opin Microbiol* **16**:262–269.

87. **Lebeer S, Vanderleyden J, De Keersmaecker SCJ.** 2010. Host interactions of probiotic bacterial surface molecules: comparison with commensals and pathogens. *Nat Rev Microbiol* **8:**171–184.

88. **Lebeer S, Vanderleyden J, De Keersmaecker SCJ.** 2008. Genes and molecules of lactobacilli supporting probiotic action. *Microbiol Mol Biol Rev* **72:**728–764.

89. **Faith JJ, McNulty NP, Rey FE, Gordon JI.** 2011. Predicting a human gut microbiota's response to diet in gnotobiotic mice. *Science* **333:**101–104.

90. **McNulty NP, Yatsunenko T, Hsiao A, Faith JJ, Muegge BD, Goodman AL, Henrissat B, Oozeer R, Cools-Portier S, Gobert G, Chervaux C, Knights D, Lozupone CA, Knight R, Duncan AE, Bain JR, Muehlbauer MJ, Newgard CB, Heath AC, Gordon JI.** 2011. The impact of a consortium of fermented milk strains on the gut microbiome of gnotobiotic mice and monozygotic twins. *Sci Trans Med* **3:**106ra106.

91. **García-Fruitós E.** 2012. Lactic acid bacteria: a promising alternative for recombinant protein production. *Microb Cell Fact* **11:**157.

92. **Rodríguez JM, Martínez MI, Horn N, Dodd HM.** 2003. Heterologous production of bacteriocins by lactic acid bacteria. *Int J Food Microbiol* **80:**101–116.

93. **de Ruyter PG, Kuipers OP, de Vos WM.** 1996. Controlled gene expression systems for *Lactococcus lactis* with the food-grade inducer nisin. *Appl Environ Microbiol* **62:**3662–3667.

94. **LeBlanc JG, Aubry C, Cortes-Perez NG, de Moreno de LeBlanc A, Vergnolle N, Langella P, Azevedo V, Chatel J-M, Miyoshi A, Bermúdez-Humarán LG.** 2013. Mucosal targeting of therapeutic molecules using genetically modified lactic acid bacteria: an update. *FEMS Microbiol Lett* **344:**1–9.

95. **Repa A, Grangette C, Daniel C, Hochreiter R, Hoffmann-Sommergruber K, Thalhamer J, Kraft D, Breiteneder H, Mercenier A, Wiedermann U.** 2003. Mucosal co-application of lactic acid bacteria and allergen induces counter-regulatory immune responses in a murine model of birch pollen allergy. *Vaccine* **22:**87–95.

96. **Round JL, Mazmanian SK.** 2009. The gut microbiota shapes intestinal immune responses during health and disease. *Nat Rev Immunol* **9:**313–323.

97. **Ianiro G, Tilg H, Gasbarrini A.** 2016. Antibiotics as deep modulators of gut microbiota: between good and evil. *Gut* **65:**gutjnl–2016–312297.

98. **Cox LM, Blaser MJ.** 2015. Antibiotics in early life and obesity. *Nat Rev Endocrinol* **11:**182–190.

99. **Russell SL, Gold MJ, Hartmann M, Willing BP, Thorson L, Wlodarska M, Gill N, Blanchet M-R, Mohn WW, McNagny KM, Finlay BB.** 2012. Early life antibiotic-driven changes in microbiota enhance susceptibility to allergic asthma. *EMBO Rep* **13:**440–447.

100. **Slimings C, Riley TV.** 2014. Antibiotics and hospital-acquired *Clostridium difficile* infection: update of systematic review and meta-analysis. *J Antimicrob Chemother* **69:**881–891.

101. **World Health Organization.** 2014. *Antimicrobial Resistance: Global Report on Surveillance.* World Health Organization, Geneva Switzerland.

102. **Lewis K.** 2013. Platforms for antibiotic discovery. *Nat Rev Drug Discov* **12:**371–387.

103. **Villa TG, Veiga-Crespo P (ed).** 2009. *Enzybiotics: Antibiotic Enzymes as Drugs and Therapeutics.* John Wiley & Sons, Inc, Hoboken, NJ.

104. **Alvarez-Sieiro P, Montalbán-López M, Mu D, Kuipers OP.** 2016. Bacteriocins of lactic acid bacteria: extending the family. *Appl Microbiol Biotechnol* **100:**2939–2951.

105. **Cotter PD, Ross RP, Hill C.** 2013. Bacteriocins: a viable alternative to antibiotics? *Nat Rev Microbiol* **11:**95–105.

106. **Riboulet-Bisson E, Sturme MHJ, Jeffery IB, O'Donnell MM, Neville BA, Forde BM, Claesson MJ, Harris H, Gardiner GE, Casey PG, Lawlor PG, O'Toole PW, Ross RP.** 2012. Effect of *Lactobacillus salivarius* bacteriocin Abp118 on the mouse and pig intestinal microbiota. *PLoS One* **7:**e31113.

107. **Kommineni S, Bretl DJ, Lam V, Chakraborty R, Hayward M, Simpson P, Cao Y, Bousounis P, Kristich CJ, Salzman NH.** 2015. Bacteriocin production augments niche competition by enterococci in the mammalian gastrointestinal tract. *Nature* **526:**719–722.

108. **Field D, Connor PMO, Cotter PD, Hill C, Ross RP.** 2008. The generation of nisin variants with enhanced activity against specific Gram-positive pathogens. *Mol Microbiol* **69:**218–230.

109. **Field D, Begley M, O'Connor PM, Daly KM, Hugenholtz F, Cotter PD, Hill C, Ross RP.** 2012. Bioengineered nisin A derivatives with enhanced activity against both Gram positive and Gram negative pathogens. *PLoS One* **7:**e46884.

110. **van Pijkeren J-P, Neoh KM, Sirias D, Findley AS, Britton RA.** 2012. Exploring optimization parameters to increase ssDNA recombineering in *Lactococcus lactis* and *Lactobacillus reuteri*. *Bioengineered* **3:**209–217.

111. **Doleyres Y, Beck P, Vollenweider S, Lacroix C.** 2005. Production of 3-hydroxypropionaldehyde using a two-step process with *Lactobacillus reuteri*. *Appl Microbiol Biotechnol* **68:**467–474.

112. **De Weirdt R, Crabbé A, Roos S, Vollenweider S, Lacroix C, van Pijkeren J-P, Britton RA, Sarker S, Van de Wiele T, Nickerson CA.** 2012. Glycerol supplementation enhances *L. reuteri*'s protective effect against *S.* Typhimurium colonization in a 3-D model of colonic epithelium. *PLoS One* **7:**e37116.

113. **Talarico TL, Casas IA, Chung TC, Dobrogosz WJ.** 1988. Production and isolation of reuterin, a growth inhibitor produced by *Lactobacillus reuteri*. *Antimicrob Agents Chemother* **32:**1854–1858.

114. **Dishisha T, Pereyra LP, Pyo S-H, Britton RA, Hatti-Kaul R.** 2014. Flux analysis of the *Lactobacillus reuteri* propanediol-utilization pathway for production of 3 hydroxypropionaldehyde, 3-hydroxypropionic acid and 1,3-propanediol from glycerol. *Microb Cell Fact* **13:**76.

115. **Schaefer L, Auchtung TA, Hermans KE, Whitehead D, Borhan B, Britton RA.** 2010. The antimicrobial compound reuterin (3-hydroxypropionaldehyde) induces oxidative stress via interaction with thiol groups. *Microbiology* **156:**1589 1599.

116. **Rakonjac J, Bennett NJ, Spagnuolo J, Gagic D, Russel M.** 2011. Filamentous bacteriophage: biology, phage display and nanotechnology applications. *Curr Issues Mol Biol* **13:**51–76.

117. **Rakonjac J, Feng J, Model P.** 1999. Filamentous phage are released from the bacterial membrane by a two-step mechanism involving a short C-terminal fragment of pIII. *J Mol Biol* **289:**1253–1265.

118. **Sheehan MM, Stanley E, Fitzgerald GF, van Sinderen D.** 1999. Identification and characterization of a lysis module present in a large proportion of bacteriophages infecting *Streptococcus thermophilus*. *Appl Environ Microbiol* **65:**569–577.

119. **Wang IN, Smith DL, Young R.** 2000. Holins: the protein clocks of bacteriophage infections. *Annu Rev Microbiol* **54:**799–825.

120. **Fischetti VA.** 2009. *Bacteriophage Lysins: The Ultimate Enzybiotic.* John Wiley & Sons, Inc, Hoboken, NJ.

121. **Cheng X, Zhang X, Pflugrath JW, Studier FW.** 1994. The structure of bacteriophage T7 lysozyme, a zinc amidase and an inhibitor of T7 RNA polymerase. *Proc Natl Acad Sci USA* **91:**4034–4038.

122. **Nelson D, Schuch R, Chahales P, Zhu S, Fischetti VA.** 2006. PlyC: a multimeric bacteriophage lysin. *Proc Natl Acad Sci USA* **103:**10765–10770.

123. **Navarre WW, Ton-That H, Faull KF, Schneewind O.** 1999. Multiple enzymatic activities of the murein hydrolase from staphylococcal phage ϕ11. Identification of a D-alanyl-glycine endopeptidase activity. *J Biol Chem* **274:**15847–15856.

124. **Becker SC, Dong S, Baker JR, Foster-Frey J, Pritchard DG, Donovan DM.** 2009. LysK CHAP endopeptidase domain is required for lysis of live staphylococcal cells. *FEMS Microbiol Lett* **294:**52–60.

125. **Sulakvelidze A, Alavidze Z, Morris JG Jr.** 2001. Bacteriophage therapy. *Antimicrob Agents Chemother* **45:**649–659.

126. **Chatain-Ly MH.** 2014. The factors affecting effectiveness of treatment in phages therapy. *Front Microbiol* **5:**51.

127. **Loessner MJ, Kramer K, Ebel F, Scherer S.** 2002. C-terminal domains of *Listeria monocytogenes* bacteriophage murein hydrolases determine specific recognition and high-affinity binding to bacterial cell wall carbohydrates. *Mol Microbiol* **44:**335–349.

128. **Porter CJ, Schuch R, Pelzek AJ, Buckle AM, McGowan S, Wilce MCJ, Rossjohn J, Russell R, Nelson D, Fischetti VA, Whisstock JC.** 2007. The 1.6 A crystal structure of the catalytic domain of PlyB, a bacteriophage lysin active against *Bacillus anthracis*. *J Mol Biol* **366:**540–550.

129. **Schuch R, Nelson D, Fischetti VA.** 2002. A bacteriolytic agent that detects and kills *Bacillus anthracis*. *Nature* **418:**884–889.

130. **Meng X, Shi Y, Ji W, Meng X, Zhang J, Wang H, Lu C, Sun J, Yan Y.** 2011. Application of a bacteriophage lysin to disrupt biofilms formed by the animal pathogen *Streptococcus suis*. *Appl Environ Microbiol* **77:**8272–8279.

131. **Loeffler JM, Nelson D, Fischetti VA.** 2001. Rapid killing of *Streptococcus pneumoniae* with a bacteriophage cell wall hydrolase. *Science* **294:**2170–2172.

132. **Entenza JM, Loeffler JM, Grandgirard D, Fischetti VA, Moreillon P.** 2005. Therapeutic effects of bacteriophage Cpl-1 lysin against *Streptococcus pneumoniae* endocarditis in rats. *Antimicrob Agents Chemother* **49:**4789–4792.

133. **Lood R, Winer BY, Pelzek AJ, Diez-Martinez R, Thandar M, Euler CW, Schuch R, Fischetti VA.** 2015. Novel phage lysin capable of killing the multidrug-resistant Gram-negative bacterium *Acinetobacter baumannii* in a mouse bacteremia model. *Antimicrob Agents Chemother* **59:**1983–1991.

134. **Oliveira H, Thiagarajan V, Walmagh M, Sillankorva S, Lavigne R, Neves-Petersen**

MT, Kluskens LD, Azeredo J. 2014. A thermostable *Salmonella* phage endolysin, Lys68, with broad bactericidal properties against Gramnegative pathogens in presence of weak acids. *PLoS One* **9:**e108376. (Erratum, doi:10.1371/journal. pone.0115267.)

135. Wu H, Lu H, Huang J, Li G, Huang Q. 2012. EnzyBase: a novel database for enzybiotic studies. *BMC Microbiol* **12:**54.

136. Zhou Y, Liang Y, Lynch KH, Dennis JJ, Wishart DS. 2011. PHAST: a fast phage search tool. *Nucleic Acids Res* **39:**W347–W352.

137. Britton RA, Young VB. 2014. Role of the intestinal microbiota in resistance to colonization by *Clostridium difficile*. *Gastroenterology* **146:**1547–1553.

138. Merrigan M, Venugopal A, Mallozzi M, Roxas B, Viswanathan VK, Johnson S, Gerding DN, Vedantam G. 2010. Human hypervirulent *Clostridium difficile* strains exhibit increased sporulation as well as robust toxin production. *J Bacteriol* **192:**4904–4911.

139. He M, Miyajima F, Roberts P, Ellison L, Pickard DJ, Martin MJ, Connor TR, Harris SR, Fairley D, Bamford KB, D'Arc S, Brazier J, Brown D, Coia JE, Douce G, Gerding D, Kim HJ, Koh TH, Kato H, Senoh M, Louie T, Michell S, Butt E, Peacock SJ, Brown NM, Riley T, Songer G, Wilcox M, Pirmohamed M, Kuijper E, Hawkey P, Wren BW, Dougan G, Parkhill J, Lawley TD. 2013. Emergence and global spread of epidemic healthcare-associated *Clostridium difficile*. *Nat Genet* **45:**109–113.

140. Baines SD, O'Connor R, Freeman J, Fawley WN, Harmanus C, Mastrantonio P, Kuijper EJ, Wilcox MH. 2008. Emergence of reduced susceptibility to metronidazole in *Clostridium difficile*. *J Antimicrob Chemother* **62:**1046–1052.

141. Freeman J, Bauer MP, Baines SD, Corver J, Fawley WN, Goorhuis B, Kuijper EJ, Wilcox MH. 2010. The changing epidemiology of *Clostridium difficile* infections. *Clin Microbiol Rev* **23:**529–549.

142. Cho I, Blaser MJ. 2012. The human microbiome: at the interface of health and disease. *Nat Rev Genet* **13:**260–270.

143. Ley RE, Bäckhed F, Turnbaugh P, Lozupone CA, Knight RD, Gordon JI. 2005. Obesity alters gut microbial ecology. *Proc Natl Acad Sci USA* **102:**11070–11075.

144. Ridaura VK, Faith JJ, Rey FE, Cheng J, Duncan AE, Kau AL, Griffin NW, Lombard V, Henrissat B, Bain JR, Muehlbauer MJ, Ilkayeva O, Semenkovich CF, Funai K, Hayashi DK, Lyle BJ, Martini MC, Ursell LK, Clemente JC, Van Treuren W, Walters WA, Knight R, Newgard CB, Heath AC, Gordon JI. 2013. Gut microbiota from twins discordant for obesity modulate metabolism in mice. *Science* **341:**1241214.

145. Alang N, Kelly CR. 2015. Weight gain after fecal microbiota transplantation. *Open Forum Infect Dis* **2:**ofv004.

146. Mayer MJ, Narbad A, Gasson MJ. 2008. Molecular characterization of a *Clostridium difficile* bacteriophage and its cloned biologically active endolysin. *J Bacteriol* **190:**6734–6740.

147. Gomaa AA, Klumpe HE, Luo ML, Selle K, Barrangou R, Beisel CL. 2014. Programmable removal of bacterial strains by use of genome-targeting CRISPR-Cas systems. *MBio* **5:** e00928-13.

148. Beisel CL, Gomaa AA, Barrangou R. 2014. A CRISPR design for next-generation antimicrobials. *Genome Biol* **15:**516.

149. Lieber MR. 2010. The mechanism of double-strand DNA break repair by the nonhomologous DNA end-joining pathway. *Annu Rev Biochem* **79:**181–211.

150. Paez-Espino D, Morovic W, Sun CL, Thomas BC, Ueda K, Stahl B, Barrangou R, Banfield JF. 2013. Strong bias in the bacterial CRISPR elements that confer immunity to phage. *Nat Commun* **4:**1430.

151. Bikard D, Euler CW, Jiang W, Nussenzweig PM, Goldberg GW, Duportet X, Fischetti VA, Marraffini LA. 2014. Exploiting CRISPR-Cas nucleases to produce sequence-specific antimicrobials. *Nat Biotechnol* **32:**1146–1150.

152. Citorik RJ, Mimee M, Lu TK. 2014. Sequence-specific antimicrobials using efficiently delivered RNA-guided nucleases. *Nat Biotechnol* **32:**1141–1145.

153. Nicoletti M, Bertani G. 1983. DNA fusion product of phage P2 with plasmid pBR322: a new phasmid. *Mol Gen Genet* **189:**343–347.

154. Gibson DG, Young L, Chuang R-Y, Venter JC, Hutchison CA III, Smith HO. 2009. Enzymatic assembly of DNA molecules up to several hundred kilobases. *Nat Methods* **6:**343–345.

155. de Ruyter PG, Kuipers OP, Meijer WC, de Vos WM. 1997. Food-grade controlled lysis of *Lactococcus lactis* for accelerated cheese ripening. *Nat Biotechnol* **15:**976–979.

156. Benbouziane B, Ribelles P, Aubry C, Martín R, Kharrat P, Riazi A, Langella P, Bermúdez-Humarán LG. 2013. Development of a stress-inducible controlled expression (SICE) system in *Lactococcus lactis* for the production and delivery of therapeutic molecules at mucosal surfaces. *J Biotechnol* **168:**120–129.

United States Regulatory Considerations for Development of Live Biotherapeutic Products as Drugs

18

SHEILA M. DREHER-LESNICK,[1] SCOTT STIBITZ,[1] and
PAUL E. CARLSON, JR.[2]

INTRODUCTION

Our expanding knowledge of the nature and importance of the human microbiota has provided additional impetus to investigate the use of beneficial bacteria to promote improved health. Recent technological developments in both next-generation DNA sequencing and novel bioinformatic analyses have advanced our understanding of the nature of our microbiome and the degree to which its makeup correlates with human health and specific disease states. It is clear that the application of these technologies has the potential to inform the mechanisms of beneficial effects and to identify potentially valuable candidates for intervention. It should be noted, however, that there is a long history of the use of bacteria, initially in the form of naturally fermented foods and later by investigation of the potential roles of individual bacterial strains in disease prevention. For example, the strain *Escherichia coli* Nissle 1917 was reportedly isolated about 100 years ago from a World War I soldier who, unlike his cohorts, appeared unaffected by bacterial dysentery, and it has remained a subject of study ever since (1).

[1]Division of Bacterial, Parasitic, and Allergenic Products, Office of Vaccines Research and Review, Center for Biologics Evaluation and Research, Food and Drug Administration, Silver Spring, MD 20993
Bugs as Drugs: Therapeutic Microbes for the Prevention and Treatment of Disease
Edited by Robert A. Britton and Patrice D. Cani
© 2018 American Society for Microbiology, Washington, DC
doi:10.1128/microbiolspec.BAD-0017-2017

The human microbiota comprises the gut microbial communities along with those of every surface or space in the human body that has a connection to the external world. As a result of the numerous publications deriving directly, or indirectly, from the Human Microbiome Project, we are starting to gain insight into the microbial species that make up these communities. Of perhaps greatest interest aside from the gut microbiota are the skin, oral, vaginal, and respiratory tract communities, due to their relevance to human health and disease. Application of live organisms to these sites may necessitate alternative modes of delivery such as topical creams, oral rinses, vaginal suppositories, and aerosol sprays, respectively. Those targeted to the gut are likely to be administered in pill form but may also be given rectally. Specialized oral formulations may also allow for delivery of live organisms to specific points within the gastrointestinal tract.

The use of bacterial strains targeting the gut is perhaps best exemplified by what are commonly known as probiotics, which are commercially available in conventional foods or dietary supplements. Hundreds of different preparations are sold with claims of improving digestive health. Many questions remain about the effectiveness of dietary supplements containing probiotics. A recent study by the Agency for Healthcare Research and Quality, commissioned by the FDA and NIH, examined 622 published studies on probiotics to assess evidence for safety. Of these, 387 addressed the presence or absence of one or more specific adverse events, although most were not designed to address safety. They found that the quality of study design varied greatly, adverse events were poorly documented, and the probiotic in question was often not specified. However, within these constraints, the investigators found that "there was no indication that the quantity of reported adverse events was increased in short-term probiotic intervention arms compared to the controls." They also stated that "future studies that explicitly monitor for

the issues of concern are needed to quantify the actual risk of specific adverse events in intervention studies" (2).

Studies designed to assess the efficacy of probiotic dietary supplements to address specific health issues have become more common (www.clinicaltrials.gov). One difference between these types of studies and the typical use of probiotic supplements by individuals is the health of the subjects. Many of those enrolled in studies assessing marketed products containing probiotics for treatment of disease may not have good gut barrier integrity and a functional mature immune system. These and other health concerns may greatly influence an individual's susceptibility to the live organism(s) included in the supplement or any contaminating microorganisms. Both of these concerns have been observed with probiotic use in compromised individuals (3, 4). Therefore an important aspect of regulatory review of proposals for the use of live biotherapeutic products (LBPs), including commercially available probiotic-containing products, in clinical trials is the vulnerability of the study's target population. An LBP, as defined by the Center for Biologics Evaluation and Research (CBER), is "a biological product that: 1) contains live organisms, such as bacteria; 2) is applicable to the prevention, treatment, or cure of a disease or condition of human beings; and 3) is not a vaccine" (5). While the vast majority of LBPs in clinical trials to date are those that are most like commercially available probiotic organisms sold over the counter (www.clinicaltrials.gov), we recognize that we are entering a new age in which investigations of novel strains will be sought.

CLINICAL INVESTIGATIONS WITH LIVE BIOTHERAPEUTIC PRODUCTS AND THE IND PROCESS

By law, any substance that is intended for use in the diagnosis, cure, mitigation, treatment, or prevention of disease meets the definition of a drug under section 201(g)[1](B) of the Food, Drug, and Cosmetic Act (6) and cannot be introduced into interstate commerce unless it is either approved for such use by the FDA or an Investigational New Drug (IND) application is in effect (6). Therefore, clinical studies investigating LBPs with the intended use to diagnose, cure, mitigate, treat, or prevent disease in humans must be pursued through the IND process. Additional FDA guidance on when an IND is required can be found in "Investigational New Drug Applications (INDs): Determining Whether Human Research Studies Can Be Conducted Without an IND" (7). The regulatory pathway for LBPs follows the standard drug and biologics development pathway. LBPs are regulated by CBER within the FDA, and licensure is attained by approval of a biologics license application.

Multiple FDA resources are available to help sponsors navigate the IND application process. In the context of IND applications, the sponsor is the investigator or company that submits the IND to the FDA. INDs are required for both clinical trials for commercial development and investigator-initiated research-only studies. The FDA has published several guidance documents regarding the IND application process, procedures, and reporting requirements. These guidance documents provide sponsors with additional information regarding how to complete their IND application and comply with the IND regulations (21 CFR Part 312).

The following FDA websites are a good place to start when planning to submit an IND application:

1. https://www.fda.gov/Drugs/Development ApprovalProcess/HowDrugsareDeveloped andApproved/ApprovalApplications/ InvestigationalNewDrugINDApplication/ default.htm
2. https://www.fda.gov/Drugs/Development ApprovalProcess/HowDrugsareDeveloped andApproved/ApprovalApplications/ InvestigationalNewDrugINDApplication/ ucm343349.htm

One important benefit of initiating the IND process is early communication with the FDA. For general inquiries contact CBER's Office of Communication, Outreach, and Development (8). The FDA also encourages sponsors planning to submit an IND to request a pre-IND meeting with the agency. The pre-IND process allows the sponsor to receive FDA feedback prior to submitting an IND application. In preparation for a pre-IND meeting, information submitted to the FDA by the sponsor is reviewed by a full review team. Sponsors submit relevant information and ask specific questions regarding their proposed clinical study and information to be included in the initial IND application, including supportive preclinical and chemistry, manufacturing, and controls (CMC) data. The FDA provides written responses to the questions asked based on the information provided in the pre-IND package ahead of the actual meeting. Additional information regarding formal meetings between the FDA and sponsors/applicants can be found in the guidance document "Formal Meetings between the FDA and Sponsor or Applicants" (9).

Several publications provide additional advice based on the authors' experiences submitting applications to the FDA. Shapiro (10) offers detailed explanations elaborating on the pre-IND process and what information to submit to the FDA for review. While the paper is written in the context of a submission for a vaccine, the information can be applied to other biologic products, including LBP candidates. Of note are the sections describing information to provide for critical issues in manufacturing. Other publications offer insights for investigators and clinicians for preparing the IND package itself, including examples of what to include for each section of the IND (11, 12). In terms of what CMC information to include in an IND for a clinical study using an LBP, CBER refers sponsors to the guidance document "Guidance for Industry Early Clinical Trials with Live Biotherapeutic Products: Chemistry, Manufacturing, and Control Information"

(5). This guidance was updated in 2016 to include a section on IND studies utilizing commercially available LPBs. The revised LBP guidance states that when certain conditions are met, the FDA may grant a waiver of the requirement to submit CMC information for INDs using commercially available conventional foods and dietary supplements. If a waiver is not applicable, CMC information must be provided in the IND application. The amount of CMC information that needs to be included depends on the phase of the investigation, the dosage form, and the amount of information otherwise available [21 CFR 312.23(a)(7)]. Additional considerations regarding CMC information for LBP IND applications are highlighted by Ross et al. (13) and discussed in more detail below.

ADDITIONAL CMC CONSIDERATIONS

For early-phase clinical investigations with live biotherapeutic products, safety assessment of the product taking into consideration the proposed subject population is the primary focus. Sponsors submitting CMC information for LBPs, particularly novel LBPs, should include enough information to allow an assessment of the safety of the product. This can be detailed in the CMC sections describing and characterizing the product and when describing product release specifications. Description of the product strain should include the biological name and strain designation for each individual strain, the original source of each strain, with information pertaining to the health status of the original donor (if available), and subsequent passage history and generation of stocks. Each of these pieces of information contributes to the safety assessment of a novel bacterial species for clinical use in humans. The general description of the drug substance (the unformulated active substance that may be subsequently formulated with excipients to produce the drug product) and final drug product (the finished dosage form of the product) should include all relevant physical, chemical, and biological components (5). Additional relevant information, including the delivery method and the identity of any excipients included in the final product composition, should also be adequately described.

Strain Characterization

Because safety is the primary concern, strain characterization information should focus on the identification of potentially undesirable traits of all bacterial strains included in the product. Among others, strain characterization information should include details about the presence of virulence factors or toxins and antibiotic resistance genes. Sponsors should also address the potential for transfer of genetic elements encoding these genes to other organisms. One approach to address these concerns is through whole-genome sequencing of each strain in a given product. The genome sequence can be analyzed for the presence of undesirable genes, including known virulence factors and antibiotic resistance genes. Having the full genome sequence could also allow for assessment of the potential for transfer of identified genes of concern to other species present in the product and host sites exposed to product colonization, whether that is transient or stable. In some cases, it may be possible to address such concerns by examining the genetic context surrounding resistance genes for mobile elements (i.e., transposable elements, plasmids, bacteriophage, etc.).

Another important part of LBP strain characterization includes determining the strain's antibiotic resistance profile. The IND submission should include information about the phenotypic characterization of the antibiotic resistance profiles for each product strain and the minimum inhibitory or minimum bactericidal concentrations for a panel of antibiotics relevant to the strain(s) of interest. It is important to establish sensitivity to clinically useful antibiotics that can be used to treat product-related infections should they arise during a clinical trial. Having both genetic and phenotypic data on antibiotic resistance within the product organism(s) can help inform rational decisions concerning the safety of a given strain for human clinical use.

Adequate information about pharmacological and toxicological studies must be submitted to support a proposed clinical trial evaluating the LBP. This information can include both *in vitro* and *in vivo* studies to support the proposed indication for which the product is being investigated for treatment, as well as any safety-related data that were gathered. Information on the hypothesized mechanism of action of a given product strain should also be provided along with data generated to support the hypothesis.

Product Release Testing

Special attention should be given to adequately describe product release testing for the drug substance (bulk) and final drug product. When describing product release specifications, descriptions of all tests and assays used in release testing of the product, as well as tentative acceptance criteria for all assays, should be included in the IND. For early-phase trials, acceptance criteria are frequently set based on limited data and manufacturing experience and are subsequently adjusted as clinical and product development proceeds in later phases. These release specifications should include tests for identity, purity, and potency of the drug substance and drug product.

The identity test is a specific measurement for each product that can adequately identify it as the specific product and distinguish it from other products being made in the same facility. The identity test should detect the microbial strain(s) in the product. Additional product characterization assays may be included in release testing and consist of biochemical or genotypic methods or a combination of both. If one or more genetic loci are known to be important for the mecha-

nism of action of a given product, product characterization tests should be developed to confirm the presence of these features. For bacterial consortia, product characterization assays need to have sufficient specificity to allow the identification of each strain included in the final product.

In testing for product purity, "purity" is defined as "relative freedom from extraneous matter in the finished product" [21 CFR 601.3 (r)]. For live biotherapeutic products this should include demonstrating the absence of contaminating bacteria and/or yeast in a given product. Purity testing of LBPs, and placebo when applicable, should include bioburden testing. CBER recommends testing for bioburden as described in the U.S. Pharmacopeia microbial limits testing (14, 15). Release specifications that CBER generally considers acceptable include <200 CFU/dose for total aerobic extraneous bacterial counts and <20 CFU/dose for total extraneous yeast and mold counts, with evidence of the absence of known pathogens as described in U.S. Pharmacopeia chapter 62. Since LBPs contain a high number of live organisms, data demonstrating system suitability of the assay should also be included. Acceptance criteria may be more stringent, and additional testing may be required, depending on the target patient population and the proposed trial. Additional microbiological testing may also be required, depending on the manufacturing facility and process and taking into consideration what other organisms are being propagated or manipulated within the manufacturing space and facility. Purity tests may also include testing for endotoxin content, residual antibiotics, or other components introduced during manufacture.

Product release testing includes an assessment of product potency. For live biotherapeutic products, potency assays are typically a measurement of product viability, which is generally measured in terms of the total viable CFU of each strain per unit or dose of product. These assays need to provide accurate and reproducible measurements of the total viable bacteria in the final product. Potency specifications should be set for release of the drug substance for downstream manufacturing and for release of the final drug product for clinical use. When designing potency assays, it is important to consider that they should be able to detect subpotent lots. Additional potency tests measuring specific mechanism(s) of action for a given product should be included if such mechanisms are known. In early stages of product development, acceptance criteria for product release may be set as a fairly wide range. As experience is gained with regard to product manufacture and testing during clinical and product development in later phases, acceptance criteria are adjusted and tightened. Additionally, for multistrain products, potency assays should be developed to allow enumeration of each strain present in the final formulation. All assays and analytical methods need to be validated prior to performing pivotal studies to demonstrate product safety and effectiveness for licensure.

In addition to release specifications, products should be assessed for stability over time. The assays developed for measurements of purity and potency should be included as part of a detailed stability plan in the IND submission. The goal of the stability program is to demonstrate that the drug substance and drug product remain within the set release specifications for both purity and potency under the proposed storage conditions for the duration of the proposed study. Available stability data should be included in the original IND submission.

Investigators preparing to submit an IND for FDA review often seek additional guidance regarding current good manufacturing practice (CGMP) requirements during the IND process. The FDA's guidance on CGMP for phase 1 investigational drugs provides additional information and recommendations regarding CGMP requirements in early-phase trials (16). The guidance notes that "adherence to CGMP during manufacture of phase 1 investigational drugs occurs mostly through:

well defined, written procedures, adequately controlled equipment and manufacturing environment, and accurately and consistently recorded data from manufacturing (including testing)" (16). This information can be addressed when describing manufacturing details in the CMC section of the IND. As already noted, requirements for the extent of CMC information submitted to the IND, which includes information regarding adherence to CGMP, increases as product development proceeds in later phases [21 CFR 312.23 (a)(7)] (17).

Additional Considerations for Genetically Modified LBPs

Genetically modified LBPs are typically assessed under the same guidelines and criteria as nonmodified strains. Strain characterization information should include detailed descriptions of all genetic modifications, discussion of the genetic stability of the modifications, and the presence of any genetic markers. Depending on the nature of the modification, some additional information may be requested to address specific questions. To assess the stability of the genetic modifications, tests should be included to show that the expected genetic modifications are present in the final product. If the genetic modification includes the addition of antibiotic resistance genes, the sponsor should provide justification for why this resistance marker remains incorporated in the genome of the product strain. The addition of antibiotic resistance genes that would preclude treatment in the event of an opportunistic infection caused by the product strain is not acceptable. As product development continues to later-phase clinical trials and licensure, CBER strongly recommends developing strains lacking such antibiotic resistance marker insertions.

CONCLUSION

When LBPs are used as drugs, sufficient CMC information must be provided to ensure safety, taking into consideration the nature of the product and the proposed clinical study. Requirements for product testing and characterization sometimes run counter to the prevailing public opinion that LBP products, particularly those containing strains found in probiotic supplements or related strains, are safe for human use and consumption. In addition to LBP strains found in conventional foods and dietary supplements being investigated for clinical use, we anticipate investigations of new LBP strains and approaches. Such organisms will presumably be identified in, and isolated from, our own microbial communities and will likely be selected on the basis of traits which are expected to be beneficial. These are also likely to be organisms for which we have limited or no experience in their use or application. While the potential benefit may arguably be greater, the unknowns, particularly with regard to safety, may be greater as well. Another approach is the genetic engineering of live biotherapeutic organisms to endow select strains with specific traits of interest. While genetic engineering alone does not increase safety concerns regarding these hypothetical new products, the newly endowed traits will make them novel entities for which basic safety questions will need to be addressed. It is our hope and expectation that the coming years will bring important new advancements in these areas with benefits for improved human health.

CITATION

Dreher-Lesnick SM, Stibitz S, Carlson PE Jr. 2017. U.S. regulatory considerations for development of live biotherapeutic products as drugs. Microbiol Spectrum 5(5):BAD-0017-2017.

REFERENCES

1. **Tannock GW.** 2002. *Probiotics and Prebiotics.* Horizon Scientific Press, Wymondham, United Kingdom.

2. **Hempel S, Newberry S, Ruelaz A, Wang Z, Miles JNV, Suttorp MJ, Johnsen B, Shanman R, Slusser W, Fu N, Smith A, Roth B, Polak J, Motala A, Perry T, Shekelle PG.** 2011. *Safety of Probiotics to Reduce Risk and Prevent or Treat Disease.* Agency for Healthcare Research and Quality, Rockville, MD.

3. **Besselink MGH, Timmerman HM, Buskens E, Nieuwenhuijs VB, Akkermans LMA, Gooszen HG, Dutch Acute Pancreatitis Study Group.** 2004. Probiotic prophylaxis in patients with predicted severe acute pancreatitis (PROPATRIA): design and rationale of a double-blind, placebo-controlled randomised multicenter trial [ISRCTN 38327949]. *BMC Surg* **4:**12.

4. **Vallabhaneni S, Walker TA, Lockhart SR, Ng D, Chiller T, Melchreit R, Brandt ME, Smith RM, Centers for Disease Control and Prevention (CDC).** 2015. Notes from the field: fatal gastrointestinal mucormycosis in a premature infant associated with a contaminated dietary supplement: Connecticut, 2014. *MMWR Morb Mortal Wkly Rep* **64:**155–156.

5. **FDA Center for Biologics Evaluation and Research.** 2016. *Guidance for industry early clinical trials with live biotherapeutic products: chemistry, manufacturing, and control information.* http://www.fda.gov/downloads/Biologics BloodVaccines/GuidanceComplianceRegulatory Information/Guidances/General/UCM292704. pdf.

6. **U.S. Government Printing Office.** 2010. Federal Food, Drug, and Cosmetic Act. *In 21—Food and Drugs,* 2010 ed; U.S. Government Printing Office: Washington, DC. http://www.gpo.gov/fdsys/pkg/ USCODE-2010-title21/html/USCODE-2010-title21-chap9-subchapII.htm.

7. **FDA.** 2013. Investigational New Drug Applications (INDs): Determining Whether Human Research Studies Can Be Conducted Without an IND. https://www.fda.gov/downloads/drugs/ guidances/ucm229175.pdf.

8. **CBER Office of Communication.** 2016. *Contacts in the Center for Biologics Evaluation & Research (CBER).* https://www.fda.gov/ AboutFDA/CentersOffices/OfficeofMedical ProductsandTobacco/CBER/ucm106001.htm.

9. **FDA.** 2009. Guidance for Industry: Formal Meetings between the FDA and Sponsor or Applicants. https://www.fda.gov/downloads/ drugs/guidances/ucm153222.pdf.

10. **Shapiro SZ.** 2002. The HIV/AIDS vaccine researchers' orientation to the process of preparing a US FDA application for an investigational new drug (IND): what it is all about and how you start by preparing for your pre-IND meeting. *Vaccine* **20:**1261–1280.

11. **Moore T, Rodriguez A, Bakken JS.** 2014. Fecal microbiota transplantation: a practical update for the infectious disease specialist. *Clin Infect Dis* **58:**541–545.

12. **Kelly CR, Kunde SS, Khoruts A.** 2014. Guidance on preparing an investigational new drug application for fecal microbiota transplantation studies. *Clin Gastroenterol Hepatol* **12:**283–288.

13. **Ross JJ, Boucher PE, Bhattacharyya SP, Kopecko DJ, Sutkowski EM, Rohan PJ, Chandler DKF, Vaillancourt J.** 2008. Considerations in the development of live biotherapeutic products for clinical use. *Curr Issues Mol Biol* **10:**13–16.

14. **U.S. Pharmacopeia.** 2009. 61. Microbiological examination of nonsterile products: microbial enumeration tests, p S3/43–S43/47. *In USP Pharmacists' Pharmacopeia.* U.S. Pharmacopeial Convention, Rockville, MD.

15. **U.S. Pharmacopeia.** 2009. 62. Microbiological examination of nonsterile products: tests for specified microorganims, p S3/47–S43/51. *In USP Pharmacists' Pharmacopeia,* U.S. Pharmacopeial Convention, Rockville, MD.

16. **FDA.** 2008. *Guidance for Industry: CGMP for Phase 1 Investigational Drugs.* https://www.fda.gov/downloads/drugs/guidances/ucm070273.pdf

17. **FDA CDER.** 2003. *Guidance for Industry INDs for Phase 2 and Phase 3 Studies Chemistry, Manufacturing, and Controls Information.* https://www.fda.gov/downloads/Drugs/Guidances/ucm070567.pdf

E. INDIRECT STRATEGIES TO TARGET MICROBIOME FUNCTION FOR HEALTH

Bacteriophage Clinical Use as Antibacterial "Drugs": Utility and Precedent

19

STEPHEN T. ABEDON[1]

INTRODUCTION

Phage therapy is the use of bacterial viruses to reduce or eliminate bacterial infections. As such, phage therapy has been employed clinically for approximately 100 years. It is possible, nevertheless, that more English-language reviews and commentaries on bacteriophage use as antibacterial agents are published yearly (e.g., for 2015 [1–19] and for approximately the first third of 2016 [20–30]), than there are people within the borders of the United States who are subject to officially sanctioned phage treatment. This contrasts with well over 100 million courses of antibiotic that are prescribed per year (31).

Phages—or bacteriophages, as phages are more formally known—more broadly can be employed as a form of biocontrol within a number of nonclinical contexts. For example, there is phage treatment of foods such as for reducing pathogen numbers, most notably of the foodborne pathogen *Listeria monocytogenes* (13, 28, 29, 32, 33). Also, for example, there is the treatment of plants for reducing the quantities of bacterial plant pathogens found in association with crops, particularly as marketed by the Utah-based company OmniLytics, Inc. (34–38). Phages especially represent alternatives as well as adjuvants to the use of small-molecule antibiotics. Notably, they are non-xenobiotic, that is, they do not consist of chemically unnatural materials, and

[1]Department of Microbiology, The Ohio State University, Mansfield, OH 44906

Bugs as Drugs: Therapeutic Microbes for the Prevention and Treatment of Disease
Edited by Robert A. Britton and Patrice D. Cani
© 2018 American Society for Microbiology, Washington, DC
doi:10.1128/microbiolspec.BAD-0003-2016

typically they are effective against antibiotic-resistant bacteria. These viruses can be useful for combating unwanted bacteria in part because they have evolved for billions of years as specifically acting antibacterial agents. Phages are highly abundant and diverse, generally easy to work with, and represent two of seven "tier 1" alternatives to antibiotics for systemic use as considered by Czaplewski et al. (39). Particularly given informed phage choice, along with appropriate purification, phages do not tend to display substantial toxicities toward, for example, human tissues, or even against nontarget portions of the human microbiome.

Notwithstanding these positive factors, phage therapy is not widely employed in clinical practice. Part of the reason for its relative absence is historical and accompanying tradition, part is due to regulatory constraints, and another part (40) is that only relatively recently has there been widespread recognition of a need for alternatives to antibiotics as antibacterial drugs. This review provides an overview of the arguments for why further development of phages as antibacterial "drugs" to supplement or in some cases even replace small-molecule antibiotics may be warranted. A related aim is to suggest that substantial clinical development already has occurred.

Glossary of Terms

Toward introducing phage therapy and related concepts, in this section I define a number of relevant terms.

Biocontrol Here this term refers to the use of phages as antibacterial agents; phage therapy is a type of phage-mediated biological control of bacteria, i.e., "biocontrol" as used here.

Crude lysate Phage lysate of host bacteria from which phages have not been substantially purified; e.g., at most a crude lysate has been subject to filter sterilization to remove intact bacteria along with relatively large pieces of bacterial debris but not removal of smaller debris or sufficient reduction of contamination with endotoxin.

Endotoxin Lipid-based component of the outer membranes of Gram-negative bacteria.

Lysate Typically fluid product of phage-induced lysis of bacterial cultures.

Lysogen Bacterial cell hosting one or more lysogenic cycles/prophages.

Lysogeny Description of a phage infection that is ongoing, usually over large numbers of bacterial generations, and which does not produce phage virions unless lysogeny is exited; lysogeny is the product of a lysogenic infection/lysogenic cycle.

Phage Virus that can productively infect bacterial cells; "phage" can refer to the virions or the virus more generally, e.g., "phage infection"; also known as bacteriophage or bacterial virus.

Phage therapy Application of phages as medicinals, particularly as used in the clinic or by veterinarians; a specific type of phage-mediated biocontrol of bacteria.

Professionally lytic phage Phage that is not temperate, nor closely related to temperate phages, and which releases phage progeny via lytic cycles; "virulent," "strictly lytic," "obligately lytic," etc. are also descriptions of phages that are both lytic and not temperate, but also that are not necessarily distantly related to temperate phages; professionally lytic phages are preferred for phage-mediated biocontrol.

Prophage Phage genome as observed during lysogenic cycles; prophages traditionally are seen as integrated into the chromosomes of their bacterial host, though plasmid prophages exist as well.

Temperate phage Phage that is capable of displaying lysogenic cycles; most temperate phages are also lytic phages, that is, releasing virions from productive infections via host-cell lysis; contrast temperate with virulent, strictly lytic, obligately lytic, professionally lytic, or obligately productive phages.

Staphage lysate Formulation consisting of phage-lysed *Staphylococcus* culture in which associated phages may or may not represent an active ingredient.

Transduction Virus-mediated movement, especially of nonviral DNA from one potential host cell to another; specialized transduction is the movement of relatively small amounts of bacterial DNA as mediated by excising prophages, whereas generalized transduction is the movement of relatively large amounts of bacterial DNA as mediated by phages which otherwise are less destructive to bacterial genomes and less selective when packaging DNA into virions.

PHAGE THERAPY AND PHAGE-MEDIATED BIOCONTROL

The use of phages as antibacterial agents can be differentiated into uses that, in their utility, are more antibiotic-like versus more disinfectant-like. Because successful introduction of phages into clinics may be informed by efforts to employ phages more widely as antibacterials, in this section I differentiate the therapeutic use of phages from a broader utility as biological control agents of undesirable bacteria. This discussion is provided in part to briefly overview this nontherapeutic antibacterial use of phages.

Phage Therapy

Phage therapy literally is the use of bacterial viruses as therapeutic agents (see Table 1 for a summary of published modern human treatment). Usually these therapeutic aspects are assumed to stem directly from phage antibacterial activity. There exist, however, other therapeutic utilities of phages, for example, as delivery vehicles of toxins or DNA (e.g., 27, 41, 42) or as immune system modulators and characterizers (43–46). Among bactericidal phage therapies, it is also possible to distinguish prophylaxes from the targeting of already contaminating, colonizing, or infecting bacteria.

Considering just phage antibacterial aspects, we can view phage therapy as a subset of phage-mediated biological control of bacteria (47), or simply "biocontrol" for short.

Elsewhere, and somewhat consistent with usage by others, I have suggested that the phrase "phage therapy," as a subset of biocontrol, should be used particularly in those circumstances where organisms, e.g., ourselves, are individually treated with phages to reduce the numbers of bacteria that in some manner are affecting the treated individual. All other uses of phages as antibacterial agents, by contrast, may be referred to as different forms of biocontrol (next section) rather than explicitly as phage therapy (48). Thus, phage-mediated removal of colonizing pathogenic bacteria from individual affected humans or from affected individual animals is unambiguously phage therapy. Given such treatment of individuals directly with phages, as though phage formulations were complex drugs, we can consider the process of phage therapy from a pharmacological perspective. Drugs, in particular, have specific chemical properties, are delivered to bodies in some manner, are able to reach and maintain different concentrations in different regions of the body, and can impact the body in both intended and unintended ways.

A number of reviews have considered various aspects of phage therapy pharmacology (e.g., 49–53). Furthermore, a diversity of pharmacologically familiar application approaches have been employed clinically or experimentally in phage therapy. These include local application, systemic application, and the attachment of phages to surfaces to prevent subsequent colonization. Local application traditionally includes application to body surfaces and wounds, inhalation into the lungs, and delivery to various mucus membranes including the oral cavity and vagina. Systemic delivery, at least in principle, may include *per os*, via suppositories, or via injection. Surgically, it is also possible to infuse phages relatively deeply into tissues. Phages, in addition, may be packaged in various ways prior to delivery, including into liposomes (54, 55) or encapsidated by various additional means (6). To minimize complications, typically, phages that are lytic, that are not capable

TABLE 1 Modern clinical or human experimental phage therapy (English-language literature)

Targets	Comment	Number treated[a]	Substantial efficacy	Authors	Year	Reference
Various	Various treatments	62	47%[b]	Łusiak-Szelachowska et al.	2017	142
S. aureus	Diabetic foot ulcers	9	100%	Fish et al.	2016	183
E. coli	Diarrhea	79	0%[c]	Sarker et al.	2016	114
S. aureus	Eye treatment	1	100%	Fadlallah et al.	2015	185
Various	Various treatments	>100	95%[d]	Kutateladze	2015	186
P. aeruginosa, S. aureus	Safety trial (topical dosing)	9	NA[e]	Rose et al.	2014	116
E. coli, Proteus	Safety trial (oral dosing)	15	NA	McCallin et al.	2013	91
Various	Various treatments	153	40%	Międzybrodzki et al.	2012	102
E. coli	Safety trial (oral dosing)	15	NA	Sarker et al.	2012	113
P. aeruginosa	Urinary tract infection	1	100%	Khawaldeh et al.	2011	188
P. aeruginosa, S. aureus	Cystic fibrosis patient	1	NA[f]	Kvachadze et al.	2011	189
NA	Cystic fibrosis patients	NA	NA	Kutateladze and Adamia	2010	144
E. faecalis	Chronic bacterial prostatitis	3	100%	Letkiewicz et al.	2009	190
E. coli, P. aeruginosa, S. aureus	Safety trial (topical dosing)	39	NA[g]	Rhoads et al.	2009	117
P. aeruginosa	Chronic otitis	12[h]	25%[i]	Wright et al.	2009	118
NA	Cystic fibrosis patient	1	NA	Kutateladze and Adamia	2008	137
S. aureus	Gastrointestinal colonization	1	100%	Leszczyński et al.	2008	191
S. aureus	Economics of methicillin-resistant S. aureus treatment	6	NA	Międzybrodzki et al.	2007	206
P. aeruginosa	Burn wound infection	1	100%	Marza et al.	2006	192
Staphylococcus spp.	Otitis media	1	0%[j]	Weber-Dąbrowska et al.	2006	207
E. coli	Safety trial (oral dosing)	15	NA	Bruttin and Brüssow	2005	112
S. aureus	Radiation burn and PhagoBioDerm	2	100%	Jikia et al.	2005	193
S. aureus	Hand-washing experiment	NA	NA	O'Flaherty et al.	2005	68
Various	Septicemia	94	85%	Weber-Dąbrowska et al.	2003	208
Various	Wounds, ulcerations, and PhagoBioDerm	96	70%	Markoishvili et al.	2002	194
S. aureus	Peripheral neutrophil functioning	37	73%	Weber-Dąbrowska et al.	2002	209

Various	Infections of cancer patients	20	100%	Weber-Dąbrowska et al.	2001	210
Various	Various treatments	1,307	96%	Weber-Dąbrowska et al.	2000	187
Various	Chronic SBI[k] of skin	31	74%	Cisło et al.	1987	211
Various	Determination of neutralizing antibody	57	77%	Kucharewicz-Krukowska and Ślopek	1987	139
Various	SBI	550	85%[l]	Ślopek et al.	1987	181
Various	SBI	56	88%	Weber-Dąbrowska et al.	1987	182
Various	SBI	370	85%	Ślopek et al.	1985	178
Various	SBI in children	114	89%	Ślopek et al.	1985	179
Staphylococcus	SBI	254	85%	Ślopek et al.	1985	180
Various	SBI	150	81%	Ślopek et al.	1984	177
Various	SBI	138	88%	Ślopek et al.	1983	103
Various	SBI	84	88%	Ślopek et al.	1983	176
S. aureus (or other)	Treatment of hidradenitis suppurativa with Staphage Lysate[m]	8	75–100%[n]	Kress et al.	1981	212

[a]Throughout this review, numbers treated refers to non-placebo-treated individuals for whom studies or treatments were completed.

[b]Clinical improvement or better.

[c]Relatively little effort in this trial appears to have been devoted to ensuring that sufficient numbers of phages of desired specificity would be present in the vicinity of target bacteria.

[d]It is not obvious what types of cases this percentage refers to, e.g., both acute and chronic or just acute.

[e]NA, either not available or not applicable.

[f]Endpoints of treatment of cystic fibrosis patients are sufficiently ambiguous that "NA," not applicable, has been assigned despite arguably positive results.

[g]Phage choice in this trial was biased toward better phage in vitro characterization rather than toward ability to treat those strains of wound-infecting bacteria encountered.

[h]Plus 12 placebo controls.

[i]Based on only single phage dosing in the course of a phase I/II clinical trial.

[j]Phage therapy had some positive impact, but clearance did not occur until subsequent lactoferrin treatment was employed.

[k]SBI, suppurative bacterial infections.

[l]This publication is an overview of previously published Ślopek et al. articles; here and in these others, results indicated as "++++" or "+++" are counted as "substantial efficacy" versus merely positive results; typically, these are treatments of chronic bacterial infections that had already been subject to antibiotic therapy, and in some cases (about one-quarter) antibiotic treatment also coincided with phage treatment.

[m]Staphylococcal phage lysate.

[n]This article is not necessarily looking at phage therapy in the sense of phages penetrating to and then directly killing target bacteria; i.e., efficacy instead may be a consequence of immune system stimulation. From the abstract: "Six of the 8 patients reported noticeable improvement in odor, consistency, and amount of drainage and considerable decreases in pain. Seven of the 8 patients reported improvement in the ability of lesions to drain spontaneously, and a decrease in the frequency of inflammatory nodules. All 8 patients reported that the inflammatory periods were definitely shorter."

of displaying lysogeny (and thus are not temperate), and that are not closely related to temperate phages are preferred for phage therapy purposes. These are phages that can be described as "professionally lytic" (56).

Phage-Mediated Biocontrol

Biocontrol, other than that which can be described unambiguously as "phage therapy" (previous section), includes the disinfection of nonliving surfaces or environments (e.g., 57–61). Representative forms of biocontrol thus are the treatment of aquatic environments to remove unwanted cyanobacteria (for references, see reference 62) or phage-mediated removal of certain bacteria during water treatment (23). So too, one can view as forms of biocontrol phage application to foods, to food animals preharvest, or to food-handling equipment, in each of these cases to remove foodborne pathogens which otherwise could affect humans (6, 13, 14, 22, 28, 29, 32, 33, 63) or, instead, to remove organisms which can affect food quality (64, 65). The treatment of biofilms is similar, particularly other than in the course of treating diseases (e.g., 1, 66). Thus, for example, the removal of biofouling biofilms from inanimate surfaces (25), e.g., membrane filters (67), would constitute of a form of biocontrol but should not be described as medicinal therapy.

More ambiguous is the disinfection of surfaces of our own bodies such as in the course of hand-washing (68). This is biocontrol, but it also, at least arguably, could be viewed as therapeutic as well, and particularly so if removal is of more than simply transient microbiota, e.g., clearance of methicillin-resistant *Staphylococcus aureus* from body surfaces prior to surgery (69). Also ambiguous is the application of phages to plants (70–73) or to fungi such as mushrooms (74) to remove bacterial pathogens affecting these organisms. These are examples simply of biocontrol to the extent that phages are applied to multiple individuals simultaneously, e.g., spraying fields to treat bacterial diseases affecting plant species versus, for example, soaking individual plants or seeds prior to planting, with the latter arguably being more therapeutic in its nature. So too is the newly explored application of phages to control bacterial disease in honey bees, which also can include phage application in feed (75) versus phage application less specifically to entire hives. This distinction can be seen with poultry as well, i.e., spraying pens to inoculate animals against, for example, colibacillosis (76) versus feeding phages directly to animals (77).

The use of phages in the context of aquaculture (e.g., 78) may be viewed similarly. Ambiguity between biocontrol and phage therapy is seen particularly with the release of phages directly into water (79) rather than more individually directed application such as feed-borne phage delivery (80), with the latter approach, toward treating or preventing disease in husbanded animals, e.g., farmed fish, more reasonably described as phage therapy rather than biocontrol. Phage treatment of invertebrate feed animals in aquaculture to remove pathogens capable of impacting farmed fish (81), however, would clearly constitute a form of biocontrol rather than therapy, just as is the case with antipathogen treatment of foods prior to human consumption (above). In each of these cases, broader phage application (biocontrol) has greater potential to impact bacteria whether or not those bacteria are directly associated with potentially negatively affected host organisms. This contrasts with phages predominantly reaching only those bacteria currently colonizing treated individuals, i.e., as seen with phage therapy, which is the primary emphasis of this review.

UTILITY

The utility of phages as antibacterial agents is derived from two basic phage properties: (i) phage virions primarily consist of proteins and nucleic acid, that is, they are not xenobiotic (59); and (ii) the mechanisms of phage antibacterial activity, by and large, are somewhat robust, consisting of multiple mechanisms per phage, and are not thought to overlap substantially in terms of molecular targets with those of existing antibiotics (e.g., 82). This section considers the safety of phages themselves, i.e., virions as well as phage infections, the safety of the formulations within which therapeutic phages are carried, the impact of phages on nontarget microbiota, and the safety track record of phage administration—preclinical, clinical, and in terms of clinical trials. Also relevant to phage utility, as nonxenobiotic pharmaceuticals, is the idea of emergent property pharmacology. For balance, this section also considers various countering issues, including discussion of the potential for phages to interact with immune systems. The latter, it should be noted upfront, and rightly or wrongly, is typically seen as much less of an issue within the phage therapy community (e.g., 83) than as typically viewed from outside of that community. Formal listings of "pros and cons of phage therapy" can be found in a number of publications (e.g., 1, 4, 59, 84–86). Issues of efficacy are addressed in the subsequent section.

Low Toxicity of Well-Chosen Phages

Despite the great genetic diversity that is seen among phages (e.g., 87), the chemical diversity of phage virions—as basically protein- and nucleic acid-based entities—pales in comparison to the chemical diversity seen among drugs generally, e.g., antibacterial drugs (88). The latter, especially at higher concentrations, can be toxic to bodies by mechanisms that can be unrelated to the drugs' mechanisms of antibacterial activity. Phages, by contrast, tend to be relatively inert within bodies other than while displaying bioactivity during their interactions with target bacteria. As a consequence, minimum toxic concentrations for phages within bodies tend, at least so far as is understood, to be somewhat higher than

minimum effective concentrations. Due to the resultantly large therapeutic index, i.e., toxic dose relative to effective dose, the application of phages to bodies tends not to result in phage-virion-associated side effects, and this is true even given the potential for phages to amplify their numbers *in situ* in the course of eradicating target bacteria. Crucially, the relative lack of chemical diversity of phage virions, i.e., their nonxenobiotic nature, can greatly simplify the process of developing specific phage products.

Despite the relative lack of direct, chemical toxicities associated with phage virions, and their comparative inertness in the absence of interaction with target bacteria, a variety of concerns typically are raised regarding the potential for phages to harm bodies. These include the prospect of phages interacting with immune systems, their potential to encode harmful gene products such as exotoxins, and their ability to modify target bacteria in ways that are potentially harmful to us, e.g., by converting bacteria to lytic products or by transducing DNA between bacteria. It is important to note, though, that especially given proper phage choice (34, 89, 90), particularly of appropriately characterized and purified professionally lytic phages, these concerns in practice have not been known to result in substantial harm to treated organisms or environments. Furthermore, Pirnay et al. (53) describe concern about transduction as "optional." Thus, an important utility as well as a safety characteristic of well-chosen phages is their generally low toxicity.

Formulated Products

Phage formulated products consist not just of phage virions, which can be viewed as active ingredients, but also of various carriage materials (34, 89). The latter most notably can include lysis products produced during phage preparation—which can be toxic and/or contribute to formulation immunogenicity—though carriage materials can also include intrinsic components of growth media as well as materials released from bacteria even in the absence of lysis. These latter issues to a degree can be controlled in the course of choosing the bacterial host and growth media used to generate phage stocks. It is especially useful to avoid, if possible, hosts for phage-stock generation that are capable of producing toxic products since those hosts not only may produce those products but will also carry potentially transducible genes that underlie that production. Included in the list of "genes" to avoid are also prophages, because these can potentially contaminate phage stocks as virions and also transduce host genes. In principle, though, it should be possible to analyze phage stocks or formulated products (91, 92) for even relatively low-level phage-virion carriage of bacterial genes (e.g. 93, 94).

In terms of intrinsic media components, a reasonable argument can be made that it can be best to avoid ingredients that are of animal origin, e.g., to avoid the introduction of prions or animal viruses into formulations (34, 85, 95). Generally, however, the most-considered carriage material-associated hazard is endotoxin. Endotoxin can be released from Gram-negative bacteria both with and without phage-induced lysis, and a variety of approaches have been developed for separating endotoxin from phage virions (34, 89, 96, 97). Such purification nevertheless is not essential under all circumstances, and indeed is generally less of a concern the further dosing is from parenteral. Thus, for example, topical dosing of wounds or oral dosing does not require nearly as much phage purification prior to use (34, 43), in contrast to intravenous (i.v.) dosing (26, 45). In general, therefore, while it is relevant to consider the toxicity of the formulations within which therapeutic phages are suspended, such toxicities tend to be mostly avoidable issues or seldom tend to be highly problematic in practice. See also Vandenheuvel et al. (17) for a recent review of issues of phage formulated products with an emphasis on enhancing stability.

Low Phage Impact on Nontarget Microbiota

The potential for phage impact on nontarget organisms is an issue predominantly because of how phages can be contrasted in this regard with nonphage antibacterial agents, that is, rather than this being an issue emanating from phage properties themselves. Further, this issue of impact on other than target bacteria can be broadened to that of low phage-virion influence on nontarget organisms more generally, that is, phage interaction with our own cells and tissues as well as our microbiome. Phages, as cytotoxic entities in particular, tend to be highly specialized in terms of what they are cytotoxic toward.

The range of bacteria that a typical phage can infect tends to be relatively narrow (98); indeed, Górski et al. (5) report, despite extensive experience, an ability to access what they call "an active specific phage" against *S. aureus*, *Enterococcus faecalis*, and *Pseudomonas aeruginosa* strains only 90%, 77%, and 72% of the time, respectively. The result is that phages tend to have relatively little impact not just on our own tissues but also on our microbiomes, beyond their impact, that is, on target bacteria. The caveat, however, is that at least in principle a phage's transductive host range might be wider than its virion-productive host range or bactericidal host range. Transduction issues can be minimized by employing professionally lytic phages, and otherwise in the course of phage characterization (92), though as previously noted there are differences of opinion over whether transduction should be a concern beyond avoiding phages which have obviously high transduction likelihoods (53, 83). The potential for additional bactericidal activity also can be minimized in the course of phage characterization using spot testing, which ideally (99) is able to detect an ability of phages to kill host bacteria even if those bacteria cannot support phage replication. Even without such effort, it at least has not been obvious that phage therapy has substantial unintended impacts on normal microbiota. Antibiotic use, by contrast, can be somewhat disruptive of microbiomes, leading to negative health consequences (100).

Low Toxicity in Use

The points discussed in the three previous sections are somewhat theoretical. That is, there are reasons to expect that therapeutic phage products can be fairly safe, thus not resulting in any more than minor side effects. An important remaining question nevertheless is whether, empirically, phages are nontoxic or otherwise not damaging to bodies or environments during actual use. This question can be framed as one of emergent property pharmacology (subsequent section). That is, despite arguments for the potential for phages to be safe upon use, are they? There are four general areas of evidence for actual phage safety: animal testing, a substantial amount of clinical use, actual (though limited in number) clinical trials (17), and the nature of our interaction with phages as normally found in our environments.

In short, with animal testing (e.g., feeding phages to rats [101]), modern clinical use (102), or in the course of clinical safety trials (next section), there have been only relatively minor side effects associated with phage application, particularly relative to the symptoms associated with the infection being treated. According to Międzybrodzki et al. (102, p. 111)—and keeping in mind that crude lysates apparently were employed for these procedures (61, 103) so the basis of noted adverse reactions cannot be readily assigned—"The most frequent adverse reactions to phage preparations found in patients subjected to PT were symptoms from the digestive tract (nausea, abdominal pain, loss of appetite), local reactions at the site of administration of a phage preparation (redness, various uncomfortable feelings, but also individual cases of atopic dermatitis, urticarial blistering, as well as purulent blistering), superinfections (as seen in 4.6% of patients), and a rise in body

temperature (3.3% subfebrile and 3.3% febrile)." Arguably, even fewer instances of side effects are seen given sufficient phage purification prior to use, particularly when avoiding more invasive application of crude phage lysates (e.g., parenteral), though use of crude lysates appears to have been the case during less modern phage use as therapeutics (e.g., references 85, 104, and 105).

Further, we are surrounded by phages. Except for those which are known to contribute to disease (e.g., exotoxin-encoding temperate phages [106, 107], which ideally will be avoided for phage therapy), so-called endogenous phages (108) with which our bodies regularly interact are not known to directly give rise to disease. For example, the human oral cavity may contain on the order of 100 billion (10^{11}) viruses, many of which are bacteriophages (109). Arguments can be made that this point simply has not been sufficiently well studied or that endogenous phages might give rise to dysbioses (e.g., 109, 110). Nonetheless, such issues can be mitigated in terms of phage therapy through proper phage choice: use of phages which display appropriately narrow host ranges and which are not temperate and do not otherwise encode potentially dangerous gene products. In general, the application of well-chosen and perhaps especially well-purified phages to bodies has not been known to result in a substantial worsening of patient health.

Safety Trials

A handful of phage therapy safety trials have been performed over the previous 20 or so years. These I review as follows. More complete discussion of phage clinical trials can be found, e.g., in references 7, 17, 61, and 111 and in a subsequent section.

Kutter et al. (61) provide a personal communication-based overview of an otherwise unpublished study from 2000 undertaken by Exponential Biotherapies, Inc. A dose of 5×10^6 anti-*Enterococcus* phages was supplied intravenously to 12 healthy volunteers, which worked out to roughly 10^3 phages per ml of blood. This is a dosage which I would argue could be many orders of magnitude too low for therapeutic purposes (51) unless *in situ* phage replication were able to raise these numbers substantially (50). Reported side effects consisted of a transient rash that was observed in one subject. No mention is made of the degree to which phages were purified prior to use, but a conservative assumption would be that they were substantially purified.

In 2005, Bruttin and Brüssow (112) published the results of a phase I phage-therapy safety trial. Phage T4 was supplied orally to 15 healthy adults in 150 ml of mineral water at concentrations of 10^3 or 10^5 per ml, thrice daily for 2 days. No side effects that the authors attributed to phage dosing were reported. In otherwise equivalent trials, similar results were seen with higher phage densities (113) as well as when treating children, the latter employing a commercially available Russian phage product (91). See too the more recent study of Sarker et al. (114), which is considered below. Brüssow (115, p. 138) noted that "as phages are considered relatively low risk when the [U.S. Food and Drug Administration] selection criteria are met, not very high numbers of treated humans are needed to demonstrate their safety."

Rose et al. (116) describe the treatment of nine volunteers in a 2007 burn-treatment phage-therapy safety trial. A phage cocktail active against both *P. aeruginosa* (two phages) and *S. aureus* (one phage) was employed. Phages were present at a titer of 10^9/ml, were separated from endotoxin prior to use, were applied only once at a density of 10^7 per cm^2, and were used in conjunction with standard protocols, i.e., other than phage treatment. The authors concluded (p. 70), "No adverse events were reported and no clinical or laboratory test abnormalities related to the application of phages were observed."

In 2009, Rhoads et al. (117) studied the impact of topical application of a cocktail of eight phages (10^9/ml diluted 12.5-fold) active individually against *Escherichia coli*, *P. aeruginosa*, and *S. aureus*. Application was topical in combination with ultrasonic debridement to chronic venous leg ulcers of 18 volunteers (plus 21 placebo controls) over a 12-week period, with one application per week. No negative impacts in terms of either side effects or interference with wound healing were observed. See also the discussion of this trial in reference 61.

Also in 2009, Wright et al. (118) published a study in which chronic otitis was treated topically in 24 volunteers, none currently undergoing antibiotic therapy, using anti-*Pseudomonas* phages (cocktail of six). Half were treated once in one ear with 10^5 phages and half with placebo. This was a phase I/II trial, that is, safety as well as preliminary efficacy were being studied. The author's conclusion regarding safety (p. 353) was that "there were no reportable side effects, and no evidence of local or systemic toxicity."

Emergent Property Pharmacology

An emergent property is a higher-level characteristic of a system that is difficult to predict from lower-level aspects. Thus, the collective properties of groups of organisms can be difficult to predict given knowledge gleaned solely from the study of individual organisms in isolation. In the case of emergent property pharmacology, the difficulty in question is prediction of the pathophysiological consequences of drug application solely from a drug's chemical or other characteristics as determined in isolation from actual use. This issue arises in pharmacology particularly because the number of possible targets of drug action within a body can be vast, and at least some of the resulting interactions can be disruptive of homeostasis. In short, it can be difficult to predict all of a drug's potential side effects prior to undertaking animal testing or clinical trials.

Emergent properties can substantially increase both the cost and duration of drug development because "most 'hits' [antibiotics] fail to proceed to clinical stages because of the subsequent discovery of mammalian toxicity" (40, p. 326). An additional consequence is the commercialization of drugs despite known toxicities, i.e., the standard package insert disclaimers associated with most pharmaceuticals. In principle, a phage which comes to display unexpected toxicities—or insufficient host range, e.g., pyophage development as discussed in reference 61—should be easily replaced given the genetic diversity of phages available for isolation. Considered instead in this section, however, is the relatively low potential for unexpected phage toxicities to begin with.

Two basic strategies can be employed to minimize a drug's emergent properties. The first is to improve the predictive power such that drug physiological properties may be more readily projected based on chemical properties. In this way, drugs which are anticipated to ultimately display toxicities may be sidelined earlier during the development process. Alternatively, one can seek out drug candidates which, independent of knowledge of chemical properties, tend to be biased toward high specificity in terms of their interaction with body tissues and toward reduced intrinsic toxicity, as indeed can be the case generally for therapeutic protein products (119). In many cases, natural products also have been honed by evolution toward substantial specificity in their physiological interactions (120).

This idea of natural products displaying greater specificity for the sake of greater if narrower effectiveness is a variation on a broader concept of what can be described as antagonistic pleiotropy, that is, the tendency for enhancement of one aspect of an organism—here, the natural product—to give rise to changes, often in some negative manner, in other phenotypic aspects of the same organism (121, 122). Thus, the evolution of increased effectiveness against a specific target, e.g., what an agent binds to, can result in decreased effectiveness against other targets.

In terms of emergent property pharmacology, the important general point is that it is a drug interacting with other body locations, or inappropriate interactions with primary targets, that often can lead to secondary pharmacodynamic consequences, i.e., side effects.

In terms of phage therapy emergent property pharmacology (59), the result of antagonistic pleiotropy is that phages, in many cases, have been honed by evolution toward limiting their physiological interactions with entities other than those bacteria with which the phage has some potential to subsequently produce phage progeny. In practice, this means phages tend to display relatively narrow host ranges, i.e., narrow spectra of activity as considered in pharmacological terms. As a consequence, phages tend *not* to be highly effective at interacting, especially in negative terms, with eukaryotic cells and tissues; see, though, the issue of lysogeny and lysogenic conversion such as the ability of certain temperate phages to encode bacterial exotoxins (106, 123).

Another way of making these points is that while phages, as viruses, can serve as highly cytotoxic agents, that cytotoxicity tends to be limited to those organisms into which phage virions can deliver their nucleic acid genomes (e.g., 124). In other words, phage virions represent vehicles of cytotoxic agent delivery, but both the delivery of those agents and, to a large extent, the cytotoxicity itself tend to be specific to an only minor subset of possible targets. Indeed, given this specificity, it is typical to not even consider phages to be cytotoxic agents.

The relative lack of emergent property pharmacology associated with phages as potential medicinals makes it possible to characterize phages *in vitro* toward use *in vivo* without substantial concern about unanticipated side effects. In this modern age of phage therapy, this characterization can include the sequencing and annotation of phage genomes, which addresses the other means of avoiding emergent properties, that of achieving substantial predictive *in vitro* characterization. Even without such sequencing, however, phages have not tended to display emergent toxicities during use (previous sections). Indeed, an argument can be made that regulatory approval of phage formulations for therapy could apply more in terms of specific approaches to characterization rather than in terms of specific phage isolates. The latter is just how annual influenza vaccines are developed, which a number of authors have suggested, discussed, and/or advocated as a model for the regulation of phage therapeutics (16, 85, 117, 125–134). Even yearly approval of new formulations, however, might unreasonably curtail phage therapy's potential to quickly respond, through development of new therapeutic phages, to the need to target newly arising pathogen strains (135). As biocontrol agents of foods, the designation of phages following proper characterization as GRAS, that is, generally recognized as safe, can result in regulatory implementation of this idea of phage interchangeability based on criteria for characterization versus completely independent trials (32). GRAS designation functions, however, within the context of biocontrol rather than of phage therapy, *sensu stricto*.

Addressing Potential Caveats

Most or all concerns with phage use as antibacterial agents, particularly within a clinical context, are either hypothetical or readily addressable. The potential for phages to encode bacterial virulence factors, for example, can be addressed with increasing bioinformatic power given phage genome sequencing. This potential, however, (i) generally has not been reported as an issue during actual phage therapy, whether clinical or preclinical, (ii) is avoidable to a large extent by avoiding the use of temperate phages for phage therapy, i.e., particularly by employing professionally lytic phages, and (iii) otherwise could become apparent in the course of toxicity testing. The potential for phages to transduce genes can be avoided by not using phage types which are known to be prone to

transduction (including temperate phages), by avoiding hosts for phage-stock generation which carry undesirable genes or prophages, by testing phage stocks for the presence of such genes, and even by testing the potential for phages to transduce from or to multiple additional strains. Toxins and other dangerous contaminants that potentially may be found in phage lysates are, as noted, not always an issue but nonetheless can be addressed through various purification approaches as well as by avoiding growth media ingredients that can potentially carry these factors.

Also relevant is the issue of presumptive treatment. Broad-spectrum antibiotics are convenient to prescribe because substantial prior knowledge of target organism susceptibility often is not required. Indeed, this convenience likely contributed in earlier decades to the rise of antibiotics to treat bacterial infections instead of phages as selectively toxic antibacterials (an abbreviated history of phage therapy is provided below). It is difficult to develop phage formulations that possess as wide a spectrum of activity as those of typical broad-spectrum antibiotics, however. Two not mutually exclusive technical solutions nonetheless exist which potentially can address phage therapy's presumptive treatment issue. The first is to employ phage cocktails as therapeutic agents since, by mixing different phage types into a single product, its spectrum of activity can be substantially broadened (126, 128, 136). The result can be an increase in the likelihood that any given formulation will cover most of the strains of a given bacterial pathogen that may be encountered. In addition, it is possible to include multiple phages to multiple species to allow the treatment of infections without first identifying target species (137), though this approach is more complicated because it involves more phages as well as more targets. Notwithstanding such complication in development, Kutter et al. (61, p. 260) report that one cocktail produced in the former Soviet Republic of Georgia contains "hundreds of different phages that together target over 28 bacterial species."

The second approach to addressing the issue of presumptive treatment is to improve diagnostics, particularly so that the phage susceptibility of target pathogens can be ascertained rapidly, ideally in minutes, as well as reasonably inexpensively (29, 138). A goal would be that precise diagnosis in terms of the phage vulnerability of presumptive pathogens could be determined relatively soon after examining patients. The need for rapidity in diagnostics as well as presumptive treatment more generally, however, is less important given the treatment of chronic versus more acute bacterial infections. This is because with chronic bacterial infections more time and resources —a hospital's versus those of stand-alone medical practices—can be available to match phages to bacterial targets prior to use.

Phages and Immune Systems

Lastly in terms of potential detriments to phage utility is the question of phage interaction with animal immune systems (139–142). An often-leveled critique of phage therapy is that phage virions predominantly consist of proteins, and proteins are immunogenic. The immunogenicity of phage virions has long been appreciated, and it raises at least two concerns vis-à-vis phage therapy: phage-immune system interactions will negatively impact patients, and phage-immune system interactions will interfere with the effectiveness of phage therapy. Both of these concerns can be relevant to protein-based therapeutics generally, of which currently over 200 are being marketed (119), and to at least some extent both of these concerns are valid for phages. Nevertheless, these issues are not necessarily "game changers" so far as the practice of phage therapy is concerned.

First, substantial negative consequences of phage-immune system interactions during therapy are relatively rare, are typically not life threatening (i.e., are easily controlled or reversed), and especially as reported in the early phage literature, are difficult to distinguish from the interaction of phage carriage material with immune systems, that is, nonphage materials found in phage lysates (above). A product consisting essentially of phage-induced *S. aureus* lysate at one time was deliberately employed clinically to at least hundreds of patients (607 reported), including both intradermally and subcutaneously, for immune-system stimulation, but no anaphylactic reactions or serum sickness were reported despite weeks and months of application (104). Note, though, that side effects were reported in at least one patient, including abdominal pain following intranasal application; in addition, known responses to staphylococcus exposure were also observed, particularly temporary liver enlargement and tenderness, which the authors categorized as "temporary discomfort," with treatment nevertheless generally continued in these cases. See too the discussion of Górski et al. (43). Second, immune system-mediated inactivation of phages does not necessarily translate into phage therapy failure (140, 142).

One circumstance in which problematic phage-immune system interactions would be expected to be greatest is with direct phage administration to the blood, i.e., intravenous (i.v.) treatment. The i.v. administration of phages is an issue because of fears of anaphylaxis and concerns about the development of humoral immune responses to phages, though it should be noted that i.v. exposure in and of itself appears to result in lower protein-based drug immunogenicity than injection into solid tissues such as intramuscular or subcutaneous injection or inhalation into the lungs (119). In addition is the potential nonspecific impact of the mononuclear phagocyte system, also known as the reticuloendothelial system. The latter has been shown to substantially reduce the duration of circulation of certain phage virions (143). Notwithstanding these issues, i.v. application of phage virions during phage therapy has substantial historical clinical precedence, which is remarkable given the crude methods of virion purification which were employed during the early decades of phage therapy. Indeed, Speck and Smithyman (26) recently made a case for the i.v. application of phages for therapy, which they suggest may be particularly effective against bacteremias along with endocarditis by *S. aureus* and as treatments for typhoid fever. See also the discussion by Kutateladze and Adamia (144) of i.v. phage application by the Eliava Institute.

PRECEDENT

The practice of phage therapy dates back to the very dawn of phage research (145, 146), and indeed, early research on the nature of phages might be reasonably viewed as a consequence of interest in phage therapy rather than the other way around. Phage therapy was explored clinically in many locations around the globe, though it persisted to differing degrees from region to region. Overall, a fairly substantial body of published research on clinical phage therapy has been built up. Not all has been published in the English-language primary literature, however, though a fair amount is English-language accessible within reviews. In this section I provide a primer on, in particular, the English-language literature on clinical phage therapy. For numerous reviews of this subject, see references 43, 61, 85, 92, 125, 147, and 148.

100 Years of Phage Therapy

Phages were "codiscovered" by Frederick Twort and Félix d'Hérelle in 1915 (149, 150) and 1917 (151, 152), respectively. Earlier studies have been cited as possibly involving phages (e.g., see references 153 and 154), particularly that of Hankin (155) from 1896, though the evidence for phage involvement in that study is not strong, given that heating bacteria-disinfecting water in unsealed tubes destroyed antibacterial activity while heating in "hermetically sealed tubes" did not (156). The first published hint of phage therapy can be found in d'Hérelle (151), including the title of that 1917 paper (emphasis mine): "On an Invisible Microbe *Antagonistic* to Dysentery Bacilli" (152). D'Hérelle's emphasis on phages serving as bacterial antagonists, versus phages simply existing, may be supported by his later claims (157, p. 45) that the simple evidence of phage existence, in the form of plaques, "was ordinary enough, so banal indeed that many bacteriologists had certainly made it before on a variety of cultures." As also reported by d'Hérelle in that same article, the notion that phages are a "filterable virus" was not even his original idea but instead was a suggestion of Charles Nicolle, at the time (probably around 1915) director of the Pasteur Institute in Tunis. Even d'Hérelle's term, "bacteriophage" ("un bactériophage obligatoire"), is suggestive of his emphasis on the antibacterial nature of phages (*phage*, from Greek, meaning "to eat" or "devour") or simply the "dissolution of bacteria" (158, p. 6), rather than on their potential viral nature, of which, as noted, he nevertheless appeared to be well aware (152, 158).

In 1918, d'Hérelle (159, p. 972) provided what may be the first suggestion of the therapeutic use of phages as antibacterial agents: "...il semble donc logique de proposer comme traitement de la dysenterie bacillaire l'administration, dès l'apparition des premiers symptômes, de cultures actives du microbe bactériophage." [Translation by Google: "...it seems logical to propose as a treatment for shigellosis administration, from the onset of symptoms, active cultures of the microbe bacteriophage."] By 1919, d'Hérelle (145, p. 934) had described the treatment of birds with phages (translation initially by Google): "...abrupt cessation of the enzootic the day of administration of the microbe bacteriophage confirms indisputably the role of the microbe as an immunity agent." By at least 1921, we have a publication of phage therapy in humans (160), in this case anti-*Staphylococcus* treatment of skin via phage injection. Indeed, the first monograph considering phage therapy, *Le Bactériophage: Son Rôle dans l'Immunité*, was published by d'Hérelle in 1921. In the 1922 English translation of that book (161, p. 266) we find mention of "ingestion of cultures of the anti-Shiga bacteriophage, this treatment was applied for therapeutic purposes to patients affected with bacillary dysentery." Thus, we are nearing the 100th anniversary of the clinical use of phages as antibacterial agents. Though it is difficult to say exactly how many individuals have been treated with phages over those years, Debarbieux et al. (162, p. 1) speculate that the number is in the "thousands if not millions."

Grab Bag of Pre-"Modern" Human Use

Summers (163) encapsulates the history of phage therapy as a sequence of four periods consisting of enthusiasm, skepticism, abandonment, and then a recent revival. Break points are roughly the early 1930s (164), mid 1940s, and mid to late 1990s. Abandonment, corresponding to the rise of antibiotics, was not complete and, indeed, varied from region to region, with substantial retention of phage use as antibacterial agents seen in the former Soviet Union as well as Europe (125, 137, 147). A recent English-language summary of work published in the Soviet Union throughout much of the abandonment period is provided in book form by Chanishvili (148). Substantial phage use as a human therapeutic continues to take place to this day, especially in association with the George Eliava Institute of Bacteriophages, Microbiology, and Virology in Tbilisi, Georgia, which was founded, with the help of d'Hérelle, in 1923 (e.g., 137, 148), as well as the Phage Therapy Unit established in 2005 in association with the Ludwik Hirszfeld Institute of Immunology and Experimental Therapy in Wrocław, Poland (43, 102). In this section I summarize various English-language studies dating from the prerevival period of phage therapy. For a more detailed exploration of the early phage-therapy literature, particularly with regard to phage treatment of lung-associated infections, see reference 105.

In 1929, Larkum (165) supplied a list of justifications for the utility as well as disadvantages of phage use as antibacterial therapeutic agents, with the disadvantage being particularly that of excessive specificity. In addition, a "problem of controls" is explicitly indicated regarding the interpretation of outcomes. A summary of 13 studies and over 450 cases in total of phage treatment of *S. aureus* infections in humans is presented. Larkum states (p. 37), "Although these results cannot be adequately summarized, it is evident that from 75 to 80% of the patients had marked and immediate improvement. The details of many of these cases are such as to convince the reader that something other than coincidence was responsible for the results reported. Nor can the enthusiasm of the individual worker be entirely responsible, for it is a noteworthy fact that whereas in bacteriophage treatment of other infections, typhoid fever and dysentery for example, many workers have given unfavorable reports, only one which is not exceedingly favorable has as yet appeared concerning staphylococcus [*sic*] treatments." Larkum presents an additional ~240 cases of phage treatment of furunculosis involving subcutaneous phage injection. Larkum describes the immediate results (p. 39) by stating, "The lesions present regress, the exudate changes from purulent to serous, the pain is promptly relieved, and the lesions start healing within 24 hours from the time of inoculation. There are exceptions to be sure, but they are exceedingly rare." Fully successful treatment was reported in 78% of cases. In 19% there was mostly mild recurrence. In 3% of cases there was no improvement.

As is the case in many of these older studies, the following statement tends to hold (165, p. 39): "...the inoculation of bacteriophage gives reactions in the majority of instances. These are as a rule extremely mild..." Note, though, that in 1% of patients the response to phages is described as severe. Both in terms of side effects and efficacy, it is important to keep in mind, however, that the formulations employed likely represented at least an approximation of crude lysates, which for *Staphylococcus* treatments may or may not function independently of the phages themselves in treating infections (104). Larkum notes, though, that some of the patients had previously received vaccines, presumably to the etiology, with no benefit, and he suggests that these patients might be viewed as controls.

In 1935, Dunlap (166) reported the successful treatment of *S. aureus* meningitis using phages, citing two previous publications by others in which three additional cases were also successfully treated using phages. The etiology was identified from a spinal tap 5 days following the beginning of symptoms, at which time antimeningococcus serum was supplied intraspinally (days 5 and 6). Treatment also consisted (p. 1595) of "copious spinal drainage by lumbar taps, approximately twice a day" along with intraspinal acriflavine administration on days 6 and 7. Phages were tested against the bacteria *in vitro* and were supplied, also intraspinally, on days 7, 8, 9, and 10, plus subcutaneously on day 16. Dunlap states (p. 1595) that "the first negative spinal fluid culture resulted after the administration of the second ampule of bacteriophage and remained negative throughout the duration of the illness." Recovery was described as complete, though it is not obvious that phage action alone was responsible for that recovery.

In 1941, MacNeal et al. (167) described a (presumably) New York-based "service" of supplying staphylococcal phages to physicians. They present detailed instructions for how to dose intravenously since (p. 550) "strange as it may seem, our records show several instances in which intravenous therapy was abandoned because of difficulty in venipuncture." They note further that "in severe sepsis, vein puncture may need to be done several times daily over long periods of time and the importance of careful preservation of the veins cannot be overemphasized." In phage treatment of septicemia they report that a "shock reaction" is expected and apparently tolerated by the patient as well

as desired by the physician, though the authors note (pp. 552–553) that it "…is rather alarming to those who have not previously observed it and is not entirely free from danger." They recommend treating with sulfamethylthiazole or sulfathiazole simultaneously with phages. Three case studies are presented in this article, two of which were successful. Of the third, in which the patient apparently succumbed to infection, the authors note retrospectively that it may have been desirable to have employed higher doses of intravenous bacteriophage prior to identification of the target etiology.

In 1946, also from MacNeal et al. (168), came the combined use of phages and penicillin against various etiologies as published near the dawn of widespread antibiotic use. Notably, concern is expressed over resistance to penicillin. They note as well, in introducing the topic, that it had been shown previously, and then confirmed by these authors, that combined use of phages and penicillin *in vitro* was more effective against "moderately resistant" staphylococci than either alone and, further, that this effect could be seen as well with the normally penicillin-resistant Gram-negative "coli." The article otherwise recounts a number of case studies —chronic osteomyelitis, facial carbuncle, bacterial endocarditis, intestinal perforation, bacteremia—in which phages and penicillin were administered both intramuscularly and intravenously, with various *Staphylococcus* and "coli" etiologies as well as *Streptococcus*, all with favorable outcomes. Unfortunately, it is not obvious that phage-only versus penicillin-only controls were sufficiently employed to conclusively rule in a synergistic effect between penicillin and phages *in vivo*. Nevertheless, as the authors suggest (pp. 980–981), "This combined action in the test tube may be designated as a potentiating, conjoined, or synergistic effect… For practical purposes it is significant that this combined action is also manifest in the clinical use of these agents in treating otherwise malignant infections, particularly those due to staphylococci, colon bacilli, and selected members of the streptococcus group."

In 1945, Morton and Engely (169) presented a review of phage use to treat dysentery. They caution that it is necessary to confirm that phage preparations are active against target organisms in order to evaluate the effectiveness of treatments and also that phage presence, whether endogenous or therapeutically supplied, can interfere with the laboratory enumeration of target bacteria. The review first considers nine clinical studies which had indicated poor phage therapeutic performance along with, in many cases, suggestions of where those specific studies may have been flawed (e.g., possible phage gastric inactivation, lack of demonstration of phage effectiveness *in vitro*, low phage titer applied, too few cases reported, and a lack of controls). The review then considers 19 clinical studies which had been cited as evidence for the effectiveness of antidysentery phage treatment, again with suggestions of how these studies in their opinion likely were flawed. While concluding that these treatment reports together are inconclusive with regard to addressing the question of phage treatment efficacy against dysentery in humans, their conclusions regarding prophylaxis are positive. From their review of experimental treatment in animals they concluded that (p. 591) "dysentery phage has demonstrated an unmistakably therapeutic action." It is important to note, however, that the animal disease models employed were not necessarily of dysentery *per se*.

In 1956, Mills (170) reported on the use of filter-sterilized *S. aureus* lysates containing between 10^8 and 10^{10} phages/ml to treat sinusitis via nasal inhalation of aerosolized phages. Initially, 0.25 ml was applied, with a gradual increase to 1.0 ml per dose and with treatments taking place over 2 to 6 weeks, involving 10 to 20 treatments. Results are reported as "excellent" in 45% of cases and "good" in 33%. Fatigue, mild aches and pain, chills and fever, etc. are described as side effects observed early during treatment, and these are attributed, in part, to successful lysis of targeted bacteria. Treatments of 60 patients are reported, with two cases described in detail.

An important overall summary is that results from clinical phage therapy have been both reported for thousands of patients as well as critically reviewed in the older literature. This literature is well worth the consideration of modern-day phage therapists because it can supply invaluable clues as to why phage treatments may or may not have worked, i.e., as toward development of phage therapy best practices (171). It should be noted as well that in many cases this earlier literature involves the initiation of phage treatment closer to the point of diagnosis of infection than is the case for more modern treatment, especially of chronic bacterial infections, a bias that we can speculate would be due to a relative lack of viable alternative treatment approaches prior to the advent of widespread antibiotic use. This would be in contrast to the more modern treatment of chronic bacterial infections (next section), that is, infections which typically have been proven over long periods prior to the initiation of phage treatment to not be susceptible to treatment using more conventional therapies, particularly antibiotics (e.g., 102).

I have been collecting over the past decade and more a list of phage therapy, biocontrol, and related publications (>1,000; see publications.phage-therapy.org), and there are few that involve human treatment between 1945 and the 1980s, that is, during Summers' period of abandonment, at least as published in English. Peitzman (164) published in 1969 an engaging history of phage therapy during the enthusiasm and skepticism periods that provides a number of clues to what went wrong to result in abandonment of the technique, especially in North America. Mostly, I believe, problems can be summed up as consisting, typically, of enthusiasm outpacing both understanding and rigor. Presumably, however, a death blow was dealt by the widespread introduction of antibiotics, which it should be noted—and to be fair—also have displayed a lag in terms of enthusiasm outpacing both understanding and rigor, i.e., as we are now coming to appreciate problems

associated with routine antibiotic use in terms of both the evolution of antibiotic resistance and the disruption of microbiomes. The story ultimately was somewhat different regarding the fate of phage therapy behind the so-called

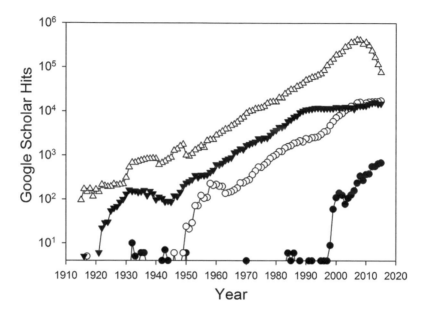

FIGURE 1 Prevalence of use of the phrase "phage therapy" in the literature. Google Scholar searches were performed without "include patents" or "include citations" checked. Shown are searches on "phage therapy" (in quotation marks, ●), "antibiotic resistant" OR "antibiotic resistance" (as written, ○), "bacteriophage" (▼), and "microbiology" (△). To limit presentation of spurious results, the y axis begins at four hits. Results and discussion: ●: "phage therapy" as a phrase is present to a small degree during the skepticism period (early 1930s through mid 1940s) and just prior to the recent revival (mid 1980s through mid to late 1990s) but then displays what appears to be renewed enthusiasm leading up to 2001. Starting from 2003 there then is a steady if less steep climb with a doubling approximately every 4 years. Relative lack of use especially prior to 1950 could reflect the popularity of alternative phrasing for "phage therapy," including in non-English publications, though this possibility was not explored. ○: Reference to antibiotic resistance goes through an initial spurt beginning around 1950 and peaking in about 1960. This is followed by a nadir in 1963 and then a steady if less steep rise with a doubling approximately every 7 years. The presented curve first comes to exceed that of "bacteriophage" in 2005. ▼: Reference to the word "bacteriophage" likely is less representative early on due to non-English publications. Nevertheless, again there is early enthusiasm that is discernible starting around 1920 and peaking in the early 1930s. This is followed by a slow decline that levels out during 1943 through 1945, i.e., toward the end of World War II. A steady climb follows that parallels the rise in the use of the term "microbiology," as indeed, so does the rise in reference to antibiotic resistance, but which to a degree plateaus for "bacteriophage" around 1990. Though not explored here, it can be speculated that the slower increase in use of "bacteriophage" starting in 1990 is a consequence of a greater prominence of the use of "phage" instead in publications, though alternatively, this switch may reflect a real decline in the rate of growth of the field; for additional data on the prevalence of bacteriophage publications, see reference 205. △: Reference to "microbiology" is presented as a general growth-in-the-literature control. The peak in 2007 and subsequent steady, ultimately multifold decline in its use is inexplicable, but similar drops are also seen with searches on "biology," "chemistry," "physics," and "physiology" (not shown), so this likely reflects indexing lags by Google.

Iron Curtain, as Chanishvili ably recounts (148). In Fig. 1 I provide my justification for labeling the mid to late 1990s to early 2000s as the point of transition to Summers' revival period of phage therapy study.

Modern Use

A substantial rekindling of interest in phage therapy began during the mid to late 1990s as reflected by a rapid surge in publications using that phrase, increasing, according to Google Scholar, from four such publications each in 1995, 1996, and 1997 to a peak of about 140 publications in 2001 (Fig. 1). This span seems to represent a second period of enthusiasm. A decline in usage followed, with about 78 publications in 2003, a drop which likely captured a second if brief period of skepticism, or at least a popping of the "bubble" of this second period of enthusiasm. I would like to suggest that Summers' (163) "recent revival," as proposed in 2011, be dubbed simply "revival" and be considered to span from the mid to late 1990s through approximately 2002. Since 2003, as noted, there has been a steady if slower increase in the use of the phrase "phage therapy." I would like to suggest, somewhat optimistically, that this increase represents a "premainstream" period of phage therapy development. That is, there seems to be an ongoing increase in enthusiasm for phage therapy but as yet only minimal expansion of its clinical use worldwide. For recent calls for such expansion, see for example, references 8 and 162.

Notwithstanding the above discussion, in hindsight and with some consensus, a modern period of phage therapy can be described in terms of English-language publication that begins during the 1980s with the animal work of H. Williams Smith and collaborators in England (172–175) and the clinical work reported by S. Slopek and collaborators in Poland (103, 139, 176–182). As above, I point especially to Chanishvili (148) for discussion of the Russian and

Georgian literature, though see also reference 61 for a broader discussion. In this section I provide overviews of recent phage therapy use in the clinic as has been published over approximately the past 10 years. These specifically are other than strictly safety trials, i.e., as were discussed above. These are published primarily in English, mostly in the primary literature, and are presented in descending-date order. Earlier as well as non-English-published clinical work has been reviewed elsewhere (e.g., 43, 85, 148). See Table 1 for a more complete listing of English-language human phage therapy articles (mostly primary literature) published since 1980.

Fish et al. (183) used an *S. aureus* phage to treat nine *S. aureus*-associated diabetic foot ulcers, specifically as found on toes, with six cases presented, one of them methicillin-resistant *S. aureus* associated. The ulcers were poorly vascularized, were not responding to antibiotic therapy including as topically applied, and toe amputation was indicated prior to phage treatment but not undertaken. Tissue was removed (debridement) in three cases, and in one case phage treatment was used to prevent infection. Topical phage application was once per week using volumes of 0.1 to 0.5 ml (of 10^7 to 10^8 phages/ml), varying with the size of the area treated, applied to gauze packed over the wound; patients were instructed to leave the dressing in place for 48 h. All ulcers healed in an average of 7 weeks. Because these were compassionate-use clinical treatments, no controls were employed other than a failure of ("poor response to") conventional treatments employed prior to initiation of phage treatment.

Sarker et al. (114) followed up previous anti-*E. coli* trials by the same group (91, 112, 113, 115, 184) involving antidiarrhea treatment of children, using oral delivery. Treatment success, however, was not achieved. It is probable that insufficient phage numbers were employed since *E. coli* densities found in the gastrointestinal tract likely were insufficient to substantially boost phage numbers *in situ* to densities required to result in adequate bacterial eradication. In addition, the host range of the phages employed may not have included the etiologies involved.

Fadlallah et al. (185) report on the use of a commercially available staphylococcal phage against chronic vancomycin-intermediate *S. aureus*. This involved treatment of interstitial keratitis and corneal abscess of a 65-year-old woman's left eye at the Phage Therapy Center in Tbilisi, Georgia. The patient had experienced various infections, vancomycin treatments, and staphylococcal carriage over an 11-year, initially postoperative period. The phage was delivered topically using eye drops as well as via a nasal spray, and also systemically intravenously. The duration of treatment was 4 weeks. As confirmed during testing 3 and 6 months later, the result was an absence of ocular and nasal carriage of the target organism.

Kutateladze (186) describes the activity of the Eliava Phage Therapy Center in Tbilisi, Georgia, from 2012 through 2014. She describes over 3,000 patient visits for phage therapy, though there is no indication that these are unique patients versus repeat visits by some of the same patients. Of these patients, 39 were described as "foreign." She also reports that phage preparations were supplied to 130 patients from abroad. Efficacy is indicated with the statement (p. 81), "more than 95% exhibiting significant improvement and recovery." In addition, a complete lack of "complications or side effects after phage application" was reported (p. 81). In the case of treatment of chronic bacterial infections, there is an indication that phage therapy was useful primarily for reducing ongoing antibiotic requirements as well as increasing the length of periods of remission rather than necessarily resulting in outright cure.

Międzybrodzki et al. (102) provide a summary of 153 patients treated from 2008 to 2010 at the Phage Therapy Unit in Wrocław, Poland. Their emphasis is on what they describe as the treatment of "otherwise untreatable chronic bacterial infections," that is, where for various reasons treatment success using antibiotics, including due to resistance, simply was not possible, and with ongoing antibiotic treatment not necessarily discontinued upon the initiation of phage treatment. Treatments did not involve surgery or hospitalization (61). The infections treated are described as orthopedic, respiratory, soft tissue, and urogenital and of 43-month median duration prior to initiation of phage treatment (thus all are chronic). Per their description (102, p. 86), "Phage preparations against *Staphylococcus, Enterococcus, E. coli, Pseudomonas, Klebsiella, Enterobacter, Proteus, Citrobacter, Salmonella,* and/or *Stenotrophomonas...* were administered to patients topically, orally, intrarectally, intravaginally, or as inhalations of aerosol." These phage preparations consistently were composed of only a single phage type, though in the case of mixed infections more than one phage type would be applied in alternation. Phage sensitivity of target organisms was determined as necessary, i.e., before treatment, in response to unsatisfactory results, and after completion of treatments, with treatments lasting a median of 55 days.

Pathogen eradication was observed in 18.3% of cases, what they describe as a "good clinical result" in another 8.5% of patients, and "clinical improvement" for a further 13.1% of patients, for a total of 39.9% "good response" to phage therapy. The largest success (65.7% good results) was seen against enterococcal infections as well as oral or intrarectal application (72.2% "good responses" and 44% eradication or recovery, respectively). There was no significant difference between rates of success with versus without use of nonphage antibacterials in conjunction with phage treatment. A pertinent observation is that statistically significant differences in outcomes were seen depending upon the site of phage administration employed, suggesting that treatments, though not blinded, nonetheless were to a degree controlled between patients. It is noted, however, that the treatment success rate is somewhat less than has been reported previously in Poland (181, 187), though one has to wonder whether the lack of the use of surgery in the treatments reported by Międzybrodzki et al. may have contributed to this difference. The authors consider the "lack of significant side effects" (p. 115) to be consistent with historical results.

Khawaldeh et al. (188) describe treatment, in Australia, of a *P. aeruginosa* urinary tract infection of a 67-year-old woman following uretic stent placement. Antibiotic treatment took place over a 2-year period. Subsequent treatment involved the use of a six-phage cocktail active against the target bacterium, obtained from the Eliava Institute (phage preparation involved filter sterilization, presumably to remove contaminating cells and larger cellular debris). Bladder instillations took place twice a day for 20 days with 20 ml of approximately 2×10^7 phages/ml. The patient was also treated with the antibiotics colistin and meropenem, starting on day 6, with the latter as had been employed previously. Bacterial viable counts were reduced from 2×10^6/ml on day 0 to roughly 10-fold lower on days 1 through 5, 50-fold lower on day 6 (prior to antibiotic treatment), 500-fold lower by day 7, and reduced to 0 on day 8. Phages alone thus appeared to contribute to at least an approximately 50-fold decline in bacterial numbers and may have contributed to the further observed reductions.

Kvachadze et al. (189) reported on the treatment of a 7-year-old cystic fibrosis patient with both anti-*Staphylococcus* and anti-*Pseudomonas* phages. Phages were delivered via nebulizer every 4 to 6 weeks. Improvement in the patient's general condition was reported as well as an ability to cut antibiotic dosing in half.

Kutateladze and Adamia (144) summarize the use of phages as supplements to standard cystic fibrosis treatments performed at the National Center of Cystic Fibrosis in Tbilisi, Georgia. Patients included both infants and adults, with phages supplied by nebulizer over spans of approximately 1 week. The authors suggest that phage use had the effect of causing "a substantial decrease in the concentration of bacterial cells" found in sputum samples (p. 4). Improvements in patient health as well as extensions of time until subsequent bacterial colonization were also attributed to phage use. No use of mock-treatment controls or details of individual cases were reported.

Letkiewicz et al. (190) describe phage treatment, at the Phage Therapy Unit in Wrocław, Poland, of three patients suffering from *E. faecalis* prostate infections which had previously resisted antibiotics and other treatment strategies. Between 10^7 and 10^9 phages/ml were present in formulations, which were matched to target bacteria (102). Phage preparations were applied rectally twice daily for 28 to 33 days, resulting in eradication of the target pathogen in all three cases.

Wright et al. (118) reported the results of a successful phase I/II clinical trial treating *P. aeruginosa* chronic otitis infections of duration prior to phage treatment ranging from up to 2 to more than 50 years. Half of the 24 volunteers were treated with phages and half with placebo. Additional treatment details—involving in all cases only a single phage dose—are described under the heading of "Safety Trials," above. Phage replication in the course of treatment was observed. No placebo-treated volunteers experienced improvement, while the blinded clinical investigator informally noted that "after 20 patients it was clear… that there was a marked effect in approximately half the patients" (p. 356). Three (of 12) phage-treated volunteers experienced substantial symptomatic improvement ("almost complete recovery") as well as elimination of the pathogen to below detectable numbers.

Leszczyński et al. (191) treated one patient orally to eliminate gastrointestinal colonization by methicillin-resistant *S. aureus* that appeared to have given rise to urinary tract infection. A sterile lysate (10 ml) of three different phages with titer of 7×10^8 phages/ml was applied three times per day. This phage application followed gastric juice neutralization (187). Treatment spanned 4 weeks but appeared to have eliminated the target organism, as determined via rectal swabs, after 1 week of phage treatment.

Marza et al. (192), in a single case study, demonstrated phage multiplication in association with a *P. aeruginosa* burn wound infection. Phage treatment coincided with elimination of the target pathogen but also a febrile episode. The latter, though, was also observed in the same patient in the absence of phage application. Intravenous ceftazidime dosing was employed as well, obscuring the phage role in the process.

Jikia et al. (193) recount the treatment, in Tbilisi, Georgia, of multiply antibiotic-resistant *S. aureus*-infected radiation burns using a phage- and antibiotic-impregnated biopolymer, PhagoBioDerm (ciprofloxacin was the antibiotic, to which the target bacteria were already resistant). Antibiotics were applied beginning 1 month prior to the start of phage treatment, but a lack of sufficient impact of those treatments resulted in the decision to employ phages. In 2 days after the start of phage treatment, wounds decreased in size along with the extent of purulent drainage, and by day 7 wounds were *S. aureus*-negative.

Markoishvili et al. (194) describe the treatment of infected wounds and/or ulcerations associated with 96 patients with PhagoBioDerm after a failure of "standard clinical therapy" (as described for 22 cases). In addition to phages, PhagoBioDerm contains ciprofloxacin and benzocaine, the latter to reduce pain. Complete recovery was indicated for 70% of individuals.

FURTHER DEVELOPMENT

Preclinical development of phages for therapeutic purposes is relevant only to the extent that useful data are obtained. Whether data are useful depends on such obvious issues as the question of whether animal or *in vitro* infection models are appropriate and whether associated phage dosing protocols are realistic, such as in terms of timing. This section briefly addresses these issues. Also considered, though not in depth, is that successful development of phage therapeutics is highly dependent on the phage therapy regulatory environment, the economics of antibacterial drug development in general, and the economics of phage therapeutic development more specifically.

Preclinical Efforts

Phage characterization prior to introduction into the clinic can involve determination of whether therapeutic phages are able to display lysogenic cycles (they should not), whether they carry potentially dangerous genes (ditto), possibly whether they are capable of effecting generalized transduction (ditto as well), and more recently whether complete genome sequencing and annotation has been achieved. In addition, monitoring for toxicity is crucial as a standard aspect of pharmaceutical development. Phage host range determination is also important, as too can be consideration of incompatibilities between different phage types or excessive overlap in antibacterial abilities during cocktail development. What these various determinations all have in common is that they are relatively independent of assay conditions. Specifically, they do not necessarily involve assessment of phage therapy efficacy as an antibacterial agent given accurate approximation of real-world conditions.

Unfortunately, in many cases preclinical efforts appear to have been expended more toward identifying experimental protocols which may give rise to what can be interpreted as efficacious results rather than toward the development of more realistic though potentially also more challenging experimental conditions. It is likely that these tendencies result from a combination of the relative ease with which laboratories can take up phage research, the duration of graduate student careers, and the duration of grants. In short, and for good reason, much preclinical phage therapy research in the modern era has tended to prioritize demonstration of phage therapy success rather than critical product development. In many instances there also has been a tendency toward only limited *in vitro* phage characterization before moving on to animal testing, tendencies which one can speculate might stem from greater experience among various researchers with handling animals versus characterizing phages.

These tendencies have several important consequences. The first is that numerous proof-of-principle results likely are of limited utility for either specific or more general phage therapy development. The second is that it really pays, as in any field of science, to understand the system being considered, here especially phage phenotypic characteristics as well as the basics of phage therapy pharmacology. The third issue, and potentially the most difficult to address, is that there exists a crucial need both to understand the real-world conditions under which phage therapy is to be undertaken and to develop realistic model systems for evaluating efficacy. For example, if chronic bacterial infections are a target, e.g., such as *Staphylococcus* infections that have resisted treatment over long time frames, then some realistic approximation of chronic bacterial infections ought to serve as the basis for experimentation both *in vitro* and *in vivo* (195). Quoting Larkum, from 1929 (165, p. 35), "It is possible to produce staphylococcus infection in many animals, and it is possible to terminate such processes through use of bacteriophage, but these infections are not to be compared with naturally acquired diseases, nor can the results of experimentation be translated into terms of human disease and treatment." Furthering this sentiment, nearly 90 years later, Czaplewski et al. (39, p. 240) noted, "Studies should define and test clear go or no-go decision points for product progression. Programmes of work that are mainly in vitro or those focused entirely on surrogate endpoints (eg, characterising cytokines rather than pathology, microbiology, or clinical response) might not be competitive for funding." Or, as noted by Debarbieux et al. (162, p. 2), "...instead of expecting basic science to run almost unlimited investigations since many molecular aspects of phage therapy are still not understood. If we had waited for immunology to be fully understood at the molecular level before the use of vaccines, most of us would not be reading this paper!"

Regulation and Economics

The other important aspect of phage therapy development is issues of regulation and economics, as has been considered by numerous authors. Regulatory issues in particular have been addressed, for example, in references 32, 115, 134, and 196–199. The economics of development of phage therapeutics have been discussed in references 39 and 115, with intellectual property rights aspects considered in reference 197. See Ventola (200) for a discussion of the economics and regulation of antibiotic development more generally, including their observation vis-à-vis the latter (p. 280) that "studies comparing antibiotics with placebo are considered to be unethical," which appears to have been an ongoing complication of phage therapy development, as too, perhaps, are expectations based on past experience that antibacterial drugs should be relatively inexpensive. As a consequence of these and other impediments to antibacterial development, 155 nonphage antibacterial agents have been approved for clinical use since 1938, of which only 62% are still in use, and only three have been approved recently, i.e., during "the current decade" (201).

Harnessing the full potential of phages and antibacterial agents more generally will require regulatory mechanisms that explicitly do not place the full economic burden of full-blown clinical trials on every possible modification of a product. The justification for this need is that, unlike many drug targets, the drug targets of phages are not static but instead are capable of evolving both individually (that is, over the course of individual infections) and across communities (with new strains entering into as well as evolving within communities). Therefore, there is reason to argue that the regulation of all antimicrobial agents should be such that it is at least recognized that there can be an ongoing need for new agents not just for the sake of generating new profits as patents expire but instead because new strains of target organisms literally represent new diseases, or at least new variants on established diseases, as viewed from a pharmacological perspective. Or, as stated by Xu et al. (18, p. 11), the problem which needs to be addressed is that "the rate of development of new antibiotics is slower than the rate of the appearance of antibiotic resistance." What phages offer that is relatively unique, given this latter perspective, is large numbers of potential candidate drugs that are relatively lacking in pharmaceutically emergent properties. Or, as De Vos and Pirnay (3) noted, the "development of new phage preparations [is] quick and cheap" (see also reference 4). Thus, given repeated emergence of pharmacologically new bacterial disease types in combination with an abundance of new potential drugs to combat those new diseases, logic at least would be consistent with seeking effective ways of addressing the former with the latter.

In light of this context, would it be reasonable for phage therapy to demand favored treatment from regulators? That is, might phages be viewed as "special" from a regulatory standpoint? To a degree the answer to that question may effectively be "Yes" because regulators do appear to "get it," that is, to understand that there can be worth in attempting to work with those phage qualities that are relatively unique rather than against those same qualities. Nevertheless, what would be the justification for carving out a relatively unique track for regulatory approval of phages? I offer four answers to

that question: phages are abundant, they are simple in structure to the point that many are uncomfortable with the suggestion that they are even organisms, they can be relatively safe, and they possess a long history of relatively rigorous clinical use. Indeed, as I have stated elsewhere (50, p. 39), "If an effectively inexhaustible supply of antibiotic types were available to which cross-resistance did not excessively occur and which displayed very high therapeutic indices (ratio of a drug's toxic to therapeutic dose), then there would not be an antibiotic crisis."

CONCLUSION

Pratt (202, p. 3) has stated, "The ideal antibiotic would have no deleterious effect on the patient but would be lethal to the organism. There is no ideal antibiotic." Penicillin G in nonallergic individuals, however, is cited as coming closest to this ideal. Perhaps phages come close as well. Indeed, to a degree, the apparent safety of phage interaction with the human body underlies the basis of phage designation as Generally Recognized As Safe (GRAS) additives to food. Within this context, the simplicity of phage development as drugs provides an advantage over many other antibacterial drug candidates, with a possible exception of certain vaccines (i.e., influenza) or monoclonal antibodies. An argument also can be made that phages exist, at least absent genetic engineering (10, 203), as naturally occurring entities and as such could, in principle, be marketed as natural products (196) or instead as probiotics (147, 197) rather than as medicinals.

A distinction between phage use as antibacterial agents versus newer, especially synthetic small-molecule antibacterials is that phages have been subject to many decades of clinical use that at least arguably has been effective, appears to have not raised significant safety concerns, and has involved large numbers of people, i.e., thousands if not millions. Without that history, phage therapy would exist simply as another "new" approach to treating bacterial infections. With that history, however, we rightly should view phage therapy as not just another new approach to treating bacterial infections but instead as a relatively mature antibacterial technology, one that is ripe for further clinical implementation and development. As has been suggested elsewhere (8, p. 685), such clinical implementation by interested physicians can be achieved in the United States via "compassionate use to lay the groundwork for physician and public acceptance as well as full-blown clinical trials." Preclinical research will still be important to furthering phage therapy development, however. Especially there is a need to put greater effort toward improving *in vitro* and *in vivo* models of chronic bacterial infections, e.g., as can require weeks of phage treatment to achieve reasonable levels of efficacy (102, 171, 204). More generally, rather than focusing on relatively facile proof-of-principle studies, instead specific impediments to antibacterial success may need to be systematically determined and then overcome in the course of rigorous experimental phage therapy exploration.

ACKNOWLEDGMENTS

The author has consulted for and served on advisory boards for companies with phage therapy interests, holds equity stake in a number of these companies, and maintains the websites phage.org and phage-therapy.org. The text presented, however, represents the perspective of the author alone, and no help was received in its writing. I would like to thank Elizabeth Kutter, who read and commented on the manuscript.

CITATION

Abedon ST. 2017. Bacteriophage clinical use as antibacterial "drugs": utility and precedent. Microbiol Spectrum 5(4):BAD-0003-2016.

REFERENCES

1. **Abedon ST.** 2015. Ecology of anti-biofilm agents. II. Bacteriophage exploitation and biocontrol of biofilm bacteria. *Pharmaceuticals (Basel)* **8:**559–589.

2. **Chan BK, Abedon ST.** 2015. Bacteriophages and their enzymes in biofilm control. *Curr Pharm Des* **21:**85–99.

3. **De Vos D, Pirnay JP.** 2015. Phage therapy: could viruses help resolve the worldwide antibiotic crisis?, p 110–114. *In* Carlet J, Upham G (ed), *AMR Control 2015: Overcoming Global Antibiotic Resistance*. World Alliance Against Antibiotic Resistance.

4. **Doffkay Z, Dömötör D, Kovács T, Ráíkhely G.** 2015. Bacteriophage therapy against plant, animal and human pathogens. *Acta Biol Szeged* **59:**291–302.

5. **Górski A, Dąbrowska K, Hodyra-Stefaniak K, Borysowski J, Międzybrodzki R, Weber-Dąbrowska B.** 2015. Phages targeting infected tissues: novel approach to phage therapy. *Future Microbiol* **10:**199–204.

6. **Hussain MA, Liu H, Wang Q, Zhong F, Guo Q, Balamurugan S.** 2017. Use of encapsulated bacteriophages to enhance farm to fork food safety. *Crit Rev Food Sci Nutr* **57:**2801–2810.

7. **Kingwell K.** 2015. Bacteriophage therapies re-enter clinical trials. *Nat Rev Drug Discov* **14:**515–516.

8. **Kutter EM, Kuhl SJ, Abedon ST.** 2015. Reestablishing a place for phage therapy in western medicine. *Future Microbiol* **10:**685–688.

9. **Nakonieczna A, Cooper CJ, Gryko R.** 2015. Bacteriophages and bacteriophage-derived endolysins as potential therapeutics to combat Gram-positive spore forming bacteria. *J Appl Microbiol* **119:**620–631.

10. **Nobrega FL, Costa AR, Kluskens LD, Azeredo J.** 2015. Revisiting phage therapy: new applications for old resources. *Trends Microbiol* **23:**185–191.

11. **Oliveira H, Sillankorva S, Merabishvili M, Kluskens LD, Azeredo J.** 2015. Unexploited opportunities for phage therapy. *Front Pharmacol* **6:**180.

12. **Patel SR, Verma AK, Verma VC, Janga MR, Nath G.** 2015. Bacteriophage therapy: looking back in to the future, p 284–294. *In* Méndez-Vilas A (ed), *The Battle Against Microbial Pathogens: Basic Science, Technology Advances and Educational Programs*. Formatex Research Center, Badajoz, Spain.

13. **Pulido RP, Grande Burgos MJ, Galvez A, López RL.** 2015. Application of bacteriophages in post-harvest control of human pathogenic

and food spoiling bacteria. *Crit Rev Biotechnol* **36**:851–861.

14. **Petsong K, Vongkamjan K.** 2015. Applications of *Salmonella* bacteriophages in the food production chain, p 275–283. *In* Méndez-Vilas A (ed), *The Battle Against Microbial Pathogens: Basic Science, Technology Advances and Educational Programs.* Formatex Research Center, Badajoz, Spain.

15. **Pires DP, Vilas Boas D, Sillankorva S, Azeredo J.** 2015. Phage therapy: a step forward in the treatment of *Pseudomonas aeruginosa* infections. *J Virol* **89**:7449–7456.

16. **Sarhan WA, Azzazy HM.** 2015. Phage approved in food, why not as a therapeutic? *Expert Rev Anti Infect Ther* **13**:91–101.

17. **Vandenheuvel D, Lavigne R, Brüssow H.** 2015. Bacteriophage therapy: advances in formulation strategies and human clinical trials. *Annu Rev Virol* **2**:599–618.

18. **Xu Y, Liu Y, Liu Y, Pei J, Yao S, Cheng C.** 2015. Bacteriophage therapy against *Enterobacteriaceae*. *Virol Sin* **30**:11–18.

19. **Young R, Gill JJ.** 2015. Phage therapy redux: what is to be done? *Science* **350**:1163–1164.

20. **Expert round table on acceptance and re-implementation of bacteriophage therapy.** 2016. Silk route to the acceptance and re-implementation of bacteriophage therapy. *Biotechnol J* **11**:595–600.

21. **Dubey K, Chandraker S, Sao S, Gupta A, Dubey SK.** 2016. Bacteriophages as an antibacterial agent: a promising alternative. *J Curr Microbiol App Sci* **5**:231–234.

22. **Grant A, Hashem F, Parveen S.** 2016. *Salmonella* and *Campylobacter*: antimicrobial resistance and bacteriophage control in poultry. *Food Microbiol* **53**(Pt B):104–109.

23. **Jassim SA, Limoges RG, El-Cheikh H.** 2016. Bacteriophage biocontrol in wastewater treatment. *World J Microbiol Biotechnol* **32**:70.

24. **Moharir RV, Khairnar K.** 2016. Bacteriophage as a bio controller: a review. *Int J Adv Res SciEng Technol* **3**:1350–1354.

25. **Motlagh AM, Bhattacharjee AS, Goel R.** 2016. Biofilm control with natural and genetically-modified phages. *World J Microbiol Biotechnol* **32**:67.

26. **Speck P, Smithyman A.** 2016. Safety and efficacy of phage therapy via the intravenous route. *FEMS Microbiol Lett* **363**:fnv242.

27. **Karimi M, Mirshekari H, Moosavi Basri SM, Bahrami S, Moghoofei M, Hamblin MR.** 2016. Bacteriophages and phage-inspired nanocarriers for targeted delivery of therapeutic cargos. *Adv Drug Deliv Rev* **106**(Pt A):45–62.

28. **Pietracha D, Misiewicz A.** 2016. Use of products containing a phage in food Industry as a new method for *Listeria monocytogenes* elimination from food (*Listeria monocytogenes* phages in food industry): a review. *Czech J Food Sci* **34**:1–8.

29. **Bai J, Kim YT, Ryu S, Lee JH.** 2016. Biocontrol and rapid detection of food-borne pathogens using bacteriophages and endolysins. *Front Microbiol* **7**:474.

30. **Brüssow H.** 2016. Targeting the gut to protect the bladder: oral phage therapy approaches against urinary *Escherichia coli* infections? *Environ Microbiol* **18**:2084–2088.

31. **Hicks LA, Taylor TH Jr, Hunkler RJ.** 2013. U.S. outpatient antibiotic prescribing, 2010. *N Engl J Med* **368**:1461–1462.

32. **Sulakvelidze A.** 2013. Using lytic bacteriophages to eliminate or significantly reduce contamination of food by foodborne bacterial pathogens. *J Sci Food Agric* **93**:3137–3146.

33. **Borysowski J, Górski A.** 2014. The use of phages as biocontrol agents in foods, p 215–235. *In* Borysowski J, Miedzybrodzki R, Górski A (ed), *Phage Therapy: Current Research and Applications.* Caister Academic Press, Norfolk, United Kingdom.

34. **Gill JJ, Hyman P.** 2010. Phage choice, isolation, and preparation for phage therapy. *Curr Pharm Biotechnol* **11**:2–14.

35. **Balogh B, Jones JB, Iriarte FB, Momol MT.** 2010. Phage therapy for plant disease control. *Curr Pharmaceut Biotechnol* **11**:48–57

36. **Sulakvelidze A, Pasternack GR.** 2010. Industrial and regulatory issues in bacteriophage applications in food production and processing, p 297–326. *In* Sabour PM, Griffiths MW (ed), *Bacteriophages in the Control of Food- and Waterborne Pathogens.* ASM Press, Washington, DC.

37. **Frampton RA, Pitman AR, Fineran PC.** 2012. Advances in bacteriophage-mediated control of plant pathogens. *Int J Microbiol* **2012**:326452.

38. **Żaczek M, Weber-Dąbrowska B, Górski A.** 2015. Phages in the global fruit and vegetable industry. *J Appl Microbiol* **118**:537–556.

39. **Czaplewski L, Bax R, Clokie M, Dawson M, Fairhead H, Fischetti VA, Foster S, Gilmore BF, Hancock RE, Harper D, Henderson IR, Hilpert K, Jones BV, Kadioglu A, Knowles D, Ólafsdóttir S, Payne D, Projan S, Shaunak S, Silverman J, Thomas CM, Trust TJ, Warn P, Rex JH.** 2016. Alternatives to antibiotics: a pipeline portfolio review. *Lancet Infect Dis* **16**:239–251.

40. **Bentley R, Bennett JW.** 2003. What is an antibiotic? Revisited. *Adv Appl Microbiol* **52**:303–331.

41. **Clark J, Abedon ST, Hyman P.** 2012. Phages as therapeutic delivery vehicles, p 86–100. *In* Hyman P, Abedon ST (ed), *Bacteriophages in Health and Disease.* CABI Press, Wallingford, United Kingdom.

42. **Pranjol MZ, Hajitou A.** 2015. Bacteriophage-derived vectors for targeted cancer gene therapy. *Viruses* **7:**268–284.

43. **Górski A, Borysowski J, Miedzybrodzki R, Weber-Dąbrowska B.** 2007. Bacteriophages in medicine, p 125–158. *In* Mc Grath S, van Sinderen D (ed), *Bacteriophage: Genetics and Microbiology.* Caister Academic Press, Norfolk, United Kingdom.

44. **Dąbrowska K, Miedzybrodzki R, Miernikiewicz P, Figura G, Górski A.** 2014. Non-bactericidal effects of phages in mammals, p 141–155. *In* Borysowski J, Miedzybrodzki R, Górski A (ed), *Phage Therapy: Current Research and Applications.* Caister Academic Press, Norfolk, United Kingdom.

45. **Olszowska-Zaremba N, Borysowski J, Dabrowska J, Górski A.** 2012. Phage translocation, safety, and immunomodulation, p 168–184. *In* Hyman P, Abedon ST (ed), *Bacteriophages in Health and Disease.* CABI Press, Wallingford, United Kingdom.

46. **Górski A, Międzybrodzki R, Borysowski J, Dąbrowska K, Wierzbicki P, Ohams M, Korczak-Kowalska G, Olszowska-Zaremba N, Łusiak-Szelachowska M, Kłak M, Jończyk E, Kaniuga E, Gołaś A, Purchla S, Weber-Dąbrowska B, Letkiewicz S, Fortuna W, Szufnarowski K, Pawełczyk Z, Rogóż P, Kłosowska D.** 2012. Phage as a modulator of immune responses: practical implications for phage therapy. *Adv Virus Res* **83:**41–71.

47. **Harper DR.** 2006. Biological control by microorganisms, p 1–10. *In The Encyclopedia of Life Sciences.* John Wiley & Sons, Chichester, United Kingdom.

48. **Abedon ST.** 2009. Kinetics of phage-mediated biocontrol of bacteria. *Foodborne Pathog Dis* **6:**807–815.

49. **Levin BR, Bull JJ.** 2004. Population and evolutionary dynamics of phage therapy. *Nat Rev Microbiol* **2:**166–173.

50. **Abedon ST, Thomas-Abedon C.** 2010. Phage therapy pharmacology. *Curr Pharm Biotechnol* **11:**28–47.

51. **Abedon ST.** 2014. Bacteriophages as drugs: the pharmacology of phage therapy, p 69–100. *In* Borysowski J, Miedzybrodzki R, Górski A (ed), *Phage Therapy: Current Research and Applications.* Caister Academic Press, Norfolk, United Kingdom.

52. **Ryan EM, Gorman SP, Donnelly RF, Gilmore BF.** 2011. Recent advances in bacteriophage therapy: how delivery routes, formulation, concentration and timing influence the success of phage therapy. *J Pharm Pharmacol* **63:** 1253–1264.

53. **Pirnay JP, Blasdel BG, Bretaudeau L, Buckling A, Chanishvili N, Clark JR, Corte-Real S, Debarbieux L, Dublanchet A, De Vos D, Gabard J, Garcia M, Goderdzishvili M, Górski A, Hardcastle J, Huys I, Kutter E, Lavigne R, Merabishvili M, Olchawa E, Parikka KJ, Patey O, Pouilot F, Resch G, Rohde C, Scheres J, Skurnik M, Vaneechoutte M, Van Parys L, Verbeken G, Zizi M, Van den Eede G.** 2015. Quality and safety requirements for sustainable phage therapy products. *Pharm Res* **32:**2173–2179.

54. **Nieth A, Verseux C, Barnert S, Süss R, Römer W.** 2015. A first step toward liposome-mediated intracellular bacteriophage therapy. *Expert Opin Drug Deliv* **12:**1411–1424.

55. **Singla S, Harjai K, Katare OP, Chhibber S.** 2015. Bacteriophage-loaded nanostructured lipid carrier: improved pharmacokinetics mediates effective resolution of *Klebsiella pneumoniae*-induced lobar pneumonia. *J Infect Dis* **212:**325–334.

56. **Hobbs Z, Abedon ST.** 2016. Diversity of phage infection types and associated terminology: the problem with 'lytic or lysogenic'. *FEMS Microbiol Lett* **363:**fnw047.

57. **Roy B, Ackermann H-W, Pandian S, Picard G, Goulet J.** 1993. Biological inactivation of adhering *Listeria monocytogenes* by listeria-phages and a quaternary ammonium compound. *Appl Environ Microbiol* **59:**2914–2917.

58. **Chanishvili N, Sharp R.** 2008. Bacteriophage therapy: experience from the Eliava Institute, Georgia. *Microbiol Aust* **29:**96–101.

59. **Curtright AJ, Abedon ST.** 2011. Phage therapy: emergent property pharmacology. *J Bioanalyt Biomed* **S6:**002.

60. **Niu YD, Stanford K, McAllister TA, Callaway TR.** 2012. Role of phages in control of bacterial pathogens in food, p 240–255. *In* Hyman P, Abedon ST (ed), *Bacteriophages in Health and Disease.* CABI Press, Wallingford, United Kingdom.

61. **Kutter E, Borysowski J, Miedzybrodzki R, Górski A, Weber-Dąbrowska B, Kutateladze M, Alavidze Z, Goderdzishvili M, Adamia R.** 2014. Clinical phage therapy, p 257–288. *In* Borysowski J, Miedzybrodzki R, Górski A (ed), *Phage Therapy: Current Research and Applications.* Caister Academic Press, Norfolk, United Kingdom.

62. **Abedon ST.** 2009. Impact of phage properties on bacterial survival, p 217–235. *In* Adams HT (ed), *Contemporary Trends in Bacteriophage*

Research. Nova Science Publishers, Hauppauge, NY.

63. **El Haddad L, Roy JP, Khalil GE, St-Gelais D, Champagne CP, Labrie S, Moineau S.** 2016. Efficacy of two *Staphylococcus aureus* phage cocktails in cheese production. *Int J Food Microbiol* **217**:7–13.

64. **Deasy T, Mahony J, Neve H, Heller KJ, van Sinderen D.** 2011. Isolation of a virulent *Lactobacillus brevis* phage and its application in the control of beer spoilage. *J Food Prot* **74**:2157–2161.

65. **Ladero V, Gómez-Sordo C, Sánchez-Llana E, Del Rio B, Redruello B, Fernández M, Martín MC, Alvarez MA.** 2016. Q69 (an *E. faecalis*-infecting bacteriophage) as a biocontrol agent for reducing tyramine in dairy products. *Front Microbiol* **7**:445.

66. **Sillankorva S, Azeredo J.** 2014. The use of bacteriophages and bacteriophage-derived enzymes for clinically relevant biofilm control, p 309–329. *In* Borysowski J, Miedzybrodzki R, Górski A (ed), *Phage Therapy: Current Research and Applications.* Caister Academic Press, Norfolk, United Kingdom.

67. **Bhattacharjee AS, Choi J, Motlagh AM, Mukherji ST, Goel R.** 2015. Bacteriophage therapy for membrane biofouling in membrane bioreactors and antibiotic-resistant bacterial biofilms. *Biotechnol Bioeng* **112**:1644–1654.

68. **O'Flaherty S, Ross RP, Meaney W, Fitzgerald GF, Elbreki MF, Coffey A.** 2005. Potential of the polyvalent anti-*Staphylococcus* bacteriophage K for control of antibiotic-resistant staphylococci from hospitals. *Appl Environ Microbiol* **71**:1836–1842.

69. **Mann NH.** 2008. The potential of phages to prevent MRSA infections. *Res Microbiol* **159**:400–405.

70. **Das M, Bhowmick TS, Ahern SJ, Young R, Gonzalez CF.** 2015. Control of Pierce's disease by phage. *PLoS One* **10**:e0128902.

71. **Rombouts S, Volckaert A, Venneman S, Declercq B, Vandenheuvel D, Allonsius CN, Van Malderghem C, Jang HB, Briers Y, Noben JP, Klumpp J, Van Vaerenbergh J, Maes M, Lavigne R.** 2016. Characterization of novel bacteriophages for biocontrol of bacterial blight in leek caused by *Pseudomonas syringae* pv. porri. *Front Microbiol* **7**:279.

72. **Balogh B, Jones JB, Iriarte FB, Momol MT.** 2010. Phage therapy for plant disease control. *Curr Pharm Biotechnol* **11**:48–57.

73. **Jones JB, Jackson LE, Balogh B, Obradovic A, Iriarte FB, Momol MT.** 2007. Bacteriophages for plant disease control. *Annu Rev Phytopathol* **45**:245–262.

74. **Munsch P, Olivier JM.** 1995. Biocontrol of bacterial blotch of the cultivated mushroom with lytic phages: some practical considerations, p 595–602. *In* Elliott TJ (ed), *Science and Cultivation of Edible Fungi.* Vol. II: Proceedings of the 14th International Congress.

75. **Yost DG, Tsourkas P, Amy PS.** 2016. Experimental bacteriophage treatment of honeybees (*Apis mellifera*) infected with *Paenibacillus larvae*, the causative agent of American foulbrood disease. *Bacteriophage* **6**:e1122698.

76. **El-Gohary FA, Huff WE, Huff GR, Rath NC, Zhou ZY, Donoghue AM.** 2014. Environmental augmentation with bacteriophage prevents colibacillosis in broiler chickens. *Poult Sci* **93**:2788–2792.

77. **Oliveira A, Sereno R, Azeredo J.** 2010. *In vivo* efficiency evaluation of a phage cocktail in controlling severe colibacillosis in confined conditions and experimental poultry houses. *Vet Microbiol* **146**:303–308.

78. **Silva YJ, Moreirinha C, Pereira C, Costa L, Rocha RJ, Cunha Â, Gomes NCM, Calado R, Almeida A.** 2016. Biological control of *Aeromonas salmonicida* infection in juvenile Senegalese sole (*Solea senegalensis*) with phage AS-A. *Aquaculture* **450**:225–233.

79. **Laanto E, Bamford JK, Ravantti JJ, Sundberg LR.** 2015. The use of phage FCL-2 as an alternative to chemotherapy against columnaris disease in aquaculture. *Front Microbiol* **6**:829.

80. **Alagappan K, Karuppiah V, Deivasigamani B.** 2016. Protective effect of phages on experimental *V. parahaemolyticus* infection and immune response in shrimp (Fabricius, 1798). *Aquaculture* **453**:86–92.

81. **Kalatzis PG, Bastías R, Kokkari C, Katharios P.** 2016. Isolation and characterization of two lytic bacteriophages, φSt2 and φGrn1; phage therapy application for biological control of *Vibrio alginolyticus* in aquaculture live feeds. *PLoS One* **11**:e0151101.

82. **Wagemans J, Lavigne R.** 2012. Phages and their hosts, a web of interactions: applications to drug design, p 119–133. *In* Hyman P, Abedon ST (ed), *Bacteriophages in Health and Disease.* CABI Press, Wallingford, United Kingdom.

83. **Thiel K.** 2004. Old dogma, new tricks: 21st century phage therapy. *Nat Biotechnol* **22**:31–36.

84. **Kutter E.** 2005. Phage therapy: bacteriophages as natural, self-limiting antibiotics, p 1147–1161. *In* Pizzorno W (ed), *Textbook of Natural Medicine*, 3rd ed. Churchill Livingston, St. Louis, MO.

85. **Sulakvelidze A, Kutter E.** 2005. Bacteriophage therapy in humans, p 381–436. *In* Kutter E, Sulakvelidze A (ed), *Bacteriophages: Biology and Application.* CRC Press, Boca Raton, FL.

86. **Loc-Carrillo C, Abedon ST.** 2011. Pros and cons of phage therapy. *Bacteriophage* **1:**111–114.

87. **Pope WH, Bowman CA, Russell DA, Jacobs-Sera D, Asai DJ, Cresawn SG, Jacobs WR Jr, Hendrix RW, Lawrence JG, Hatfull GF, Science Education Alliance Phage Hunters Advancing Genomics and Evolutionary Science, Phage Hunters Integrating Research and Education, Mycobacterial Genetics Course.** 2015. Whole genome comparison of a large collection of mycobacteriophages reveals a continuum of phage genetic diversity. *eLife* **4:**e06416.

88. **Pratt WB, Fekety R.** 1986. *The Antimicrobial Drugs.* Oxford University Press, New York, NY.

89. **Lobocka M, Hejnowicz MS, Gagala U, Weber-Dąbrowska B, Wegrzyn G, Dadlez M.** 2014. The first step to bacteriophage therapy: how to choose the correct phage, p 23–67. *In* Borysowski J, Międzybrodzki R, Górski A (ed), *Phage Therapy: Current Research and Applications.* Caister Academic Press, Norfolk, United Kingdom.

90. **Krylov V, Shaburova O, Pleteneva E, Krylov S, Kaplan A, Burkaltseva M, Polygach O, Chesnokova E.** 2015. Selection of phages and conditions for the safe phage therapy against *Pseudomonas aeruginosa* infections. *Virol Sin* **30:**33–44.

91. **McCallin S, Alam Sarker S, Barretto C, Sultana S, Berger B, Huq S, Krause L, Bibiloni R, Schmitt B, Reuteler G, Brüssow H.** 2013. Safety analysis of a Russian phage cocktail: from metagenomic analysis to oral application in healthy human subjects. *Virology* **443:**187–196.

92. **Górski A, Miedzybrodzki R, Borysowski J, Weber-Dąbrowska B, Lobocka M, Fortuna W, Letkiewicz S, Zimecki M, Filby G.** 2009. Bacteriophage therapy for the treatment of infections. *Curr Opin Investig Drugs* **10:**766–774.

93. **Roux S, Krupovic M, Debroas D, Forterre P, Enault F.** 2013. Assessment of viral community functional potential from viral metagenomes may be hampered by contamination with cellular sequences. *Open Biol* **3:**130160.

94. **Quirós P, Colomer-Lluch M, Martínez-Castillo A, Miró E, Argente M, Jofre J, Navarro F, Muniesa M.** 2014. Antibiotic resistance genes in the bacteriophage DNA fraction of human fecal samples. *Antimicrob Agents Chemother* **58:**606–609.

95. **Goodridge L, Abedon ST.** 2008. Bacteriophage biocontrol: the technology matures. *Microbiol Aust* **29:**48–49.

96. **Branston SD, Wright J, Keshavarz-Moore E.** 2015. A non-chromatographic method for the removal of endotoxins from bacteriophages. *Biotechnol Bioeng* **112:**1714–1719.

97. **Szermer-Olearnik B, Boratyński J.** 2015. Removal of endotoxins from bacteriophage preparations by extraction with organic solvents. *PLoS One* **10:**e0122672.

98. **Hyman P, Abedon ST.** 2010. Bacteriophage host range and bacterial resistance. *Adv Appl Microbiol* **70:**217–248.

99. **Mirzaei MK, Nilsson AS.** 2015. Isolation of phages for phage therapy: a comparison of spot tests and efficiency of plating analyses for determination of host range and efficacy. *PLoS One* **10:**e0118557. (Erratum, **10:**e0127606. doi:10.1371/journal.pone.0127606.)

100. **Langdon A, Crook N, Dantas G.** 2016. The effects of antibiotics on the microbiome throughout development and alternative approaches for therapeutic modulation. *Genome Med* **8:**39.

101. **Hwang JY, Kim JE, Song YJ, Park JH.** 2016. Safety of using *Escherichia coli* bacteriophages as a sanitizing agent based on inflammatory responses in rats. *Food Sci Biotechnol* **25:**355–360.

102. **Międzybrodzki R, Borysowski J, Weber-Dąbrowska B, Fortuna W, Letkiewicz S, Szufnarowski K, Pawełczyk Z, Rogóż P, Kłak M, Wojtasik E, Górski A.** 2012. Clinical aspects of phage therapy. *Adv Virus Res* **83:**73–121.

103. **Slopek S, Durlakowa I, Weber-Dąbrowska B, Kucharewicz-Krukowska A, Dabrowski M, Bisikiewicz R.** 1983. Results of bacteriophage treatment of suppurative bacterial infections. I. General evaluation of the results. *Arch Immunol Ther Exp (Warsz)* **31:**267–291.

104. **Salmon GG Jr, Symonds M.** 1963. Staphage lysate therapy in chronic staphylococcal infections. *J Med Soc N J* **60:**188–193.

105. **Abedon ST.** 2015. Phage therapy of pulmonary infections. *Bacteriophage* **5:**e1020260.

106. **Christie GE, Allison HA, Kuzio J, McShan M, Waldor MK, Kropinski AM.** 2012. Prophage-induced changes in cellular cytochemistry and virulence, p 33–60. *In* Hyman P, Abedon ST (ed), *Bacteriophages in Health and Disease.* CABI Press, Wallingford, United Kingdom.

107. **Kuhl S, Abedon ST, Hyman P.** 2012. Diseases caused by phages, p 21–32. *In* Hyman P, Abedon ST (ed), *Bacteriophages in Health and Disease.* CABI Press, Wallingford, United Kingdom.

108. **Górski A, Weber-Dąbrowska B.** 2005. The potential role of endogenous bacteriophages in controlling invading pathogens. *Cell Mol Life Sci* **62:**511–519.

109. **Edlund A, Santiago-Rodriguez TM, Boehm TK, Pride DT.** 2015. Bacteriophage and their

potential roles in the human oral cavity. *J Oral Microbiol* **7:**27423.

110. **De Paepe M, Leclerc M, Tinsley CR, Petit MA.** 2014. Bacteriophages: an underestimated role in human and animal health? *Front Cell Infect Microbiol* **4:**39.

111. **Sansom C.** 2015. Phage therapy for severe infections tested in the first multicentre trial. *Lancet Infect Dis* **15:**1384–1385.

112. **Bruttin A, Brüssow H.** 2005. Human volunteers receiving *Escherichia coli* phage T4 orally: a safety test of phage therapy. *Antimicrob Agents Chemother* **49:**2874–2878.

113. **Sarker SA, McCallin S, Barretto C, Berger B, Pittet AC, Sultana S, Krause L, Huq S, Bibiloni R, Bruttin A, Reuteler G, Brüssow H.** 2012. Oral T4-like phage cocktail application to healthy adult volunteers from Bangladesh. *Virology* **434:**222–232.

114. **Sarker SA, Sultana S, Reuteler G, Moine D, Descombes P, Charton F, Bourdin G, McCallin S, Ngom-Bru C, Neville T, Akter M, Huq S, Qadri F, Talukdar K, Kassam M, Delley M, Loiseau C, Deng Y, El Aidy S, Berger B, Brüssow H.** 2016. Oral phage therapy of acute bacterial diarrhea with two coliphage preparations: a randomized trial in children from Bangladesh. *EBioMedicine* **4:**124–137.

115. **Brüssow H.** 2012. What is needed for phage therapy to become a reality in Western medicine? *Virology* **434:**138–142.

116. **Rose T, Verbeken G, Vos DD, Merabishvili M, Vaneechoutte M, Lavigne R, Jennes S, Zizi M, Pirnay JP.** 2014. Experimental phage therapy of burn wound infection: difficult first steps. *Int J Burns Trauma* **4:**66–73.

117. **Rhoads DD, Wolcott RD, Kuskowski MA, Wolcott BM, Ward LS, Sulakvelidze A.** 2009. Bacteriophage therapy of venous leg ulcers in humans: results of a phase I safety trial. *J Wound Care* **18:**237–238, 240–243.

118. **Wright A, Hawkins CH, Anggård EE, Harper DR.** 2009. A controlled clinical trial of a therapeutic bacteriophage preparation in chronic otitis due to antibiotic-resistant *Pseudomonas aeruginosa*; a preliminary report of efficacy. *Clin Otolaryngol* **34:**349–357.

119. **Yin L, Chen X, Vicini P, Rup B, Hickling TP.** 2015. Therapeutic outcomes, assessments, risk factors and mitigation efforts of immunogenicity of therapeutic protein products. *Cell Immunol* **295:**118–126.

120. **Teichert RW, Olivera BM.** 2010. Natural products and ion channel pharmacology. *Future Med Chem* **2:**731–744.

121. **Williams GC.** 1957. Pleiotropy, natural selection, and the evolution of senescence. *Evolution* **11:**398–411.

122. **Elena SF, Sanjuán R.** 2003. Evolution. Climb every mountain? *Science* **302:**2074–2075.

123. **Los M, Kuzio J, McConnell MR, Kropinski AM, Wegrzyn G, Christie GE.** 2010. Lysogenic conversion in bacteria of importance to the food industry, p 157–198. *In* Sabour PM, Griffiths MW (ed), *Bacteriophages in the Control of Food- and Waterborne Pathogens.* ASM Press, Washington, DC.

124. **Khan Mirzaei M, Haileselassie Y, Navis M, Cooper C, Sverremark-Ekström E, Nilsson AS.** 2016. Morphologically distinct *Escherichia coli* bacteriophages differ in their efficacy and ability to stimulate cytokine release *in vitro*. *Front Microbiol* **7:**437.

125. **Kutter E, De Vos D, Gvasalia G, Alavidze Z, Gogokhia L, Kuhl S, Abedon ST.** 2010. Phage therapy in clinical practice: treatment of human infections. *Curr Pharm Biotechnol* **11:**69–86.

126. **Chan BK, Abedon ST, Loc-Carrillo C.** 2013. Phage cocktails and the future of phage therapy. *Future Microbiol* **8:**769–783.

127. **Petty NK, Evans TJ, Fineran PC, Salmond GPC.** 2007. Biotechnological exploitation of bacteriophage research. *Trends Biotechnol* **25:**7–15.

128. **Pirnay JP, De Vos D, Verbeken G, Merabishvili M, Chanishvili N, Vaneechoutte M, Zizi M, Laire G, Lavigne R, Huys I, Van den Mooter G, Buckling A, Debarbieux L, Pouillot F, Azeredo J, Kutter E, Dublanchet A, Górski A, Adamia R.** 2011. The phage therapy paradigm: prêt-à-porter or sur-mesure? *Pharm Res* **28:**934–937.

129. **Gill JJ, Young R.** 2011. Therapeutic applications of phage biology: history, practice and recommendations, p 367–410. *In* Miller AA, Miller PF (ed), *Emerging Trends in Antibacterial Discovery: Answering the Call to Arms.* Caister Academic Press, Norfolk, United Kingdom.

130. **Harper DR, Enright MC.** 2011. Bacteriophages for the treatment of *Pseudomonas aeruginosa* infections. *J Appl Microbiol* **111:**1–7.

131. **Keen EC.** 2012. Phage therapy: concept to cure. *Front Microbiol* **3:**238.

132. **Henein A.** 2013. What are the limitations on the wider therapeutic use of phage? *Bacteriophage* **3:**e24872.

133. **Kaźmierczak Z, Górski A, Dąbrowska K.** 2014. Facing antibiotic resistance: *Staphylococcus aureus* phages as a medical tool. *Viruses* **6:**2551–2570.

134. **Pelfrene E, Willebrand E, Cavaleiro Sanches A, Sebris Z, Cavaleri M.** 2016. Bacteriophage therapy: a regulatory perspective. *J Antimicrob Chemother* **71:**2071–2074.

135. **Pirnay J-P, Verbeken G, Rose T, Jennes S, Zizi M, Huys I, Lavigne R, Merabishvili M, Vaneechoutte M, Buckling A, De Vos D.** 2012. Introducing yesterday's phage therapy in today's medicine. *Future Virol* **7:**379–390.

136. **Chan BK, Abedon ST.** 2012. Phage therapy pharmacology phage cocktails. *Adv Appl Microbiol* **78:**1–23.

137. **Kutateladze M, Adamia R.** 2008. Phage therapy experience at the Eliava Institute. *Med Mal Infect* **38:**426–430.

138. **Cox CR.** 2012. Bacteriophage-based methods of baterial detection and identification, p 134–152. *In* Hyman P, Abedon ST (ed), *Bacteriophages in Health and Disease*. CABI Press, Wallingford, United Kingdom.

139. **Kucharewicz-Krukowska A, Slopek S.** 1987. Immunogenic effect of bacteriophage in patients subjected to phage therapy. *Arch Immunol Ther Exp (Warsz)* **35:**553–561.

140. **Lusiak-Szelachowska M, Zaczek M, Weber-Dąbrowska B, Międzybrodzki R, Kłak M, Fortuna W, Letkiewicz S, Rogóż P, Szufnarowski K, Jończyk-Matysiak E, Owczarek B, Górski A.** 2014. Phage neutralization by sera of patients receiving phage therapy. *Viral Immunol* **27:**295–304.

141. **Hodyra-Stefaniak K, Miernikiewicz P, Drapała J, Drab M, Jończyk-Matysiak E, Lecion D, Kaźmierczak Z, Beta W, Majewska J, Harhala M, Bubak B, Kłopot A, Górski A, Dąbrowska K.** 2015. Mammalian host-versus-phage immune response determines phage fate *in vivo*. *Sci Rep* **5:**14802.

142. **Lusiak-Szelachowska M, Zaczek M, Weber-Dabrowska B, Miedzybrodzki R, Letkiewicz S, Fortuna W, Rogoz P, Szufnarowski K, Jonczyk-Matysiak E, Olchawa E, Walaszek KM, Gorski A.** 2016. Antiphage activity of sera during phage therapy in relation to its outcome. *Future Microbiol* **12:**109–117.

143. **Merril CR.** 2008. Interaction of bacteriophages with animals, p 332–352. *In* Abedon ST (ed), *Bacteriophage Ecology*. Cambridge University Press, Cambridge, United Kingdom.

144. **Kutateladze M, Adamia R.** 2010. Bacteriophages as potential new therapeutics to replace or supplement antibiotics. *Trends Biotechnol* **28:**591–595.

145. **d'Hérelle F.** 1919. Sur le rôle du microbe bactériophage dans la typhosa aviaire [On the role of the microbe bacteriophage in the avian typhoid]. *Compt.rend. Acad Sci* **169:**932–934.

146. **Summers WC.** 1999. *Felix d'Herelle and the Origins of Molecular Biology*. Yale University Press, New Haven, CT.

147. **Abedon ST, Kuhl SJ, Blasdel BG, Kutter EM.** 2011. Phage treatment of human infections. *Bacteriophage* **1:**66–85.

148. **Chanishvili N.** 2012. *A Literature Review of the Practical Application of Bacteriophage Research*. Nova Publishers, Hauppauge, NY.

149. **Twort FW.** 1915. An investigation on the nature of ultra-microscopic viruses. *Lancet* **186:**1241–1243.

150. **Twort FW.** 2011. An investigation on the nature of ultra-microscopic viruses. *Bacteriophage* **1:**127–129.

151. **d'Hérelle F.** 1917. Sur un microbe invisible antagoniste des bacilles dysentériques. *C RAcad Sci Ser D* **165:**373–375.

152. **d'Hérelle F.** 2011. On an invisible microbe antagonistic to dysentery bacilli. *Bacteriophage* **1:**3–5.

153. **Chanishvili N.** 2012. Phage therapy: history from Twort and d'Herelle through Soviet experience to current approaches. *Adv Virus Res* **83:**3–40.

154. **van Helvoort T.** 1992. Bacteriological and physiological research styles in the early controversy on the nature of the bacteriophage phenomenon. *Med Hist* **36:**243–270.

155. **Hankin ME.** 1896. L'action bactéricide des eaux de la Jumna et du Gange sur le vibrion du choléra. *Ann Inst Pasteur (Paris)* **10:**511–523.

156. **Abedon ST, Thomas-Abedon C, Thomas A, Mazure H.** 2011. Bacteriophage prehistory: is or is not Hankin, 1896, a phage reference? *Bacteriophage* **1:**174–178.

157. **d'Hérelle F.** 1949. The bacteriophage. *Sci News* **14:**44–59.

158. **d'Hérelle F, Smith GH.** 1930. *The Bacteriophage and Its Clinical Application*. Charles C. Thomas, Publisher, Springfield, IL.

159. **d'Hérelle F.** 1918. Sur le rôle du microbe filtrant bactériophage dans la dysentérie bacillaire. *Compt Rend Acad Sci* **167:**970–972.

160. **Bruynoghe R, Maisin J.** 1921. Essais de thérapeutique au moyen du bactériophage du Staphylocoque. *Compt Rend Soc Biol* **85:**1120–1121.

161. **d'Hérelle F.** 1922. *The Bacteriophage: Its Role in Immunity*. Williams and Wilkins Co, Waverly Press, Baltimore, MD.

162. **Debarbieux L, Pirnay JP, Verbeken G, De Vos D, Merabishvili M, Huys I, Patey O, Schoonjans D, Vaneechoutte M, Zizi M, Rohde C.** 2016. A bacteriophage journey at the European Medicines Agency. *FEMS Microbiol Lett* **363:**fnv225.

163. **Summers WC.** 2001. Bacteriophage therapy. *Annu Rev Microbiol* **55:**437–451.

164. **Peitzman SJ.** 1969. Felix d'Herelle and bacteriophage therapy. *Trans Stud Coll Physicians Phila* **37:**115–123.

165. **Larkum NW.** 1929. Bacteriophage treatment of *Staphylococcus* infections. *J Infect Dis* **45:**34–41.

166. **Dunlap JE.** 1935. Staphylococcic meningitis with recovery. *J Am Med Assoc* **104:**1594–1595.

167. **MacNeal WJ, Frisbee FC, McRae MA.** 1941. Bacteriophage service in staphylococcal infections. *Am J Clin Pathol* **11:**549–561.

168. **MacNeal WJ, Filak L, Blevins A.** 1946. Conjoined action of penicillin and bacteriophages. *J Lab Clin Med* **31:**974–981.

169. **Morton HE, Engely EB.** 1945. Dysentery bacteriophage: review of the literature on its prophylactic and therapeutic uses in man and in experimental infections in animals. *J Am Med Assoc* **127:**584–591.

170. **Mills AE.** 1956. *Staphylococcus* bacteriophage lysate aerosol therapy of sinusitis. *Laryngoscope* **66:**846–858.

171. **Abedon ST.** 2012. Phage therapy best practices, p 256–272. *In* Hyman P, Abedon ST (ed), *Bacteriophages in Health and Disease.* CABI Press, Wallingford, United Kingdom.

172. **Smith HW, Huggins MB.** 1982. Successful treatment of experimental *Escherichia coli* infections in mice using phage: its general superiority over antibiotics. *J Gen Microbiol* **128:**307–318.

173. **Smith HW, Huggins MB.** 1983. Effectiveness of phages in treating experimental *Escherichia coli* diarrhoea in calves, piglets and lambs. *J Gen Microbiol* **129:**2659–2675.

174. **Smith HW, Huggins MB, Shaw KM.** 1987. The control of experimental *Escherichia coli* diarrhoea in calves by means of bacteriophages. *J Gen Microbiol* **133:**1111–1126.

175. **Smith HW, Huggins MB, Shaw KM.** 1987. Factors influencing the survival and multiplication of bacteriophages in calves and in their environment. *J Gen Microbiol* **133:**1127–1135.

176. **Slopek S, Durlakowa I, Weber-Dąbrowska B, Kucharewicz-Krukowska A, Dabrowski M, Bisikiewicz R.** 1983. Results of bacteriophage treatment of suppurative bacterial infections. II. Detailed evaluation of the results. *Arch Immunol Ther Exp (Warsz)* **31:**293–327.

177. **Slopek S, Durlakowa I, Weber-Dąbrowska B, Dabrowski M, Kucharewicz-Krukowska A.** 1984. Results of bacteriophage treatment of suppurative bacterial infections. III. Detailed evaluation of the results obtained in further 150 cases. *Arch Immunol Ther Exp (Warsz)* **32:**317–335.

178. **Slopek S, Kucharewicz-Krukowska A, Weber-Dąbrowska B, Dabrowski M.** 1985. Results of bacteriophage treatment of suppurative bacterial infections. IV. Evaluation of the results obtained in 370 cases. *Arch Immunol Ther Exp (Warsz)* **33:**219–240.

179. **Slopek S, Kucharewicz-Krukowska A, Weber-Dąbrowska B, Dabrowski M.** 1985. Results of bacteriophage treatment of suppurative bacterial infections. V. Evaluation of the results obtained in children. *Arch Immunol Ther Exp (Warsz)* **33:**241–259.

180. **Slopek S, Kucharewicz-Krukowska A, Weber-Dąbrowska B, Dabrowski M.** 1985. Results of bacteriophage treatment of suppurative bacterial infections. VI. Analysis of treatment of suppurative staphylococcal infections. *Arch Immunol Ther Exp (Warsz)* **33:**261–273.

181. **Slopek S, Weber-Dąbrowska B, Dabrowski M, Kucharewicz-Krukowska A.** 1987. Results of bacteriophage treatment of suppurative bacterial infections in the years 1981–1986. *Arch Immunol Ther Exp (Warsz)* **35:**569–583.

182. **Weber-Dąbrowska B, Dabrowski M, Slopek S.** 1987. Studies on bacteriophage penetration in patients subjected to phage therapy. *Arch Immunol Ther Exp (Warsz)* **35:**563–568.

183. **Fish R, Kutter E, Wheat G, Blasdel B, Kutateladze M, Kuhl S.** 2016. Bacteriophage treatment of intransigent diabetic toe ulcers: a case series. *J Wound Care* **25**(Suppl 7)**:**S27–S33.

184. **Brussow H.** 2007. Phage therapy: the Western perspective, p 159–192. *In* Mc Grath S, van Sinderen D (ed), *Bacteriophage: Genetics and Microbiology.* Caister Academic Press, Norfolk, United Kingdom.

185. **Fadlallah A, Chelala E, Legeais JM.** 2015. Corneal infection therapy with topical bacteriophage administration. *Open Ophthalmol J* **9:**167–168.

186. **Kutateladze M.** 2015. Experience of the Eliava Institute in bacteriophage therapy. *Virol Sin* **30:**80–81.

187. **Weber-Dąbrowska B, Mulczyk M, Górski A.** 2000. Bacteriophage therapy of bacterial infections: an update of our institute's experience. *Arch Immunol Ther Exp (Warsz)* **48:**547–551.

188. **Khawaldeh A, Morales S, Dillon B, Alavidze Z, Ginn AN, Thomas L, Chapman SJ, Dublanchet A, Smithyman A, Iredell JR.** 2011. Bacteriophage therapy for refractory *Pseudomonas aeruginosa* urinary tract infection. *J Med Microbiol* **60:**1697–1700.

189. **Kvachadze L, Balarjishvili N, Meskhi T, Tevdoradze E, Skhirtladze N, Pataridze T, Adamia R, Topuria T, Kutter E, Rohde C, Kutateladze M.** 2011. Evaluation of lytic activity

of staphylococcal bacteriophage Sb-1 against freshly isolated clinical pathogens. *Microb Biotechnol* **4:**643–650.

190. **Letkiewicz S, Miedzybrodzki R, Fortuna W, Weber-Dąbrowska B, Górski A.** 2009. Eradication of *Enterococcus faecalis* by phage therapy in chronic bacterial prostatitis: case report. *Folia Microbiol (Praha)* **54:**457–461.

191. **Leszczyński P, Weber-Dąbrowska B, Kohutnicka M, Luczak M, Górecki A, Górski A.** 2006. Successful eradication of methicillin-resistant Staphylococcus aureus (MRSA) intestinal carrier status in a healthcare worker: case report. *Folia Microbiol (Praha)* **51:**236–238.

192. **Marza JAS, Soothill JS, Boydell P, Collyns TA.** 2006. Multiplication of therapeutically administered bacteriophages in *Pseudomonas aeruginosa* infected patients. *Burns* **32:**644–646.

193. **Jikia D, Chkhaidze N, Imedashvili E, Mgaloblishvili I, Tsitlanadze G, Katsarava R, Glenn Morris J Jr, Sulakvelidze A.** 2005. The use of a novel biodegradable preparation capable of the sustained release of bacteriophages and ciprofloxacin, in the complex treatment of multidrug-resistant *Staphylococcus aureus*-infected local radiation injuries caused by exposure to Sr^{90}. *Clin Exp Dermatol* **30:**23–26.

194. **Markoishvili K, Tsitlanadze G, Katsarava R, Morris JG Jr, Sulakvelidze A.** 2002. A novel sustained-release matrix based on biodegradable poly(ester amide)s and impregnated with bacteriophages and an antibiotic shows promise in management of infected venous stasis ulcers and other poorly healing wounds. *Int J Dermatol* **41:**453–458.

195. **Abedon ST.** 2016. Commentary: phage therapy of staphylococcal chronic osteomyelitis in experimental animal model. *Front Microbiol* **7:**1251.

196. **Verbeken G, Pirnay JP, Lavigne R, Jennes S, De Vos D, Casteels M, Huys I.** 2014. Call for a dedicated European legal framework for bacteriophage therapy. *Arch Immunol Ther Exp (Warsz)* **62:**117–129.

197. **De Vos D, Verbeken G, Ceulemans C, Huys I, Pirnay J-P.** 2014. Reintroducing phage therapy in modern medicine: the regulatory and intellectual property hurdles, p 289–307. *In* Borysowski J, Miedzybrodzki R, Górski A (ed), *Phage Therapy: Current Research and Applications.* Caister Academic Press, Norfolk, United Kingdom.

198. **Parracho HM, Burrowes BH, Enright MC, McConville ML, Harper DR.** 2012. The role of regulated clinical trials in the development of bacteriophage therapeutics. *J Mol Genet Med* **6:**279–286.

199. **Cooper CJ, Khan Mirzaei M, Nilsson AS.** 2016. Adapting drug approval pathways for bacteriophage-based therapeutics. *Front Microbiol* **7:**1209.

200. **Ventola CL.** 2015. The antibiotic resistance crisis. Part 1. Causes and threats. *P&T* **40:**277–283.

201. **Kinch MS, Patridge E, Plummer M, Hoyer D.** 2014. An analysis ofFDA-approved drugs for infectious disease: antibacterial agents. *Drug Discov Today* **19:**1283–1287.

202. **Pratt WB.** 1977. *Chemotherapy of Infection.* Oxford University Press, New York, NY.

203. **Pires DP, Cleto S, Sillankorva S, Azeredo J, Lu TK.** 2016. Genetically engineered phages: a review of advances over the last decade. *Microbiol Mol Biol Rev* **80:**523–543.

204. **Abedon ST.** 2016. Bacteriophage exploitation of bacterial biofilms: phage preference for less mature targets? *FEMS Microbiol Lett* **363:** fnv246.

205. **Kropinski AM, Clokie MRJ.** 2009. Methods in molecular biology. Introduction. *Methods Mol Biol* **502:**xiii–xxii.

206. **Miedzybrodzki R, Fortuna W, Weber-Dąbrowska B, Górski A.** 2007. Phage therapy of staphylococcal infections (including MRSA) may be less expensive than antibiotic treatment. *Postepy Hig Med Dosw (Online)* **61:**461–465.

207. **Weber-Dąbrowska B, Zimecki M, Kruzel M, Kochanowska I, Lusiak-Szelachowska M.** 2006. Alternative therapies in antibiotic-resistant infection. *Adv Med Sci* **51:**242–244.

208. **Weber-Dąbrowska B, Mulczyk M, Górski A.** 2003. Bacteriophages as an efficient therapy for antibiotic-resistant septicemia in man. *Transplant Proc* **35:**1385–1386.

209. **Weber-Dąbrowska B, Zimecki M, Mulczyk M, Górski A.** 2002. Effect of phage therapy on the turnover and function of peripheral neutrophils. *FEMS Immunol Med Microbiol* **34:**135–138.

210. **Weber-Dąbrowska B, Mulczyk M, Górski A.** 2001. Bacteriophage therapy for infections in cancer patients. *Clin Appl Immunol Rev* **1:**131–134.

211. **Cisło M, Dabrowski M, Weber-Dąbrowska B, Woytoń A.** 1987. Bacteriophage treatment of suppurative skin infections. *Arch Immunol Ther Exp (Warsz)* **35:**175–183.

212. **Kress DW, Graham WP III, Davis TS, Miller SH.** 1981. A preliminary report on the use of Staphage Lysate for treatment of hidradenitis suppurativa. *Ann Plast Surg* **6:**393–395.

Modulation of the Gastrointestinal Microbiome with Nondigestible Fermentable Carbohydrates To Improve Human Health

20

EDWARD C. DEEHAN,[1] REBBECA M. DUAR,[1] ANISSA M. ARMET,[1]
MARIA ELISA PEREZ-MUÑOZ,[1] MINGLIANG JIN,[2] and JENS WALTER[1,3]

THE GI MICROBIOME AND CHRONIC NONCOMMUNICABLE DISEASES

Vertebrates have evolved with dense microbial populations in their gastrointestinal (GI) tract (referred to as the GI microbiome) that contribute to performance and health of the host (1). Although symbiotic in nature, animal experiments have established that the GI microbiota plays a causative role in the development of chronic noncommunicable diseases (CNCDs) such as obesity, diabetes, cardiovascular disease, colon cancer, autism, autoimmune diseases, allergies, and other atopic diseases including asthma (Fig. 1) (2). CNCDs are often associated with microbial dysbiosis, which is typically characterized by a reduced diversity, a bloom of facultative taxa (such as enterobacteria), and a lower output of beneficial metabolites (3). These associations provide a clear rationale for the development of strategies that modulate GI microbiome structure and function for the prevention of CNCDs (4).

Various strategies have been developed for the introduction of live microbes to modulate the GI ecosystem, through either probiotics, live biotherapeutics, or fecal transplants. These approaches have generated tremendous interest (5).

[1]Department of Agricultural, Food and Nutritional Science, University of Alberta, Edmonton, Alberta, Canada T6G 2E1; [2]Department of Microbiology and Immunology, Northwestern Polytechnical University, Xi'an, Shaanxi, China 710065; [3]Department of Biological Sciences, University of Alberta, Edmonton, Alberta, Canada T6G 2E1

Bugs as Drugs: Therapeutic Microbes for the Prevention and Treatment of Disease
Edited by Robert A. Britton and Patrice D. Cani
© 2018 American Society for Microbiology, Washington, DC
doi:10.1128/microbiolspec.BAD-0019-2017

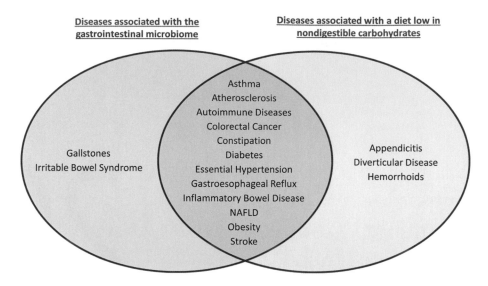

FIGURE 1 CNCDs that are associated with the GI microbiome and diets low in NDC. An industrialized lifestyle is associated with an increased prevalence of multiple CNCDs (15). Most of these diseases have now clearly been associated with the GI microbiome (pathology in animal models is dramatically different under germfree conditions, and the GI microbiome displays a dysbiosis in humans suffering from the disease). The Venn diagram designates CNCDs that are associated with the GI microbiome (2, 221, 247, 248) and a diet low in NDCs (13, 107, 244). NAFLD, nonalcoholic fatty liver disease.

However, diet has also been shown to readily alter GI microbiome structure and function (6–8), making it a particularly promising modifiable lifestyle factor of interest for the treatment of CNCDs. In addition, dietary supplements that employ nondigestible carbohydrates (NDCs) have been developed for several decades as prebiotics, targeted to support growth of beneficial GI microbiota in an attempt to improve health (9).

Interestingly, the incidence of most microbiota-associated CNCDs has substantially increased in recent decades in industrialized countries (10, 11), suggesting that practices associated with industrialized lifestyles predispose to disease. Although the exact factors that drive disease development are unknown and likely complex, the lack of NDCs is one contributing factor (12, 13). Humans likely evolved consuming more than 100 grams of NDCs daily, and nonindustrialized communities still exist today that have intakes that parallel those of our ancestors

(14). In the 1970s, Denis Burkitt and colleagues compared industrialized (United States and United Kingdom) and nonindustrialized (rural Africa) populations and found strong epidemiological links between urbanization and a reduction of dietary NDC intake (13, 15). These lifestyle shifts were associated with increased prevalence of CNCDs (13, 15). Recent research demonstrated that a diet low in NDCs that are accessible to the GI microbiota (i.e., nondigestible fermentable carbohydrates [NDFCs]) resulted in reduced production of fermentation end products that provide important physiological and immunological functions to the host (16, 17). Moreover, a diet low in NDFCs has been implicated in the depletion of microbiome diversity observed in industrialized societies (18–22) and the loss of bacterial species that rely on them for growth (23). Therefore, a possible explanation for the rise in CNCDs is that by shifting away from a diet in which our human-microbiota interrelationship evolved, we have essentially disrupted this symbiosis, ultimately reducing or removing the evolutionary routed benefits provided by the microbes (12).

The connections described above provide a rationale for the application of NDFCs to modulate the composition and/or function of the GI microbiome to benefit host health. In this article, we discuss (i) the concepts by which the GI microbiome can be modulated through the intake of NDCs that are fermentable (or accessible to the microbes), (ii) the effects of these strategies on GI microbiota, (iii) the mechanisms by which these strategies promote health, and (iv) the future research needed to optimize these strategies for their use in the field of human nutrition. We will focus on strategies that allow the systematic increase of NDFCs in the human adult diet by means of supplements such as prebiotics, fermentable dietary fiber, and microbiota-accessible carbohydrates (MACs), and not through whole-food sources such as fruits and vegetables. Supplemental NDFCs could provide a promising avenue for targeted modulation of the GI microbiota once they are understood at a mechanistic level (24). They could also provide an applicable strategy for increasing NDFC consumption within the context of an industrialized lifestyle, since current whole-food-focused strategies encouraged by nutritional organizations have shown little success in increasing NDFC intake (25, 26). Furthermore, even though NDFCs such as human milk oligosaccharides are important for infant growth and development and have tremendous potential to be included in infant formula (27), we will focus this article on the application of NDFCs in weaned children and adults.

MODULATION OF THE GI MICROBIOME THROUGH NDFCS: THREE CONCEPTS

Prebiotics

Although the potential to modulate the human GI microbiome through NDFCs had

been recognized decades earlier (especially in Japan), the term "prebiotics" was coined by Gibson and Roberfroid in 1995. A prebiotic was initially defined as a "nondigestible food ingredient that beneficially affects the host by selectively stimulating the growth and/or activity of one or a limited number of bacteria already resident in the colon, and thus attempt to improve host health" (9). The definition has been adjusted various times (28), with the International Scientific Association for Probiotics and Prebiotics (ISAPP) consensus panel proposing the most recent definition: "a substrate that is selectively utilized by host microorganisms conferring a health benefit" (29). Currently, the most commonly used definition is "a selectively fermented ingredient that results in specific changes in the composition and/or activity of the gastrointestinal microbiota, thus conferring benefit(s) upon host health" (30). Although most definitions do not restrict prebiotics to carbohydrates, currently only lactulose, inulin-type fructans, and trans-galactooligosaccharides are considered prebiotics (30). Polydextrose, glucooligosaccharides, lactosucrose, soybean oligosaccharides, and xylooligosaccharides have been further proposed as "candidate prebiotics" (30). However, the criteria that these carbohydrates would have to fulfill to move beyond the status of mere candidates have not been clearly established (28).

To date, most definitions, including the recent definition brought forward by the ISAPP consensus panel (29), require that prebiotics have to be "specific" for or "selective" toward health-promoting taxonomic groups. Conceptually, the idea is to shift the GI microbial community toward a more "healthy" state. This concept is derived from early findings from culture-based and later probe- and primer-based studies that found bifidobacteria and lactobacilli (putatively health-promoting organisms) to be selectively stimulated through prebiotics such as inulin and galactooligosaccharides (31). However, even though there is a strong rationale to specifically target the beneficial components and functional attributes of the GI microbiome, the prebiotic concept as it currently stands has been repeatedly criticized for being poorly defined (28, 32–34) and/or scientifically outdated (28, 35, 36). Some scientists have suggested revisions to the concept (36), while others consider it completely obsolete (5, 35). Criticism is primarily focused on the concept of selectivity and the question of how to identify beneficial microbiota that should be targeted (28, 36).

First, based on the most current scientific understanding, it is too simplistic to categorize GI microbes as either "good" or "bad." Microbes can possess both beneficial and detrimental traits, strains of one species can differ widely in their attributes, and their role is highly context-dependent (e.g., host genetic predisposition, host physiology, GI microbial ecology, diet, etc.). Second, it has been argued that the specific targets should go beyond that of *Bifidobacterium* and *Lactobacillus* species, because many bacterial genera (*Akkermansia*, *Eubacterium*, and *Fecalibacterium*) have been linked to health benefits (37–40), including taxa previously considered to be detrimental, such as *Clostridia* and *Bacteroides* (41, 42). Third, given that the GI microbiota functions as a complex community, it may be imperative to support community characteristics such as diversity, stability, and ecosystem functionality (e.g., short-chain fatty acid [SCFA] output), which have all been positively correlated with health (43–45). To this end, the formation of SCFAs does not rely on selective fermentation. Moreover, although some strains of bifidobacteria and lactobacilli have been reported to produce butyrate and propionate (46), which are the SCFAs with the most evidence for health effects (17), from the metabolism of amino acids, the amounts produced (<150 μM) are less than 1% of what bacteria produce from the fermentation of carbohydrates (46, 47). Bifidobacteria and lactobacilli lack the biosynthetic pathways to produce butyrate and propionate from the fermentation of carbohydrates (48–51) and therefore cannot be the target of prebiotics that aim at boosting these

SCFAs. Fourth, human studies using next-generation sequencing have shown that the response of the GI microbiome to NDFCs that are currently regarded as prebiotics, such as inulin, is not as selective as previously believed (52), while NDFCs that were considered to be broadly fermented result in restricted shifts of the GI microbiome (53–55). In this respect, it is important to consider that no carbohydrate is fermented solely by one or two species (partially because bacterial traits are shared between bacteria through horizontal gene transfer [56]), and no carbohydrate is broadly fermented, especially not under the competitive conditions within the GI tract (57). So the recent proposition by the ISAPP consensus panel that selectivity "could extend to several microbial groups, just not all" (29), would essentially mean that any carbohydrate would qualify as a prebiotic.

The notion that carbohydrates currently accepted as prebiotics are not utilized differently by the GI microbiota when compared to "regular" dietary fibers has recently been demonstrated using *in vitro* fecal fermentations of inulin (a well-described prebiotic) and pectin (not considered a prebiotic) (58). Both carbohydrates induced multiple substrate-specific compositional shifts. The fermentation of inulin resulted in the increased abundance of five taxa, while the fermentation of pectin resulted in the enrichment of seven different taxa. Nevertheless, both carbohydrates resulted in comparable amounts of SCFAs (58). This illustrates that both inulin and pectin can lead to a specific enrichment of different bacterial species among the GI microbiome, which would allow targeted modulation of GI microbiota. In spite of this, the rationale for why only one of them is considered a prebiotic is not obvious from these findings, especially considering that selectivity, according to the ISAPP consensus panel, "could extend to several microbial groups" (29). What constitutes a specific fermentation therefore remains ill-defined.

In this respect, it is important to point out that specificity of a prebiotic has, to date, been exclusively established only by the determination of compositional shifts. However, species that utilize a prebiotic might produce metabolites without becoming enriched. For example, *Bacteroides* numbers often decrease after the administration of prebiotics even if they are able to utilize them (59, 60), likely since their growth is negatively affected through a reduction in pH that results from the production of SCFAs (58, 61, 62). To truly establish whether a prebiotic is selectively fermented would require the use of techniques such as stable isotope probing (63) that allow for the identification of all microbes that are able to utilize the substrate within a complex microbial community, including those that do not become enriched. Finally, there are often substantially different inter-individual responses within the GI microbiome toward a prebiotic, yet this variation has not been considered in the concept at all (36).

Overall, we agree with recently published statements that the prebiotic concept is ill defined and based on outdated scientific views (5, 28, 32–35). To address these inconsistencies, Bindels and colleagues proposed updating the definition of a prebiotic to "a non-digestible compound that, through its metabolization by microorganisms in the GI tract, modulates composition and/or activity of the GI microbiota, thus conferring a beneficial physiological effect on the host" (28). By removing the requirement of specificity, this definition embraces the complexity of host-microbe metabolic interactions and focuses on ecological and functional features of the microbiota that are more likely to be relevant for host physiology, such as the production of SCFAs. Still, consensus on the definition of a prebiotic has not been reached (32), and some scientists prefer to abandon the term altogether (35). However, it is the opinion of the authors that the term remains helpful, as it has become well known in the scientific community and is recognized by regulators, industry, consumers, and health care professionals. Therefore, the prebiotic

concept could remain valuable after the inconsistencies in the definition have been resolved.

Fermentable Dietary Fiber

Based on current definitions, most prebiotic carbohydrates are dietary fibers, but not all dietary fibers are considered to be prebiotics (64, 65). Nonetheless, a clear-cut distinction between prebiotics and nonprebiotic dietary fiber is not possible (33), and it is increasingly recognized that the fermentation of dietary fiber by the colonic microbiota contributes to human health.

The term "dietary fiber" was coined in 1953 by Eben Hipsley to describe the nondigestible components of the plant cell wall (66). Later, in the mid-1970s, Trowell and colleagues refined the definition to "remnants of plant cells resistant to hydrolysis by the alimentary enzymes of man, the group of substances that remain in the ileum but are partially hydrolyzed by bacteria in the colon" (67). Since then, the definition has undergone several revisions. The most widely used definition was put forth in 2009 by the Codex Alimentarius Commission, a joint principal branch of the Food and Agriculture Organization and the World Health Organization, which defines dietary fiber as "carbohydrate polymers with ten or more monomeric units, which are not hydrolyzed by the endogenous enzymes in the human small intestine and belong to the following categories:

1. Edible carbohydrate polymers naturally occurring in the food as consumed,
2. Carbohydrate polymers which have been obtained from raw materials by physical, enzymatic, or chemical means and which have been shown to have a physiological effect of benefit to health as demonstrated by generally accepted scientific evidence to competent authorities, and
3. Synthetic carbohydrate polymers which have been shown to have a physiological

effect of benefit to health as demonstrated by generally accepted scientific evidence to competent authorities" (68).

The decision to consider carbohydrates with three to nine monomeric units (oligosaccharides) as dietary fiber was left to individual country's authorities (26). Recently, the Food and Drug Administration in the United States updated its food labeling regulations to model the Codex definition by requiring that "isolated" and "synthetic" NDCs added to foods must first demonstrate a beneficial physiological effect in humans prior to being permitted as a dietary fiber on a food label (69).

Dietary fibers can be found in plants, bacteria, and fungi and can be chemically synthesized (Fig. 2) (70, 71). Plant-derived nonstarch polysaccharides display a substantial variety of chemical structures due to the diverse functional roles that they play in plants (71). Dietary fibers also include starches that are resistant to human digestion (resistant starches [RSs]), which are divided into five subtypes based on the mechanism responsible for their inaccessibility to host digestion (72). Given the heterogenic chemical structures found in dietary fibers, their utilization within the GI tract often requires a diverse array of enzymes distributed among various microbial members. The extent by which different fiber types are utilized or fermented by the GI microbiota is therefore structure-dependent and relies on the metabolic capabilities of an individual's microbiome, which ultimately determines the bacterial metabolites produced from the fermentation (24).

The chemical structure of a dietary fiber also determines other important physicochemical properties such as solubility and viscosity (73), which influence its accessibility to microbes. Most linear fibers form crystalline structures (such as cellulose), which significantly reduces their solubility in water. Meanwhile, dietary fibers with charged moieties or structural irregularities in the sugar

backbone and side chains (such as β-glucan) tend to increase in solubility, which is often correlated with fermentability (74). However, one common exception is RSs, which are typically insoluble in water yet highly fermentable (33). Furthermore, most soluble dietary fibers tend to also be viscous in water (33), which relates to their ability to render a solution gelatinous via the absorption of water (74). Solubility and viscosity are important characteristics that influence the functionality of a dietary fiber, but for the purpose of modulating the GI microbiota, fermentability is of particular relevance.

"Dietary fiber" is a widely accepted and useful term to describe NDCs that influence health benefits. Most consumers recognize the term, because it is a required part of the nutrition facts label of processed food. However, to describe NDFCs that are intended to modulate the GI microbiome, the term has obvious limitations. Various mechanisms (e.g., reduced absorption through viscosity, bile acid binding, stool bulking, etc.) have been identified by which dietary fiber can benefit human health completely independently of their effects on the GI microbiome (73). In addition, as described above, not all dietary fibers are fermented by the microbiota. The definition of a prebiotic proposed by Bindels and colleagues would encompass dietary fibers for which there is evidence that they improve health via the GI microbiota (28), but as described above, there is no agreement on the definition of a prebiotic (32). What is clear is that the portion of dietary fiber that is fermentable or "accessible" by an individual's microbiota is what determines its ability to modulate the GI microbiome. This notion is central to the concept of microbiota-accessible carbohydrates (MACs).

MACs

To address the limitations of the concepts discussed above, especially as they relate to the inter-individual differences of the human GI

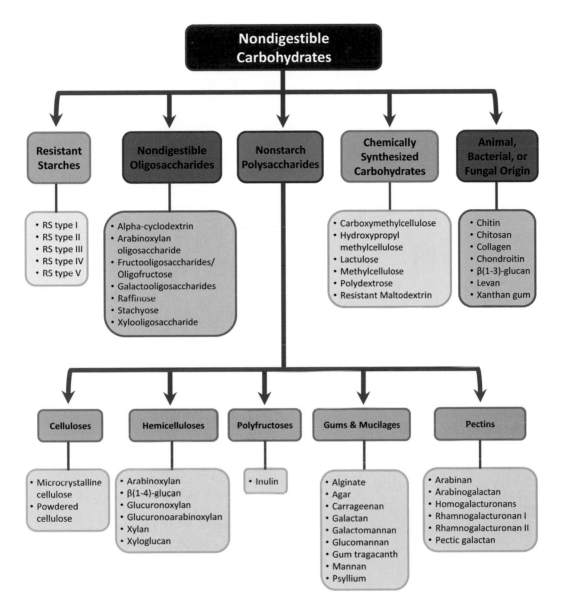

FIGURE 2 Categories of NDCs. NDCs are a heterogeneous group of compounds that display diverse chemical structures, which is the basis for their categorization alongside their origin (24, 70, 71). Nondigestible oligosaccharides are NDCs composed of three to nine monosaccharides and are from either plant or animal origin, as well as chemically synthesized.

microbiome, Sonnenburg and Sonnenburg introduced the concept of MACs (16). MACs can be divided into dietary MACs (NDFCs such as prebiotics and dietary fiber) and host-derived MACs (such as mucosal glycans) (16). Determining whether an NDFC is considered a MAC is not entirely dependent on the NDFC's physicochemical characteristics, because an individual's GI microbiota must also have the enzymatic capacity to metabolize it (75, 76). For example, cellulose does not qualify as a MAC for humans, because the capacity of the human GI microbiota to ferment cellulose is extremely low (77), while it would qualify as a MAC for other host species (e.g., hindgut and foregut fermenters). On the other hand, RS type 3 would be considered a MAC for most individuals, as it is readily metabolized by their GI microbiota. However, individuals who lack the keystone species *Ruminococcus bromii* do not have the enzymatic capacity to metabolize RS type 3, and thus for these individuals, it would not be considered a MAC (75). The concept of MACs is therefore particularly applicable to efforts aimed at personalizing human nutrition, which could customize dietary recommendations toward the goal of incorporating specific NDFCs that are known to be accessible to an individual's GI microbiota.

The concept of dietary MACs is essentially equivalent to that of fermentable dietary fiber, with the additional criterion regarding the individuality of the GI microbiota in their capacity to utilize certain NDFCs. Both concepts include the same types of NDFCs (16), and according to Bindels and colleagues, these carbohydrates could be considered prebiotic if they exert a health benefit via the GI microbiota (28). Because there is currently no unifying concept that describes NDFCs that target the GI microbiota for health purposes, we will continue to refer to these carbohydrates as NDFCs for the purpose of this review.

HOW DO NDFCs MODULATE GI MICROBIOTA COMPOSITION AND FUNCTION?

Modulation of GI Microbiota Composition and Diversity

Consumption of NDFCs has the potential to improve human health by changing both the composition (structure and diversity) and the function (metabolism) of the microbial communities that reside in the GI tract. Dietary administration of NDFCs alters the

nutritional niches in the GI tract by providing substrates for microbial growth. Thus, in general, species that are able to utilize these substrates can expand their populations (78). For example, administration of RS has been shown to enrich specific bacterial groups (*Bifidobacterium adolescentis*, *R. bromii*, and *Eubacterium rectale*) in a subset of individuals (53–55). The taxa shown to be enriched differ between RS type 2 (which appears to be similar to RS type 3 [75]) and RS type 4 (55), indicating that shifts are dependent on the carbohydrate's chemical structure. Accordingly, the consumption of galactooligosaccharides mainly induces *Bifidobacterium* species that possess the enzymatic machinery to efficiently utilize this substrate (60). In addition to its enzymatic capacity, the ability of a microbe to "adhere" to a substrate and to tolerate the environmental conditions generated from fermentation (e.g., low pH) determines whether a microbe can become enriched. Although RS is utilized by many members of the human GI microbiota (57, 79, 80), the species that become enriched under competition (*B. adolescentis*, *R. bromii*, and *E. rectale*) have been shown to directly adhere to this substrate in the human GI tract (80).

Furthermore, the degradation of many complex NDFCs does require a different species with complementary enzymatic repertoires for their degradation, which establishes syntrophic interrelationships within the GI microbiota (81–83). Primary fermenters directly degrade NDFCs, leading to the release of partial breakdown products and the production of metabolites that can benefit themselves, as well as be beneficial or inhibitory (e.g., through acidity) to other taxa (84). Secondary fermenters benefit through cross-feeding on these partial carbohydrate breakdown products and the metabolic end products released by primary fermenters (82, 85). Through coculture experiments, *R. bromii* has been identified as a primary fermenter of RS types 2 and 3, whereupon RS degradation-reducing sugars are released that support the growth of secondary fermenters that are not able to degrade RS directly, including *B. adolescentis*, *E. rectale*, and *Bacteroides thetaiotaomicron* (75). Another cross-feeding relationship exists for hydrogen-consuming species such as *Blautia hydrogenotrophica*, which flourish in the mouse GI tract only if in bi-association with *B. thetaiotaomicron* by utilizing the hydrogen generated as an end product of fermentation by the latter (86). Removal of hydrogen maintains the redox balance (NAD^+/NADH ratio) in the GI tract, providing conditions favorable for fermentation, and can result in the formation of methane by methanogens (such as *Methanobrevibacter smithii*) and acetate by acetogens (such as *B. hydrogenotrophica*), which is further converted to butyrate by other taxa, including *Roseburia intestinalis* (87–89). Lactate is another metabolic end product of NDFC fermentation that can also be converted to butyrate through cross-feeding between lactate-producing species and lactate-utilizing butyrogenic species (83, 90).

While the processes described above lead to the enrichment of GI microbes through the fermentation of NDFCs, with different species being either directly or indirectly stimulated, there are taxa that simultaneously become inhibited through the metabolites produced. For instance, *Bacteroides* species often decrease in number after the administration of NDFCs (37, 59, 60), even though this group of bacteria is well equipped to utilize these substrates. These inhibitory effects are due to *Bacteroides* having a low tolerance for acidic conditions generated from the SCFAs produced during the fermentation of NDFCs (58, 62).

The impact of NDFCs on the GI microbiome composition displays several consistent characteristics that are important for therapeutic applications. First, the magnitude of the induced changes can be substantial, with specific species becoming enriched to constitute more than 30% of the fecal microbiota (54, 55, 60), thus providing a potential strategy for the enrichment of minority members of the GI microbiome to become dominant members. However, these changes are only maintained as long as the substrate is consumed. Once the substrate is no longer available, resilience of the microbiota results in a return to the original state. Second, the microbial response to NDFCs is highly individualized, with some individuals showing substrate-specific shifts, while others do not respond at all (55, 60). The reason for this individuality is not yet understood. Individuals might lack keystone species (75) or contain strains with varying enzymatic capacity for the substrate (91). Third, although individualized, compositional changes observed after administration of NDFCs remain restricted to certain groups of microbes. This is true for classic prebiotics such as inulin and galactooligosaccharides that are supposed to be selectively fermented (60, 92), but it also applies to substrates that were assumed to be broadly utilized, such as RSs and pectin (54, 55, 58). The reason for these observations stems from the highly competitive conditions within the human GI tract, which allow for only certain microbes to benefit directly from the NDFCs (87). Although central to the original prebiotic concept (30), whether such specific shifts are related to health outcomes still remains to be established.

Most CNCDs are associated with a dysbiosis that displays decreases in bacterial diversity and/or genetic richness of the GI microbiome (3, 43, 44). Although it is difficult to prove whether these patterns are the cause or an effect of disease, community ecology theory postulates high diversity as a beneficial trait that is attributed to stability and functionality of the ecosystem (45, 93). Several independent research groups have consistently shown that individuals from non-industrialized populations in various parts of the world have greater GI microbiome diversity when compared to individuals from industrialized regions (94). This increased diversity is reflected not only in the number of bacterial species (or operational taxonomic units) (18–22), but also in the abundance of genetic functions encoded in the GI microbiome (20). While there are many possible factors that could cause reduced GI microbial diversity through industrialization (e.g., sanitization and antibiotic use), dietary diversity is considered a key mediator (16, 95). Research using humanized mice (mice that have been colonized with a human GI microbiota) demonstrated that a maternal diet low in MACs induced significant depletions in the GI microbiota diversity of the offspring within only a few generations and that this depletion was irreversible even after the reintroduction of MACs (23). Enrichment of the maternal diet with MACs maintained the GI microbiota diversity in the offspring over multiple generations (23). Moreover, the transition of non-human primates from wild to semicaptive to captive conditions led to a reduction in bacterial operational taxonomic unit richness. An in-depth analysis of the chloroplast sequences found within the 16S sequences obtained from fecal samples suggested that this depletion was in part driven by a reduction in the diversity of dietary plant content, and particularly by a reduction in the consumption of NDFCs (96).

Overall, there is convincing evidence that a depletion of NDFCs in the diet results in a reduction of microbial diversity within the human GI microbiome, thus providing a rationale for targeting microbial diversity through dietary modulations. An enrichment of both the amount and structural diversity of NDFCs could in theory enhance microbial diversity and gene richness by generating niche opportunities (24). Cross-sectional assessments of long-term dietary intake in overweight humans have shown that long-term consumption of fruit and vegetables, and therefore NDFCs, is associated with higher GI microbial gene richness and diversity (44, 97). Conversely, short-term dietary intervention studies have produced conflicting results (37, 98, 99). Studies supplementing fiber-rich whole foods have been shown to increase GI microbial diversity (37, 93), while most short-term feeding trials with purified NDFCs (55, 60, 98, 100) or even whole-plant-based diets (6) had no effect.

In summary, although clear associations exist between the consumption of NDFCs, GI microbial diversity, and improved metabolic and inflammatory markers of CNCDs, rigorously controlled human intervention studies with NDFCs that assess well-defined clinical and microbial endpoints are needed to determine (i) if diversity can be enhanced by NDFCs and (ii) to what extent this constitutes a microbial-dependent mechanism by which NDFCs can improve human health.

Impact of NDFCs on GI Microbiome Function

The provision of NDFCs not only impacts microbiota composition as described above, but also changes the profile of microbial-derived metabolites within the GI tract (101). The fermentation of NDFCs results in the production of beneficial metabolites (e.g., SCFAs) and microbial gases (H_2, CO_2, CH_4), with SCFAs being the main focus of recent research (17, 101). Acetate, propionate, and butyrate are the dominant SCFAs (at >95%) (102). A significant portion of acetate (around 24%) can support the production of butyrate through microbial cross-feeding (103). The total amount and proportion of individual SCFAs produced is dependent on the type of NDFC (104), as well as the individual microbiota (105), further reinforcing that the response of human GI microbiota to NDFCs is individualized.

Fermentation of NDFCs within the GI tract leads to various systemic effects on the host, including an influence on energy homeostasis and metabolism (17). A majority of the SCFAs produced are rapidly absorbed in the GI tract, with only around 5 to 10% being excreted in the feces (101). Upon absorption, the majority of butyrate is metabolized by the colonocytes and serves as their major form of energy (106). Propionate reaches the liver via portal circulation, where it is primarily utilized for hepatic gluconeogenesis (GNG). Acetate, on the other hand, reaches peripheral circulation at extensively higher concentrations than the other SCFAs, where it is metabolized by peripheral tissues for energy, in addition to being utilized by the liver for lipogenesis (101–103). NDCs provide the host with 0 to 2.5 kcal/g (with digestible carbohydrates providing 4 kcal/g), dependent on their level of fermentability by the GI microbiota (107).

A low intake of NDFCs leads not only to a reduction in SCFAs, but also to shifts in GI microbiota metabolism toward the utilization of less favorable nutrients, particularly dietary and endogenously supplied proteins (108). For instance, moving the diet of human volunteers from a weight-maintenance diet to a high-protein, low-carbohydrate diet not only significantly reduced the production of total SCFAs and butyrate (109), but also led to an increase in potentially detrimental metabolites derived from the fermentation of amino acids, including branched chain fatty acids, ammonia, amines, N-nitroso compounds, phenolic compounds including p-Cresol, and sulfides (Fig. 3) (110, 111). These metabolites are thought to directly contribute to the development of CNCDs, particularly colon cancer (111). In addition, depletion of NDFCs within the diet subsequently causes the GI microbiota to shift their glycan-foraging behavior toward utilizing host-derived substrates such as mucins by upregulating the expression of bacterial genes necessary for the metabolization of mucosal glycoproteins (112). This shift toward the fermentation of mucosal glycans leads to a significant depletion of the epithelial mucus layer (113), which can cause GI inflammation and increases the host's susceptibility to pathogen invasion (114).

In summary, the metabolic effect of NDFCs is central to their importance in human nutrition and their effects when used as supplements (115) in the form of prebiotics or fermentable dietary fiber (65). Although the fermentation of NDFCs is considered beneficial, this subject is not without its controversies. Individuals with obesity tend to have increased fecal SCFAs when compared to their lean counterparts (116), and SCFAs might contribute to weight gain by providing energy. In addition, butyrate has a controversial role in the induction of colon cancer, because it has been shown to fuel the hyperproliferation of colon epithelial cells in a mouse model of the disease (117, 118). However, epidemiological studies consistently report a negative association between dietary fiber consumption, which would increase SCFAs, and both obesity (119) and colon cancer (120, 121). Furthermore, as discussed below, the majority of the physiological effects associated with SCFAs are considered beneficial.

PHYSIOLOGICAL EFFECTS OF NDFCs ON THE HOST

Two primary signaling mechanisms have been described by which SCFAs influence the biological responses of the host. First, SCFAs can impose epigenetic regulation through direct inhibition of histone deacetylase activity and expression (122). Histone deacetylase inhibition has been indicated as a central mechanism by which SCFAs modulate the immune system and inhibit the development of colon cancer (122). Second, SCFAs can bind to G-protein-coupled receptors (GPRs), with the primary receptors activated by SCFAs being GPR41, GPR43, and GPR109A (122). GPR41 and GPR43 are coexpressed locally on colonic enteroendocrine L-cells (46, 47), as well as systemically expressed in white adipose tissue, skeletal muscle, and the liver (46–48). GPR109A (which is also commonly referred to as niacin receptor 1 since niacin is its primary ligand [123]) has been shown to be expressed on ileal and colonic enterocytes, adipocytes, and immune cells (123–125). Agonists for GPR41 can be ranked in the following order based on potency: propionate greater than or equal to butyrate, butyrate greater than acetate; however, these SCFAs exhibit similar potencies for GPR43 (126, 127). Butyrate, on the other hand, is the only SCFA known to bind

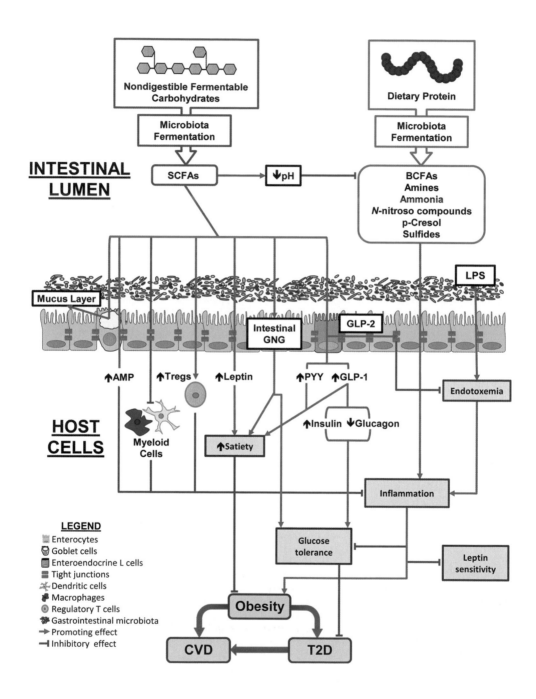

to GPR109A. Overall, SCFAs are a primary microbiota-dependent mechanism by which NDFCs modulate host health (17) through the regulation of satiety, glucose and lipid metabolism, as well as systemic inflammation (Fig. 3).

Regulation of Satiety

The regulation of the balance between hunger and satiety, which ultimately impacts energy intake, is highly complex and is influenced by multiple physiological, psychological, and environmental factors (128). SCFAs act as physiological regulators of satiety by primarily functioning as signaling molecules through the enhanced production of key anorectic hormones such as peptide tyrosine tyrosine (PYY) and glucagon-like peptide-1 (GLP-1) (Fig. 3) (47). By means of activating GPR41 and GPR43, SCFAs induce the release of both PYY and GLP-1 from colonic enteroendocrine L-cells into systemic circulation (129, 130). PYY has been shown to promote satiety by acting on the arcuate nucleus within the hypothalamus to suppress neuropeptide Y neurons and activate pro-opiomelanocortin neurons while also delaying gastric emptying (131, 132). GLP-1 similarly influences the hypothalamus by binding to the GLP-1 receptor (133, 134) while also inhibiting gastric empty-ing and the secretion of gastric acid (135, 136). Furthermore, the SCFAs acetate and propionate have been shown to act on white adipose tissue to stimulate the production of leptin, another anorectic hormone involved in the regulation of satiety (Fig. 3) (137, 138).

SCFAs can also regulate the interplay between hunger and satiety independent of anorectic hormones. Acetate has been shown to induce satiety through directly eliciting hypothalamic appetite suppression (139). Furthermore, propionate and butyrate promote an upregulation of intestinal GNG gene expression, which positively influences energy homeostasis and promotes satiety by portal vein glucose sensors (140, 141). Besides influencing energy intake, SCFAs may also affect energy expenditure. In rodents, SCFA supplementation promoted an increased rate of oxygen consumption while also enhancing mitochondrial function, adaptive thermogenesis, and fat oxidation (142, 143). However, the extent of this influence and its relevance to humans is not currently known.

Glucose and Lipid Metabolism

Obesity, cardiovascular disease, type 2 diabetes, and other CNCDs are associated with an altered glucose and lipid metabolism (144, 145). Human intervention studies have shown

---

FIGURE 3 Mechanisms by which the metabolism of NDFCs by the GI microbiota modulates host health. NDFCs are fermented by the GI microbiota to SCFAs, which upon absorption into enterocytes can activate intestinal GNG, leading to improved satiety and glucose homeostasis. SCFAs can further stimulate enteroendocrine L-cells to secrete PYY, GLP-1, and GLP-2. Both PYY and GLP-1 act as satiety hormones, while GLP-1 also promotes glucose tolerance. Meanwhile, the secretion of GLP-2 enhances intestinal barrier function by upregulating the expression of tight junction proteins. SCFAs further enhance the intestinal barrier by stimulating mucin secretion from goblet cells, which aids in reducing the translocation of LPS through the intestinal epithelium, consequently reducing inflammation. Additionally, SCFAs exert immunomodulatory effects by regulating the production of antimicrobial peptides, the expansion of regulatory T-cells, and myeloid cell function to inhibit inflammation. Moreover, SCFAs signal to organs distant from the GI tract, such as white adipose tissue, where they may act on adipocytes promoting the secretion of leptin, another anorectic hormone. Furthermore, the presence of NDFCs inhibits the production of potentially detrimental metabolites from the fermentation of dietary proteins through lowering intestinal pH. AMP, antimicrobial peptides; BCFAs, branched-chain fatty acids; CVD, cardiovascular disease; GLP, glucagon-like peptide; GNG, gluconeogenesis; LPS, lipopolysaccharides; PYY, peptide tyrosine tyrosine; SCFAs, short-chain fatty acids; T2D, type 2 diabetes; Tregs, regulatory T-cells.

that increased consumption of NDFCs can improve glucose and lipid metabolism (146–148), thereby providing a mechanism by which they reduce the risk of developing cardiovascular disease, type 2 diabetes, and other CNCDs (149, 150). As discussed above, activation of enteroendocrine L-cells by SCFAs stimulates the release of GLP-1, which directly acts on pancreatic β-cells to promote insulin and inhibit glucagon secretion (133, 151, 152). GLP-1 is also known to improve β-cell responsiveness to glucose, even in glucose-resistant β-cells (153, 154). Additionally, SCFAs themselves, specifically propionate, have recently been shown to act directly on β-cells to stimulate insulin secretion, independent of GLP-1 (155). This would subsequently increase the uptake of glucose by skeletal muscle and adipose tissues while also decreasing hepatic-associated GNG (156). Further, SCFAs have been shown to inhibit hepatic-associated GNG via upregulation of intestinal GNG (140). This reduction in hepatic GNG is critical, because enhanced hepatic production of glucose is linked to insulin resistance and the development of some CNCDs (157, 158).

SCFAs may also directly act on the liver to further influence hepatic glucose and lipid metabolism, which may in part be mediated by GPR41 and GPR43 signaling (127). Dietary administration of SCFAs decreased lipid accumulation within the liver in mice by means of increased lipid utilization (159). This occurred primarily by downregulation of peroxisome-proliferator-activated receptor-γ expression and activity, which stimulated AMP-activated protein kinase-associated fatty acid oxidation within the liver. This SCFA-induced increase in fat oxidation was also observed in adipose tissue (159). SCFAs may play a further role in lipid metabolism by acting on adipose tissue through both intracellular and extracellular mechanisms. The acute administration of acetate and propionate in humans led to a significant reduction in serum free fatty acid levels (160). This may be in part due to a GPR43-dependent decrease in the intracellular lipolytic activity of adipocytes (161). In addition to this, propionate may also have extracellular lipolytic properties by enhancing the activity of adipose tissue lipoprotein lipase (162). Collectively, the mechanistic involvement of SCFAs in modulating glucose and lipid metabolism has been well established in animal and *in vitro* models, although further research is needed to clarify if these findings translate to humans.

Systemic Inflammation

Most CNCDs are characterized by a state of systemic, low-grade inflammation, which contributes to disease progression (144, 145, 163). Although the findings are to some degree variable, recent research indicates that NDFCs have anti-inflammatory effects (164, 165), primarily through SCFA-dependent mechanisms involving intestinal barrier function and regulation of immune cell responses (17).

Barrier function and endotoxemia

Diminished GI barrier function enhances the translocation of lipopolysaccharide (LPS) and other microbial-derived proinflammatory molecules across the GI epithelial layer. LPS interacts with LPS-binding protein and CD14 to stimulate Toll-like receptor-4 and subsequently promotes a proinflammatory response, including a systemic increase in acute-phase proteins and proinflammatory cytokines (166). Elevated plasma LPS in humans (endotoxemia) is positively correlated with percent body fat, excessive energy intake, metabolic inflammation, insulin resistance, and dyslipidemia (37, 167–169). In mice, endotoxemia has been demonstrated to cause obesity and insulin resistance without influencing food intake (170). Considering this, promoting GI mucosal barrier function could constitute a strategy to address CNCD-associated metabolic abnormalities.

SCFAs have been shown to enhance GI barrier function through upregulating the expression of tight junction proteins, which occurs through at least two mechanisms. First, NDFC-induced SCFA production increases GLP-2 secretion by enteroendocrine L-cells (171, 172), which leads to an upregulation in the expression of tight junction proteins (zonula occludens-1 and occludin) and, concomitantly, a reduction in LPS and systemic inflammation (Fig. 3) (173). Recently, Kelly and colleagues illustrated another mechanism by which SCFA metabolism (mainly butyrate) within intestinal epithelial cells creates a state of hypoxia, which enhances intestinal barrier integrity (174), likely through enhanced tight junction protein expression (175).

Other mechanisms by which SCFAs have been shown to improve GI barrier function include butyrate-driven upregulation of epithelial cell proliferation and differentiation (176), enhanced production of antimicrobial peptides including secretory immunoglobulin A (IgA) and intestinal alkaline phosphatase (177), stimulation of goblet cells to secrete mucus that fortifies the GI mucus layer (178, 179), and GPR109A-dependent regulation of enterocyte-derived interleukin-18, which is essential to maintain mucosal homeostasis and ultimately GI barrier function (180, 181).

Immunoregulation

Subpopulations of immunosuppressive regulatory T-cells (Tregs) play an essential role in both the maintenance of immunotolerance and, ultimately, the prevention of many CNCDs (182, 183). Microbiota-derived SCFAs, particularly butyrate and propionate, have been demonstrated to encourage immunotolerance through expansion and differentiation of Tregs (182). This process has been shown to occur through GPR43-dependent signaling (184), as well as through the epigenetic regulation of the Foxp3 promoter through inhibition of histone deacetylase (185, 186). This systemic immunoregulatory effect is thought to be determined largely by the immunologic context. For example, in a

state of infection, SCFAs enhance the differentiation of proinflammatory T-helper cell subsets (i.e., Th1 and Th17 cells) instead of Tregs (187). This suggests that SCFA production from the fermentation of NDFCs may play an intricate role in host immune responses to infection beyond lowering intestinal pH, which inhibits colonization by pathogens (9).

The immunoregulatory effect of SCFAs is, however, not solely reliant upon an expansion of Tregs and can occur in organ systems throughout the body (e.g., lungs, skin) (188, 189). SCFAs have also been shown to regulate immune cells of the myeloid lineage (Fig. 3) through facilitating the polarization of macrophages toward an M2 phenotype involved in downregulating an inflammatory response (190), specifically that of GI macrophages to LPS (191). Moreover, SCFAs modulate neutrophil activity through suppressing their migratory behavior (192) while shifting their microbial killing phenotype toward increased phagocytic activity with diminished proinflammatory cytokine production (193, 194). The activity of dendritic cells has similarly been shown to be influenced by SCFAs, primarily through enhancing their ability to induce the differentiation of Tregs (180) and to promote the production of IgA by plasma cells (195). Furthermore, SCFAs act directly on β-cells to enhance the production of IgA, both by acting as an energy source and by upregulating the expression of genes necessary for plasma cell differentiation (196). SCFAs can also act on nonimmune cells to stimulate the release of antimicrobial peptides. Within the pancreas, SCFAs act on pancreatic β-cells in a GPR-dependent manner to enhance the secretion of cathelicidin-related antimicrobial peptide, which ultimately induces Treg cell expansion and protects against the development of autoimmune diabetes (197). Although additional research is needed, these animal and *in vitro* models elegantly illustrate the central mechanisms by which microbiota-derived SCFAs reduce inflammation.

EVIDENCE FOR MICROBIOTA-MEDIATED HEALTH EFFECTS OF NDFCs

There is substantial evidence from well-designed animal studies that NDFCs, or the metabolic products that result from their fermentation (e.g., SCFAs), have beneficial effects and that these effects are in part due to the GI microbiota. Work originating from Patrice Cani and Nathalie Delzenne's research groups has repeatedly demonstrated, although primarily through associations and not causal assessments, that the GI microbiota is implicated in the ability of NDFCs to improve obesity-associated low-grade inflammation and insulin resistance (40, 171–173, 198). Research employing fecal microbiota transplantation methodology supports these findings and further suggests a causative link, in that upon transferring the GI microbiota from mice fed an NDFC (resistant maltodextrin) to antibiotic-treated *db/db* mice (a model of type 2 diabetes), the improved glucose homeostatic phenotype was likewise transferred (199).

Work with GPR41 and GPR43 knockout (KO) mice, or their specific receptor antagonists, provides additional evidence that the NDFC-associated metabolic health effects described above are mediated by the GI microbiota and specifically through the production of SCFAs. For instance, the ability of SCFAs to stimulate insulin secretion through increased GLP-1 release (200, 201), promote satiety through enhanced PYY secretion (202), reduce systemic free fatty acid levels (161), or regulate blood pressure (203) is lost in GPR41 and/or GPR43 KO mice. Moreover, the combination of GPR41 KO mice with a model of allergic asthma showed that the production of SCFAs was essential for NDFCs to protect against allergic airway inflammation, which occurred by impairing the ability of lung dendritic cells to promote allergen-reactive Th2 responses (188). A similarly designed study compared the effect of guar gum, a viscous NDFC, in wild-type, GPR43 KO, and GPR109A KO mice treated with dextran sulfate sodium, which induces colitis. The study showed that signaling through GPR43 and GPR109A was essential for the NDFC to protect against the development of colitis (204).

Although these animal studies do illustrate a clear causative link between NDFCs, host health, and GI microbiota composition and function (e.g., SCFAs), knowledge of the exact role of the GI microbiota in the health effects of NDFCs remains incomplete. One experimental approach by which this could be resolved is through the comparison of the physiological effects of NDFCs in conventionalized and germfree animals (28). However, germfree animals are not without limitations since there are important physiological features that differ from their conventional counterparts, including an immune system that is not fully developed (205, 206). Furthermore, the pathological progression of CNCD-like symptoms in several animal models is often vastly different under germfree conditions, preventing direct comparison between germfree and conventional animals (207, 208). To address these limitations, one could alternatively test if the phenotypic effects of NDFCs are able to be transferred through cohousing or fecal microbial transfers. This is based on the premise that if the beneficial effect of the NDFC is caused by a shift in the microbiome, then the same beneficial effect should be seen in the recipient animal (28).

In humans, most microbiota-associated CNCDs are also linked to a low intake of dietary NDFCs, with a substantial degree of overlap between the two (Fig. 1). This suggests that NDFCs may prevent CNCDs through modulation of the GI microbiome (209). Epidemiological studies have established convincing associations between dietary fiber intake and health (149, 150, 210), and although findings from human intervention studies are less consistent (210), health claims have been approved for dietary fibers (cancer and cardiovascular disease) (211) and prebiotics (constipation) (212).

Moreover, multiple human intervention studies have been conducted that assess the effect of NDFCs on well-defined clinical outcomes while also characterizing the microbiome for compositional and functional signatures that correlate with these health outcomes (37, 52, 98, 213–216). For instance, treatment with the prebiotic inulin led to an increase in both *Bifidobacterium* and *Faecalibacterium prausnitzii*, which was inversely correlated with serum LPS levels, indicating that the prebiotic enhanced GI barrier function through modulating the GI microbiota (52). Furthermore, systematic meta-analyses have shown that prebiotic supplementation is capable of restoring bowel function (217), while also reversing multiple metabolic abnormalities associated with CNCDs, including reducing fasting insulin, triglycerides, and low-density lipoprotein cholesterol levels (146, 148, 218, 219). Supplementation with lupin kernel fiber, a viscous NDFC, also led to a significant reduction in low-density lipoprotein cholesterol levels, and this response was inversely correlated with the fecal excretion of SCFAs (220). Although these studies do detect microbial signatures that closely correlate with clinical outcomes of NDFC supplementation, they do not provide direct evidence for a causative role of the GI microbiota (28, 221).

Still, some studies have been conducted that do indicate a causative link between the GI microbiota and NDFCs. Work from Fredrik Bäckhed's group paired a human study with a humanized germfree mouse model to demonstrate that improved glucose metabolism due to whole-grain barley intake was dependent on the presence of *Prevotella copri* within the participant's GI tract (222). Furthermore, by providing SCFAs directly through colonic infusions, studies have demonstrated that SCFAs do promote a systematic increase in PYY and GLP-1, while also benefiting markers of inflammation (223, 224).

Clinical research that establishes clear connections between the health benefits of NDFCs and the GI microbiota, as well as clear evidence for the role of the GI microbiota in the health effects of NDFCs, including the underlying mechanisms involved, is altogether limited. As described above, NDFCs can exert health benefits through microbiota-independent mechanisms such as a reduction in nutrient absorption through viscosity or binding of bile acids and cholesterol (73). This clearly illustrates a need for future studies that pair rigorously designed human studies with animal models, because this would constitute a unique tool to assess causation in humans (209, 222).

FUTURE DIRECTIONS

Assessing the Clinical Efficacy of NDFCs and the Role of the GI Microbiome

Until now, most of the clinical evaluation of NDFCs has occurred through one-sided studies that solely assess either the GI microbiome or the host while completely overlooking the other (59, 225). Clinical research is needed that assesses the effect of NDFCs in rigorously designed randomized controlled trials with relevant clinical endpoints and a parallel characterization of the role of the GI microbiota in these effects. Doing so would require close collaborations between nutritionally and microbiologically focused research groups to facilitate truly interdisciplinary research.

Despite clear evidence of the benefits of NDFCs from epidemiological studies, results from human intervention studies remain inconsistent (210). These inconsistencies could stem from a variety of reasons. Most of the dietary fiber assessed in epidemiological studies is derived from whole foods (fruits, vegetables, and whole grains), in which the NDFCs are consumed intact within a food matrix that also includes components such as phytochemicals and bioactive lipids (226). These bioactive compounds are likely to act synergistically within the food matrix (227, 228), and once purified to be used as a supplement, the health effects of the NDFC might be lost or reduced (229). However, purified fibers and prebiotics, as well as their fermentation products (SCFAs), have been repeatedly shown to be beneficial in mouse models (209). The variability in human intervention studies could arise from both the highly inter-individualized nature of the human GI microbiome (53, 55, 60) and the variability in the host's metabolic response to NDFCs (39, 222). These two factors are inherently higher in humans, because mouse colonies are often composed of inbred mice housed in a highly standardized environment and are fed homogeneous diets. Given that the GI microbiotas of human subjects differ in the degree by which they are able to utilize specific NDFCs (75, 76), inter-individual variation is likely to be more pronounced in studies using a single purified substrate instead of a mixture of substrates or a whole food containing multiple fiber chemistries. In this respect, studies should characterize the chemical structure of the NDFCs to establish structure-function relationships between NDFC-chemistry and GI microbiome gene content, because this could be used to personalize approaches (24).

What is needed are human intervention studies with clinical endpoints that compare single NDFCs and their mixtures to those effects observed from whole foods, while also including a multi-omics approach for the analysis of the GI microbiome. Metagenomic analyses can identify specific shifts in GI microbiome composition and structure (e.g., diversity) that correlate with health outcomes. Such shifts, if they exist, would suggest that health benefits are due to selective changes of the GI microbiota in accordance with the original prebiotic concept (30). However, such studies should also include predictive modeling to determine how inter-individual differences in microbiome composition and functional capacity impact clinical outcomes. These studies could provide an explanation for the high variation observed in intervention studies with NDFCs and would establish a basis for personalized NDFC applications.

Pairing this approach with a metabolomic analysis can further identify the compounds that are associated with health outcomes, which could range from microbial metabolites that originate from the fermentation of NDFCs to phytochemicals and their metabolic derivatives. Research has shown that phytochemicals present in fruits, vegetables, whole grains, and many fiber extracts are also metabolically transformed by the GI microbiota and absorbed by the host, correlating with health benefits (230).

Considering that the human-microbiota symbiosis evolved with a supply of NDCs beyond 100 g/day, future human intervention studies should clearly be performed with more physiologically relevant doses (14). Supplementation of 10 to 15 grams in intervention studies ensures that participants meet current dietary fiber recommendations of around 30 g/day (26), but this intake is still far below that of our ancestors (12, 14), potentially hindering the opportunity to detect evolutionary routed interrelationships between NDFCs, the GI microbiota, and health. Although experiments in nonindustrialized populations are clearly confounded by the possibility that specific fiber-degrading bacteria have been lost (16, 23), human studies that used NDC doses greater than 50 g/day did detect health benefits through the assessment of CNCD markers. For instance, by switching African Americans over to a more traditional South African diet that consisted of 55 g/day of NDCs, markers of colon cancer were improved in only 2 weeks (231). Furthermore, following a 2-week dietary intervention that resembled an ancestral diet, with around 143 g/d of NDCs provided as green leafy vegetables, fruit, and nuts, a 25% reduction in total cholesterol was observed, which is a response comparable to cholesterol-lowering medications (232, 233). These studies clearly provide a rationale for the use of higher doses of fiber in clinical research.

The approach described in this paragraph would ultimately help to identify putative mechanisms by which NDFCs exert their health effects, which would allow the formation of hypotheses that would inform the design of clinical studies and assist in the development of dietary strategies and targeted applications of NDFCs to improve human health.

Elucidating the Exact Mechanisms

Although well-conducted human studies with clinical endpoints would be sufficient to establish efficiency of NDFCs and obtain health claims for dietary fibers or prebiotics (28, 234), it is important to point out that such research would establish only correlations and not causation. Correlations can be misleading, because directionality cannot be established, especially since host parameters altered through NDFCs (e.g., inflammation, metabolic outcomes) can in themselves have an effect on the GI microbiota (235, 236). In addition, intake of RS has clearly established that the health effects of an NDFC can be completely independent of the GI microbiota, even though clear correlations between diet-induced shifts in the microbiome and host markers exist (237).

In this respect, it is important to consider that human studies have unavoidable limitations when it comes to establishing mechanisms, because the health effects of NDFCs can be completely microbiota-independent. For example, NDCs increase fecal bulk and decrease colonic transit time (238), which in turn influences GI microbiota composition (239). Ingestion of viscous NDCs may also increase the viscosity of digesta, interrupting the rate of nutrient absorption and ultimately promoting an improvement in clinical markers, especially postprandial glycemic response (240, 241). Furthermore, NDCs sequester compounds such as sterols, bile acids, and carcinogens (242–244), inhibiting their absorbance and enhancing their excretion. Modulation of the bile acid pool alone may have systemic implications for glucose and lipid metabolism, as well as systemic inflammation through action on the farnesoid X

receptor and the GPR TGR5 (245). These microbiota-independent mechanisms can be difficult to distinguish from microbiota-dependent mechanisms, especially because they still might lead to strong correlations between diet-induced shifts in microbiome composition and host markers (237).

Elucidation of the role of the GI microbiota in the health effects of NDFCs and the underlying mechanisms will require innovative experimental approaches such as utilizing animal studies in parallel with human intervention studies to directly test the role of the GI microbiota in health outcomes (209, 222). Although establishing the contribution of the GI microbiota in the health outcomes of an NDFC would in theory be required to establish its prebiotic action, such studies would be extremely difficult and costly, and probably an unrealistic demand for the purpose of defining if an NDFC qualifies as a prebiotic. Therefore, despite the limitations discussed above, the establishment of correlations between the microbiome features and health benefits of an NDFC should probably be considered sufficient from a practical standpoint to establish which NDFCs constitute prebiotics (28). Establishing the causal role of the GI microbiota and the underlying mechanisms would remain essential information for the development of improved nutritional strategies. Only an in-depth mechanistic understanding will allow for the selection of NDFCs, or mixtures thereof, to systematically target specific features of the GI microbiome (i.e., specific taxa, diversity, metabolites) with the goal of correcting both immunometabolic abnormalities and dysbiotic features that underlie CNCDs.

CONCLUSION

The human diet has clearly changed over the last millennia, resulting in diminished potential to support our GI microbial community with growth substrates due to the dramatic reduction in the intake of NDFCs to a mere fraction of what was present in the diet of our ancestors (14). Evidence points to this "fiber gap" as being one prominent driving force behind the increased prevalence of CNCDs (13, 26). Although increased consumption of NDFC-rich whole foods such as fruits, vegetables, and whole grains is preferable from a nutritional perspective, efforts to increase their consumption have been ineffective to date, because dietary fiber levels remain low despite substantial efforts from nutritional agencies (25). Humans resist long-term changes of their dietary habits (246), illustrating a need for NDFC sources that can readily enrich the standard western diet (12). A broad array of NDFCs, which have vast potential to enhance the food supply, already exist on the market; however, product development and consumer research, in combination with clinical research, is needed to determine practical and cost-effective means by which these NDFCs can be incorporated into the food supply (12).

We know that there is a high degree of inter-individual variation in GI microbial response to NDFCs (53, 55, 60), and we have the tool set available to determine to what degree this individuality affects health outcomes in clinical studies (39). This essential knowledge would ultimately support the development of a framework by which interventions with NDFCs could be personalized. This ensures tremendous potential for growth within this field, promising exciting new developments as the focus of human nutrition shifts toward targeted nourishment of our symbiotic microbial communities as a way of preventing and treating CNCDs through supplementation with NDFCs.

CITATION

Deehan EC, Duar RM, Armet AM, Perez-Muñoz ME, Jin M, Walter J. 2017. Modulation of the gastrointestinal microbiome with nondigestible fermentable carbohydrates to improve human health. Microbiol Spectrum 5(5):BAD-0019-2017.

REFERENCES

1. **Walter J, Ley R.** 2011. The human gut microbiome: ecology and recent evolutionary changes. *Annu Rev Microbiol* **65:**411–429.
2. **Schroeder BO, Bäckhed F.** 2016. Signals from the gut microbiota to distant organs in physiology and disease. *Nat Med* **22:**1079–1089.
3. **Walker AW, Lawley TD.** 2013. Therapeutic modulation of intestinal dysbiosis. *Pharmacol Res* **69:**75–86.
4. **Brahe LK, Astrup A, Larsen LH.** 2016. Can we prevent obesity-related metabolic diseases by dietary modulation of the gut microbiota? *Adv Nutr* **7:**90–101.
5. **Olle B.** 2013. Medicines from microbiota. *Nat Biotechnol* **31:**309–315.
6. **David LA, Maurice CF, Carmody RN, Gootenberg DB, Button JE, Wolfe BE, Ling AV, Devlin AS, Varma Y, Fischbach MA, Biddinger SB, Dutton RJ, Turnbaugh PJ.** 2014. Diet rapidly and reproducibly alters the human gut microbiome. *Nature* **505:**559–563.
7. **Wu GD, Chen J, Hoffmann C, Bittinger K, Chen Y-Y, Keilbaugh SA, Bewtra M, Knights D, Walters WA, Knight R, Sinha R, Gilroy E, Gupta K, Baldassano R, Nessel L, Li H, Bushman FD, Lewis JD.** 2011. Linking long-term dietary patterns with gut microbial enterotypes. *Science* **334:**105–108.
8. **Wu GD, Compher C, Chen EZ, Smith SA, Shah RD, Bittinger K, Chehoud C, Albenberg LG, Nessel L, Gilroy E, Star J, Weljie AM, Flint HJ, Metz DC, Bennett MJ, Li H, Bushman FD, Lewis JD.** 2016. Comparative metabolomics in vegans and omnivores reveal constraints on diet-dependent gut microbiota metabolite production. *Gut* **65:**63–72.
9. **Gibson GR, Roberfroid MB.** 1995. Dietary modulation of the human colonic microbiota: introducing the concept of prebiotics. *J Nutr* **125:**1401–1412.
10. **Bach J-F.** 2002. The effect of infections on susceptibility to autoimmune and allergic diseases. *N Engl J Med* **347:**911–920.
11. **Bickler SW, DeMaio A.** 2008. Western diseases: current concepts and implications for pediatric surgery research and practice. *Pediatr Surg Int* **24:**251–255.
12. **Deehan EC, Walter J.** 2016. The fiber gap and the disappearing gut microbiome: implications for human nutrition. *Trends Endocrinol Metab* **27:**239–242.
13. **Burkitt DP, Walker ARP, Painter NS.** 1974. Dietary fiber and disease. *JAMA* **229:**1068–1074.
14. **Eaton SB, Eaton SB III, Konner MJ.** 1997. Paleolithic nutrition revisited: a twelve-year

retrospective on its nature and implications. *Eur J Clin Nutr* **51**:207–216.

15. **Burkitt DP.** 1973. Some diseases characteristic of modern Western civilization. *BMJ* **1**:274–278.

16. **Sonnenburg ED, Sonnenburg JL.** 2014. Starving our microbial self: the deleterious consequences of a diet deficient in microbiota-accessible carbohydrates. *Cell Metab* **20**:779–786.

17. **Koh A, De Vadder F, Kovatcheva-Datchary P, Bäckhed F.** 2016. From dietary fiber to host physiology: short-chain fatty acids as key bacterial metabolites. *Cell* **165**:1332–1345.

18. **Martínez I, Stegen JC, Maldonado-Gómez MX, Eren AM, Siba PM, Greenhill AR, Walter J.** 2015. The gut microbiota of rural Papua New Guineans: composition, diversity patterns, and ecological processes. *Cell Reports* **11**:527–538.

19. **Schnorr SL, Candela M, Rampelli S, Centanni M, Consolandi C, Basaglia G, Turroni S, Biagi E, Peano C, Severgnini M, Fiori J, Gotti R, De Bellis G, Luiselli D, Brigidi P, Mabulla A, Marlowe F, Henry AG, Crittenden AN.** 2014. Gut microbiome of the Hadza hunter-gatherers. *Nat Commun* **5**:3654.

20. **Clemente JC, Pehrsson EC, Blaser MJ, Sandhu K, Gao Z, Wang B, Magris M, Hidalgo G, Contreras M, Noya-Alarcón Ó, Lander O, McDonald J, Cox M, Walter J, Oh PL, Ruiz JF, Rodriguez S, Shen N, Song SJ, Metcalf J, Knight R, Dantas G, Dominguez-Bello MG.** 2015. The microbiome of uncontacted Amerindians. *Sci Adv* **1**:e1500183.

21. **Yatsunenko T, Rey FE, Manary MJ, Trehan I, Dominguez-Bello MG, Contreras M, Magris M, Hidalgo G, Baldassano RN, Anokhin AP, Heath AC, Warner B, Reeder J, Kuczynski J, Caporaso JG, Lozupone CA, Lauber C, Clemente JC, Knights D, Knight R, Gordon JI.** 2012. Human gut microbiome viewed across age and geography. *Nature* **486**:222–227.

22. **De Filippo C, Cavalieri D, Di Paola M, Ramazzotti M, Poullet JB, Massart S, Collini S, Pieraccini G, Lionetti P.** 2010. Impact of diet in shaping gut microbiota revealed by a comparative study in children from Europe and rural Africa. *Proc Natl Acad Sci USA* **107**:14691–14696.

23. **Sonnenburg ED, Smits SA, Tikhonov M, Higginbottom SK, Wingreen NS, Sonnenburg JL.** 2016. Diet-induced extinctions in the gut microbiota compound over generations. *Nature* **529**:212–215.

24. **Hamaker BR, Tuncil YE.** 2014. A perspective on the complexity of dietary fiber structures and their potential effect on the gut microbiota. *J Mol Biol* **426**:3838–3850.

25. **King DE, Mainous AG III, Lambourne CA.** 2012. Trends in dietary fiber intake in the United States, 1999–2008. *J Acad Nutr Diet* **112**:642–648.

26. **Jones JM.** 2014. CODEX-aligned dietary fiber definitions help to bridge the 'fiber gap'. *Nutr J* **13**:34.

27. **Hill DR, Newburg DS.** 2015. Clinical applications of bioactive milk components. *Nutr Rev* **73**:463–476.

28. **Bindels LB, Delzenne NM, Cani PD, Walter J.** 2015. Towards a more comprehensive concept for prebiotics. *Nat Rev Gastroenterol Hepatol* **12**:303–310.

29. **Gibson GR, Hutkins R, Sanders ME, Prescott SL, Reimer RA, Salminen SJ, Scott K, Stanton C, Swanson KS, Cani PD, Verbeke K, Reid G.** 2017. Expert consensus document: the International Scientific Association for Probiotics and Prebiotics (ISAPP) consensus statement on the definition and scope of prebiotics. *Nat Rev Gastroenterol Hepatol* **14**:491–502.

30. **Gibson GR, Scott KP, Rastall RA, Tuohy KM, Hotchkiss A, Dubert-Ferrandon A, Gareau M, Murphy EF, Saulnier D, Loh G, Macfarlane S, Delzenne N, Ringel Y, Kozianowski G, Dickmann R, Lenoir-Wijnkoop I, Walker C, Buddington R.** 2010. Dietary prebiotics: current status and new definition. *Food Sci Tech Bull Funct Foods* **7**:1–19.

31. **Roberfroid M.** 2007. Prebiotics: the concept revisited. *J Nutr* **137**(Suppl 2):830S–837S.

32. **Katsnelson A.** 2016. Core concept: prebiotics gain prominence but remain poorly defined. *Proc Natl Acad Sci USA* **113**:14168–14169.

33. **Verspreet J, Damen B, Broekaert WF, Verbeke K, Delcour JA, Courtin CM.** 2016. A critical look at prebiotics within the dietary fiber concept. *Annu Rev Food Sci Technol* **7**:167–190.

34. **Suez J, Elinav E.** 2017. The path towards microbiome-based metabolite treatment. *Nat Microbiol* **2**:17075.

35. **Shanahan F.** 2015. Fiber man meets microbial man. *Am J Clin Nutr* **101**:1–2.

36. **Louis P, Flint HJ, Michel C.** 2016. How to manipulate the microbiota: prebiotics. *Adv Exp Med Biol* **902**:119–142.

37. **Martínez I, Lattimer JM, Hubach KL, Case JA, Yang J, Weber CG, Louk JA, Rose DJ, Kyureghian G, Peterson DA, Haub MD, Walter J.** 2013. Gut microbiome composition is linked to whole grain-induced immunological improvements. *ISME J* **7**:269–280.

38. **Quévrain E, Maubert M-A, Michon C, Chain F, Marquant R, Tailhades J, Miquel S, Carlier L, Bermúdez-Humarán LG, Pigneur B, Lequin O, Kharrat P, Thomas G, Rainteau**

D, Aubry C, Breyner N, Afonso C, Lavielle S, Grill JP, Chassaing G, Chatel J-M, Trugnan G, Xavier R, Langella P, Sokol H, Seksik P. 2016. Identification of an anti-inflammatory protein from *Faecalibacterium prausnitzii*, a commensal bacterium deficient in Crohn's disease. *Gut* **65**:415–425.

39. Zeevi D, Korem T, Zmora N, Israeli D, Rothschild D, Weinberger A, Ben-Yacov O, Lador D, Avnit-Sagi T, Lotan-Pompan M, Suez J, Mahdi JA, Matot E, Malka G, Kosower N, Rein M, Zilberman-Schapira G, Dohnalová L, Pevsner-Fischer M, Bikovsky R, Halpern Z, Elinav E, Segal E. 2015. Personalized nutrition by prediction of glycemic responses. *Cell* **163**:1079–1094.

40. Everard A, Belzer C, Geurts L, Ouwerkerk JP, Druart C, Bindels LB, Guiot Y, Derrien M, Muccioli GG, Delzenne NM, de Vos WM, Cani PD. 2013. Cross-talk between *Akkermansia muciniphila* and intestinal epithelium controls diet-induced obesity. *Proc Natl Acad Sci USA* **110**:9066–9071.

41. Atarashi K, Tanoue T, Oshima K, Suda W, Nagano Y, Nishikawa H, Fukuda S, Saito T, Narushima S, Hase K, Kim S, Fritz JV, Wilmes P, Ueha S, Matsushima K, Ohno H, Olle B, Sakaguchi S, Taniguchi T, Morita H, Hattori M, Honda K. 2013. Treg induction by a rationally selected mixture of *Clostridia* strains from the human microbiota. *Nature* **500**:232–236.

42. Round JL, Lee SM, Li J, Tran G, Jabri B, Chatila TA, Mazmanian SK. 2011. The Toll-like receptor 2 pathway establishes colonization by a commensal of the human microbiota. *Science* **332**:974–977.

43. Le Chatelier E, et al, MetaHIT Consortium. 2013. Richness of human gut microbiome correlates with metabolic markers. *Nature* **500:** 541–546.

44. Cotillard A, Kennedy SP, Kong LC, Prifti E, Pons N, Le Chatelier E, Almeida M, Quinquis B, Levenez F, Galleron N, Gougis S, Rizkalla S, Batto J-M, Renault P, Doré J, Zucker JD, Clément K, Ehrlich SD, ANR MicroObes Consortium. 2013. Dietary intervention impact on gut microbial gene richness. *Nature* **500**:585–588.

45. Lozupone CA, Stombaugh JI, Gordon JI, Jansson JK, Knight R. 2012. Diversity, stability and resilience of the human gut microbiota. *Nature* **489**:220–230.

46. LeBlanc JG, Chain F, Martín R, Bermúdez-Humarán LG, Courau S, Langella P. 2017. Beneficial effects on host energy metabolism of short-chain fatty acids and vitamins produced by commensal and probiotic bacteria. *Microb Cell Fact* **16**:79.

47. Canfora EE, Jocken JW, Blaak EE. 2015. Short-chain fatty acids in control of body weight and insulin sensitivity. *Nat Rev Endocrinol* **11**:577–591.

48. Zheng J, Ruan L, Sun M, Gänzle M. 2015. A genomic view of lactobacilli and pediococci demonstrates that phylogeny matches ecology and physiology. *Appl Environ Microbiol* **81**:7233–7243.

49. Makras L, Falony G, Van der Meulen R, De Vuyst L. 2006. Letter to the editor. *J Appl Microbiol* **100**:1388–1389.

50. Klijn A, Mercenier A, Arigoni F. 2005. Lessons from the genomes of bifidobacteria. *FEMS Microbiol Rev* **29**:491–509.

51. Flint HJ, Duncan SH, Scott KP, Louis P. 2015. Links between diet, gut microbiota composition and gut metabolism. *Proc Nutr Soc* **74**:13–22.

52. Dewulf EM, Cani PD, Claus SP, Fuentes S, Puylaert PGB, Neyrinck AM, Bindels LB, de Vos WM, Gibson GR, Thissen J-P, Delzenne NM. 2013. Insight into the prebiotic concept: lessons from an exploratory, double blind intervention study with inulin-type fructans in obese women. *Gut* **62**:1112–1121.

53. Venkataraman A, Sieber JR, Schmidt AW, Waldron C, Theis KR, Schmidt TM. 2016. Variable responses of human microbiomes to dietary supplementation with resistant starch. *Microbiome* **4**:33.

54. Walker AW, Ince J, Duncan SH, Webster LM, Holtrop G, Ze X, Brown D, Stares MD, Scott P, Bergerat A, Louis P, McIntosh F, Johnstone AM, Lobley GE, Parkhill J, Flint HJ. 2011. Dominant and diet-responsive groups of bacteria within the human colonic microbiota. *ISME J* **5**:220–230.

55. Martínez I, Kim J, Duffy PR, Schlegel VL, Walter J. 2010. Resistant starches types 2 and 4 have differential effects on the composition of the fecal microbiota in human subjects. *PLoS One* **5**:e15046.

56. El Kaoutari A, Armougom F, Gordon JI, Raoult D, Henrissat B. 2013. The abundance and variety of carbohydrate-active enzymes in the human gut microbiota. *Nat Rev Microbiol* **11**:497–504.

57. Flint HJ, Bayer EA, Rincon MT, Lamed R, White BA. 2008. Polysaccharide utilization by gut bacteria: potential for new insights from genomic analysis. *Nat Rev Microbiol* **6**:121–131.

58. Chung WSF, Walker AW, Louis P, Parkhill J, Vermeiren J, Bosscher D, Duncan SH, Flint HJ. 2016. Modulation of the human gut

microbiota by dietary fibres occurs at the species level. *BMC Biol* **14:**3.

59. **Sawicki CM, Livingston KA, Obin M, Roberts SB, Chung M, McKeown NM.** 2017. Dietary fiber and the human gut microbiota: application of evidence mapping methodology. *Nutrients* **9:**125.

60. **Davis LMG, Martínez I, Walter J, Goin C, Hutkins RW.** 2011. Barcoded pyrosequencing reveals that consumption of galactooligosaccharides results in a highly specific bifidogenic response in humans. *PLoS One* **6:**e25200.

61. **Walker AW, Duncan SH, McWilliam Leitch EC, Child MW, Flint HJ.** 2005. pH and peptide supply can radically alter bacterial populations and short-chain fatty acid ratios within microbial communities from the human colon. *Appl Environ Microbiol* **71:**3692–3700.

62. **Duncan SH, Louis P, Thomson JM, Flint HJ.** 2009. The role of pH in determining the species composition of the human colonic microbiota. *Environ Microbiol* **11:**2112–2122.

63. **Tannock GW, Lawley B, Munro K, Sims IM, Lee J, Butts CA, Roy N.** 2014. RNA-stable-isotope probing shows utilization of carbon from inulin by specific bacterial populations in the rat large bowel. *Appl Environ Microbiol* **80:**2240–2247.

64. **Holscher HD.** 2017. Dietary fiber and prebiotics and the gastrointestinal microbiota. *Gut Microbes* **8:**172–184.

65. **Slavin J.** 2013. Fiber and prebiotics: mechanisms and health benefits. *Nutrients* **5:**1417–1435.

66. **Hipsley EH.** 1953. Dietary "fibre" and pregnancy toxaemia. *BMJ* **2:**420–422.

67. **Trowell HC.** 1974. Editorial: definitions of dietary fibre. *Lancet* **1:**503.

68. **Joint FAO/WHO Food Standards Programme.** 2010. *Secretariat of the CODEX Alimentarius Commission: CODEX Alimentarius (CODEX) guidelines on nutrition labeling CAC/GL 2-1985 as last amended 2010.* FAO, Rome, Italy.

69. **Food and Drug Administration.** 2016. *Food Labeling: Revision of the Nutrition and Supplement Facts Labels. Report no. RIN 0910-AF22.* FDA, College Park, MD.

70. **Fuller S, Beck E, Salman H, Tapsell L.** 2016. New horizons for the study of dietary fiber and health: a review. *Plant Foods Hum Nutr* **71:**1–12.

71. **Tungland BC, Meyer D.** 2002. Nondigestible oligo- and polysaccharides (dietary fiber): their physiology and role in human health and food. *Compr Rev Food Sci Food Saf* **1:**90–109.

72. **Raigond P, Ezekiel R, Raigond B.** 2015. Resistant starch in food: a review. *J Sci Food Agric* **95:**1968–1978.

73. **Mudgil D, Barak S.** 2013. Composition, properties and health benefits of indigestible carbohydrate polymers as dietary fiber: a review. *Int J Biol Macromol* **61:**1–6.

74. **Guillona F, Champ M.** 2000. Structural and physical properties of dietary fibres, and consequences of processing on human physiology. *Food Res Int* **33:**233–245.

75. **Ze X, Duncan SH, Louis P, Flint HJ.** 2012. *Ruminococcus bromii* is a keystone species for the degradation of resistant starch in the human colon. *ISME J* **6:**1535–1543.

76. **Hehemann J-H, Correc G, Barbeyron T, Helbert W, Czjzek M, Michel G.** 2010. Transfer of carbohydrate-active enzymes from marine bacteria to Japanese gut microbiota. *Nature* **464:**908–912.

77. **Chassard C, Delmas E, Robert C, Bernalier-Donadille A.** 2010. The cellulose-degrading microbial community of the human gut varies according to the presence or absence of methanogens. *FEMS Microbiol Ecol* **74:**205–213.

78. **Walter J.** 2015. Murine gut microbiota-diet trumps genes. *Cell Host Microbe* **17:**3–5.

79. **Kovatcheva-Datchary P, Egert M, Maathuis A, Rajilić-Stojanović M, de Graaf AA, Smidt H, de Vos WM, Venema K.** 2009. Linking phylogenetic identities of bacteria to starch fermentation in an *in vitro* model of the large intestine by RNA-based stable isotope probing. *Environ Microbiol* **11:**914–926.

80. **Leitch ECM, Walker AW, Duncan SH, Holtrop G, Flint HJ.** 2007. Selective colonization of insoluble substrates by human faecal bacteria. *Environ Microbiol* **9:**667–679.

81. **Rakoff-Nahoum S, Coyne MJ, Comstock LE.** 2014. An ecological network of polysaccharide utilization among human intestinal symbionts. *Curr Biol* **24:**40–49.

82. **Flint HJ, Scott KP, Duncan SH, Louis P, Forano E.** 2012. Microbial degradation of complex carbohydrates in the gut. *Gut Microbes* **3:**289–306.

83. **Belenguer A, Duncan SH, Calder AG, Holtrop G, Louis P, Lobley GE, Flint HJ.** 2006. Two routes of metabolic cross-feeding between *Bifidobacterium adolescentis* and butyrate-producing anaerobes from the human gut. *Appl Environ Microbiol* **72:**3593–3599.

84. **Coyte KZ, Schluter J, Foster KR.** 2015. The ecology of the microbiome: networks, competition, and stability. *Science* **350:**663–666.

85. **Koropatkin NM, Cameron EA, Martens EC.** 2012. How glycan metabolism shapes the human gut microbiota. *Nat Rev Microbiol* **10:**323–335.

86. **Rey FE, Faith JJ, Bain J, Muehlbauer MJ, Stevens RD, Newgard CB, Gordon JI.** 2010.

Dissecting the *in vivo* metabolic potential of two human gut acetogens. *J Biol Chem* **285:** 22082–22090.

87. **Fischbach MA, Sonnenburg JL.** 2011. Eating for two: how metabolism establishes interspecies interactions in the gut. *Cell Host Microbe* **10:**336–347.

88. **Barcenilla A, Pryde SE, Martin JC, Duncan SH, Stewart CS, Henderson C, Flint HJ.** 2000. Phylogenetic relationships of butyrate-producing bacteria from the human gut. *Appl Environ Microbiol* **66:**1654–1661.

89. **Chassard C, Bernalier-Donadille A.** 2006. H2 and acetate transfers during xylan fermentation between a butyrate-producing xylanolytic species and hydrogenotrophic microorganisms from the human gut. *FEMS Microbiol Lett* **254:**116–122.

90. **Duncan SH, Louis P, Flint HJ.** 2004. Lactate-utilizing bacteria, isolated from human feces, that produce butyrate as a major fermentation product. *Appl Environ Microbiol* **70:**5810–5817.

91. **Lozupone CA, Hamady M, Cantarel BL, Coutinho PM, Henrissat B, Gordon JI, Knight R.** 2008. The convergence of carbohydrate active gene repertoires in human gut microbes. *Proc Natl Acad Sci USA* **105:**15076–15081.

92. **Vandeputte D, Falony G, Vieira-Silva S, Wang J, Sailer M, Theis S, Verbeke K, Raes J.** 2017. Prebiotic inulin-type fructans induce specific changes in the human gut microbiota. *Gut.* [Epub ahead of print.]

93. **Tap J, Furet J-P, Bensaada M, Philippe C, Roth H, Rabot S, Lakhdari O, Lombard V, Henrissat B, Corthier G, Fontaine E, Doré J, Leclerc M.** 2015. Gut microbiota richness promotes its stability upon increased dietary fibre intake in healthy adults. *Environ Microbiol* **17:**4954–4964.

94. **Segata N.** 2015. Gut microbiome: westernization and the disappearance of intestinal diversity. *Curr Biol* **25:**R611–R613.

95. **Heiman ML, Greenway FL.** 2016. A healthy gastrointestinal microbiome is dependent on dietary diversity. *Mol Metab* **5:**317–320.

96. **Clayton JB, Vangay P, Huang H, Ward T, Hillmann BM, Al-Ghalith GA, Travis DA, Long HT, Tuan BV, Minh VV, Cabana F, Nadler T, Toddes B, Murphy T, Glander KE, Johnson TJ, Knights D.** 2016. Captivity humanizes the primate microbiome. *Proc Natl Acad Sci USA* **113:**10376–10381.

97. **Kong LC, Holmes BA, Cotillard A, Habi-Rachedi F, Brazeilles R, Gougis S, Gausserès N, Cani PD, Fellahi S, Bastard J-P, Kennedy SP, Doré J, Ehrlich SD, Zucker J-D, Rizkalla SW, Clément K.** 2014. Dietary patterns differ-

ently associate with inflammation and gut microbiota in overweight and obese subjects. *PLoS One* **9:**e109434.

98. **Upadhyaya B, McCormack L, Fardin-Kia AR, Juenemann R, Nichenametla S, Clapper J, Specker B, Dey M.** 2016. Impact of dietary resistant starch type 4 on human gut microbiota and immunometabolic functions. *Sci Rep* **6:** 28797.

99. **West NP, Christophersen CT, Pyne DB, Cripps AW, Conlon MA, Topping DL, Kang S, McSweeney CS, Fricker PA, Aguirre D, Clarke JM.** 2013. Butyrylated starch increases colonic butyrate concentration but has limited effects on immunity in healthy physically active individuals. *Exerc Immunol Rev* **19:**102–119.

100. **Hooda S, Boler BMV, Serao MCR, Brulc JM, Staeger MA, Boileau TW, Dowd SE, Fahey GCJ Jr, Swanson KS.** 2012. 454 pyrosequencing reveals a shift in fecal microbiota of healthy adult men consuming polydextrose or soluble corn fiber. *J Nutr* **142:**1259–1265.

101. **Wong JM, de Souza R, Kendall CW, Emam A, Jenkins DJ.** 2006. Colonic health: fermentation and short chain fatty acids. *J Clin Gastroenterol* **40:**235–243.

102. **Cummings JH, Pomare EW, Branch WJ, Naylor CP, Macfarlane GT.** 1987. Short chain fatty acids in human large intestine, portal, hepatic and venous blood. *Gut* **28:**1221–1227.

103. **Boets E, Gomand SV, Deroover L, Preston T, Vermeulen K, De Preter V, Hamer HM, Van den Mooter G, De Vuyst L, Courtin CM, Annaert P, Delcour JA, Verbeke KA.** 2017. Systemic availability and metabolism of colonic-derived short-chain fatty acids in healthy subjects: a stable isotope study. *J Physiol* **595:**541–555.

104. **Yang J, Martínez I, Walter J, Keshavarzian A, Rose DJ.** 2013. *In vitro* characterization of the impact of selected dietary fibers on fecal microbiota composition and short chain fatty acid production. *Anaerobe* **23:**74–81.

105. **Yang J, Rose DJ.** 2014. Long-term dietary pattern of fecal donor correlates with butyrate production and markers of protein fermentation during *in vitro* fecal fermentation. *Nutr Res* **34:**749–759.

106. **Roediger WE.** 1980. Role of anaerobic bacteria in the metabolic welfare of the colonic mucosa in man. *Gut* **21:**793–798.

107. **Dahl WJ, Stewart ML.** 2015. Position of the Academy of Nutrition and Dietetics: Health Implications of Dietary Fiber. *J Acad Nutr Diet* **115:**1861–1870.

108. **Cummings JH, Macfarlane GT.** 1991. The control and consequences of bacterial fer-

mentation in the human colon. *J Appl Bacteriol* **70**:443–459.

109. **Duncan SH, Belenguer A, Holtrop G, Johnstone AM, Flint HJ, Lobley GE.** 2007. Reduced dietary intake of carbohydrates by obese subjects results in decreased concentrations of butyrate and butyrate-producing bacteria in feces. *Appl Environ Microbiol* **73**:1073–1078.

110. **Russell WR, Gratz SW, Duncan SH, Holtrop G, Ince J, Scobbie L, Duncan G, Johnstone AM, Lobley GE, Wallace RJ, Duthie GG, Flint HJ.** 2011. High-protein, reduced-carbohydrate weight-loss diets promote metabolite profiles likely to be detrimental to colonic health. *Am J Clin Nutr* **93**:1062–1072.

111. **Windey K, De Preter V, Verbeke K.** 2012. Relevance of protein fermentation to gut health. *Mol Nutr Food Res* **56**:184–196.

112. **Sonnenburg JL, Xu J, Leip DD, Chen C-H, Westover BP, Weatherford J, Buhler JD, Gordon JI.** 2005. Glycan foraging *in vivo* by an intestine-adapted bacterial symbiont. *Science* **307**:1955–1959.

113. **Earle KA, Billings G, Sigal M, Lichtman JS, Hansson GC, Elias JE, Amieva MR, Huang KC, Sonnenburg JL.** 2015. Quantitative imaging of gut microbiota spatial organization. *Cell Host Microbe* **18**:478–488.

114. **Desai MS, Seekatz AM, Koropatkin NM, Kamada N, Hickey CA, Wolter M, Pudlo NA, Kitamoto S, Terrapon N, Muller A, Young VB, Henrissat B, Wilmes P, Stappenbeck TS, Núñez G, Martens EC.** 2016. A dietary fiber-deprived gut microbiota degrades the colonic mucus barrier and enhances pathogen susceptibility. *Cell* **167**:1339–1353.e21.

115. **Lambeau KV, McRorie JWJ Jr.** 2017. Fiber supplements and clinically proven health benefits: how to recognize and recommend an effective fiber therapy. *J Am Assoc Nurse Pract* **29**:216–223.

116. **Schwiertz A, Taras D, Schäfer K, Beijer S, Bos NA, Donus C, Hardt PD.** 2010. Microbiota and SCFA in lean and overweight healthy subjects. *Obesity (Silver Spring)* **18**:190–195.

117. **Belcheva A, Irrazabal T, Robertson SJ, Streutker C, Maughan H, Rubino S, Moriyama EH, Copeland JK, Kumar S, Green B, Geddes K, Pezo RC, Navarre WW, Milosevic M, Wilson BC, Girardin SE, Wolever TMS, Edelmann W, Guttman DS, Philpott DJ, Martin A.** 2014. Gut microbial metabolism drives transformation of MSH2-deficient colon epithelial cells. *Cell* **158**:288–299.

118. **Lupton JR.** 2004. Microbial degradation products influence colon cancer risk: the butyrate controversy. *J Nutr* **134**:479–482.

119. **Du H, van der A DL, Boshuizen HC, Forouhi NG, Wareham NJ, Halkjaer J, Tjønneland A, Overvad K, Jakobsen MU, Boeing H, Buijsse B, Masala G, Palli D, Sørensen TI, Saris WH, Feskens EJ.** 2010. Dietary fiber and subsequent changes in body weight and waist circumference in European men and women. *Am J Clin Nutr* **91**:329–336.

120. **Ben Q, Sun Y, Chai R, Qian A, Xu B, Yuan Y.** 2014. Dietary fiber intake reduces risk for colorectal adenoma: a meta-analysis. *Gastroenterology* **146**:689–699.e6.

121. **Kunzmann AT, Coleman HG, Huang W-Y, Kitahara CM, Cantwell MM, Berndt SI.** 2015. Dietary fiber intake and risk of colorectal cancer and incident and recurrent adenoma in the Prostate, Lung, Colorectal, and Ovarian Cancer Screening Trial. *Am J Clin Nutr* **102**:881–890.

122. **Tan J, McKenzie C, Potamitis M, Thorburn AN, Mackay CR, Macia L.** 2014. The role of short-chain fatty acids in health and disease. *Adv Immunol* **121**:91–119.

123. **Thangaraju M, Cresci GA, Liu K, Ananth S, Gnanaprakasam JP, Browning DD, Mellinger JD, Smith SB, Digby GJ, Lambert NA, Prasad PD, Ganapathy V.** 2009. GPR109A is a G-protein-coupled receptor for the bacterial fermentation product butyrate and functions as a tumor suppressor in colon. *Cancer Res* **69**:2826–2832.

124. **Wanders D, Graff EC, Judd RL.** 2012. Effects of high fat diet on GPR109A and GPR81 gene expression. *Biochem Biophys Res Commun* **425**:278–283.

125. **Cresci GA, Thangaraju M, Mellinger JD, Liu K, Ganapathy V.** 2010. Colonic gene expression in conventional and germfree mice with a focus on the butyrate receptor GPR109A and the butyrate transporter SLC5A8. *J Gastrointest Surg* **14**:449–461.

126. **Le Poul E, Loison C, Struyf S, Springael J-Y, Lannoy V, Decobecq M-E, Brezillon S, Dupriez V, Vassart G, Van Damme J, Parmentier M, Detheux M.** 2003. Functional characterization of human receptors for short chain fatty acids and their role in polymorphonuclear cell activation. *J Biol Chem* **278**:25481–25489.

127. **Brown AJ, Goldsworthy SM, Barnes AA, Eilert MM, Tcheang L, Daniels D, Muir AI, Wigglesworth MJ, Kinghorn I, Fraser NJ, Pike NB, Strum JC, Steplewski KM, Murdock PR, Holder JC, Marshall FH, Szekeres PG, Wilson S, Ignar DM, Foord SM, Wise A, Dowell SJ.** 2003. The Orphan G protein-coupled receptors GPR41 and GPR43 are activated by propionate and other short chain carboxylic acids. *J Biol Chem* **278**:11312–11319.

128. **Blundell J, de Graaf C, Hulshof T, Jebb S, Livingstone B, Lluch A, Mela D, Salah S, Schuring E, van der Knaap H, Westerterp M.** 2010. Appetite control: methodological aspects of the evaluation of foods. *Obes Rev* **11:**251–270.

129. **Samuel BS, Shaito A, Motoike T, Rey FE, Bäckhed F, Manchester JK, Hammer RE, Williams SC, Crowley J, Yanagisawa M, Gordon JI.** 2008. Effects of the gut microbiota on host adiposity are modulated by the short-chain fatty-acid binding G protein-coupled receptor, Gpr41. *Proc Natl Acad Sci USA* **105:** 16767–16772.

130. **Tolhurst G, Heffron H, Lam YS, Parker HE, Habib AM, Diakogiannaki E, Cameron J, Grosse J, Reimann F, Gribble FM.** 2012. Short-chain fatty acids stimulate glucagon-like peptide-1 secretion via the G-protein-coupled receptor FFAR2. *Diabetes* **61:**364–371.

131. **Savage AP, Adrian TE, Carolan G, Chatterjee VK, Bloom SR.** 1987. Effects of peptide YY (PYY) on mouth to caecum intestinal transit time and on the rate of gastric emptying in healthy volunteers. *Gut* **28:**166–170.

132. **Batterham RL, Cowley MA, Small CJ, Herzog H, Cohen MA, Dakin CL, Wren AM, Brynes AE, Low MJ, Ghatei MA, Cone RD, Bloom SR.** 2002. Gut hormone PYY(3-36) physiologically inhibits food intake. *Nature* **418:**650–654.

133. **Wei Y, Mojsov S.** 1995. Tissue-specific expression of the human receptor for glucagon-like peptide-I: brain, heart and pancreatic forms have the same deduced amino acid sequences. *FEBS Lett* **358:**219–224.

134. **Merchenthaler I, Lane M, Shughrue P.** 1999. Distribution of pre-pro-glucagon and glucagon-like peptide-1 receptor messenger RNAs in the rat central nervous system. *J Comp Neurol* **403:**261–280.

135. **Schjoldager BT, Mortensen PE, Christiansen J, Ørskov C, Holst JJ.** 1989. GLP-1 (glucagon-like peptide 1) and truncated GLP-1, fragments of human proglucagon, inhibit gastric acid secretion in humans. *Dig Dis Sci* **34:**703–708.

136. **Näslund E, Bogefors J, Skogar S, Grybäck P, Jacobsson H, Holst JJ, Hellström PM.** 1999. GLP-1 slows solid gastric emptying and inhibits insulin, glucagon, and PYY release in humans. *Am J Physiol* **277:**R910–R916.

137. **Xiong Y, Miyamoto N, Shibata K, Valasek MA, Motoike T, Kedzierski RM, Yanagisawa M.** 2004. Short-chain fatty acids stimulate leptin production in adipocytes through the G protein-coupled receptor GPR41. *Proc Natl Acad Sci USA* **101:**1045–1050.

138. **Zaibi MS, Stocker CJ, O'Dowd J, Davies A, Bellahcene M, Cawthorne MA, Brown AJH,** Smith DM, Arch JRS. 2010. Roles of GPR41 and GPR43 in leptin secretory responses of murine adipocytes to short chain fatty acids. *FEBS Lett* **584:**2381–2386.

139. **Frost G, Sleeth ML, Sahuri-Arisoylu M, Lizarbe B, Cerdan S, Brody L, Anastasovska J, Ghourab S, Hankir M, Zhang S, Carling D, Swann JR, Gibson G, Viardot A, Morrison D, Louise Thomas E, Bell JD.** 2014. The short-chain fatty acid acetate reduces appetite via a central homeostatic mechanism. *Nat Commun* **5:**3611.

140. **De Vadder F, Kovatcheva-Datchary P, Goncalves D, Vinera J, Zitoun C, Duchampt A, Bäckhed F, Mithieux G.** 2014. Microbiota-generated metabolites promote metabolic benefits via gut-brain neural circuits. *Cell* **156:**84–96.

141. **Delaere F, Duchampt A, Mounien L, Seyer P, Duraffourd C, Zitoun C, Thorens B, Mithieux G.** 2013. The role of sodium-coupled glucose co-transporter 3 in the satiety effect of portal glucose sensing. *Mol Metab* **2:**47–53.

142. **Kimura I, Inoue D, Maeda T, Hara T, Ichimura A, Miyauchi S, Kobayashi M, Hirasawa A, Tsujimoto G.** 2011. Short-chain fatty acids and ketones directly regulate sympathetic nervous system via G protein-coupled receptor 41 (GPR41). *Proc Natl Acad Sci USA* **108:**8030–8035.

143. **Gao Z, Yin J, Zhang J, Ward RE, Martin RJ, Lefevre M, Cefalu WT, Ye J.** 2009. Butyrate improves insulin sensitivity and increases energy expenditure in mice. *Diabetes* **58:**1509–1517.

144. **Freitag J, Berod L, Kamradt T, Sparwasser T.** 2016. Immunometabolism and autoimmunity. *Immunol Cell Biol* **94:**925–934.

145. **Hajer GR, van Haeften TW, Visseren FLJ.** 2008. Adipose tissue dysfunction in obesity, diabetes, and vascular diseases. *Eur Heart J* **29:**2959–2971.

146. **Kellow NJ, Coughlan MT, Reid CM.** 2014. Metabolic benefits of dietary prebiotics in human subjects: a systematic review of randomised controlled trials. *Br J Nutr* **111:**1147–1161.

147. **Whitehead A, Beck EJ, Tosh S, Wolever TMS.** 2014. Cholesterol-lowering effects of oat β-glucan: a meta-analysis of randomized controlled trials. *Am J Clin Nutr* **100:**1413–1421.

148. **Beserra BTS, Fernandes R, do Rosario VA, Mocellin MC, Kuntz MGF, Trindade EBSM.** 2014. A systematic review and meta-analysis of the prebiotics and synbiotics effects on glycaemia, insulin concentrations and lipid parameters in adult patients with overweight or obesity. *Clin Nutr* **34:**845–858.

149. **Ning H, Van Horn L, Shay CM, Lloyd-Jones DM.** 2014. Associations of dietary fiber intake

with long-term predicted cardiovascular disease risk and C-reactive protein levels (from the National Health and Nutrition Examination Survey Data [2005–2010]). *Am J Cardiol* **113:**287–291.

150. **Yao B, Fang H, Xu W, Yan Y, Xu H, Liu Y, Mo M, Zhang H, Zhao Y.** 2014. Dietary fiber intake and risk of type 2 diabetes: a dose-response analysis of prospective studies. *Eur J Epidemiol* **29:**79–88.

151. **Kreymann B, Williams G, Ghatei MA, Bloom SR.** 1987. Glucagon-like peptide-1 7-36: a physiological incretin in man. *Lancet* **2:**1300–1304.

152. **Komatsu R, Matsuyama T, Namba M, Watanabe N, Itoh H, Kono N, Tarui S.** 1989. Glucagonostatic and insulinotropic action of glucagonlike peptide I-(7-36)-amide. *Diabetes* **38:**902–905.

153. **Farilla L, Bulotta A, Hirshberg B, Li Calzi S, Khoury N, Noushmehr H, Bertolotto C, Di Mario U, Harlan DM, Perfetti R.** 2003. Glucagon-like peptide 1 inhibits cell apoptosis and improves glucose responsiveness of freshly isolated human islets. *Endocrinology* **144:**5149–5158.

154. **Holz GGI IV, Kühtreiber WM, Habener JF.** 1993. Pancreatic beta-cells are rendered glucose-competent by the insulinotropic hormone glucagon-like peptide-1(7-37). *Nature* **361:**362–365.

155. **Pingitore A, Chambers ES, Hill T, Maldonado IR, Liu B, Bewick G, Morrison DJ, Preston T, Wallis GA, Tedford C, Castañera González R, Huang GC, Choudhary P, Frost G, Persaud SJ.** 2017. The diet-derived short chain fatty acid propionate improves beta-cell function in humans and stimulates insulin secretion from human islets *in vitro*. *Diabetes Obes Metab* **19:**257–265.

156. **Röder PV, Wu B, Liu Y, Han W.** 2016. Pancreatic regulation of glucose homeostasis. *Exp Mol Med* **48:**e219.

157. **Clore JN, Stillman J, Sugerman H.** 2000. Glucose-6-phosphatase flux *in vitro* is increased in type 2 diabetes. *Diabetes* **49:**969–974.

158. **Magnusson I, Rothman DL, Katz LD, Shulman RG, Shulman GI.** 1992. Increased rate of gluconeogenesis in type II diabetes mellitus. A 13C nuclear magnetic resonance study. *J Clin Invest* **90:**1323–1327.

159. **den Besten G, Bleeker A, Gerding A, van Eunen K, Havinga R, van Dijk TH, Oosterveer MH, Jonker JW, Groen AK, Reijngoud D-J, Bakker BM.** 2015. Short-chain fatty acids protect against high-fat diet-induced obesity via a PPARγ-dependent switch from lipogenesis to fat oxidation. *Diabetes* **64:**2398–2408.

160. **Wolever TM, Spadafora P, Eshuis H.** 1991. Interaction between colonic acetate and propionate in humans. *Am J Clin Nutr* **53:**681–687.

161. **Ge H, Li X, Weiszmann J, Wang P, Baribault H, Chen J-L, Tian H, Li Y.** 2008. Activation of G protein-coupled receptor 43 in adipocytes leads to inhibition of lipolysis and suppression of plasma free fatty acids. *Endocrinology* **149:**4519–4526.

162. **Al-Lahham S, Roelofsen H, Rezaee F, Weening D, Hoek A, Vonk R, Venema K.** 2012. Propionic acid affects immune status and metabolism in adipose tissue from overweight subjects. *Eur J Clin Invest* **42:**357–364.

163. **Gregor MF, Hotamisligil GS.** 2011. Inflammatory mechanisms in obesity. *Annu Rev Immunol* **29:**415–445.

164. **Jiao J, Xu J-Y, Zhang W, Han S, Qin L-Q.** 2015. Effect of dietary fiber on circulating C-reactive protein in overweight and obese adults: a meta-analysis of randomized controlled trials. *Int J Food Sci Nutr* **66:**114–119.

165. **North CJ, Venter CS, Jerling JC.** 2009. The effects of dietary fibre on C-reactive protein, an inflammation marker predicting cardiovascular disease. *Eur J Clin Nutr* **63:**921–933.

166. **Piya MK, Harte AL, McTernan PG.** 2013. Metabolic endotoxaemia: is it more than just a gut feeling? *Curr Opin Lipidol* **24:**78–85.

167. **Lassenius MI, Pietiläinen KH, Kaartinen K, Pussinen PJ, Syrjänen J, Forsblom C, Pörsti I, Rissanen A, Kaprio J, Mustonen J, Groop P-H, Lehto M, FinnDiane Study Group.** 2011. Bacterial endotoxin activity in human serum is associated with dyslipidemia, insulin resistance, obesity, and chronic inflammation. *Diabetes Care* **34:**1809–1815.

168. **Hawkesworth S, Moore SE, Fulford AJ, Barclay GR, Darboe AA, Mark H, Nyan OA, Prentice AM.** 2013. Evidence for metabolic endotoxemia in obese and diabetic Gambian women. *Nutr Diabetes* **3:**e83.

169. **Amar J, Burcelin R, Ruidavets JB, Cani PD, Fauvel J, Alessi MC, Chamontin B, Ferriéres J.** 2008. Energy intake is associated with endotoxemia in apparently healthy men. *Am J Clin Nutr* **87:**1219–1223.

170. **Cani PD, Amar J, Iglesias MA, Poggi M, Knauf C, Bastelica D, Neyrinck AM, Fava F, Tuohy KM, Chabo C, Waget A, Delmée E, Cousin B, Sulpice T, Chamontin B, Ferrières J, Tanti J-F, Gibson GR, Casteilla L, Delzenne NM, Alessi MC, Burcelin R.** 2007. Metabolic endotoxemia initiates obesity and insulin resistance. *Diabetes* **56:**1761–1772.

171. **Everard A, Lazarevic V, Derrien M, Girard M, Muccioli GG, Neyrinck AM, Possemiers**

S, Van Holle A, François P, de Vos WM, Delzenne NM, Schrenzel J, Cani PD. 2011. Responses of gut microbiota and glucose and lipid metabolism to prebiotics in genetic obese and diet-induced leptin-resistant mice. *Diabetes* **60**:2775–2786.

172. Neyrinck AM, Possemiers S, Druart C, Van de Wiele T, De Backer F, Cani PD, Larondelle Y, Delzenne NM. 2011. Prebiotic effects of wheat arabinoxylan related to the increase in bifidobacteria, *Roseburia* and *Bacteroides/Prevotella* in diet-induced obese mice. *PLoS One* **6**:e20944.

173. Cani PD, Possemiers S, Van de Wiele T, Guiot Y, Everard A, Rottier O, Geurts L, Naslain D, Neyrinck A, Lambert DM, Muccioli GG, Delzenne NM. 2009. Changes in gut microbiota control inflammation in obese mice through a mechanism involving GLP-2-driven improvement of gut permeability. *Gut* **58**:1091–1103.

174. Kelly CJ, Zheng L, Campbell EL, Saeedi B, Scholz CC, Bayless AJ, Wilson KE, Glover LE, Kominsky DJ, Magnuson A, Weir TL, Ehrentraut SF, Pickel C, Kuhn KA, Lanis JM, Nguyen V, Taylor CT, Colgan SP. 2015. Crosstalk between microbiota-derived short-chain fatty acids and intestinal epithelial HIF augments tissue barrier function. *Cell Host Microbe* **17**:662–671.

175. Saeedi BJ, Kao DJ, Kitzenberg DA, Dobrinskikh E, Schwisow KD, Masterson JC, Kendrick AA, Kelly CJ, Bayless AJ, Kominsky DJ, Campbell EL, Kuhn KA, Furuta GT, Colgan SP, Glover LE. 2015. HIF-dependent regulation of claudin-1 is central to intestinal epithelial tight junction integrity. *Mol Biol Cell* **26**:2252–2262.

176. Peng L, He Z, Chen W, Holzman IR, Lin J. 2007. Effects of butyrate on intestinal barrier function in a Caco-2 cell monolayer model of intestinal barrier. *Pediatr Res* **61**:37–41.

177. Chen H, Wang W, Degroote J, Possemiers S, Chen D, De Smet S, Michiels J. 2015. Arabinoxylan in wheat is more responsible than cellulose for promoting intestinal barrier function in weaned male piglets. *J Nutr* **145**: 51–58.

178. Gaudier E, Jarry A, Blottière HM, de Coppet P, Buisine M-P, Aubert J-P, Laboisse C, Cherbut C, Hoebler C. 2004. Butyrate specifically modulates MUC gene expression in intestinal epithelial goblet cells deprived of glucose. *Am J Physiol Gastrointest Liver Physiol* **287**: G1168–G1174.

179. Burger-van Paassen N, Vincent A, Puiman PJ, van der Sluis M, Bouma J, Boehm G, van Goudoever JB, van Seuningen I, Renes IB. 2009. The regulation of intestinal mucin MUC2

expression by short-chain fatty acids: implications for epithelial protection. *Biochem J* **420**: 211–219.

180. Singh N, Gurav A, Sivaprakasam S, Brady E, Padia R, Shi H, Thangaraju M, Prasad PD, Manicassamy S, Munn DH, Lee JR, Offermanns S, Ganapathy V. 2014. Activation of Gpr109a, receptor for niacin and the commensal metabolite butyrate, suppresses colonic inflammation and carcinogenesis. *Immunity* **40**:128–139.

181. Nowarski R, Jackson R, Gagliani N, de Zoete MR, Palm NW, Bailis W, Low JS, Harman CCD, Graham M, Elinav E, Flavell RA. 2015. Epithelial IL-18 equilibrium controls barrier function in colitis. *Cell* **163**:1444–1456.

182. Zeng H, Chi H. 2015. Metabolic control of regulatory T cell development and function. *Trends Immunol* **36**:3–12.

183. Cipolletta D. 2014. Adipose tissue-resident regulatory T cells: phenotypic specialization, functions and therapeutic potential. *Immunology* **142**:517–525.

184. Smith PM, Howitt MR, Panikov N, Michaud M, Gallini CA, Bohlooly-Y M, Glickman JN, Garrett WS. 2013. The microbial metabolites, short-chain fatty acids, regulate colonic Treg cell homeostasis. *Science* **341**:569–573.

185. Arpaia N, Campbell C, Fan X, Dikiy S, van der Veeken J, deRoos P, Liu H, Cross JR, Pfeffer K, Coffer PJ, Rudensky AY. 2013. Metabolites produced by commensal bacteria promote peripheral regulatory T-cell generation. *Nature* **504**:451–455.

186. Furusawa Y, Obata Y, Fukuda S, Endo TA, Nakato G, Takahashi D, Nakanishi Y, Uetake C, Kato K, Kato T, Takahashi M, Fukuda NN, Murakami S, Miyauchi E, Hino S, Atarashi K, Onawa S, Fujimura Y, Lockett T, Clarke JM, Topping DL, Tomita M, Hori S, Ohara O, Morita T, Koseki H, Kikuchi J, Honda K, Hase K, Ohno H. 2013. Commensal microbe-derived butyrate induces the differentiation of colonic regulatory T cells. *Nature* **504**:446–450.

187. Park J, Kim M, Kang SG, Jannasch AH, Cooper B, Patterson J, Kim CH. 2015. Short-chain fatty acids induce both effector and regulatory T cells by suppression of histone deacetylases and regulation of the mTOR-S6K pathway. *Mucosal Immunol* **8**:80–93.

188. Trompette A, Gollwitzer ES, Yadava K, Sichelstiel AK, Sprenger N, Ngom-Bru C, Blanchard C, Junt T, Nicod LP, Harris NL, Marsland BJ. 2014. Gut microbiota metabolism of dietary fiber influences allergic airway disease and hematopoiesis. *Nat Med* **20**:159–166.

189. Schwarz A, Bruhs A, Schwarz T. 2017. The short-chain fatty acid sodium butyrate func-

tions as a regulator of the skin immune system. *J Invest Dermatol* **137:**855–864.

190. **Ji J, Shu D, Zheng M, Wang J, Luo C, Wang Y, Guo F, Zou X, Lv X, Li Y, Liu T, Qu H.** 2016. Microbial metabolite butyrate facilitates M2 macrophage polarization and function. *Sci Rep* **6:**24838.

191. **Chang PV, Hao L, Offermanns S, Medzhitov R.** 2014. The microbial metabolite butyrate regulates intestinal macrophage function via histone deacetylase inhibition. *Proc Natl Acad Sci USA* **111:**2247–2252.

192. **Kamp ME, Shim R, Nicholls AJ, Oliveira AC, Mason LJ, Binge L, Mackay CR, Wong CHY.** 2016. G protein-coupled receptor 43 modulates neutrophil recruitment during acute inflammation. *PLoS One* **11:**e0163750.

193. **Vinolo MAR, Rodrigues HG, Hatanaka E, Sato FT, Sampaio SC, Curi R.** 2011. Suppressive effect of short-chain fatty acids on production of proinflammatory mediators by neutrophils. *J Nutr Biochem* **22:**849–855.

194. **Maslowski KM, Vieira AT, Ng A, Kranich J, Sierro F, Yu D, Schilter HC, Rolph MS, Mackay F, Artis D, Xavier RJ, Teixeira MM, Mackay CR.** 2009. Regulation of inflammatory responses by gut microbiota and chemoattractant receptor GPR43. *Nature* **461:**1282–1286.

195. **Wu W, Sun M, Chen F, Cao AT, Liu H, Zhao Y, Huang X, Xiao Y, Yao S, Zhao Q, Liu Z, Cong Y.** 2017. Microbiota metabolite short-chain fatty acid acetate promotes intestinal IgA response to microbiota which is mediated by GPR43. *Mucosal Immunol* **10:**946–956.

196. **Kim M, Qie Y, Park J, Kim CH.** 2016. Gut microbial metabolites fuel host antibody responses. *Cell Host Microbe* **20:**202–214.

197. **Sun J, Furio L, Mecheri R, van der Does AM, Lundeberg E, Saveanu L, Chen Y, van Endert P, Agerberth B, Diana J.** 2015. Pancreatic β-cells limit autoimmune diabetes via an immunoregulatory antimicrobial peptide expressed under the influence of the gut microbiota. *Immunity* **43:**304–317.

198. **Cani PD, Neyrinck AM, Fava F, Knauf C, Burcelin RG, Tuohy KM, Gibson GR, Delzenne NM.** 2007. Selective increases of bifidobacteria in gut microflora improve high-fat-diet-induced diabetes in mice through a mechanism associated with endotoxaemia. *Diabetologia* **50:**2374–2383.

199. **He B, Nohara K, Ajami NJ, Michalek RD, Tian X, Wong M, Losee-Olson SH, Petrosino JF, Yoo S-H, Shimomura K, Chen Z.** 2015. Transmissible microbial and metabolomic remodeling by soluble dietary fiber improves metabolic homeostasis. *Sci Rep* **5:**10604.

200. **Priyadarshini M, Villa SR, Fuller M, Wicksteed B, Mackay CR, Alquier T, Poitout V, Mancebo H, Mirmira RG, Gilchrist A, Layden BT.** 2015. An acetate-specific GPCR, FFAR2, regulates insulin secretion. *Mol Endocrinol* **29:**1055–1066.

201. **Psichas A, Sleeth ML, Murphy KG, Brooks L, Bewick GA, Hanyaloglu AC, Ghatei MA, Bloom SR, Frost G.** 2015. The short chain fatty acid propionate stimulates GLP-1 and PYY secretion via free fatty acid receptor 2 in rodents. *Int J Obes* **39:**424–429.

202. **Brooks L, Viardot A, Tsakmaki A, Stolarczyk E, Howard JK, Cani PD, Everard A, Sleeth ML, Psichas A, Anastasovskaj J, Bell JD, Bell-Anderson K, Mackay CR, Ghatei MA, Bloom SR, Frost G, Bewick GA.** 2017. Fermentable carbohydrate stimulates FFAR2-dependent colonic PYY cell expansion to increase satiety. *Mol Metab* **6:**48–60.

203. **Natarajan N, Hori D, Flavahan S, Steppan J, Flavahan NA, Berkowitz DE, Pluznick JL.** 2016. Microbial short chain fatty acid metabolites lower blood pressure via endothelial G-protein coupled receptor 41. *Physiol Genomics* **48:**826–834.

204. **Macia L, Tan J, Vieira AT, Leach K, Stanley D, Luong S, Maruya M, Ian McKenzie C, Hijikata A, Wong C, Binge L, Thorburn AN, Chevalier N, Ang C, Marino E, Robert R, Offermanns S, Teixeira MM, Moore RJ, Flavell RA, Fagarasan S, Mackay CR.** 2015. Metabolite-sensing receptors GPR43 and GPR109A facilitate dietary fibre-induced gut homeostasis through regulation of the inflammasome. *Nat Commun* **6:**6734.

205. **Belkaid Y, Hand TW.** 2014. Role of the microbiota in immunity and inflammation. *Cell* **157:**121–141.

206. **Coates ME.** 1975. Gnotobiotic animals in research: their uses and limitations. *Lab Anim* **9:**275–282.

207. **Bäckhed F, Manchester JK, Semenkovich CF, Gordon JI.** 2007. Mechanisms underlying the resistance to diet-induced obesity in germ-free mice. *Proc Natl Acad Sci USA* **104:**979–984.

208. **Schwabe RF, Jobin C.** 2013. The microbiome and cancer. *Nat Rev Cancer* **13:**800–812.

209. **Sonnenburg JL, Bäckhed F.** 2016. Diet-microbiota interactions as moderators of human metabolism. *Nature* **535:**56–64.

210. **Buyken AE, Goletzke J, Joslowski G, Felbick A, Cheng G, Herder C, Brand-Miller JC.** 2014. Association between carbohydrate quality and inflammatory markers: systematic review of observational and interventional studies. *Am J Clin Nutr* **99:**813–833.

211. **Food and Drug Administration.** 2016. *Code of Federal Regulations Title 21. Subpart E: Specific*

Requirements for Health Claims. Report no. 21CFR101. FDA, College Park, MD.

212. **EFSA Panel on Dietetic Products Nutrition and Allergies.** 2015. Scientific opinion on the substantiation of a health claim related to "native chicory inulin" and maintenance of normal defecation by increasing stool frequency pursuant to Article 13.5 of Regulation (EC) No 1924/2006. *EFSA J* **13**:3951.

213. **Clarke ST, Green-Johnson JM, Brooks SPJ, Ramdath DD, Bercik P, Avila C, Inglis GD, Green J, Yanke LJ, Selinger LB, Kalmokoff M.** 2016. β2-1 fructan supplementation alters host immune responses in a manner consistent with increased exposure to microbial components: results from a double-blinded, randomised, cross-over study in healthy adults. *Br J Nutr* **115**:1748–1759.

214. **Lambert JE, Parnell JA, Tunnicliffe JM, Han J, Sturzenegger T, Reimer RA.** 2017. Consuming yellow pea fiber reduces voluntary energy intake and body fat in overweight/obese adults in a 12-week randomized controlled trial. *Clin Nutr* **36**:126–133.

215. **Vanegas SM, Meydani M, Barnett JB, Goldin B, Kane A, Rasmussen H, Brown C, Vangay P, Knights D, Jonnalagadda S, Koecher K, Karl JP, Thomas M, Dolnikowski G, Li L, Saltzman E, Wu D, Meydani SN.** 2017. Substituting whole grains for refined grains in a 6-wk randomized trial has a modest effect on gut microbiota and immune and inflammatory markers of healthy adults. *Am J Clin Nutr* **105**:635–650.

216. **Nicolucci AC, Hume MP, Martínez I, Mayengbam S, Walter J, Reimer RA.** 2017. Prebiotic reduces body fat and alters intestinal microbiota in children with overweight or obesity. *Gastroenterology.* [Epub ahead of print.]

217. **Collado Yurrita L, San Mauro Martín I, Ciudad-Cabañas MJ, Calle-Purón ME, Hernández Cabria M.** 2014. Effectiveness of inulin intake on indicators of chronic constipation; a meta-analysis of controlled randomized clinical trials. *Nutr Hosp* **30**:244–252.

218. **Brighenti F.** 2007. Dietary fructans and serum triacylglycerols: a meta-analysis of randomized controlled trials. *J Nutr* **137**(Suppl):2552S–2556S.

219. **Liu F, Prabhakar M, Ju J, Long H, Zhou HW.** 2017. Effect of inulin-type fructans on blood lipid profile and glucose level: a systematic review and meta-analysis of randomized controlled trials. *Eur J Clin Nutr* **71**:9–20.

220. **Fechner A, Kiehntopf M, Jahreis G.** 2014. The formation of short-chain fatty acids is positively associated with the blood lipid-lowering effect of lupin kernel fiber in mod-erately hypercholesterolemic adults. *J Nutr* **144**:599–607.

221. **Buttó LF, Haller D.** 2017. Functional relevance of microbiome signatures: the correlation era requires tools for consolidation. *J Allergy Clin Immunol* **139**:1092–1098.

222. **Kovatcheva-Datchary P, Nilsson A, Akrami R, Lee YS, De Vadder F, Arora T, Hallen A, Martens E, Björck I, Bäckhed F.** 2015. Dietary fiber-induced improvement in glucose metabolism is associated with increased abundance of *Prevotella. Cell Metab* **22**:971–982.

223. **Freeland KR, Wolever TMS.** 2010. Acute effects of intravenous and rectal acetate on glucagon-like peptide-1, peptide YY, ghrelin, adiponectin and tumour necrosis factor-alpha. *Br J Nutr* **103**:460–466.

224. **van der Beek CM, Canfora EE, Lenaerts K, Troost FJ, Olde Damink SWM, Holst JJ, Masclee AAM, Dejong CHC, Blaak EE.** 2016. Distal, not proximal, colonic acetate infusions promote fat oxidation and improve metabolic markers in overweight/obese men. *Clin Sci (Lond)* **130**:2073–2082.

225. **Livingston KA, Chung M, Sawicki CM, Lyle BJ, Wang DD, Roberts SB, McKeown NM.** 2016. Development of a publicly available, comprehensive database of fiber and health outcomes: rationale and methods. *PLoS One* **11**: e0156961.

226. **Saura-Calixto F.** 2011. Dietary fiber as a carrier of dietary antioxidants: an essential physiological function. *J Agric Food Chem* **59**:43–49.

227. **Vitaglione P, Mennella I, Ferracane R, Rivellese AA, Giacco R, Ercolini D, Gibbons SM, La Storia A, Gilbert JA, Jonnalagadda S, Thielecke F, Gallo MA, Scalfi L, Fogliano V.** 2015. Whole-grain wheat consumption reduces inflammation in a randomized controlled trial on overweight and obese subjects with unhealthy dietary and lifestyle behaviors: role of polyphenols bound to cereal dietary fiber. *Am J Clin Nutr* **101**:251–261.

228. **Quirós-Sauceda AE, Palafox-Carlos H, Sáyago-Ayerdi SG, Ayala-Zavala JF, Bello-Perez LA, Alvarez-Parrilla E, de la Rosa LA, González-Córdova AF, González-Aguilar GA.** 2014. Dietary fiber and phenolic compounds as functional ingredients: interaction and possible effect after ingestion. *Food Funct* **5**:1063–1072.

229. **Jacobs DR Jr, Tapsell LC.** 2007. Food, not nutrients, is the fundamental unit in nutrition. *Nutr Rev* **65**:439–450.

230. **Cardona F, Andrés-Lacueva C, Tulipani S, Tinahones FJ, Queipo-Ortuño MI.** 2013. Benefits of polyphenols on gut microbiota and implications in human health. *J Nutr Biochem* **24**:1415–1422.

231. O'Keefe SJD, Li JV, Lahti L, Ou J, Carbonero F, Mohammed K, Posma JM, Kinross J, Wahl E, Ruder E, Vipperla K, Naidoo V, Mtshali L, Tims S, Puylaert PGB, DeLany J, Krasinskas A, Benefiel AC, Kaseb HO, Newton K, Nicholson JK, de Vos WM, Gaskins HR, Zoetendal EG. 2015. Fat, fibre and cancer risk in African Americans and rural Africans. *Nat Commun* **6:** 6342.

232. Jenkins DJ, Kendall CW, Popovich DG, Vidgen E, Mehling CC, Vuksan V, Ransom TP, Rao AV, Rosenberg-Zand R, Tariq N, Corey P, Jones PJ, Raeini M, Story JA, Furumoto EJ, Illingworth DR, Pappu AS, Connelly PW. 2001. Effect of a very-high-fiber vegetable, fruit, and nut diet on serum lipids and colonic function. *Metabolism* **50:**494–503.

233. Kendall CW, Esfahani A, Jenkins DJ. 2010. The link between dietary fibre and human health. *Food Hydrocoll* **24:**42–48.

234. Delcour JA, Aman P, Courtin CM, Hamaker BR, Verbeke K. 2016. Prebiotics, fermentable dietary fiber, and health claims. *Adv Nutr* **7:**1–4.

235. Martínez I, Perdicaro DJ, Brown AW, Hammons S, Carden TJ, Carr TP, Eskridge KM, Walter J. 2013. Diet-induced alterations of host cholesterol metabolism are likely to affect the gut microbiota composition in hamsters. *Appl Environ Microbiol* **79:**516–524.

236. Carding S, Verbeke K, Vipond DT, Corfe BM, Owen LJ. 2015. Dysbiosis of the gut microbiota in disease. *Microb Ecol Health Dis* **26:** 26191.

237. Bindels LB, Segura Munoz RR, Gomes-Neto JC, Mutemberezi V, Martínez I, Salazar N, Cody EA, Quintero-Villegas MI, Kittana H, de Los Reyes-Gavilán CG, Schmaltz RJ, Muccioli GG, Walter J, Ramer-Tait AE. 2017. Resistant starch can improve insulin sensitivity independently of the gut microbiota. *Microbiome* **5:**12.

238. Burkitt DP, Walker ARP, Painter NS. 1972. Effect of dietary fibre on stools and the transit-times, and its role in the causation of disease. *Lancet* **2:**1408–1411.

239. Falony G, Joossens M, Vieira-Silva S, Wang J, Darzi Y, Faust K, Kurilshikov A, Bonder MJ, Valles-Colomer M, Vandeputte D, Tito RY, Chaffron S, Rymenans L, Verspecht C, De Sutter L, Lima-Mendez G, D'hoe K, Jonckheere K, Homola D, Garcia R, Tigchelaar EF, Eeckhaudt L, Fu J, Henckaerts L, Zhernakova A, Wijmenga C, Raes J. 2016. Population-level analysis of gut microbiome variation. *Science* **352:**560–564.

240. Cameron-Smith D, Collier GR, O'Dea K. 1994. Effect of soluble dietary fibre on the viscosity of gastrointestinal contents and the acute glycaemic response in the rat. *Br J Nutr* **71:**563–571.

241. Dikeman CL, Murphy MR, Fahey GCJ Jr. 2006. Dietary fibers affect viscosity of solutions and simulated human gastric and small intestinal digesta. *J Nutr* **136:**913–919.

242. Ferguson LR, Harris PJ. 2001. Adsorption of carcinogens by dietary fiber, p 207–213. *In* Cho SS, Dreher ML (ed), *Hand-book of Dietary Fiber*. Marcel Dekker, New York, NY.

243. Gunness P, Gidley MJ. 2010. Mechanisms underlying the cholesterol-lowering properties of soluble dietary fibre polysaccharides. *Food Funct* **1:**149–155.

244. Anderson JW, Baird P, Davis RHJ Jr, Ferreri S, Knudtson M, Koraym A, Waters V, Williams CL. 2009. Health benefits of dietary fiber. *Nutr Rev* **67:**188–205.

245. Li T, Chiang JYL. 2014. Bile acid signaling in metabolic disease and drug therapy. *Pharmacol Rev* **66:**948–983.

246. Shepherd R, Shepherd R. 2002. Resistance to changes in diet. *Proc Nutr Soc* **61:**267–272.

247. Yang L, Lu X, Nossa CW, Francois F, Peek RM, Pei Z. 2009. Inflammation and intestinal metaplasia of the distal esophagus are associated with alterations in the microbiome. *Gastroenterology* **137:**588–597.

248. Wu T, Zhang Z, Liu B, Hou D, Liang Y, Zhang J, Shi P. 2013. Gut microbiota dysbiosis and bacterial community assembly associated with cholesterol gallstones in large-scale study. *BMC Genomics* **14:**669.

Index